Fundamentals of
Maternal Pathophysiology

Fundamentals of
Maternal Pathophysiology

EDITED BY

Claire Leader, MA PGCAP BSc (Hons) RN RM FHEA

**Faculty Director of Inter-professional Education and Assistant Professor
in Nursing and Midwifery at Northumbria University.
Editorial Board Member for the British Journal of Midwifery.**

Ian Peate, OBE FRCN EN(G) RGN DipN(Lond) RNT BEd (Hons) MA(Lond) LLM

**Editor in Chief, British Journal of Nursing; Consultant Editor, Journal of Paramedic Practice; Consultant Editor,
International Journal for Advancing Practice; Visiting Professor, Northumbria University; Visiting Professor,
St Georges University of London and Kingston University London; Professorial Fellow, Roehampton University;
Visiting Senior Clinical Fellow, University of Hertfordshire.**

WILEY Blackwell

This edition first published 2024
© 2024 by John Wiley & Sons Ltd

The right of Claire Leader and Ian Peate to be identified as the authors of the editorial material in this work has been asserted in accordance with law.

Registered Offices
John Wiley & Sons, Inc., 111 River Street, Hoboken, NJ 07030, USA
John Wiley & Sons Ltd, The Atrium, Southern Gate, Chichester, West Sussex, PO19 8SQ, UK

For details of our global editorial offices, customer services, and more information about Wiley products visit us at www.wiley.com.

Wiley also publishes its books in a variety of electronic formats and by print-on-demand. Some content that appears in standard print versions of this book may not be available in other formats.

Limit of Liability/Disclaimer of Warranty
The contents of this work are intended to further general scientific research, understanding, and discussion only and are not intended and should not be relied upon as recommending or promoting scientific method, diagnosis, or treatment by physicians for any particular patient. In view of ongoing research, equipment modifications, changes in governmental regulations, and the constant flow of information relating to the use of medicines, equipment, and devices, the reader is urged to review and evaluate the information provided in the package insert or instructions for each medicine, equipment, or device for, among other things, any changes in the instructions or indication of usage and for added warnings and precautions. While the publisher and authors have used their best efforts in preparing this work, they make no representations or warranties with respect to the accuracy or completeness of the contents of this work and specifically disclaim all warranties, including without limitation any implied warranties of merchantability or fitness for a particular purpose. No warranty may be created or extended by sales representatives, written sales materials or promotional statements for this work. This work is sold with the understanding that the publisher is not engaged in rendering professional services. The advice and strategies contained herein may not be suitable for your situation. You should consult with a specialist where appropriate. The fact that an organization, website, or product is referred to in this work as a citation and/or potential source of further information does not mean that the publisher and authors endorse the information or services the organization, website, or product may provide or recommendations it may make. Further, readers should be aware that websites listed in this work may have changed or disappeared between when this work was written and when it is read. Neither the publisher nor authors shall be liable for any loss of profit or any other commercial damages, including but not limited to special, incidental, consequential, or other damages.

Library of Congress Cataloging-in-Publication Data
Names: Leader, Claire, editor. | Peate, Ian, editor.
Title: Fundamentals of maternal pathophysiology / edited by Claire Leader, Ian Peate.
Description: Hoboken, NJ : Wiley-Blackwell, 2024. | Includes bibliographical references and index.
Identifiers: LCCN 2024000519 (print) | LCCN 2024000520 (ebook) | ISBN 9781119864684 (paperback) | ISBN 9781119864691 (adobe pdf) | ISBN 9781119864707 (epub)
Subjects: MESH: Pregnancy Complications–physiopathology | Reproductive Physiological Phenomena | Pregnancy–physiology | Female Urogenital Diseases–physiopathology | Perinatal Care–methods
Classification: LCC RG525 (print) | LCC RG525 (ebook) | NLM WQ 240 | DDC 618.2–dc23/eng/20240205
LC record available at https://lccn.loc.gov/2024000519
LC ebook record available at https://lccn.loc.gov/2024000520

Cover Image: © magicmine/Adobe Stock Photos
Cover Design by Wiley

Set in 9.5/12.5pt Source Sans Pro by Straive, Pondicherry, India
Printed and bound by CPI Group (UK) Ltd, Croydon, CR0 4YY

C9781119864684_220324

This book is dedicated to my late brother Marc Davenport

Contents

Antiphospholipid Syndrome   152
Rheumatoid Arthritis   153
Inflammatory Bowel Disease   154
Myasthenia Gravis   154
Multiple Sclerosis   155
Conclusion   156
References   156
Further Resources   157
Glossary   157

Chapter 9   **Cardiovascular System and Associated Disorders**   159
                 Komal Bhatt and Leo Gurney

                 Maternal Medicine Network   160
                 Cardiovascular Physiology   161
                 Approach to Heart Disease in Pregnancy   162
                 Acute Presentations in Pregnancy   163
                 Pre-existing Cardiac Disease   165
                 Disease Arising in Pregnancy   168
                 Care of Women with Cardiac Conditions   169
                 Conclusion   172
                 References   172
                 Further Resources   173
                 Glossary   173

Chapter 10   **Shock**   174
                 Claire Leader

                 Pathophysiology of Shock   175
                 Stages of Shock   175
                 Types of Shock   177
                 Primary Assessment   185
                 Conclusion   189
                 References   190
                 Further Resources   191
                 Glossary   191

Chapter 11   **The Nervous System and Associated Disorders**   192
                 Abbie Tomson and Kristian Tomson

                 Anatomy and Physiology of the Nervous System   193
                 Structure of the Nervous System   193
                 Epilepsy   198
                 Multiple Sclerosis   201
                 Eclampsia   203
                 Stroke   206
                 Conclusion   210
                 References   210
                 Further Resources   212
                 Glossary   212

Chapter 12   **The Vascular System and Associated Disorders**   213
                 Annabel Jay and Cathy Hamilton

                 Structure and Function of the Cardiovascular System   214
                 Overview of Blood Pressure   219
                 Changes to the Cardiovascular System in Pregnancy, Labour and the Puerperium   221

Alison Anderson, BSc (Hons), PGCE, MA Ed., BSc (Hons), RM, MSc
Practice Development Midwife and Specialist BAC Midwife, South Tees NHS Foundation Trust, Middlesbrough
Convenor, Virtual International Day of the Midwife Committee
Alison enjoyed thirteen years as a secondary science teacher, specialising in Biology before re-training as a midwife through Teesside University and Darlington Memorial Hospital. Alison began her career as a midwife at South Tees NHS Foundation Trust where she became the Specialist BAC (Birth After Caesarean) Midwife and then Practice Development Midwife. Alison's passions are the humanisation of childbirth and psychological safety in maternity. Alison also has a great interest in global midwifery and is convenor for the Virtual International Day of the Midwife committee and annual 24-hour virtual conference.

Komal Bhatt, BMBS, BMedSci
Obstetrics and gynaecology registrar, Birmingham Women's Hospital
Komal completed her medical training in 2017 from the University of Nottingham before starting Obstetrics and Gynaecology training in 2019. She is currently working as an obstetrics and gynaecology registrar in the West Midlands deanery.

Suzanne Britt, RM, FHEA, ADM, BA (Hons), BMedSci Midwifery (Hons), MSc Midwifery Studies, PGCHE
Postgraduate Researcher, University of Nottingham
After a teaching career in modern foreign languages, Sue qualified as a midwife in 2002. She has worked in all areas of midwifery practice, beginning her career at Chesterfield Royal Hospital before moving to Sherwood Forest Hospital in 2008 for a community midwifery post. In 2011 she completed her Master's degree and started a secondment as a research midwife at Nottingham University Hospital. In 2013 she moved into midwifery education, working as an Assistant Professor of Midwifery at the University of Nottingham, where she received global and local recognition for teaching. She has delivered on all areas of the curriculum, leading modules on public health, perinatal mental health and contemporary midwifery care. Her interest and knowledge around the musculoskeletal system span her personal and professional life, and she has qualifications in both fitness and nutrition. In 2022 she left her teaching role to start a full-time PhD at the University of Nottingham, focusing on healthcare professional response to domestic abuse.

James Castleman, MA, MD, MRCOG
Consultant in Maternal and Fetal Medicine, Birmingham Women's and Children's NHS Foundation Trust
James is a Consultant Obstetrician at Birmingham Women's and Children's Hospital, UK. He graduated with distinction from the University of Cambridge and completed Foundation training in the East of England before moving home to the Midlands for his Obstetrics and Gynaecology clinical and research training. James has subspecialty accreditation in Maternal and Fetal Medicine from the Royal College of Obstetricians and Gynaecologists. He has a monthly prenatal genomics clinic alongside a clinical geneticist and is part of the regional multidisciplinary team providing this service. His other interests include fetal therapy and obstetric cardiology, as well as maintaining a passion for delivering high-quality intrapartum care alongside midwifery colleagues.

Suzanne Crozier, DBA, SFHEA, RGN, RM
Associate Professor in Midwifery, Edinburgh Napier University
Suzanne studied nursing in Leeds before returning to Newcastle to become a midwife in 1984. She worked as a midwife at the Princess Mary Maternity Hospital for eight years, during which time she completed an Advanced Diploma in

Midwifery before moving into midwifery education. Suzanne completed an MSc and was promoted to principal lecturer at Northumbria University, where she remained for many years undertaking the role of Lead Midwife for Education as well as acting as an educational consultant for the Nursing and Midwifery Council and the Office for Students. In 2021 she took up a post as Associate Professor at Edinburgh Napier University and has recently completed a professional doctorate exploring employability in midwifery.

Claire Ford, PGCap, PhD, FHEA, PGDip, RN, BSc

Assistant Professor Northumbria University
Co-creator and Leader for Skills for Practice Website

Claire joined the teaching team at Northumbria University in 2013, having spent time working within perioperative care and completing a Postgraduate Diploma in Midwifery. She studied for her BSc (Hons) and PG Dip at Northumbria University and won academic awards for both and the Heath Award in 2009. As an Assistant Professor she teaches a range of national/international healthcare programmes and is also a joint Programme Leader for the MSc Nursing Programme. She has a passion for pain management, clinical skills, women's health, gynaecology, perioperative care, simulation and immersive technologies. She has published many articles and is actively involved in several research projects examining the use of media and technology to facilitate deep learning. She is the co-founder of the 'Skills for Practice' website, which was shortlisted for the Student Nursing Times Awards 2016 – Teaching Innovation of the Year.

Clare Gordon, RM, SCPHN – SN, BSc (Hons), MSc (S'ton), MSc (UWL), PG Cert Academic Practice, SFHEA

Senior Lecturer in Midwifery, Programme Leader – Berkshire – Midwifery, University of West London

Clare began her midwifery career in at the North Hampshire Hospital, becoming a qualified midwife in 2005. She practised as a Registered Midwife at Frimley Park Hospital, where she gained a wide range of experience before setting up a specialist weight management clinic for pregnant women. She also undertook the Specialist Community Public Health Nurse – School Nurse training and was awarded an MSc in Public Health Practice from University of Southampton in 2010. She has always enjoyed learning and educating others and joined the Midwifery team at the University of West London in 2013. She has subsequently been awarded an MSc with distinction in Professional Practice with Healthcare Education. She is a Senior Midwifery Lecturer and programme lead with a specialist interest in public health, the normality of pregnancy and birth and the foundations for safe midwifery practice.

Deborah Gurney, RN, RM, BSc, MA (Med ed), FHEA

Senior Midwifery Lecturer

Debbie began her career in healthcare by training as an adult nurse at the University of Hertfordshire in 2000. Midwifery training followed and once qualified, Debbie worked in a rotational midwifery post at the QE2 Hospital in Welwyn Garden City. Debbie developed a passion for education and worked within NHS practice development teams while undertaking a master's degree in Medical Education before securing a post as a lecturer. Debbie's key areas of interest include bridging the theory–practice gap, preceptorship, high-risk maternity care and perineal repair.

Leo Gurney, MBBS, MD, MRCOG

Consultant in Fetal and Maternal Medicine
Sub-speciality Trained Consultant in Fetal and Maternal Medicine
Clinical Lead for Fetal Medicine/Day Assessment Unit at Birmingham Women's Hospital West Midlands Fetal Medicine Network Clinical Lead

Leo is a Consultant Obstetrician and sub-specialist in maternal and fetal medicine (MFM) at Birmingham Women's Hospital. He graduated and trained in O&G in North East England and sub-specialised in MFM in Birmingham. He is the clinical lead for fetal medicine for the hospital and the West Midlands fetal medicine network and has a specialist clinical interest in fetal anomaly, fetal intervention and complex twin pregnancy, stillbirth and maternal cardiac disease.

Rosalind Haddrill, PhD, MA, BSc (Hons), PGCE, RM, SFHEA

Lecturer in Midwifery, Edinburgh Napier University

Roz trained in Sheffield and qualified as a midwife in 2005, after previous careers as a landscape architect and lecturer. She worked clinically in a variety of midwifery roles until 2019 and has worked as a midwifery lecturer since 2010 in a number of British universities. Her PhD explored delayed access to antenatal care. Her areas of interest include women's perceptions of maternity care, gestational diabetes, postnatal care and infant feeding. Roz is currently programme leader for the Master's in Midwifery programme at Edinburgh Napier University.

Cathy Hamilton, DHres, MSc, DipHE, Bsc (Hons), RN, RM
Associate Dean Academic Quality Assurance Practice Enhancement, School of Health and Social Work, University of Hertfordshire

Cathy completed her Registered General Nurse (RGN) training at St Bartholomew's Hospital London in 1984 having undertaken an integrated degree programme at the City University leading to a Bsc (Hons) Psychology and registration as an adult nurse. In 1987 she qualified as a midwife at the West Hertfordshire School of Midwifery based at Watford Maternity Unit. She worked in all areas of Hemel Hempstead and St Albans Maternity Units and as a research assistant before becoming a lecturer at the University of Hertfordshire in 2001. She gained an MSc in Midwifery at Southbank University, London in 2001 and a postgraduate diploma in teaching and learning in higher education in 2003. She completed a Doctorate in Heath Research at the University of Hertfordshire in August 2018. The title of her thesis was 'A qualitative study of midwifery practices during the second stage of labour'. She was Professional Lead (Midwifery) and Lead Midwife for Education at the University of Hertfordshire from January 2018. Since January 2023 she has been Associate Dean Academic Quality Assurance Practice Enhancement in the School of Health and Social Work, University of Hertfordshire.

Annabel Jay, DHRes, MA, PGDip (HE), DipHE, BA(Hons), RM
Visiting lecturer (Midwifery), University of Hertfordshire
Principal lecturer (Retd.), University of Hertfordshire

Annabel qualified as a direct-entry midwife at the University of Hertfordshire in 1997. She worked clinically in all areas of midwifery care at Hemel Hempstead General Hospital until 2001, when she moved into midwifery education. She continued to work part-time for West Herts Hospitals NHS Trust and East and North Herts NHS Trust until 2014. Annabel gained a doctorate in health education in 2014 and has published extensively over the past 15 years. Annabel retired in 2020, but continues to work as a visiting lecturer and PhD supervisor.

Claire Leader, MA, PGCAP, BSc (hons), RN, RM, FHEA
Faculty Director of Inter-professional Education and Assistant Professor in the Department of Nursing, Midwifery and Health at Northumbria University, Newcastle Upon Tyne.
Editorial board member for the British Journal of Midwifery.

Claire qualified as a Registered Nurse from York University in 1998, after which she moved to Leeds, working in the areas of cardiothoracic surgery and emergency nursing. In 2003 she commenced her midwifery education at Huddersfield University where she was awarded a First Class BSc (Hons). Working initially at Sheffield Teaching hospitals, she later moved to the North East where she commenced her role as a staff midwife before moving into the area of research as a research nurse and midwife, developing and delivering a range of research in the specialty of Reproductive Health and Childbirth. She was awarded a distinction for the MA in Sociology and Social Research at Newcastle University in 2012. Claire moved to Northumbria University in 2018 and is now Assistant Professor for Adult Nursing and Midwifery, while also studying for her PhD in the area of leadership in healthcare.

Sarah Malone, MBBS, MRCOG, FRANZCOG, CertClinRes, DDU (O&G)
Consultant Obstetrician: The Royal Women's Hospital, Parkville, Australia

Sarah Malone is an obstetrician with specialist training in Maternal and Fetal Medicine. She began her medical career in North East England and after spending a year working in Auckland, New Zealand, was inspired to complete training in Obstetrics and Gynaecology in Melbourne, Australia. Sarah undertook additional subspecialty training in Maternal Fetal Medicine, which included time spent working in Fetal Medicine in Birmingham, UK. Sarah is experienced in the management of complex pregnancy with particular emphasis in diagnostic ultrasound, fetal anomalies, multiple pregnancy and genetics.

Jacinta H. Martin, PhD, B. Biotechnology (Hons Class I)
Lecturer, School of Environmental and Life Sciences, College of Engineering, Science and Environment, University of Newcastle, Australia
Postdoctoral Researcher, Infertility and Reproduction Research Program, Hunter Medical Research Institute (HMRI), Australia

Jacinta is a dual Lecturer and Postdoctoral Researcher at the University of Newcastle in Australia and an HMRI fellow within the Infertility and Reproduction Research Program. Jacinta works with a multidisciplinary group of researchers using human and animal models to explore the effects of reproductive toxicants on reproduction and offspring development. Her current focus centres on exploring the biological impacts of perfluoroalkyl and polyfluoroalkyl substances. Prior to this, Jacinta was a Postdoctoral Research Fellow at the McGill University Health Centre and McGill University in Montreal, Canada.

Thomas McEwan, FRCM SFHEA RM, DipHE, BSc, TCH, PgCert (TLHE), V300, PgDip (ANNP), MSc
Consultant Editor, British Journal of Midwifery
Honorary Advanced Neonatal Nurse Practitioner, NHS Greater Glasgow and Clyde
Tom has practised as a team midwife delivering caseload-based care, a senior charge midwife within a neonatal unit and an advanced neonatal nurse practitioner. He is currently a Head of Programme for the Women's, Children, Young People and Families team within NHS Education for Scotland (NES) and has been a midwife since 1999. He is the strategic lead for the Scottish Multiprofessional Maternity Development Programme (SMMDP) and has additional responsibility for national midwifery, maternity and neonatal workforce and educational developments. He is a board member for the Scottish Cot Death Trust, and he has contributed internationally to evidence-based guidance for newborn skin care and taught neonatal nurses in Vietnam. He has also published numerous peer-reviewed articles and book chapters. He was awarded a fellowship of the Royal College of Midwives in 2023.

Janet G. Migliozzi, RGN, BSc (Hons), MSc (London), PGDEd, FHEA
Principal Lecturer in Public Health, School of Life & Medical Sciences, University of Hertfordshire
Janet commenced her nursing career in London. She has worked at a variety of hospitals across London, predominantly in vascular, orthopaedic and high-dependency surgery, before specialising in infection prevention and control. Janet has worked in nurse education since 1999 and her key interests include microbiology, particularly in relation to healthcare-associated infections, vascular/surgical nursing, public health and nurse education. Janet is currently a Principal Lecturer and a member of the Infection Prevention Society & European Federation of Nurses Associations.

Kate Nash, RGN, RM, BSc (Hons), MSc, Practice Educator/Lecturer, Doctorate in Clinical Practice
Lead Midwife for Education, University of Winchester
Kate began her nursing career at the Royal Free Hospital in 1991 and later trained as a midwife in 2000 at the University of Hertfordshire. Kate is an experienced clinician and professional midwifery advocate, having held varied roles and responsibilities within midwifery in London, the Midlands and the South East of England. Kate has worked within midwifery education since 2012 and is a passionate advocate for the safe personalised care of women, birthing people, babies and families. Kate is committed to enabling the development of attitudes, skills and knowledge to ensure this.

Maria Noonan, PhD, MSc, BSc (Hons), RNT, RM, RGN
Associate Professor in Midwifery, Department of Nursing and Midwifery, University of Limerick, Ireland
Maria began her nursing career in Beaumont Hospital. She then undertook her midwifery training and practised as a midwife in the University Maternity Hospital, Limerick. She has worked in education since 2006. Maria's key areas of interest are optimising women's and families' psychological health and care during the continuum of pregnancy, childbirth and parenthood, systematic review methodology and midwifery education, and she has published widely in the area of perinatal mental health.

Matthew Robertson, BSc (Hons) Operating Department Practice
Lecturer, Department of Nursing, Midwifery and Health
Matthew is a registered Operating Department Practitioner with the HCPC. He is also a member of the College of Operating Department Practitioners. Matthew completed his BSc (Hons) at the University of Central Lancashire in Operating Department Practice, where he was able to experience a range of complex surgical specialities. Once qualified, Matthew was employed by Newcastle Hospitals within the Cardiothoracic Surgical Department where he undertook the role of the scrub practitioner, specialising in paediatric and congenital cardiac surgery. Matthew commenced employment at Northumbria University in 2017 and since then he has developed a specialist interest in human factors within the perioperative environment and is completing a PhD on this topic, focusing on staff well-being and stress management. Recently, Matthew has had several publications regarding the care of the surgical patient and has written two book chapters

on the use of analgesics in practice and other related pharmacology. Matthew also sits as a registrant panel member for the Health and Care Professionals Tribunal Service and provides expertise on the disciplinary cases that are presented.

Vikki Smith, PhD, MSc, PgCert, BSc, RM, FHEA
Clinical Academic Midwife Sonographer

Vikki is a Clinical Academic Midwife Sonographer at Northumbria University and has a joint role at the Newcastle upon Tyne Hospitals NHS Foundation Trust (NUTH). She has been a midwife for 30 years, with most of her career based in antenatal and fetal medicine settings. Vikki completed a Postgraduate Certificate in Obstetric Ultrasound in 1999 and has extensive experience of providing pregnancy ultrasound scans. She joined the department of Nursing, Midwifery and Health at Northumbria University in 2018 and contributes to midwifery undergraduate and postgraduate teaching and supervision. Vikki is the midwife sonographer lead for a regional Placenta Accreta Spectrum screening service, and is the Programme Lead for the MSc Midwifery Studies programme. Vikki completed a PhD in 2012 and her specific research interests include antenatal ultrasound, the use of technology in maternity services and the organisation of antenatal care.

Joyce Targett, RN (Adult) HND Nursing Studies, RM BSc (HONS) Midwifery Studies, Postgraduate Certificate in Medical Ultrasound
Registered Midwife, Registered Nurse

Joyce started her career as a Medical Assistant in the Royal Air Force before commencing three years' nurse training with the University of York in 1994. During her nurse training her exposure to maternity care inspired her to become a midwife, training with the University of Northumbria. On qualifying, Joyce worked as a staff midwife in a consultant-led unit and in the community setting. In 2005, Joyce completed her training as a sonographer with the University of Teesside and continues to work as a Midwife Sonographer in a clinical setting. She primarily works within a Maternity Day Unit alongside a midwifery-led unit, where Joyce also has an active role as a Professional Midwifery Advocate.

Abbie Tomson, RM BSc (Hons), MSc
Midwife at University Hospitals Plymouth NHS Trust

Abbie trained and currently works as a midwife at University Hospitals Plymouth NHS Trust, working in both the hospital and community settings. Following her Bachelor's degree in midwifery, Abbie commenced a Master's in Advanced Professional Practice at the University of Plymouth, widening her knowledge in an array of health areas and training as a Professional Midwifery Advocate. Abbie is currently a Midwifery Ambassador and a strong advocate for the midwifery profession. Abbie has a keen interest in both anatomy and physiology, and has deepened her knowledge through completion of her yoga teacher training qualification and is now working on specialising in pregnancy and postnatal yoga.

Kristian Tomson, BSc (Hons), McPara
Enhanced Paramedic with Bosvenna Health
Bank Paramedic with South Western Ambulance Service NHS Foundation Trust

Kristian began his career as an emergency call handler with South East Coast Ambulance Service while applying to study paramedicine. Kristian trained as a paramedic in South West Ambulance Service, spending the first few years of his career in Plymouth. Over the last year Kristian has changed clinical setting from full-time pre-hospital care to primary care, working in a GP practice in Cornwall and through the Primary Care First Contact Practitioner Pathway. He has completed a number of MSc modules in Advanced Practice, including advance assessment and minor injuries and illnesses. He has interests in anatomy and physiology, maternal care, as well as pre-hospital and primary care.

Raya Vinogradov, BA, PgD, MClinRes
Senior Research Sonographer/Radiographer, Newcastle upon Tyne NHS Hospitals Foundation Trust
In-practice Fellow for the National Institute for Health and Care Research (NIHR) Applied Research Collaboration (ARC) North East and North Cumbria (NENC)
PhD Fellow at Newcastle Upon Tyne NHS Hospitals Foundation Trust Researcher Development Institute

Raya is a radiographer with a broad clinical experience in obstetric ultrasound and reproductive health research within NHS settings. Her clinical expertise evolved around antenatal care of women at increased risk of pre-eclampsia and fetal renal anomalies. Raya's research interests focus on prevention of adverse outcomes of pregnancy and on delivery of a high standard of antenatal care. In particular, Raya's work involves co-production of a behaviour intervention aiming to support women to adhere to aspirin prophylactic treatment in pregnancies at increased risk of pre-eclampsia.

Amanda Waterman, BSc (Hons), RM, MClinRes, PgCert, FHEA

Senior Lecturer in Midwifery, University of Hertfordshire

Amanda is a Senior Lecturer in Midwifery at the University of Hertfordshire and has previously worked as a Registered Midwife at West Hertfordshire Trust and University College London Hospital. She gained her BSc (Hons) in Medical Biochemistry at the University of Birmingham in 1997, before gaining a BSc (Hons) Pre-registration Midwifery degree at University of Hertfordshire in 2015. In 2019, Amanda completed her masters in Clinical Research at King's College London. Amanda's interests include lecturing in research. She was a member of the James Lind Alliance Priority Setting Partnership Steering Committee and contributed to the publication in the *British Journal of Haematology* (2019) of 'The top 10 research priorities in bleeding disorders: a James Lind Alliance Priority Setting Partnership'. Other publications include the 'Antibiotics and Antibacterials' chapter in the *Fundamentals of Pharmacology for Midwives.*

Preface

Maternal pathophysiology refers to the study of abnormal physiological processes that occur in pregnant individuals. It focuses on understanding the changes in the maternal body that may arise during pregnancy and the impacts they can have on maternal health and the well-being of the developing fetus. Pregnancy involves significant physiological adaptations to support the growth and development of the fetus. Maternal pathophysiology explores the alterations that occur in various body systems during pregnancy and any deviations from the normal physiological processes. This field of study aims to identify and understand the underlying mechanisms of maternal health conditions, complications and diseases that can arise during pregnancy. Pathophysiology involves examining the alterations in cellular, tissue and organ functions, as well as the interactions between different body systems, to gain insight into the progression and impact of disease. By studying pathophysiology, midwifery students and healthcare professionals can better comprehend the underlying causes and mechanisms of diseases, which in turn helps inform diagnostic and treatment approaches.

The intricacies of human reproduction, pregnancy and childbirth intersect with the fascinating field of disease processes. *Fundamentals of Maternal Pathophysiology* helps readers unravel the complex web of physiological changes and pathological conditions that affect the health of women and birthing people and their babies with confidence and competence.

Pregnancy is an incredible journey that brings with it profound physiological transformations. However, alongside these remarkable changes there exist numerous challenges and potential risks that can arise during this unique period in a woman's life. Understanding the fundamental mechanisms behind the pathophysiology of these complications is crucial for midwifery students and those healthcare professionals who are involved in maternal care.

Fundamentals of Maternal Pathophysiology serves as a comprehensive guide, providing readers with a deep exploration of the maternal pathophysiological processes that can disrupt the normal course of pregnancy. We delve into the intricate workings of the reproductive system, hormonal fluctuations, placental physiology and the impact of maternal health conditions on the developing fetus.

There are 21 chapters in *Fundamentals of Maternal Pathophysiology*, taking readers on an enlightening journey through the major categories of maternal pathophysiology. We discuss the normal physiology of reproduction and the astonishing event of fertilisation. Building on this foundation, we explore the physiological adaptations that occur during pregnancy, examining the changes in the cardiovascular, respiratory, endocrine, immune and other systems.

With a solid understanding of the normal processes, we then turn our attention to the disorders and complications that can arise during pregnancy. Maternal conditions such as gestational diabetes, hypertensive disorders and autoimmune diseases are addressed in detail, providing insight into their underlying mechanisms, diagnostic criteria and management approaches.

Our overall aim is to equip the student midwife with the knowledge necessary to recognise, diagnose and manage these conditions effectively, ultimately promoting optimal outcomes for both mother and baby. It is important to note that this book is not intended to replace clinical experience or professional guidance. It serves however as a companion to extend your existing knowledge and offer a solid foundation in maternal pathophysiology. Each chapter is designed to present the information in a clear and concise manner, with an emphasis on clinical relevance and evidence-based practices.

We are grateful to the authors, clinician and academics, who are experts in their respective fields, whose contributions have made this book a reality. Their expertise, dedication and passion for maternal health are evident through these pages and we hope their expertise and insight will inspire and empower midwives in their ongoing pursuit of excellence in maternal care.

We sincerely hope that *Fundamentals of Maternal Pathophysiology* will serve as a valuable resource for midwifery students, academics and healthcare professionals alike. May it provoke in you a curiosity and thirst for knowledge, fostering a deeper understanding of the intricate world of maternal pathophysiology as we strive towards improving the health and well-being of pregnant individuals and their families.

Finally, a note on language. Inclusive language in health and care is crucial for promoting equality, respecting diversity and ensuring that everyone feels represented and valued. It involves using language that is inclusive of all individuals, regardless of their gender identity, sexual orientation, race, ethnicity, disability or other characteristics. By employing inclusive language, we can foster a more inclusive and accessible environment for readers, patients and professionals alike.

When discussing gender and sex, one of the significant challenges is the complexity and fluidity of the terminology that is and that can be used. The concept of gender is multifaceted and may vary across cultures, communities and individuals. Understanding and navigating this terminology requires sensitivity, open-mindedness and a willingness to learn and adapt to evolving perspectives. It is recognised that not all birthing people will identify with their biological sex and a 'gender additive' approach to language has been advocated in the context of contemporary maternity services. This acknowledges that women may be negatively affected by reproductive health inequalities. The terms 'woman' and 'women' are used in this book along with a range of terms to identify and describe those people to whom we have the privilege to offer maternal care.

Claire Leader, Northumbria
Ian Peate, London

Acknowledgements

Claire would like to thank her husband Gavin for all the support and encouragement over the years.

Ian thanks his partner Jussi for his continued support.

We would like to thank the amazing contributors who gave of their time to help the text come to fruition.

We are grateful to the team at Wiley who were receptive and encouraged us to take this project forward.

About the Companion Website

This book is accompanied by a companion website.

www.wiley.com/go/leader/maternalpatho

This website includes:

- Multiple choice questions

CHAPTER 1

Learning the Language: Terminology

Joyce Targett

Midwife Sonographer, UK

AIM

This chapter aims to provide insight and understanding with regard to the terminology used in the provision of healthcare related to anatomy, physiology and pathophysiology.

LEARNING OUTCOMES

On completion of this chapter the reader will be able to:

- Discuss the terms and context around anatomy, physiology and pathophysiology
- Further understand prefixes and suffixes used in anatomy, physiology and pathophysiology
- Understand directional terms
- Describe the anatomical planes, the anatomical regions of the body and the body cavities

Test Your Prior Knowledge

1. What do you understand by the term pathology?
2. What is the difference between a sign and a symptom?
3. How is the root word altered by a prefix or a suffix?
4. Name and define the nine regions of the abdomen.

Science, particularly in terms used in the provision of healthcare, is inundated with Latin and Greek terminology. For all parts of the body Latin names are used and Greek terms are also common, as the Greeks are said to be the founders of modern medicine. Healthcare staff use pathophysiological concepts as they work with people to whom they offer care and as they offer treatment to those who are experiencing some type of health condition or disease.

Fundamentals of Maternal Pathophysiology, First Edition. Edited by Claire Leader and Ian Peate.
© 2024 John Wiley & Sons Ltd. Published 2024 by John Wiley & Sons Ltd.
Companion website: www.wiley.com/go/leader/maternalpatho

Red Flag

Like any country with its own language(s), the medical field has its own language too. This is important so that communication between healthcare professionals can take place quickly and efficiently without the need for too much explanation. It is a specific language that is not just used by midwives, nurses, doctors and other people who are actively involved in the medical arena. It is important for all those who work in healthcare, for example pharmacists, physiologists and dentists. Its correct use can have a significant impact on ensuring the best care.

What is important is that we are all speaking the same language. Failure to do so or making assumptions about what is meant can lead to error and mistakes.

Anatomy and Physiology

Anatomy is the study of the structure and location of body parts, while physiology is the study of the function of body parts. Both of these terms are interlinked. Understanding where the body parts are located can help you understand how they function. McGuiness (2010) explains that when thinking of the various functions of the heart and the four chambers along with the valves, this is the anatomy. Visualising these many structures can assist in understanding how blood flows through the heart and how the heart beats, which are related to its function and as such its physiology.

Anatomy

The Body Map

Learning anatomical terminology is like learning a new language. When your learning has developed and you understand more and add different terms to your vocabulary, this can help you talk confidently about the body. The anatomical directional terms and body planes present a universally recognised language of anatomy.

Red Flag

When undertaking the study of anatomy and physiology, it is essential that you have key or directional terminology so that you can give a precise description when you or others refer to the location of a body part or structure.

Learning Event

When you are next on placement, identify how many times during a shift you hear the various clinicians describe and discuss anatomy, physiology and pathophysiology. Note the terminology being used and how between the team there is a clear understanding when using one language – anatomical and physiological terminology.

All parts of the body are described in relation to other body parts and a standardised body position, known as the anatomical position, is used in anatomical terminology. An anatomical position is established from an imaginary central line that runs down the centre or midline of the body.

Orange Flag

While you are encouraged to use the correct anatomical and physiological terms when conversing with other colleagues, caution must be exercised when speaking in front of and with families. Midwives and other healthcare professionals can inadvertently use words and jargon that are strange, and they may not realise that the meaning is not clear. There are some concepts that are familiar and obvious to the multidisciplinary team but may be alien to patients.

Try first to establish what the woman knows and understands before launching into a discussion that begins at a level that is either too complex or too simple. Too often, our healthcare environments fail to recognise the needs of people with different levels of understanding about their health, and this can mean that they may fail to receive the right care at the right time.

Using jargon can instil fear, cause confusion and result in poor care.

The standard body 'map' or anatomical position (just like a map) is that of the body standing upright (orientated with the north at the top). When in this position the body is erect and faces forwards, with the arms to the side, the palms face forwards with the thumbs to the side, and the feet are slightly apart with the toes pointing forwards (see Figure 1.1). Humans are usually bilaterally symmetrical. This position is used to describe body parts and positions of patients irrespective of whether they are lying down, lying on their side or facing down.

As well as understanding the anatomy and the physiology (the structure and the function), you also need to understand directional terms and the position of the various structures. Table 1.1 lists common anatomical descriptive terms that you will need to become acquainted with. Figure 1.2 gives a more detailed depiction of anatomical positions.

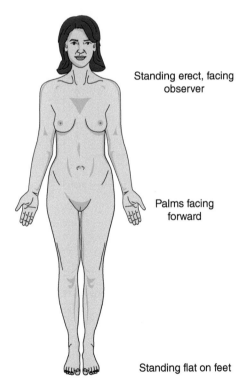

Standing erect, facing observer

Palms facing forward

Standing flat on feet

FIGURE 1.1 Anatomical position: anterior view of the body.

TABLE 1.1   Anatomical descriptive terms.

Anatomical term	Relationship to the body
Anterior	Front surface of the body or structure
Posterior	Back surface of the body or structure
Deep	Further from the surface
Superficial	Close to the surface
Internal	Nearer the inside
External	Nearer the outside
Lateral	Away from the midline
Median	Midline of the body
Medial	In the direction of the midline
Superior	Located above or towards the upper part
Inferior	Located below or towards the lower part
Proximal	Nearest to the point of reference
Distal	Furthest away from the point of reference
Prone	Lying face down in a horizontal position
Supine	Lying face up in a horizontal position

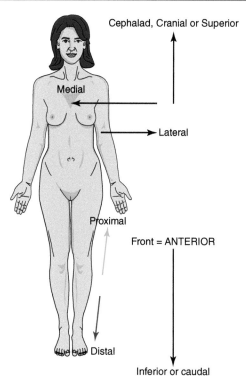

FIGURE 1.2   Anatomical position.

Anatomical Planes of the Body

A plane is an imaginary two-dimensional surface that passes through the body. There are three planes that are generally referred to in anatomy and healthcare (see Figure 1.3):

- Sagittal
- Frontal
- Transverse

The sagittal plane, the vertical plane, is the plane that divides the body or an organ vertically into right and left sides. If this vertical plane runs directly down the middle of the body, this is known as the midsagittal or median plane. If it divides the body into unequal right and left sides, then it is called a parasagittal plane.

The frontal plane is the plane dividing the body or an organ into an anterior portion and a posterior portion. The frontal plane is often referred to as a coronal plane (the word *corona* is Latin for crown).

The transverse plane divides the body or organ horizontally into the upper (superior) and lower (inferior) portions.

Anatomical Regions of the Body

The body is divided up into regions, again like a map, which compartmentalises the body into the following sections:

- Head and neck
- Trunk (thorax and abdomen)

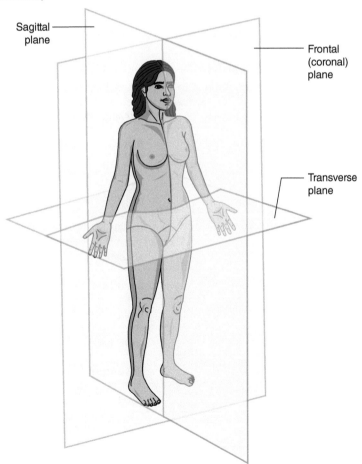

FIGURE 1.3 Anatomical planes.

- Upper limbs (arms)
- Lower limbs (legs)

Tables 1.2–1.5 outline the correct terminology for each region.

TABLE 1.2 Anatomical regions of the head and neck.

Anatomical phrase	Area of the body
Cephalic	Head
Cervical	Neck
Cranial	Skull
Frontal	Forehead
Occipital	Back of head
Ophthalmic	Eyes
Oral	Mouth
Nasal	Nose

TABLE 1.3 Anatomical regions of the trunk (thorax and abdomen).

Anatomical phrase	Area of the body
Axillary	Armpit
Costal	Ribs
Mammary	Breast
Pectoral	Chest
Vertebral	Backbone
Abdominal	Abdomen
Gluteal	Buttocks
Inguinal	Groin
Lumbar	Lower back
Pelvic	Pelvis/lower part of abdomen
Umbilical	Navel
Perineal	Between anus and external genitalia
Pubic	Pubis

TABLE 1.4 Anatomical regions of the upper limbs.

Anatomical phrase	Area of the body
Brachial	Upper arm
Carpal	Wrist
Cubital	Elbow
Forearm	Lower arm
Palmar	Palm
Digital	Fingers (also relates to toes)

TABLE 1.5 Anatomical regions of the lower limbs (legs).

Anatomical phrase	Area of the body
Femoral	Thigh
Patellar	Front of knee
Pedal	Foot
Plantar	Sole of foot
Popliteal	Hollow behind knee
Digital	Toes (also relates to fingers)

Body Cavities

Body cavities are spaces within the body that contain the internal organs. The cavity can be filled with air or with organs. Minor body cavities include the oral cavity (mouth), the nasal cavity, the orbital cavity (eye), the middle ear cavity, the uterine cavity and the synovial cavities (these are spaces within synovial joints).

There are two main cavities in the body (Figure 1.4):

- The dorsal cavity, located in the posterior region of the trunk.
- The ventral cavity, which occupies the anterior region of the trunk.

The dorsal cavity is subdivided into two:

- The cranial cavity, which encloses the brain and is protected by the cranium (skull).
- The vertebral/spinal cavity, which contains the spinal cord and is protected by the vertebrae.

The ventral cavity is subdivided into three:

- The thoracic cavity, which is surrounded by the ribs and muscles of the thoracic cavity containing the lungs, heart, trachea, oesophagus and thymus. It is separated from the abdominal cavity by the diaphragm muscle.
- The abdominal cavity, which contains the stomach, spleen, liver, gallbladder, pancreas, small intestine and most of the large intestine. The abdominal cavity is protected by the muscles of the abdominal wall and partly by the diaphragm and ribcage.
- The abdominopelvic cavity, which contains the urinary bladder, some of the reproductive organs and the rectum. The pelvic cavity is protected by the bones of the pelvis, the sacral promontory posteriorly and the symphysis pubis anteriorly.

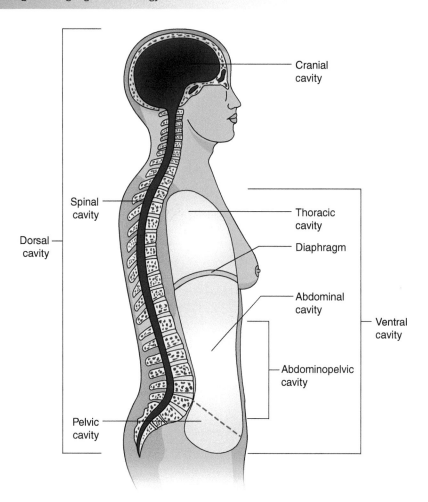

FIGURE 1.4   The cavities of the body.

Case Study 1.1

Lauren, a 22-year-old multiparous woman, presents at the early pregnancy unit complaining of a small amount of vaginal bleeding and a sharp stabbing left iliac fossa (LIF) pain for two hours. She also reports some shoulder tip and rectal pain. Her pain score is 5/10, and she has taken paracetamol (1 g) one hour prior to admission with moderate effect.

History

Gravida 2, para 1, previous full-term normal vaginal delivery (NVD)
Postnatal insertion of an intrauterine contraceptive device (IUCD) 12 months ago. Stopped breastfeeding eight weeks ago.
Last menstrual period (LMP) was six weeks ago, positive urine pregnancy test yesterday.
No significant gynaecological or medical history has been disclosed.

Red Flag

The practitioner caring for Lauren will require an understanding of the anatomy and physiology of the reproductive system (Figure 1.5).

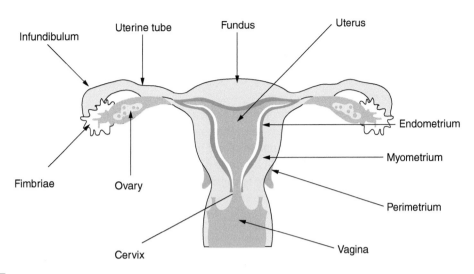

FIGURE 1.5 Anatomy and physiology of the reproductive system.

On Examination

Lauren is alert and can communicate clearly. She appears pale and clammy, her breathing is normal rate and her observations reveal she is haemodynamically stable: blood pressure 110/80 mm/Hg, pulse 96 beats/min and regular, respiratory rate 17 breaths/min and regular, temperature (tympanic) 36.4°C. There is minimal loss per vagina (PV). On abdominal palpation obvious LIF guarding but no rebound tenderness identified.

Ultrasound Examination Findings

Anteverted uterus, IUCD sited at the fundus.

Right ovary of normal appearance. Left ovary contains a corpus luteum.

Adjacent but separate to the left ovary is a mixed echo mass measuring 15 × 12 × 10 mm. The pouch of Douglas contains anechoic free fluid measuring 50 × 30 × 70 mm.

Suspected ectopic pregnancy in the left adnexa, with cervical excitation noted on examination.

Learning Event

Look through the information provided in Case Study 1.1 and highlight the information that is associated with anatomy, physiology and pathophysiology. Highlight and find the anatomical and physiological terms and determine their meaning.

Physiology

Human physiology is concerned with the study of the function of the body. Anatomy and physiology therefore relate to the study of the structure and the function of the human body.

The human body is organised in a most precise way whereby atoms combine appropriately to form molecules in the chemical organisation of the body. The molecules combine to form cells and cells organise themselves collectively as functioning masses that are known as tissues and then organs and systems. Chapter 2 describes cells and the organisation of tissues within the body.

Terminology

Already in this chapter you may have come across some complex terms. It is important to learn the language (the terminology) that is used in the provision of healthcare. This is an important part of safe, effective, woman-centred care. While it is not a pre-course requirement to be proficient in Latin or Greek in order to learn anatomical terminology, it is essential that you understand and are able to use the correct words.

There are three basic parts associated with medical terms, as described in Table 1.6.

The word root is the core of the word and this provides the basic meaning, the subject. The prefixes and suffixes modify the word root. In the term hepatitis, for example, the word root is *hepa*, which means liver. When the suffix *itis* (which means inflammation) is added to the word root it becomes hepatitis – inflammation of the liver.

A prefix can be added to the beginning of a word root to construct a different word. If the root word is *nutrition* and the prefix *mal* (meaning bad) is added, it becomes malnutrition, which means bad or poor nutrition.

Take a look at this example:

Hypothermia

The word root is *therm* (heat).

Hypo means low (this is the prefix).

The suffix is *-ia*, pertaining to a medical condition or disease process.

Hypothermia = low heat

Question: What do you think hypertension means?

Take a look at this word:

myocarditis

Now let us break it up:

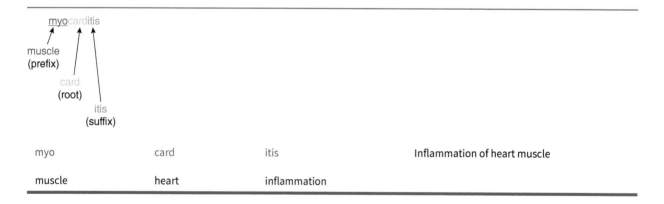

myo	card	itis	Inflammation of heart muscle
muscle	heart	inflammation	

TABLE 1.6   Basic components of a word.

Component	Description
Word root	This is usually found in the middle of the word and is its central meaning
Prefix	The prefix comes at the beginning of the word and it usually identifies some subdivision or part of the central meaning
Suffix	The suffix comes at the end of the word and modifies the central meaning in terms of what or who is interacting with it or what is happening to it

A prefix can change a word:

> Myocarditis – myo = inflammation of heart muscle
> Endocarditis – endo = inflammation of the inner layer of the heart
> Pericarditis – peri = inflammation of the outer layer of the heart

Question: Can you explain the difference between polyhydramnios and oligohydramnios?

A suffix can also alter a word:

> Cardiologist – ologist = a practitioner specialising in the heart
> Cardiomyopathy – myopathy = damage to the heart muscle
> Cardiomegaly – megaly = enlargement of the heart

In this examples the prefix and suffix changed the word but the root *card/cardio* stayed the same.

There are many frequently used prefixes and suffixes and you will already know some of them. See Table 1.7 for a list of some prefixes and suffixes that are used to make up a number of medical terms.

As is the case when learning any language, it can take time to learn all the words and, indeed, the learning will be lifelong. When you are in practice you will be able to reinforce your learning, using your new vocabulary with confidence. Take your time, seek clarification if needed and be patient with yourself.

Knowing the different anatomical terms can make it easier to understand the various pathophysiological concepts that can help you provide care that is woman centred, safe and effective.

TABLE 1.7   Some prefixes and suffixes, their meanings and examples.

Prefix/ suffix	Meanings	Examples
a/an	No, not, without, lack of	Anoxia (without oxygen) Anuria (without urine) Asepsis (without sepsis) Asymptomatic (without symptoms) Anhydramnios (without amniotic fluid) Anencephalic (without parts of brain and skull)
ab	Away from	Abduction (to move away from the midline) Abnormal (away from normal)
ad	Towards	Adduction (to move towards the midline) Adrenal (towards the kidney) Addiction (drawn towards or a strong dependence on a drug or substance)
aemia	Of blood	Leukaemia (cancer of blood cells) Anaemia (lack of red blood cells)
algia	Pain	Cephalgia (headache) Mastalgia (breast pain) Myalgia (muscle pain)
ante	Before/in front of	Antepartum/antenatal (before birth) Anterior (to the form of the body) Anteprandial (before meals)

(Continued)

TABLE 1.7   (*Continued*)

Prefix/suffix	Meanings	Examples
arthro	Joint	Arthroscope (an instrument used to look into a joint) Arthritis (joint inflammation) Arthrotomy (incision of a joint)
baro	Pressure/weight	Isobaric (having equal measure of pressure) Bariatrics (the field of medicine that offers treatment to people who are overweight) Baroreceptor (a sensor reacting to pressure changes)
brady	Slow/delayed	Bradycardia (slow heart rate) Bradykinesia (slowness in movement) Bradylalia (abnormally slow speech)
cyto	Cell	Leucocyte (white blood cell) Erythrocyte (red blood cell) Cytology (study and function of cells) Cytogenetics (study of structure and function of chromosomes)
derm	Skin	Dermatitis (inflammation of the skin) Dermatome (a surgical instrument used for cutting slices of skin) Dermatology (the study of skin)
dys	Difficulty/impaired	Dysphasia (difficulty swallowing) Dyspepsia (disordered digestion) Dysuria (difficulty in urination) Shoulder dystocia (the infant's shoulders are impacted by the pelvic bones during vaginal delivery)
ectomy	To cut out	Appendectomy (removal of the appendix) Mastectomy (removal of the breast) Prostatectomy (removal of the prostate) Hysterectomy (removal of the uterus)
endo	Inner	Endocardium (lining of the heart) Endocarditis (inflammation of the heart) Endotracheal (within the trachea) Endometriosis (a condition where tissue similar to the endometrium grows outside of the uterus)
erythro	Red	Erythrocyte (red blood cell) Erythropenia (reduction in the number of red blood cells) Erythema (reddening of the skin)
haem	Blood	Haematogenesis (formation of blood) Haematology (study of blood) Haemarthrosis (bleeding within the joint)
hydro	Water	Hydrophobia (abnormal dread of water) Hydrocephalus (accumulation of fluid within the cranium)

TABLE 1.7 (*Continued*)

Prefix/suffix	Meanings	Examples
hyper	Above/beyond/excessive	Hypertension (high blood pressure) Hyperflexion (movement of a muscle beyond its normal limit) Hyperglycaemia (high blood glucose)
hypo	Below/under/deficient	Hypotension (low blood pressure) Hypothermia (low temperature) Hypoglycaemia (low blood glucose) Hypothyroidism (underactive thyroid gland) Hypospadias (the opening of the penis is not at the tip)
intra	Within	Intravenous (within the veins) Intraocular (within the eye) Intracerebral (within the brain) Intrauterine (within the uterus)
ism	Condition/disease	Hirsutism (heavy/abnormal growth of hair) Hyperthyroidism (overactivity of the thyroid gland)
itis	Inflammation	Appendicitis (inflammation of the appendix) Mastitis (inflammation of the breast) Myocarditis (inflammation of heart muscle)
macro	Large	Macroscopic (large enough to be seen with the naked eye) Macrocytic (an abnormally large cell) Macroglossia (an abnormally large tongue) Macrosomia (fetal, large for gestational age)
mega/megaly	Enlarged	Cardiomegaly (enlarged heart) Splenomegaly (enlarged spleen) Hepatomegaly (enlarged heart)
micro	Small	Microscopic (so small can only be seen with a microscope) Microcephaly (small brain) Microsomia (small body)
myo	Muscle	Myocardium (heart muscle) Myocyte (muscle cell) Myometrium (uterine muscle)
neo	New	Neonate (newborn) Neoplasm (new growth [tumour])
nephro	Kidney	Nephritis (inflammation of the kidneys) Nephrostomy (an incision made into the kidney)
neuro	Nerve	Neuroma (a tumour growing from a nerve) Neuralgia (pain felt along the length of a nerve) Neuritis (inflammation of a nerve)

13

(*Continued*)

TABLE 1.7   (*Continued*)

Prefix/suffix	Meanings	Examples
ology	Study of	Gynaecology (study of the female reproductive system) Dermatology (study of the skin) Neurology (study of the nervous system) Cardiology (study of the heart)
oma	Tumour (swelling)	Melanoma (cancer of melanocytes) Carcinoma (type of cancer) Retinoblastoma (tumour of the eye)
ophth	Eye	Ophthalmology (study of the eye) Ophthalmoscope (instrument used to examine the inside of the eye) Ophthalmotomy (incision made into the eye)
osteo	Bone	Osteomyelitis (bone infection) Osteosarcoma (bone cancer) Osteoarthritis (inflammation of the joints)
ostomy	To make an opening (a mouth)	Colostomy (an opening into the colon) Jejunostomy (an opening into the jejunum)
oto	Ear	Otology (the study of the ear) Otosclerosis (abnormal bone growth inside the ear)
otomy	To cut into	Tracheotomy (cutting into the trachea) Craniotomy (a hole made into the skull) Thoracotomy (cutting into the chest)
para	Beside/alongside	Parathyroid (adjacent to the thyroid) Paraumbilical (alongside the umbilicus)
patho	Disease	Neuropathy (disease of the nervous system) Nephropathy (disease of the kidney) Retinopathy (disease of the retina)
penia	Deficiency	Leucopenia (deficiency of white cells) Thrombocytopenia (deficiency of thrombocytes)
peri	Around	Pericardium (serous membrane around the heart) Periosteum (covering enveloping the bones) Peritoneum (serous membrane lining the walls of the abdominal and pelvic cavities)
plasm	Substance	Plasma (liquid part of blood and lymphatic fluid) Cytoplasm (substance of a cell lying outside of the nucleus)
plasty	Repair	Arthroplasty (surgical repair or replacement of a joint) Myoplasty (surgical repair of a muscle)

TABLE 1.7 *(Continued)*

Prefix/suffix	Meanings	Examples
pneumo	Breathing/air	Pneumonia (type of chest infection) Pneumothorax (collapsed lung) Pneumograph (device used for recording respiratory movement)
poly	Many/much	Polyhydramnios (increased amniotic fluid in the uterus) Polycystic (many cysts), polyuria (much urine), polyarthritis (arthritis affecting more than four joints)
rhino	Nose	Rhinitis (inflammation of the mucous membrane of the nose) Rhinoplasty (surgical repair of the nose)
rrhoea	Discharge	Diarrhoea (frequently discharged faeces) Rhinorrhoea (excessive discharge of mucus from the nose) Galactorrhoea (excessive production of breast milk)
sclero	Toughened/hard	Sclera (hard/tough layer of the eyeballs) Scleroderma (hardening and contraction of the skin and connective tissue) Sclerosis (abnormal hardening of body tissue)
sub	Under	Subcutaneous (under the skin) Sublingual (underneath the tongue) Subarachnoid (underneath the arachnoid [layer of the brain]) Submucosa (tissue below mucus membrane)
tachy	Fast/rapid	Tachycardia (fast heart rate) Tachypnoea (fast respiratory rate),
toxo	Poison	Cytotoxic (having a destructive action on cells) Toxaemia (blood poisoning resulting from the presence of toxins) Ototoxic (being toxic to the ear)
uria	Urine	Proteinuria (protein in urine) Haematuria (presence of blood in the urine) Nocturia (passing urine at night) Pyuria (pus in the urine)
Vaso	Vessel	Vasovagal syncope (reflex syncope) Vasoconstriction (narrowing the vessel) Vasodilation (widening of the vessel) Vasospasm (sudden contraction of a vessel)

15

Pathophysiology

Pathophysiology brings together a blend of pathology and physiology that considers the connection between disordered physiology and disease or illness. Pathology defines the illness itself and physiology examines how injuries or diseases change natural biological processes. The study of pathophysiology requires the use of clinical reasoning that is then used to make a diagnosis and prescribe treatment to address the effects of disease. Learning how pathology and physiology and anatomy interconnect can ensure that the care provided is appropriate, safe and effective.

TABLE 1.8   Terms and definitions related to pathophysiology.

Term	Definition
Pathology	Study of structural alterations in cells, tissues and organs that help to identify the cause of disease
Pathogenesis	Pattern of tissue changes that are associated with the development of disease
Aetiology	Study of the cause(s) of disease and/or injury
Idiopathic	Diseases with no identifiable cause
Iatrogenic	Diseases and/or injury that occur as a result of medical (or midwifery) intervention
Clinical manifestations	Also known as signs and symptoms
Nosocomial	Diseases that are acquired as a consequence of being in a hospital environment
Diagnosis	Naming or identification of a disease
Prognosis	Expected outcome of a disease
Acute disease	Sudden appearance of signs and symptoms that last a short time
Chronic disease	Develops more slowly, lasting a long time or a lifetime
Remissions	Periods when clinical manifestations disappear or diminish significantly
Exacerbations	Periods when clinical manifestations become worse or more severe
Sequelae	Any abnormal conditions that follow on and are the result of a disease, treatment or injury

There are several terms and definitions that used and are related to pathophysiology (see Table 1.8).

Pathophysiology, according to Singh et al. (2017), is the study of the changes of normal mechanical, physical and biochemical functions, caused by a disease or resulting from an abnormal syndrome. The chapters in this text address these key pathophysiological concepts, which medical terminology is used to express and describe.

Pathophysiology is a key component of practice, enabling the midwife to take on a number of important responsibilities, such as understanding and ordering diagnostic tests, care for and treating women with acute and chronic illnesses, managing medications and managing general health and well-being, as well as disease prevention. Midwives who can recognise the pathophysiological signs and symptoms of various conditions will be able to provide a higher quality of safe and effective care to women and their families. Asking questions such as 'Why is the woman experiencing this?' assists you in understanding what is going on in a woman's body at the cellular level so that you can know how to help them.

Pathophysiology is used to understand the progression of disease so as to identify the disease and implement treatment options. Information gathered is used to identify the next course of the disease so that the most suitable mode of action can be provided to deliver the appropriate care the woman needs. The medical procedures and medications that are administered will depend very much on the nature of the disease and the needs of the woman. The main objectives when understanding pathophysiology are to assist you with the following:

- Using critical thinking to understand the pathophysiological principles for care provision.
- Analysing and explaining the effects of disease processes at systemic and cellular levels.
- Discussing the many variables that may be at play affecting the healing of the organ and tissue systems.
- Analysing the environmental risks of the progression and development of particular diseases.
- Explaining how compensatory mechanisms can be used to create a response to physiological alterations.

- Comparing and contrasting the effects of culture, ethics and genetics and how these can have an impact on disease progression, treatment and health promotion as well as disease prevention.
- Evaluating and reviewing diagnostic tests and determining if the evaluation and review have any relationship to signs and symptoms that the patient is experiencing.

Determinants of Health

While it is important to understand the pathophysiological changes that a woman may be experiencing, the midwife must also appreciate the socioeconomic and cultural factors that can have an impact on outcomes.

Orange Flag

These 'non-medical' factors are as important as whether the most appropriate test or diagnostic tool is being used or treatment prescribed. It is important to understand the molecular and genetic determinants of disease, but non-biological factors also have the potential to influence interactions with a woman and her family.

There are many factors that come together to influence the health of individuals and communities. Regardless of whether people are healthy or not, health is determined by a person's circumstances and environment. To a large extent, factors such as where we live, the state of our environment, our genetics, our income and education level and our relationships with friends and family all have significant impacts on health. The more commonly considered factors, for example access to and use of healthcare services, may in fact have less of an impact.

The social determinants of health are outlined in Figure 1.6. The determinants of health include political, social, economic, environmental and cultural factors, which shape the conditions in which we are born, grow up, live, work and age. Creating a healthy population requires action on these factors, not simply on treating ill health.

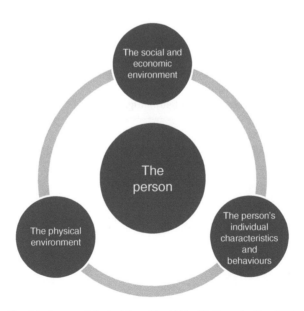

FIGURE 1.6 The determinants of health. Source: Adapted from World Health Organization (2020).

17

Case Study 1.2

Ema has attended the maternity day unit complaining of reduced fetal movements.

Ema is a gravida 1, para 0, who booked for routine antenatal care at eight weeks' gestation. The 23-year-old recently moved from Fiji to live with her husband, who is in the army and posted at a local military base. Ema has no significant medical or family history, and no known allergies or co-morbidities. She is a non-smoker and has a normal body mass index (BMI 27). Ema has accepted all routine antenatal screening as well as combined screening for Down's, Edwards' and Patau's syndromes and a glucose tolerance test.

Ema and her husband have attended all routine appointments. Nothing abnormal has been detected (NAD) at any investigation or examination and no concerns have been expressed. The primiparous is 38 weeks' gestation based on her estimated due date (EDD) from an ultrasound dating scan in the first trimester.

Prior Investigations

Serology results for HIV, hepatitis and syphilis are not detected.
Blood group A rhesus positive and antibody screen negative.
No haemoglobinopathy detected.
All haematology and biochemical markers within normal range.
Microscopy and culture of the midstream urine has no growth.
Booking blood pressure 110/70 mmHg
Routine anomaly scan found no fetal abnormality, placenta reported as anterior and not low lying.
Maternal weight gain 15 kg since booking.

On Admission

Ema is alert but does not make eye contact. She is mobilising well without any assistance. She states she is worried as she has not felt baby move for four hours. She reports no abdominal pain or loss PV. Ema states her mood is good, she is eating and drinking as normal, but has had a headache for 24 hours, which has not been eased by paracetamol. She indicates that the headache is a frontal headache, she has not experienced any visual disturbances or epigastric pain but has swollen ankles.

On Examination

Exposure appropriate for vital signs and palpation. Blood pressure 150/95 mmHg, proteinuria in the midstream urine. Heart rate 90 beats/min. Rhythm: regular. Quality: palpable radial pulse. Skin: normal skin temperature, apyrexial with a tympanic thermometer. Capillary refill time: 2 seconds. No evidence of cyanosis. O_2 saturation 98% in air. Maternal Early Warning Score (MEWS) = 2. Pitting ankle oedema.

On Palpation

Ema is semi-recumbent, the light in the room is ambient and she is comfortable.

On palpation, the uterus is soft and non-tender. The symphysis–fundal height measurement is 32 cm, which is static since previously measured at 36 weeks. The fetus presents in a longitudinal lie, cephalic presentation, 4/5 of the presenting part is palpable and the fetal heart is heard, it is regular at 140 beats/min.

The blood pressure is then repeated and recorded at 140/90 mmHg.

Learning Event

Determine the symptoms Ema is experiencing.

Looking at the information given in the case study, what would be your concerns?

- Reduced fetal movements?
- Pregnancy-induced hypertension?
- Intrauterine growth retardation?
- Social isolation and lack of support?

What would be your management plan for Ema?
Consider which investigations you would order and/or perform.

Using a Medical Dictionary: Hints and Tips

Learning to use a medical dictionary and other resources (be these electronic or hard copy) to help find the definition of a term is an important aspect of understanding the correct use of the numerous medical terms. When starting to work with an unfamiliar resource (print or otherwise), spend some time reviewing its user guide. The time invested at this stage can help later when you are looking up unfamiliar terms.

Accuracy in spelling medical terms is extremely important. Changing just one or two letters has the potential to completely change the meaning of a word and the consequences of this can be grave. Some frequently used terms and word parts are confusing because they look and sound alike, but their meanings are very different (see Table 1.9). Beware: you may encounter alternative spellings used in the United Kingdom, Australia, Canada and the United States.

If You Know How to Spell the Word

- With the first letter of the word, start in the appropriate section of the dictionary. Look at the top of the page for clues (there may be catch words there). The top left word is the first term on the page and the top right word is the last term on that page.
- Now, search alphabetically for words that begin with the first and second letters of the word you are searching for. Continue looking through each letter until you have found the term that you are looking for.
- When you think you have found it, be sure to check the spelling, letter by letter, working from left to right. Terms with similar spellings have very different meanings (for example, prostrate and prostate).
- When you have located the term, carefully check all of the definitions.

If You Do Not Know How to Spell the Word

- Listen carefully to the term and then write it down.
- If you cannot find the word on the basis of your spelling, begin to look for alternative spellings based on the beginning sound. For example, F can sound like F but the word may begin with Ph (such as pharynx, phlegm). K can sound

TABLE 1.9 Confusing terminology.

Term/word	Means	Comments
arteri/o	Artery	Endarterial means pertaining to the interior or lining of an artery (end- means within, arteri means artery, and -al means pertaining to)
ather/o	Plaque or fatty substance	An atheroma is a fatty deposit within the wall of an artery (ather means fatty substance, and -oma means tumour)
arthr/o	Joint	Arthralgia means pain in a joint or joints (arthr means joint, and -algia means pain)
-ectomy	Surgical removal	An appendectomy is surgical removal of the appendix (append means appendix, and -ectomy means surgical removal)
-ostomy	Surgical creation of an artificial opening to the body surface	A colostomy is the surgical creation of an artificial excretory opening between the colon and the body surface (col means colon, and -ostomy means the surgical creation of an artificial opening)
-otomy	Cutting or a surgical incision	A colotomy is a surgical incision into the colon (col means colon, and -otomy means a surgical incision)

Source: Stansfield et al. (2015) / Jones & Bartlett Learning.

like K but the word may begin with Ch (cholestasis for example) or C (crepitus). Psychologist begins with P but it sounds like it should begin with S.

Look Under Categories

Medical dictionaries may use categories such as diseases and syndromes so as to group disorders with these terms in their titles:

- Venereal disease would be found under Disease, venereal.
- Fetal alcohol syndrome would be found under Syndrome, fetal alcohol.

Multiple-Word Terms

When searching for a term that includes more than one word, begin the search with the last term. If you do not find it there, then move forward to the next word. Congestive heart failure, for example, is sometimes listed under heart failure, congestive. Information pertaining to gestational diabetes may be within a text about diabetes as well as in literature on the complications of pregnancy.

Searching for Definitions on the Internet and Handheld Devices

Internet search engines are helpful resources in locating definitions and details about medical conditions and terms. It is important, however, that you use a site such as the National Institute for Health and Care Excellence (NICE; www.nice.org.uk) or Scottish Intercollegiate Guidelines Network (SIGN; www.sign.ac.uk), which is known to be a reputable information source.

Beware of suggested search terms. If you do not spell a term correctly, a website might take a guess at what you are searching for. Be sure to double-check that the term you are defining is the term you intended.

Medications Management

Recent examples of medicine names that have been confused, resulting in medication errors, include:

- mercaptamine and mercaptopurine
- sulfadiazine and sulfasalazine
- risperidone and ropinirole
- zuclopenthixol decanoate and zuclopenthixol acetate

Some of these errors could result in life-threatening conditions. It is important to ensure that you do the following:

- Be extra vigilant when dispensing medicines with commonly confused drug names to ensure that the intended medicine is supplied.
- If there are any doubts about which medicine is intended, contact the prescriber before dispensing the drug.
- Adhere to local and professional guidance in relation to checking that the right medicine has been dispensed to the correct person.

Learning Event

Drugs are administered in a variety of dosages, preparations and routes. Next time you are on placement, review a drug kardex (or drug chart) and pay attention to the prescribed administration of medicines, the route, dose, frequency, interactions and contra-indications.

> ## Take-Home Points
>
> - Use the appropriate anatomical terminology to identify key body structures, body regions and directions in the body.
> - A standard reference position for mapping the body's structures is the normal anatomical position.
> - The terminology used in anatomy, physiology and pathophysiology can be bewildering. However, the purpose of this language is not to confuse, but rather to increase precision and reduce errors.
> - Anatomical terms are very often derived from ancient Greek and Latin words.
> - Anatomical terms are made up of roots, prefixes and suffixes.
> - Without doubt it is important to understand pathophysiological changes, but the socioeconomic and cultural factors that can have an impact on outcomes must also be appreciated. These are the determinants of health.
> - Learning how to use a medical dictionary and other resources to find the definition of a term is an important aspect of understanding the correct use of the numerous medical terms. The time that is spent at this stage can help later when looking up any unfamiliar terms.

Conclusion

Medical terminology may appear very intimidating and complicated. A number of terms used in midwifery, healthcare and medicine are derived from Latin and Greek. In order to understand the terminology used, it is essential to learn to break it down into its parts. When this is done you can see how it all fits together – like the carriages of a train. In translating midwifery terms, it is important to understand the word root (the foundation of the term), which can then have a prefix and/or a suffix attached to it.

In order to communicate safely with other midwives and healthcare professionals, it is imperative that there is consistency in the language being used so as to reduce any risk of confusion. Learning the language requires practice.

It is vital to understand the pathophysiological changes so as to provide the most appropriate care intervention. It is equally important to have an understanding of the impact of socioeconomic and cultural factors, the 'non-medical' factors, which can influence the outcomes.

References

McGuiness, H. (2010). *Anatomy and Physiology: Therapy Basics*, 4e. London: Hodder Education.

Singh, I., Weston, A., Kundur, A., and Dobie, G. (2017). *Haematology Case Studies with Blood Cell Morphology and Pathophysiology*. London: Academic Press/Elsevier.

Stansfield, P., Hui, Y.H., and Cross, N. (2015). *Essential Medical Terminology*, 4e. Chicago: Jones and Bartlett.

World Health Organization (2020). Health impact assessment. https://www.who.int/health-topics/health-impact-assessment (accessed November 2023).

Further Resources

British National Formulary (BNF). www.bnf.nice.org.uk (accessed November 2023).

Health Information and Quality Authority. www.hiqa.ie (accessed November 2023).

National Health Service (NHS). Abbreviations commonly found in medical records. www.nhs.uk/nhs-app/nhs-app-help-and-support/health-records-in-the-nhs-app/abbreviations-commonly-found-in-medical-records (accessed November 2023).

21

National Health Service (NHS). England Saving Babies' Lives Version Two. www.england.nhs.uk/wp-content/uploads/2019/03/Saving-Babies-Lives-Care-Bundle-Version-Two-Updated-Final-Version.pdf (accessed November 2023).

National Institute for Health and Care Excellence (NICE). Hypertension in pregnancy: diagnosis and management. www.nice.org.uk/guidance/NG133 (accessed November 2023).

Royal College of Obstetricians and Gynaecologists (RCOG). Diagnosis and management of ectopic pregnancy. www.rcog.org.uk/guidance/browse-all-guidance/green-top-guidelines/diagnosis-and-management-of-ectopic-pregnancy-green-top-guideline-no-21 (accessed November 2023).

Glossary

Anatomy	The study of the structure of living organisms and their parts
Auscultation	The act of listening to internal body sounds using a stethoscope or other listening device
Blood pressure	The force of blood against the walls of arteries, expressed in millimetres of mercury (mmHg)
Fetal alcohol syndrome	A condition in a child that results from alcohol exposure during the mother's pregnancy
Haemoglobinopathy	A term used to describe a group of blood disorders that affect red blood cells
Intrauterine	Inside the uterus
Organ	A structure composed of different tissues that work together to perform specific functions
Palpation	Using the hands and fingers to touch and feel the body, usually to examine its physical characteristics or to assess certain structures or conditions
Physiology	The branch of biology that deals with the normal functions and processes of living organisms and their parts
Pitting oedema	The accumulation of excess fluid in the body's tissues
Proteinuria	Elevated protein in the urine, may also be called albuminuria
Semi-recumbent	An upright positioning of the head and torso at an angle of 30–45°
Social determinants of health	The economic and social conditions that influence individual and group differences in health status

CHAPTER 2

Cell and Body Tissue Physiology

Annabel Jay and Cathy Hamilton

University of Hertfordshire, Hatfield, UK

AIM

The aim of this chapter is to provide an overview of the physiology of cells and tissues, including disorders that cause cell changes or damage during pregnancy, childbirth and the postnatal period. It will offer the reader some insight into the implications for caring for the mother and the developing fetus.

LEARNING OUTCOMES

On completion of this chapter the reader will be able to:

- Outline the structure and function of a human cell
- Explain the phases of a cell reproductive cycle
- Describe the structure and function of the four tissue types
- Explain the process of tissue repair (inflammation).

Test Your Prior Knowledge

1. What are the three main parts of a human cell?
2. Name the four tissue types.
3. What is the difference between mitosis and meiosis?
4. List the main symptoms of the inflammatory response to cell damage.

All living organisms are composed of one or more cells. Despite the fact that cells in different organisms may have different functions, there are many similarities between them. For example, there are similarities in their chemical composition, their chemical and biochemical behaviour and their detailed structure. All cells have the following characteristics:

- Cells carry out certain specific functions.
- Cells need to consume food to live and to perform their functions.

- Cells can grow and repair.
- Cells can reproduce.
- Cells can become damaged.
- Cells have a finite life: some live for just a few days, while others live for years.

Cell Anatomy

Each cell has a structure that is almost as complex as the human body (Figure 2.1). There is no such thing as a typical cell. However, each cell is surrounded by a membrane and contains protoplasm. This protoplasm consists of a nucleus, which is kept separate from the rest of the cell by a nuclear membrane and an opaque substance called cytoplasm (Watson 2005). The cells themselves consist of water, proteins, lipids, carbohydrates and various ions such as potassium (K^+) and magnesium (Mg^{2+}). Within the cytoplasm, there are also many complex protein structures called organelles. Cells vary in size from 2 to 20 µm. For example, a lymphocyte (a type of white blood cell) is about 8–10 µm in diameter. All the cells in the body, apart from those on the surface of the body, are surrounded by a fluid known as extracellular fluid.

The Cell Membrane

The cell membrane varies from 7.5 to 10 nm in thickness. It acts like a 'skin' that protects the cell from the outside environment. It regulates the movement of water, nutrients and waste products into and out of the cell. The cell membrane is made up of a double layer of phospholipid (fatty) molecules with protein molecules interspersed between them (Figure 2.2). A phospholipid molecule consists of a polar 'head' that is hydrophilic (water loving) and 'tails' that are hydrophobic (water hating). It is the central part of the plasma membrane, consisting of the hydrophobic 'tails', that makes the cell membrane impermeable to water-soluble molecules, and so prevents the passage of these molecules into and out of

24

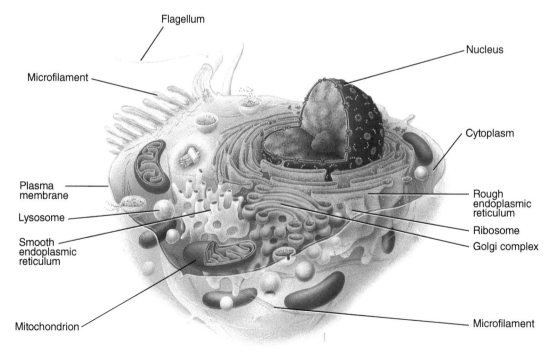

Sectional view

FIGURE 2.1   Basic structure of a cell.

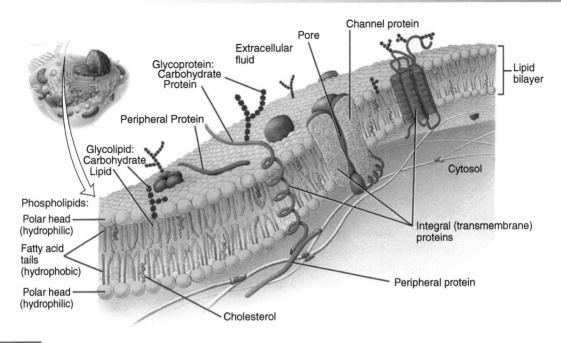

FIGURE 2.2 Anatomy of the cell membrane.

the cell (Marieb and Keller 2017). Within the cell membrane there are also plasma membrane proteins. Subunits of some of these proteins can form channels that allow the transportation of materials into and out of the cell. Other subunits are receptors for hormones and other chemicals.

Transport Across the Cell Membrane

One of the key properties of the cell membrane is its 'selective permeability'. This refers to its ability to let certain materials pass through while preventing others from doing so. This selective permeability is based on the hydrophobicity (water hatred) of its component molecules. Because the phospholipid tails in the centre of the cell membrane are composed entirely of hydrophobic fatty acid chains, it is very difficult for water-soluble (hydrophilic) molecules to penetrate to the membrane interior. The result is a very effective permeability barrier. However, this barrier can be penetrated by specific transport systems. These control what goes into and out of the cell. For example, cell membranes control metabolism by restricting the flow of glucose and other water-soluble metabolites into and out of cells. Large molecules cannot pass through the membrane proteins, but small ones such as water and amino acids can. Also, substances that easily dissolve in lipids (fats) can pass through the membrane more easily than non-lipid-soluble substances. Lipid-soluble substances include oxygen, carbon dioxide and steroid hormones.

There are numerous ways in which substances can cross the cell membrane. The most commonly cited are diffusion and osmosis. Diffusion is a form of passive transport, in which a substance of higher concentration moves to an area where there is a lower concentration of that substance (Colbert et al. 2019). This difference between the areas of high concentration and of low concentration is known as a concentration gradient. This process of diffusion is essential for respiration. It is through diffusion that oxygen is transported from the lungs to the red blood cells, and carbon dioxide makes the opposite journey from the blood to the lungs (Colbert et al. 2019).

Osmosis is the process by which water travels through a selectively permeable membrane from an area of low concentration of a solute (a substance soluble in water) to one of higher concentration. The result is that concentrations of the solute are equal on both sides of that membrane. Examples of osmosis occur in the renal system, ensuring that fluid levels within the body remain stable.

Cytoplasm

Cytoplasm is a thick, semi-transparent, elastic fluid containing suspended particles. Cytoplasm consists of 75–90% water plus solid compounds – mainly carbohydrates, lipids and inorganic substances. The cytoplasm receives raw materials from the external environment (such as from digested food) and converts them into usable energy by breaking them down to make energy. The cytoplasm is also the site where new substances are synthesised (produced) for the use of the cell. It is also where various chemicals are packaged for transport to other parts of the cell, or to other cells in the body. Chemicals in the cytoplasm facilitate the excretion of waste materials.

Nucleus

The nucleus may be likened to the brain of the cell. Most cells have a nucleus, but some do not, for example red blood cells. The lack of a nucleus means the red blood cell can adopt a concave shape, allowing it to pass through narrow capillaries. Some cells can have more than one nucleus, such as some muscle fibre cells. See Figure 2.3 for a depiction of the cell nucleus. All nuclei (the plural of nucleus) have the following characteristics:

- The nucleus is the largest structure in the cell.
- It is surrounded by a nuclear membrane, which has two layers and is selectively permeable.
- The substance within the nucleus is not called cytoplasm – it is called nucleoplasm.
- The nucleus assumes great responsibility for cell reproduction.

Most nuclei contain one or more nucleoli. These bodies contain genetic material, consisting principally of deoxyribonucleic acid (DNA). When a cell is not reproducing, the genetic material is a threadlike mass called chromatin. Before cell division, the chromatin shortens and coils into rod-shaped bodies called chromosomes.

The basic structural unit of a chromosome is a nucleosome – composed of DNA and protein (see Figure 2.4).

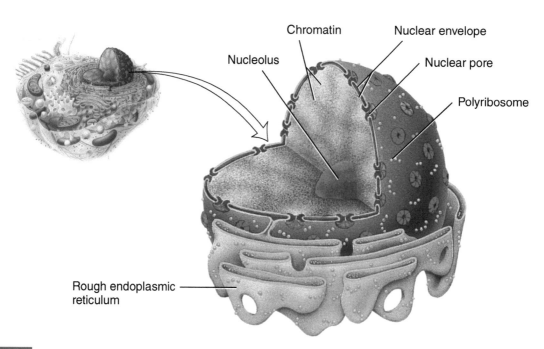

Chromatin
Nuclear envelope
Nucleolus
Nuclear pore
Polyribosome
Rough endoplasmic reticulum

FIGURE 2.3   Cell nucleus. Source: Reproduced by permission from Tortora and Derrickson 2017 / Wiley.

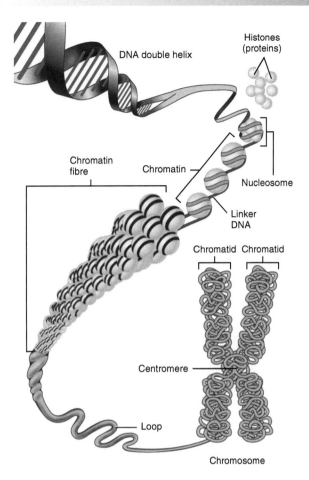

FIGURE 2.4 Chromosome and DNA. Source: Reproduced by permission from Tortora and Derrickson 2017 / Wiley.

DNA

DNA has two main functions:

- It provides the genetic 'blueprint' ensuring that the next generation of cells is identical to existing ones.
- It provides the plans for the synthesis of protein by the cell. All this information is stored in genes. The nucleus contains small, spherical bodies called nucleoli, which are responsible for the production of ribosomes from ribosomal ribonucleic acid (rRNA). Humans have 23 pairs of chromosomes in each nucleus-containing cell, with the exception of the spermatozoa and ova (sperm and eggs). Sperm and ova (collectively known as gametes) only have 23 single chromosomes (i.e. one of each pair). The chromosomes are the same for males and females except for one pair – the X and Y chromosomes. These determine whether a baby is going to be male or female. Females have two X chromosomes and males have one X and one Y chromosome.

Learning Event

In some rare instances, a fetus inherits either more or fewer chromosomes than is normal. This can result in serious health problems. Name one syndrome that is caused by the wrong number of chromosomes and find out about this using medical or midwifery/nursing textbooks or websites.

Cell Reproduction: Mitosis and Meiosis

Most human cells reproduce asexually by mitosis, but the spermatozoa and ova reproduce by meiosis. Whereas the cells reproducing by mitosis finish up as exact copies of the parent cells with a pair of each of the 23 chromosomes, the cells reproducing by meiosis finish up with one each of the 23 chromosomes.

Mitosis

In order for the body to grow, and also for the replacement of body cells that die, cells need to reproduce. They must be able to reproduce themselves identically, so that genetic information is not lost. They do this by cloning themselves. This process of cell reproduction is called mitosis, in which the number of chromosomes in the new (daughter) cells has to be the same as in the original (parent) cell. Mitosis can be divided into four stages (see Figure 2.5):

- **Prophase**: During this phase the chromosomes become shorter, fatter and more easily visible. Each chromosome now consists of two chromatids, each containing the same genetic information. The nucleolus and nuclear membrane disappear, leaving the chromosomes in the cytoplasm.
- **Metaphase**: The 46 chromosomes (two of each of the 23 chromosomes), each consisting of two chromatids, become attached to the spindle fibres.
- **Anaphase**: The chromatids in each chromosome are separated. One chromatid from each chromosome then moves towards each pole of the spindle.
- **Telophase**: There are now 46 chromatids at each pole and these will form the chromosomes of the daughter cells. The cell membrane constricts in the centre of the cell, dividing it into two cells. The nuclear spindle disappears and a nuclear membrane forms around the chromosomes in each of the daughter cells. The chromosomes become long and threadlike again and are very difficult to see. Cell division is now complete.

Before and after it has divided, the cell enters a stage known as interphase. During this phase, the cell builds up a store of energy to enable the process of division.

Meiosis

When the spermatozoon (sperm) penetrates the ovum, it releases its DNA to combine with the DNA of the ovum. If each gamete passed on the full complement of chromosomes from each parent, it would result in an embryo with 46 pairs of

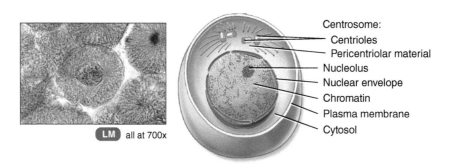

LM   all at 700x

Centrosome:
Centrioles
Pericentriolar material
Nucleolus
Nuclear envelope
Chromatin
Plasma membrane
Cytosol

FIGURE 2.5   Mitotic cell division.

chromosomes in its cells, instead of the normal 23 pairs. To prevent this happening, the gametes undergo a process known as meiosis to ensure that the resulting embryo will only carry two copies of each chromosome in each cell.

For descriptive purposes, meiosis can be divided into eight stages. They have the same names as in the mitotic process but are known as either I or II. However, there are differences as well as similarities between mitosis and meiosis.

First Meiotic Stage
- **Prophase I:** This is similar to prophase in mitosis but, instead of being scattered randomly, the chromosomes are arranged in 23 pairs. For example, the two chromosome number ones will pair up, as will the two chromosome number twos. Within each pair of chromosomes, genetic material may be exchanged between the two chromosomes. It is these exchanges that are partly responsible for the differences between children of the same parents. This process is called 'gene crossover'.
- **Metaphase I:** As in mitosis, the chromosomes become arranged on the spindles at the equator (see Figure 2.6). However, they remain in pairs.
- **Anaphase I:** One chromosome from each pair moves to each pole, so that there are now 23 chromosomes at each end of the spindle.
- **Telophase I:** The cell membrane now divides the cell into two halves, as in mitosis. Each daughter cell now has half the number of chromosomes that each parent cell had.

Second Meiotic Stage
The cells produced by the first meiotic division now divide again. Prophase II, metaphase II, anaphase II and telophase II are all similar to their equivalent stage in mitosis, with the exception that the DNA has not been replicated before prophase II, so there are only 23 single chromosomes in each of the granddaughter cells.

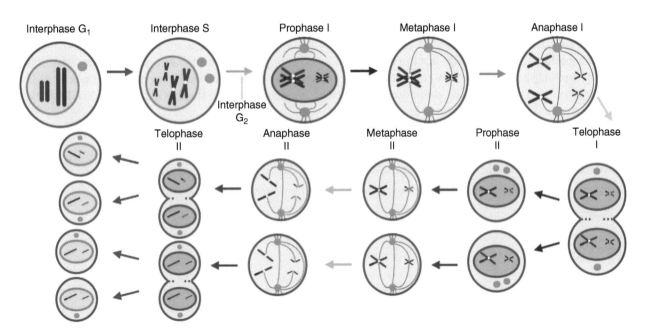

FIGURE 2.6 Meiotic cell division. Credit: Fundamentals of Anatomy and Physiology: For Nursing and Healthcare Students 3rd Edition.

Fusion of the Gametes

When the gametes, each with 23 chromosomes, fuse together, a cell known as a zygote with 23 paired chromosomes (i.e. 46 in all) is formed. One chromosome in each pair comes from the mother and one from the father. The zygote then divides many times (by mitosis) to form the embryo. The embryo thus has a full complement of genetic material, which will determine its biological characteristics as it develops.

The Organelles

All cells contain many organelles (little organs) that provide various functions. These include the following:

- **Endoplasmic reticulum** (ER): It is believed that the ER is formed from the nuclear membrane. The ER consists of membranes that form a series of channels that divide the cytoplasm into compartments. These channels are used to transport proteins. They also contain a number of enzymes of importance in cell metabolism, such as digestive enzymes.
- **Golgi apparatus:** The Golgi apparatus is a collection of membranous tubes and elongated sacs. It plays a part in concentrating and packaging some of the substances that are made in the cell, e.g. some enzymes. They also have a role in assembling substances for secretion from the cell. The Golgi are also involved in the formation of glycoproteins.
- **Lysosomes:** These are organelles bound to the membrane and contain a variety of enzymes. Lysosomes have a number of functions, including digestion of pathogenic (harmful) organisms and the breakdown of cells that are no longer needed. After a baby's birth, the uterus, which weighs around 2 kg at full term, is invaded by phagocytic cells that are rich in lysosomes – these reduce the uterus to its non-pregnant weight of around 50 g within about nine days. Lysosomes also contribute to the production of some hormones, e.g. thyroxine.
- **Mitochondria:** Often known as the powerhouses of the cell, mitochondria are often found concentrated in regions of the cell associated with intense metabolic activity. They consist of three membranes. The function of mitochondria is to generate the energy needed by the cell (in the form of ATP, adenosine triphosphate) by converting the chemical energy contained in food. The production of ATP requires the breakdown of food molecules and occurs in several stages, each requiring an appropriate enzyme. The enzymes in the mitochondria are stored in the membranes. Mitochondria are self-replicating – just like the cells. Unlike other organelles, mitochondria have their own DNA. This is inherited only from the mother. Mitochondrial DNA contains 37 genes, some of which provide instructions for making enzymes and proteins. Some chromosomal conditions are associated with changes in mitochondrial DNA and are thus only passed down the female line of inheritance.

Learning Event

Using a midwifery, nursing or medical textbook, look up and read about one disorder that is inherited via mitochondrial DNA.

Tissues

A human begins as a single cell – the zygote. As soon as fertilisation takes place, the zygote begins to divide and does so continuously. These cells divide and grow in such a way that they become specialised into muscle cells, skin cells, blood cells and so on (Marieb and Keller 2017). Cells group together to become tissues – groups of cells that are similar in structure and generally perform the same functions (McCance et al. 2018). There are four primary types of tissue, each with a specific function:

- Epithelial tissue – for covering
- Connective – for supporting

- Muscle – for movement
- Nervous – for controlling (Wheeldon 2016)

Epithelial Tissue

Epithelial tissue lines and covers most of the internal and external surface areas of the body, as well as forming the glandular tissue. For example, skin is an epithelial tissue that covers the exterior of the body, while the endometrium is an epithelial tissue that lines the uterus. Epithelial tissue is classified in two ways:

- By the number of cell layers: Simple epithelium consists of a single layer of cells. Stratified epithelium has two or more cell layers.
- By shape: Squamous, cuboidal or columnar.

Simple epithelial tissues are mostly concerned with absorption, secretion and filtration. Simple squamous epithelial cells fit very closely together to form a thin sheet of tissue. It is this type of epithelial tissue that is found in the alveoli of the lungs and the walls of capillaries. Oxygen and carbon dioxide exchange takes place through the thin layer of epithelial tissue lining the alveoli of the lungs. Nutrients and gases can pass through the epithelial tissue from the cells into and out of the capillaries (Wheeldon 2016). Figure 2.7 provides a diagrammatic representation of the types of epithelial tissue.

Cuboidal epithelial cells are thicker than squamous epithelial cells. They are found in different places of the body and perform different functions. For example, cuboidal epithelial tissue is found in glands as well as forming the walls of kidney tubules and covering the surface of the ovaries (Marieb and Keller 2017). Simple columnar epithelium is made up of a single layer of tall cells that, like the other two types, fit closely together. This tissue lines the entire length of the digestive tract from the stomach to the anus and contains goblet cells, which produce mucus. Mucous membranes are tissues formed from simple columnar epithelial that line all the body cavities that open to the exterior, including the vagina and urethra (Marieb and Keller 2017). Stratified epithelial tissue, unlike simple epithelial tissue, consists of two or more cell layers. This makes it stronger and more robust than simple epithelial tissues. Squamous epithelium is found in places that are most at risk of everyday damage, including the oesophagus, the mouth and the outer layer of the skin (Marieb and Keller 2017).

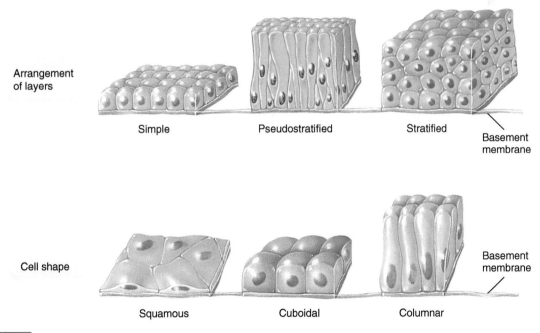

FIGURE 2.7 Types of epithelial tissue. Source: Reproduced by permission from Tortora and Derrickson 2017 / Wiley.

Expert Midwife

What is the effect of water immersion on the skin of the perineum during a waterbirth?

There are conflicting theories around the effect on the skin of the perineum and associated anatomical structures, with reports of increased, reduced or unchanged rates of perineal trauma for women who have given birth in the water (Papoutsis 2020). There are some studies reporting that a waterbirth may reduce the chance of a woman sustaining a second-degree perineal tear. In these studies the underlying physiological mechanisms contributing to this include the buoyancy of the water reducing the weight of the infant on the perineal tissues during delivery (Ulfsdottir et al. 2019), increased vasodilation and perineal blood supply resulting from the immersion in warm water (Asahieijm et al. 2017) and the support for women who give birth in the water generally being more conservative in nature, with spontaneous pushing and a slower delivery (Garland 2017).

Other studies have noted an increased risk for anal sphincter damage (known as a third- or fourth-degree perineal tear) during a waterbirth (McPherson et al. 2014). Studies exploring the potential effect of water immersion on tissue integrity on other areas of the body have noted a 'waterlogging' effect on the foot, leading to softening of the skin after 45 minutes of being in the water (Schmidt et al. 2018). Another study found that immersion of the arm in water for three hours led to significant changes in the permeability of the skin and the fine cellular structure of the outer skin layer (the stratum cornea). Shape and structural changes were noted in the intercellular spaces and more water content found throughout the skin (Ogawa-Fuse et al. 2019). Prolonged water immersion may lead to the development of inter- and intracellular aqueous inclusions (fluid bubbles) within the skin (Kalra et al. 2016). This research also found that high hydration levels in the skin may result in increased collagen, leading to reduced tensile strength of the skin (Kalra et al. 2016). Tensile strength is defined as the most stress that a material (the skin) can bear before breaking when it is stretched or pulled. It was estimated that the amount of mechanical force needed to cause the same degree of skin damage decreases up to three orders of magnitude with an increase in skin hydration, meaning that less force is required for the skin to break when it is wet.

These theories relating to the underlying physiological mechanisms associated with water immersion might explain why some women are less likely to have an intact perineum following a waterbirth when compared to giving birth in the dry (Papoutsis et al. 2021). They may also explain why women giving birth for the first time and having a waterbirth have a higher risk of sustaining severe perineal damage and anal sphincter damage than multiparous women, as they tend to stay immersed in water longer as labour is usually lengthier.

Despite these theories, the latest Cochrane Database systematic review on this topic (Cluett et al. 2018) demonstrated that waterbirth had no significant effect on the rate of severe perineal trauma. This review concluded that evidence was of moderate to low quality and that further research is needed. Papoutsis et al. (2021) recommend that future research should include taking tissue samples from the perineum and then investigating their physiological properties as a function of time of water immersion.

The establishment of some clear evidence on this topic area is important, as perineal trauma may lead to significant damage to the perineal muscles and the rectovaginal fascia, which could result in pelvic organ prolapse in later life leading to an adverse effect on a woman's sexual function. In view of this impact on quality of life, it is imperative that women are provided with robust evidence on which to base their decisions around birth.

Points for Reflection

- Based on the information presented here, what information will you provide to a woman who is considering a waterbirth?
- Consider undertaking your own review of the literature to locate the most recent research studies associated with this topic area.

Glandular Epithelium

Glandular epithelial tissue is found within glands – structures that make and secrete certain products such as saliva, sweat, enzymes and hormones. Two major types of glands develop from epithelial sheets:

- Exocrine glands have ducts leading from them, and their secretions empty through these ducts to the surface of the epithelium. Examples of exocrine glands include the sweat glands, the liver and the pancreas.
- Endocrine glands do not possess ducts. Instead, their secretions diffuse directly into the blood vessels that are found within the glands. All endocrine glands secrete hormones. These glands include the adrenal glands, the pituitary gland and the gonads (ovaries and testes).

Connective Tissue

Connective tissue is found everywhere in the body, and it connects body parts to one another. It is the most abundant and widely distributed of all four primary tissue types. It varies considerably in structure and has several functions, including protection and support (Marieb and Keller 2017). However, the most common function of connective tissue is to act as the framework on which the epithelial cells gather in order to form the organs of the body (McCance et al. 2018). Connective tissue contains three types of fibres:

- Collagen (white) fibres, which have great strength.
- Elastic (yellow) fibres, which can stretch and recoil.
- Reticular fibres, which form the internal 'skeleton' of organs such as the spleen.

Connective tissue forms a 'packing' around organs of the body and so protects them. It is able to bear weight and to withstand stretching and various traumas, such as abrasions. There is a wide variation in types of connective tissue, including fat tissue, which is soft, and bone tissue, which is hard and strong (Marieb and Keller 2017).

Orange Flag: Mastitis

Mastitis is a fairly common condition that can affect a woman postnatally, whether or not she is breastfeeding. It is characterised by localised redness, heat and pain and can cause pyrexia (raised temperature) and a general feeling of malaise. If untreated, it can result in an abscess or even sepsis in extreme cases (Wilson et al. 2020). Mastitis is usually caused by milk stasis, leading to engorgement of one or more lobes of breast tissue. This sets off an inflammatory response. This is non-infective mastitis and can be resolved by ensuring that the affected breast is drained, either by the baby suckling or by hand expression. Cool compresses and oral paracetamol can help relieve the symptoms. Antibiotics are not needed, unless there is suspicion of a bacterial infection in the breast (e.g. nipple damage), which can also be a cause of mastitis. Since it is not always possible to identify whether mastitis is infective or non-infective, women are often prescribed antibiotics as a precaution.

Bone

Bone is the most rigid of the connective tissues, and it is composed of bone cells surrounded by a very hard matrix containing calcium and large numbers of collagen fibres. Because of their hardness, bones provide protection, support and muscle attachment (Marieb and Keller 2017).

Cartilage

Cartilage, which is softer but more flexible than bone, is found in only a few places in the body, for example covering the ends of the bones where they form joints (Marieb and Hoehn 2019). Cartilage is found between the two pelvic bones, forming part of the symphysis pubis. This cushions the bones and allows a small amount of movement in the pelvis as the uterus grows.

Dense Connective Tissue

Dense connective tissue forms strong, stringy structures such as tendons (which attach skeletal muscles to bones) and the more elastic ligaments (that connect bones to other bones at joints). Dense connective tissue also makes up the lower layers of the skin (known as the dermis). A condition known as pelvic girdle pain (previously referred to as symphysis pubis dysfunction) can occur in late pregnancy, in which the ligaments connecting the two pelvic bones relax too much, causing pain and difficulty with walking. This normally resolves spontaneously during the puerperium.

Case Study 2.1   Pelvic Girdle Pain

From 30 weeks' gestation in her second pregnancy, Talia started to experience backache that steadily got worse, much worse than the backache she had experienced during her first pregnancy. This was accompanied by pain in her pubic region that got worse when she stood up. Talia described the pain as a burning, bruising sensation that radiated down to the middle of her upper thigh and got particularly bad whenever she stooped down to pick up her daughter. It also increased in severity when she lifted or parted her legs, which made climbing the stairs difficult, and Talia avoided doing this wherever possible.

Talia tried hard to continue with her daily life, putting her pain down to a pregnancy-related discomfort that she had to put up with. However, as the days passed the pain became so severe that it was interrupting her sleep, as she was unable to find a comfortable position in bed. She felt tired all the time and struggled to care for her daughter without help from her partner. This put an extra strain on their relationship as he had a demanding full-time job and was unable to do much to help her. Talia now described the pain as excruciating and at times like a stabbing pain between her legs. She was reluctant to take any form of pain relief as she was worried about the effect on her baby.

After some weeks of the pain getting more debilitating, and with Talia feeling exhausted and depressed, she reported her symptoms to the midwife. When Talia entered the room, the midwife had already noted that she was visibly in pain and walked slowly with a waddling gait, dragging her left foot slightly.

The midwife referred Talia to her GP. The doctor agreed that from her symptoms it was likely that Talia was suffering from pelvic girdle pain (PGP) related to her pregnancy. However, it was important to exclude other obstetric or medical reasons for the pain such as a urinary tract infection (UTI), a pelvic infection, the onset of preterm labour or a lumbar spine problem that would need referral to a physiotherapist.

The midwife explained the condition of PGP and gave Talia some general guidance on management of the condition and strategies that might help:

- Pain control. Simple analgesics such as paracetamol and low-potency opiates (for example codeine and dihydrocodeine or a combination of the two, co-codamol) are safe to take during pregnancy.
- Use of a transcutaneous electrical nerve stimulation (TENS) device.
- Referral to a pain clinic at the local hospital to discuss alternative options for controlling the pain.
- General advice regarding changes to daily activities. For example, it was suggested that Talia sit down to get dressed and to undertake household chores such as ironing and washing-up; that she should take as much rest as she could, seeking help from family and friends wherever possible; that she should go up and downstairs one leg at a time, leading with the most pain-free leg; and that lifting heavy weights should be avoided, as should carrying her daughter around on one hip. Talia was advised to try lying in bed on her side with a pillow between her legs, to turn under in bed rather than over or to turn over with knees together, squeezing her buttocks together as she did this.
- Advice was given to undertake gentle pelvic floor and abdominal exercises in order to increase the capacity of her muscles to maintain good posture (core stability).

After this discussion with her midwife, Talia felt reassured that she had a known condition that could be managed.

Loose Connective Tissue

Loose connective tissue is softer and contains more cells, but fewer fibres, than other types of connective tissue (with the exception of blood). There are four types of loose connective tissue:

- Areolar tissue is a soft, pliable tissue that cushions and protects the body organs that it surrounds. It helps to hold the internal organs together. It provides a reservoir of water and salts for the surrounding tissues.
- Adipose tissue, commonly known as 'fat', is areolar tissue with a high proportion of fat cells. It forms the subcutaneous tissue lying beneath the skin where it insulates the body and can protect it from the extremes of both heat and cold (Marieb and Hoehn 2019).
- Reticular tissue consists of a delicate network of reticular fibres. It forms an internal framework to support many free blood cells – mainly the lymphocytes – in the lymphoid organs, such as the lymph nodes, spleen and bone marrow (Marieb and Hoehn 2019).

- Blood is considered a connective tissue because it consists of blood cells, surrounded by a non-living, fluid matrix called blood plasma (Marieb and Hoehn 2019). Blood transports nutrients, waste material, respiratory gases (such as oxygen and carbon dioxide) and many other substances throughout the body.

Muscle Tissue

There are three types of muscle tissue (see Figure 2.8):

- Skeletal muscle is attached to bones and is involved in the movement of the skeleton. These muscles can be controlled voluntarily. The cells of skeletal muscle are long, cylindrical and have several nuclei. In addition, they appear striated (have stripes). They work by contracting and relaxing, with pairs working antagonistically: one muscle contracts and the opposite muscle relaxes. So, for example, if the muscles in the front of the arm contract and the ones at the back of the arm relax, then the arm bends.
- Cardiac muscle is only found in the heart and it pumps blood around the body by contracting and relaxing. Like skeletal muscle, it is striated. However, unlike skeletal muscles, its action is involuntary. The cells of cardiac muscle do not have a nucleus.
- Smooth muscle is found in the walls of hollow organs, such as the stomach, bladder, uterus and blood vessels. Smooth muscle has no striations and like cardiac muscle it works by involuntary action. Smooth muscle causes movement in the hollow organs; that is, as it contracts the cavity of an organ becomes smaller (constricted), and when it relaxes the organ becomes larger (dilated). This allows substances to be propelled through the organ in the right direction. Smooth muscle contracts and relaxes slowly, in a wave-like motion. During labour, the uterine muscles contract and retract; that is, they do not fully relax between contractions. As a result, the uterine cavity gradually reduces in capacity, forcing the fetus downwards, through the birth canal.

35

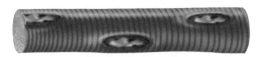

Skeletal muscle

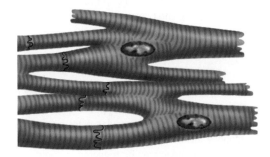

Cardiac muscle

Smooth muscle

FIGURE 2.8 Muscle cells. Source: Adapted from https://in.pinterest.com/pin/656681189392007577.

Health Promotion: Smoking During Pregnancy

The risks of smoking to general health and during pregnancy are well documented. Many chemicals contained in tobacco smoke are known to be harmful to the smoker and can also cross the placenta, causing further harm to the developing fetus. These include polycystic aromatic hydrocarbons, carbon monoxide, cyanide, lead and cadmium, all of which are inhaled in cigarette smoke (Rankin 2017).

During pregnancy, these chemicals cross the placenta and enter the fetal blood stream. Some of them may lead to reduced vascularisation (meaning a reduced development of blood vessels), internal swelling of the blood capillaries and a broadening of the basement membrane of the placental villi. This affects the efficiency of placental function, leading to a potential increase in pregnancy complications such as bleeding, miscarriage, stillbirth, preterm labour and reduced fetal growth.

Medicines Management: Syntocinon

Uterine stimulants (known as oxytocics or uterotonics) are drugs administered to women during childbirth that cause the uterine muscle to contract. They may also be used to augment labour by increasing the length, strength and frequency of existing uterine contractions and during active management of the third stage of labour. The most commonly used oxytocic drug is syntocinon. This is a synthetic substance almost identical to the natural hormone oxytocin, which is released from the posterior pituitary gland into the woman's circulation in response to the beginning of the labour and/or the infant sucking at the breast. Oxytocin has the effect of stimulating the smooth muscle contained within the uterus and has the most powerful effect towards the end of pregnancy, during labour and during the immediate postnatal period.

Nervous Tissue

Nervous tissue is concerned with control and communication within the body by means of electrical signals. The main type of cell forming nervous tissue is the neuron (Figure 2.9), which receives and conducts electrochemical impulses around the body. The structure of neurons is very different from that of other cells and they can be up to a metre long. Neurons receive and transmit electrical impulses very rapidly from one to the other across synapses (junctions). It is at the synapses that the electrical impulse can pass from neuron to neuron, or from a neuron to a muscle cell. The total number of neurons is fixed at birth and they cannot be replaced if they are damaged (McCance et al. 2018).

The neurons and supporting cells make up the structures of the nervous system, which includes the brain, the spinal cord and the nerves. Neurons play a major role in the sensation of pain. Some forms of analgesia used in childbirth, such as pethidine, affect the sensation of pain by blocking the transmission of impulses from one neuron to another.

Orange Flag: Perception of Body Image During Pregnancy

Significant changes at cellular level occur during pregnancy as the woman's body adapts physiologically to the demands of the developing fetus and impending delivery. Changes include physical changes such as weight gain, alterations to skin pigmentation, hyperflexibility of joints and significant changes within the cardiovascular, digestive and respiratory systems. There are also psychological changes associated with the pregnancy, including reports of low self-esteem, fatigue, anxiety and stress.

As a result, there is a risk that a negative body image may be triggered in some women as they are dissatisfied with the changes their body undergoes during and after pregnancy. Riesco-González (2022) demonstrated that dissatisfaction with body image led to increased reports of postnatal depression for some women. This highlights the importance of midwives explaining possible anatomical and physiological changes associated with pregnancy and the postpartum period in order to prepare women for the transformations ahead, to understand why they are occurring and that they are a necessary and a natural part of becoming a mother.

List the physiological and anatomical changes associated with pregnancy and the postpartum period that might lead to a woman feeling dissatisfied with her body image.

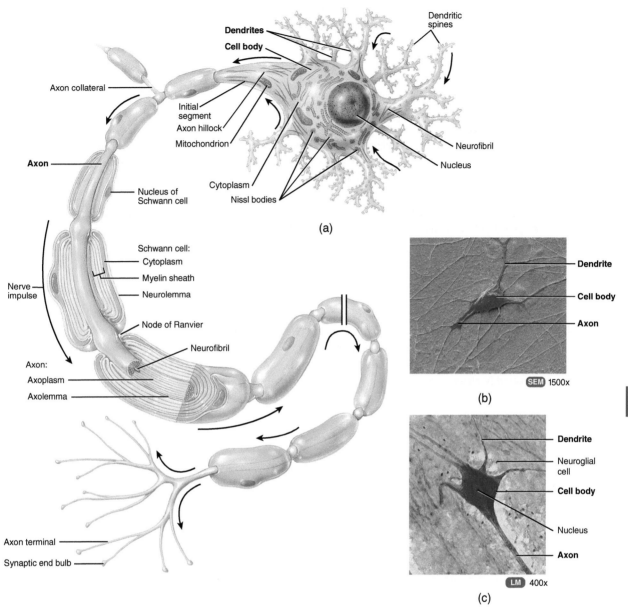

FIGURE 2.9 Nerve cells (neurons). (a) Parts of a neuron. (b, c) Motor neurons. Source: Reproduced by permission from Tortora and Derrickson 2017 / Wiley.

Tissue Damage and the Healing Process

The process of wound healing, by which the tissues repair themselves, occurs in four stages: haemostasis, inflammation, proliferation and remodelling. All of these occur simultaneously, but in a synchronised manner (Wallace et al. 2023).

Haemostasis

When injury occurs, lymphatic fluid and blood are released from the wound site. Coagulation pathways are activated in order to stop bleeding and achieve homeostasis. Vasoconstriction occurs at the wound site and clotting factors and platelets move into the area. Platelets clump together (aggregate) to form a thrombus (clot), which traps bacteria that have entered the wound. Vasoconstriction is followed by vasodilation, allowing white blood cells to enter the site to attack any pathogens and increasing the movement of plasma proteins and blood cells into the tissues in the area. This causes oedema (swelling).

Inflammation

There are four major signs and symptoms of an inflammatory response: pain, swelling, heat and redness. In severe cases, nausea, sweating, a raised pulse, lowered blood pressure and even loss of consciousness may occur. These symptoms are the body's response to pain and shock. Histamine is released from the damaged cells into the tissues. Histamine aids the inflammatory response to injury by making the capillaries more permeable to white blood cells and some proteins. This allows them to attack any pathogens in the affected tissues. Immunoglobulins are released to help destroy bacteria. Phagocytes and lymphocytes (types of white blood cells) move into the area and start to destroy any infectious organisms found there. These blood cells remain in the area until tissue regeneration (repair) takes place.

Proliferation (Granulation)

This phase starts approximately 3–10 days after injury and takes days or weeks to complete, depending on the severity of the wound. It consists of the formation of new tissues and restoration of the damaged vascular network (Ozgok Kangal and Regan 2023). During this phase new blood vessels are formed and new epithelial cells develop, starting at the wound edges. Initially only a thin layer of epithelial cells is laid down, but over time a thicker and more durable layer of cells will grow to cover the wound (Wallace et al. 2023)

Remodelling

The maturational or remodelling phase starts around week 3 and can last for up to a year in a healthy person. During the remodelling phase, the proliferation of new tissue ends, the wound contracts and the maturation of the wound begins. The tensile strength of the wound gradually increases; however, the resulting scar tissue will never be as strong as the surrounding (uninjured) tissue and will have only about 80% of its tensile strength (Ozgok Kangal and Regan 2023).

Learning Event

Consider the different types of tissue damage that commonly occur during childbirth. Where are they located? Which types of tissue are they?

Using a current midwifery textbook, read about how such damage can be minimised or even avoided.

Factors That Influence Wound Healing

In a healthy person, the healing process is usually straightforward. However, bacterial infection of a wound can delay the healing process: the term 'wound breakdown' is commonly used in midwifery to describe a perineal or abdominal wound that has become infected and is not healing normally. Other factors can interfere with wound healing, including the following:

- **Malnutrition:** Inadequate protein intake, low carbohydrate stores and low levels of vitamins C, A, B_1 and zinc can delay the healing process and result in weaker scar tissue.

- **Low oxygen perfusion:** Smokers and people with chronic lung conditions may have reduced O_2 saturation. This can impede the inflammatory process and the proliferation of new cells.
- **Some medication:** Anti-inflammatory drugs, corticosteroids and immunosuppressant drugs are among those that may impede wound healing.
- **Co-morbidities:** In women of childbearing age, diabetes mellitus can cause poor perfusion and decreased immune function, which raise the risk of infection and can delay wound healing.
- **Age:** The efficiency of wound healing decreases with age (Ozgok Kangal and Regan 2023).

Red Flag: Signs of Infections in Caesarean Wounds

Some pain, redness, swelling and heat are normal and are part of the tissue repair process. These symptoms should gradually disappear within a few days. However, excessive pain, which does not respond to over-the-counter analgesia, an offensive smell, a gaping wound and oozing exudate (pus) are suggestive of wound breakdown due to bacterial infection. If not treated quickly, infected wounds can lead to sepsis, which is a medical emergency. Women with symptoms of infection should be referred promptly to their GP for antibiotic treatment.

Woman-Centred Care: Using an Aseptic Non-touch Technique

An aseptic non-touch technique (ANNT) is a process designed to prevent the transfer of potentially harmful microorganisms to a site on the body that may be susceptible to infection (Wilson 2019). In midwifery this may include a surgical wound associated with caesarean section, a perineal wound sustained during childbirth or a damaged nipple. An aseptic technique will be required for clinical procedures that midwives may undertake, including urinary catheterisation, venous cannulation, phlebotomy, administration of intravenous drugs or fluids and the dressing of a surgical wound. It is important for midwives to involve women in discussions around when and how to undertake these procedures to alleviate anxiety, put the woman at ease and ensure they provide informed consent. Women should also be aware of the principles involved in reducing contamination so that they can play their own part in ensuring that the transfer of pathogenic organisms is reduced.

The principles of ANTT include:

- The protection of key elements of equipment that need to remain free from microorganisms (for example the barrel of a needle, or the inside of a sterile dressing).
- Risk assessment prior to undertaking the procedure to direct the midwife as to whether the key parts and sites can be protected by non-touch alone or whether the use of sterile gloves might be needed (for example during the insertion of a urinary catheter).
- A medical or standard aseptic technique can be used for procedures that are considered simple and are short in duration (taking less than 20 minutes), involve small sites (such as a puncture site) and have a smaller number of key parts.
- Surgical aseptic technique should be undertaken for complex invasive procedures lasting longer than 20 minutes and involving large and numerous key parts.

Learning Event

- Review your local policies for infection control and prevention, including use of personal protective equipment and when ANTT should be used.
- Find out what sterile equipment is available in the clinical areas and where and how it is stored.
- When might you need to use an aseptic technique in your midwifery practice? Give three examples.
- What is the role and responsibility of the midwife when undertaking ANNT?
- Review the National Institute for Health and Care Excellence guideline on prevention and control of healthcare-associated infections in primary and community care (updated 2017): www.nice.org.uk/guidance/cg139/resources/healthcareassociated-infections-prevention-and-control-in-primary-and-community-care-35109518767045.

Cells are extremely complicated parts of the body, but it is important to understand them and their functions in order to understand how the human body itself functions. Cells form tissues, which then form all the structures, systems and organs of the body. Therefore, it is necessary also to understand tissues. The remainder of this book will look at the various systems, structures and organs of the body – how they function as well as what can go wrong with them.

Conditions Associated with Cell and Tissue Damage

There follows a list of conditions that are associated with cell and tissue damage. Take some time and write notes about each of the conditions. Think about the anatomy and physiology associated these conditions. Remember to include aspects of care. If you are making notes about people you have offered care and support to, you must not include their names or any identifying details.

The condition	Your notes
Dehiscence (breakdown) of caesarean scar	
Nipple soreness in breastfeeding women	
Episiotomy	
Neonatal caput succedaneum	

Take-Home Points

- The cells are the basic living, structural and functional units of the body.
- Humans are multicellular beings.
- Each cell can take in nutrients, convert those nutrients into energy, undertake specialised functions and reproduce as required.
- Cells arise from existing cells, as one cell divides into two identical cells.
- The different types of cells carry out unique roles supporting homeostasis and provide assistance for the many functional capabilities of the human organism.
- Cell structure and function are closely related.
- Cells carry out an assortment of chemical reactions, creating and maintaining life processes.
- The types of chemical reactions within specialised cellular structures are coordinated to maintain life in a cell, tissue, organ, system and organism.

Conclusion

Understanding cellular function is crucial for midwives due to its significant implications for pregnancy, childbirth and postnatal care. Incorporating knowledge of cellular biology and function into midwifery practice has the potential to enhance the quality of care provided to pregnant women and new mothers, equipping midwives with a deeper understanding of the physiological processes that underlie pregnancy, childbirth and postpartum care. This knowledge enhances the midwife's ability to provide evidence-based, holistic care that promotes the well-being of mothers and the newborn. It bridges the gap between the microscopic world of cells and the transformative journey of childbirth, ultimately contributing to positive maternal and fetal outcomes.

References

Aasheim, V., Nilsen, A.B.V., Reinar, L.M., and Lukasse, M. (2017). Perineal techniques during the second stage of labour for reducing perineal trauma. *Cochrane Database of Systematic Reviews* 6 (6): CD006672. https://doi.org/10.1002/14651858.CD006672.pub3.

Cluett, E.R., Burns, E., and Cuthbert, A. (2018). Immersion in water during labour and birth. *Cochrane Database of Systematic Reviews* 5 (5): CD000111. https://doi.org/10.1002/14651858.CD000111.pub4.

Colbert, B.J., Ankney, J., and Lee, K.T. (2019). *Anatomy and Physiology for Health Professionals: An Interactive Journey*, 4e. Boston: Pearson.

Garland, D. (2017). *Revisiting Waterbirth: An Attitude to Care*. London: Bloomsbury.

Kalra, A., Lowe, A., and Jumaily, A.A.I. (2016). An overview of factors affecting the skin's Young's modulus. *Journal of Ageing Science* 4: 156. https://doi.org/10.4172/2329-8847.1000156.

Marieb, E.N. and Hoehn, K.N. (2019). *Human Anatomy and Physiology*, 11e. Boston: Pearson.

Marieb, E.N. and Keller, S. (2017). *Essentials of Human Anatomy and Physiology*, 12e. Harlow: Pearson.

McCance, K.L., Huether, S.E., Brashers, V.L., and Rote, N.S. (2018). *Pathophysiology: The Biologic Basis for Disease in Adults and Children*, 8e. St Louis: Elsevier.

McPherson, K.C., Beggs, A.D., Sultan, A.H. et al. (2014). Can the risk of obstetric anal sphincter injuries (OASIs) be predicted using a risk-scoring system? *BMC Research Notes* 7: 471. https://doi.org/10.1186/1756-0500-7-471.

Ogawa-Fuse, C., Morisaki, N., Shima, K. et al. (2019). Impact of water exposure on skin barrier permeability and ultrastructure. *Contact Dermatitis* 80 (4): 228–233. https://doi.org/10.1111/cod.13174.

Ozgok Kangal, M.K. and Regan, J.P. (2023). Wound healing. In: *StatPearls*. Treasure Island, FL: StatPearls Publishing https://www.ncbi.nlm.nih.gov/books/NBK535406.

Papoutsis, D. (2020). Novel insights on the possible effects of water exposure on the structural integrity of the perineum during a waterbirth. *European Journal of Midwifery* 4: 40. https://doi.org/10.18332/ejm/127263.

Papoutsis, D., Antoniou, A., Gornall, A., and Tzavara, C. (2021). The incidence of and predictors for severe perineal trauma and intact perineum in women having a waterbirth in England: a hospital-based study. *Journal of Women's Health* 30 (5): 681–688. https://doi.org/10.1089/jwh.2019.8244.

Rankin, J. (2017). *Physiology in Childbearing: With Anatomy and Related Biosciences*. St Louis: Elsevier.

Riesco-González, F.J., Antúnez-Calvente, I., Vázquez-Lara, J.M. et al. (2022). Body image dissatisfaction as a risk factor for postpartum depression. *Medicina (Kaunas, Lithuania)* 58 (6): 752. https://doi.org/10.3390/medicina58060752.

Schmidt, D., Germano, A.M.C., and Milani, T.L. (2018). Effects of water immersion on sensitivity and plantar skin properties. *Neuroscience Letters* 686: 41–46. https://doi.org/10.1016/j.neulet.2018.08.048.

Tortora, G.J. and Derrickson, B. (2017). *Tortora's Principles of Anatomy & Physiology*. Singapore: Wiley.

Ulfsdottir, H., Saltvedt, S., and Georgsson, S. (2019). Women's experiences of waterbirth compared with conventional uncomplicated births. *Midwifery* 79: 102547. https://doi.org/10.1016/j.midw.2019.102547.

Wallace, H.A., Basehore, B.M., and Zito, P.M. (2023). Wound healing phases. In: *StatPearls*. Treasure Island,FL: StatPearls Publishing https://pubmed.ncbi.nlm.nih.gov/29262065.

Watson, R. (2005). Cell structure and function, growth and development. In: *Physiology for Nursing Practice*, 3e (ed. S.E. Montague, R. Watson, and R.A. Herbert), 49–69. Edinburgh: Elsevier.

Wheeldon, A. (2016). Tissue. In: *Fundamentals of Anatomy and Physiology for Student Nurses* (ed. I. Peate and M. Nair). Chichester, UK: Wiley-Blackwell.

Wilson, J. (2019). *Infection Control in Clinical Practice*, 95–120. St Louis: Elsevier.

Wilson, E., Wood, S.L., and Benova, L. (2020). Incidence of and risk factors for lactational mastitis: a systematic review. *Journal of Human Lactation* 36 (4): 673–686. https://doi.org/10.1177/0890334420907898.

Further Resource

Peate, I. and Hamilton, C. (2022). *Fundamentals of Pharmacology for Midwives*. Chichester, UK: Wiley.

Glossary

Active transport	The process by which substances are moved along their concentration gradient (i.e. from an area with of concentration to one of higher concentration) and which requires energy
Adenosine triphosphate (ATP)	The source of energy for use and storage at the cellular level
Cytoplasm	The fluid and contents of a cell
Diffusion	The process by which substances move down their concentration gradients from a higher to a lower concentration
Hydrophilic	Water-loving substance, soluble in water
Hydrophobic	Water-hating substance, insoluble in water and soluble in lipids
Interstitial	Between cells
Intracellular	Inside the cell
Organelles	'Mini organs' that perform the vital functions of the cell
Osmosis	Movement of water through a selectively permeable membrane to equalise the solute concentration on either side of the membrane
Osmotic pressure	The pressure that must be exerted on a solution into which water is flowing by osmosis in order to completely oppose that osmotic movement
Passive transport	The process by which substances move down a concentration gradient without requiring energy
Plasma membrane	Outer layer of the cell

CHAPTER 3

Embryo Development and Fetal Growth

Vikki Smith[1] and Jacinta H. Martin[2,3]

[1] *Department of Nursing, Midwifery and Health, Northumbria University, Newcastle upon Tyne, UK*

[2] *School of Environmental and Life Sciences, College of Engineering, Science and Environment, University of Newcastle, Australia*

[3] *Infertility and Reproduction Research Program, Hunter Medical Research Institute (HMRI), Newcastle, Australia*

AIM

The aim of this chapter is to provide an in-depth overview of the early events of embryonic and fetal development.

LEARNING OUTCOMES

On completion of this chapter the reader will be able to:

- Describe the phases of pre-implantation embryo development
- Define the stages of implantation and early placental development
- Describe key events that occur to the mother and child during the fetal period
- Understand the different types of pregnancy loss and their characteristic timing

Test Your Prior Knowledge

1. At what stage is an embryo considered a fetus?
2. At which gestational week(s) is a pregnancy loss considered a miscarriage, a spontaneous abortion or a stillbirth?
3. Define the range of gestational weeks that characterise each trimester.
4. Which hormone does the modern-day pregnancy test recognise?

This chapter will explore the processes from conception to early embryonic development, implantation, early placentation and fetal development through to birth. Aspects of pathophysiology that can arise during this period of development will also be addressed.

Fundamentals of Maternal Pathophysiology, First Edition. Edited by Claire Leader and Ian Peate.
© 2024 John Wiley & Sons Ltd. Published 2024 by John Wiley & Sons Ltd.
Companion website: www.wiley.com/go/leader/maternalpatho

Note that in clinical care cases, health professionals calculate gestational stage based on a woman's last menstrual period, approximately two weeks prior to fertilisation. However, when following the development of an embryo, the date of fertilisation or conception gives us the start of embryonic development. This therefore means that there may be a two-week disparity between embryonic age and gestational age. In this chapter we have attempted to clarify these two scales.

The Germinal Stage

The germinal stage refers to the period from fertilisation through the development of the early embryo until implantation is completed in the uterus. The entire germinal stage takes approximately 10 days.

Fertilisation/Conception

Using the embryonic time scale, fertilisation or 'conception' is considered day 1. While this topic will be considered further in Chapter 5, we will briefly discuss the key concepts here to facilitate a better understanding of the remaining topics in this chapter. Conception involves the union of a haploid egg and a haploid sperm, usually in the ampulla of the fallopian tube. The result of this merger is to reconstitute diploidy in the form of a zygote, or fertilised egg. This process involves egg activation and the triggering of a series of coordinated molecular events, including mitotic divisions, that result in cell differentiation and embryo development.

Of these molecular events, arguably the most important is the fusion of the male and female pronuclei (the nuclei of a sperm or egg cell during fertilisation), also known as syngamy (Figure 3.1). During syngamy, the nuclear membranes of the male and female pronuclei are broken down and the chromosomes condense separately before lining up along the metaphase plate of the first mitotic spindle (~12–18 hours from fertilisation). At this point, the newly formed embryo contains a unique constitution of chromosomes. Following syngamy, the zygote cytoplasm will then divide in half, via a process known as cleavage. This will give rise to two identical daughter cells, each with a complete diploid set of chromosomes, generating what is now termed a two-cell embryo (by 24 hours).

Pre-implantation Development: Cleavage (Embryonic Days 2–5)

Now that cleavage has begun, the pre-implantation embryo will continue to divide such that the first two cells divide into four cells, then into eight cells and so on. Each division takes 12–24 hours. Despite the rapidly increasing number of these daughter cells (also called blastomeres), the embryo does not undergo an increase in overall size. Instead, with each successive subdivision, the ratio of nuclear to cytoplasmic material increases (Figure 3.2).

Coinciding with cleavage, the embryo travels through the oviduct into the uterine cavity (Figure 3.3). This journey is facilitated by currents created by the cilia of the uterine epithelium lining and the coordinated contractions of the uterine muscular layer.

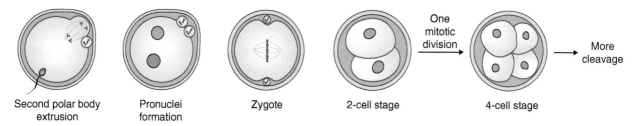

FIGURE 3.1   Fertilisation and early embryo development. Source: Reproduced with permission from Webster and de Wreede (2016) / Wiley.

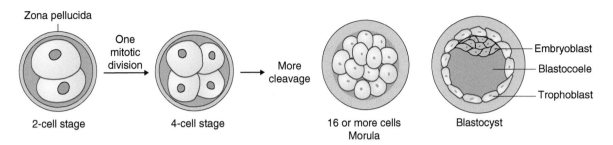

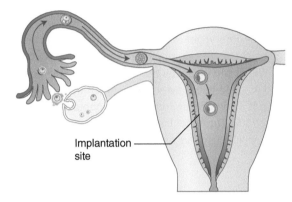

FIGURE 3.2 Pre-implantation development. Source: Reproduced with permission from Webster and de Wreede (2016) / Wiley.

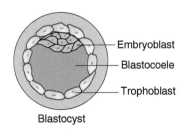

FIGURE 3.3 Pre-implantation development and implantation. Source: Reproduced with permission from Webster and de Wreede (2016) / Wiley.

After approximately three days from fertilisation, the embryo completes the journey through the fallopian tube and reaches the uterus. At this stage it now consists of approximately 16–32 blastomeres and is known as a morula. Here the first major morphological change occurs within the embryo, where the outermost cells become bound tightly together by desmosomes and gap junctions (intracellular connections). At this stage, the cells are nearly indistinguishable from one another and are undergoing a process known as 'compaction' (Figure 3.2). On day 4, the human morula begins to accumulate fluid into an internal cavity (blastocoele) around which the cells organise themselves (Figure 3.4). The fluid comes about from the uterus as sodium-potassium pumps (on the trophoblasts, see later) create a concentration gradient favouring the uptake of fluid into the embryo.

As these cells reorganise around the newly forming cavity, they become polarised and begin to differentiate based on their location: those on the 'outside' become differentially fated into trophoblast (early placental cells) and those on the 'inside' become the progenitors of the inner cell mass or embryoblast destined to become the fetus (Figure 3.4). At this stage, the embryo is now termed a blastocyst and contains around 70–100 cells that make up these two distinct cell lines.

FIGURE 3.4 Human blastocyst and the two progenitor lineages. Source: Reproduced with permission from Webster and de Wreede (2016) / Wiley.

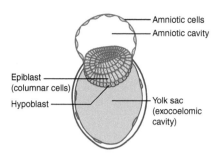

FIGURE 3.5   The bilaminar disk of the early embryo. Source: Reproduced with permission from Webster and de Wreede (2016) / Wiley.

The next stage is implantation. Here, as embryogenesis continues, the cells of the trophectoderm continue to differentiate to form the extra-embryonic structures, the chorionic sac and the fetal portion of the placenta. These play a supporting role for the embryo proper. Within the inner cell mass, further polarisation of the embryo dictated by the spatial arrangement of these cells around the fluid-filled cavity further determines their fate. Those cells directly exposed to the fluid cavity (the lowest portion) adopt a primitive endoderm (or hypoblast) fate, while the remaining cells adopt a primitive ectoderm (or epiblast) fate (Figure 3.5). The hypoblast cooperates with the trophectoderm to produce the extra-embryonic membranes, while the epiblast will largely give rise to the fetus.

Hatching (Day 6), Implantation (Day 10) and Early Placentation (Day 12)

Implantation occurs during a brief window of uterine receptivity otherwise known as the 'implantation window'. During this time the blastocyst sheds its zona pellucida (the outermost layer of the embryo) in a process known as 'hatching'. Until now, the role of the zona pellucida was to provide structural support to the oocyte and embryo, aid in species-specific binding (more important in external fertilisers), prevent polyspermy (fertilisation by more than one sperm) and prevent premature implantation and consequential establishment of an ectopic pregnancy (implantation outside of the uterus). The act of hatching requires a coordinated process of enzymatic lysis by proteases, and hydrostatic pressure exerted by the expanding blastocoel that causes the zona to rupture. Once liberated, the trophectoderm attaches (apposition and adhesion stages of implantation) to the luminal epithelium of the uterus and acquires invasive properties (invasion stage) to mediate its penetration and engulfment into the uterus (Bischof and Campana 1997). In humans, the implantation site is usually in the upper and posterior wall in the midsagittal plane of the uterus.

Appropriate attachment and invasion of the blastocyst requires coordinated modifications in the endometrial stroma in a process known as 'decidualisation' (Ramathal et al. 2010). In humans, decidualisation is the result of post-ovulatory remodelling of the endometrium and involves transformation of uterine glands, an influx of macrophages and specialised uterine natural killer cells, stromal vascular remodelling, angiogenesis and stromal glycogen accumulation (Gellersen et al. 2007). Following successful implantation, the decidua continues to develop to promote complete placentation. Once complete, the decidua consists of several sublayers, the decidua basalis (the endometrium immediately beneath the implantation site), the decidua capsularis (the overlying endometrial stroma) and the decidua parietalis (the endometrium lining the rest of the uterine cavity); each has a different role during gestation (Figure 3.6). Altogether, these processes are essential for providing an early supply of nutrients to the embryo, modulating the maternal immune system to prevent rejection and remodelling the maternal spiral arteries for the provision of adequate blood flow to the placenta later in pregnancy (Lowe and Anderson 2015).

Implantation signals the end of the pre-embryonic stage of development and the beginning of placental formation (see Chapter 7). It is at this stage that the synthesis of the hormone human chorionic gonadotropin (hCG) by the syncytiotrophoblast layer begins. hCG is essential in early pregnancy as the corpus luteum (an endocrine structure produced within the ovary following ovulation) requires hCG to sustain progesterone production and, subsequently, the uterine endometrium for successful implantation. It is also hCG that is used to detect pregnancy in a clinical setting.

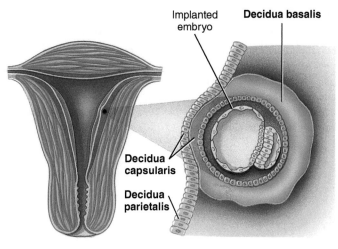

Regions of the decidua

FIGURE 3.6 The sublayers of the decidua. Source: Reproduced with permission from Webster and de Wreede (2016) / Wiley.

This window of endometrial receptivity is restricted to days 16–22 of a normal 28-day menstrual cycle, 5–10 days after the luteinising hormone surge (Navot et al. 1991). If implantation does not occur during this window, the uterus will move into the non-receptive period for the remainder of the cycle, the late luteal phase, until menstruation occurs, and the embryo (or oocyte if fertilisation does not occur) will be shed with the uterine lining.

Medical Management: Pregnancy Test

A pregnancy is confirmed by the presence of hCG in a woman's urine or blood. hCG from the implanting blastocyst first appears in blood around six to eight days following fertilisation. Blood tests are usually more sensitive than urine tests (99.5–100% vs 98%) and are able to estimate the age of a pregnancy. For a blood hCG test, venous blood must be collected by a health professional and sent away for laboratory analysis; urine tests, however, may be conducted on site or at home.

Early diagnosis of pregnancy enables early preventative interventions to ensure maternal and fetal health. This can include antenatal care and the avoidance of substances such as alcohol and nicotine that can disrupt embryonic/fetal development. A blood hCG test can distinguish between a normally progressing and an abnormal pregnancy (e.g. a molar pregnancy) and allow for appropriate intervention if needed. Early detection is also beneficial for those who do not wish to proceed with their pregnancy, as it enables termination in the early stages, when it is safest.

Red Flag: Inadequate Invasion

During the invasion stage of implantation, small, high-resistance vessels are replaced with large, low-resistance vessels in a process known as maternal spiral arterial remodelling (Bronsens et al. 1967). This remodelling process is driven by specialised trophoblast cells that invade into the nearby spiral arteries and alter the vessel walls by removing vascular smooth muscle cells and replacing endothelial cells with endovascular extra-villus trophoblast cells. It also involves the deposition of extra-cellular fibrinoid (Cartwright et al. 2010). Many of these changes can be detected in decidual vessels from 8 weeks, with deep invasion of the myometrial sections seen after 15 weeks (Pijnenborg et al. 2006). Importantly, it is now recognised that the extent of trophoblastic invasion determines later placental efficiency and fetal viability. Deficiencies in trophoblastic invasion give rise to adverse pregnancy outcomes such as intra-uterine growth restriction and pre-eclampsia.

Source: Adapted from Hunkapiller et al. (2011).

Orange Flag: Teenage Pregnancy

Teenage pregnancy is surrounded by a significant amount of stigma that can have negative impacts on the health and well-being of the pregnant teenager, who is likely to be experiencing intense and mixed feelings about the pregnancy and parenting. Those under 19 years of age also require additional care during this time, as they have unique health concerns that can make pregnancy difficult or especially taxing. If the pregnancy is unplanned or the result of a sexual assault, psychological support should also be provided. Early and regular antenatal care should also be available. These services should be equipped to deal with the intricacies of a pregnant teenager's special physical and emotional needs.

The Embryonic Stage

The embryonic stage refers to the period encompassing the third through to the eighth week of gestation. This period of development sees gastrulation, neurulation and organogenesis.

Post-Implantation Development (Embryonic Weeks 2–4 and Gestational Weeks 4–6): Gastrulation

The second and third weeks of embryological development are crucial, involving the establishment of three distinct germ layers: the mesoderm, endoderm and ectoderm via the process of gastrulation (Figure 3.7). The endoderm goes on to form the epithelium of the digestive tract, lungs, liver, pancreas and thyroid. The mesoderm gives rise to muscle, cartilage and bone, as well as the heart and circulatory system, gonads and urogenital system. The ectoderm forms to the outer components of the body, including the skin, hair and mammary glands, as well as other parts of the nervous system. During this time frame neurulation also begins. This process results in the development of the central nervous system and the neural tube, which goes on to form the early brain and spine. This is an especially crucial period of development as defects in primary neurulation are implicated in anencephaly, spina bifida and craniorachischisis.

Medicines Management: Folic Acid Supplementation

Folate or folic acid is also known as vitamin B_9. Many foods are naturally rich in vitamin B_9, including green vegetables, shellfish and nuts. Other foods may be fortified by adding folic acid during production (e.g. bread). Folate plays essential roles in producing DNA and RNA and is involved in protein metabolism. It is also required to produce red blood cells and is critical during periods of rapid growth, such as pregnancy and fetal development.

Folic acid supplementation is recommended for all women prior to conception and up to 12 weeks' gestation to reduce the risk of fetal neural tube defects (NTDs; spina bifida and anencephaly). A woman's risk of having a fetus with an NTD should be assessed, ideally before conception. The current recommendation is for women with a usual risk for NTD to take 400 µg daily. Woman with a higher NTD risk should be offered 5 mg/d.

A pregnancy is considered to have an increased chance of an NTD if:

- Either parent has an NTD or previously had a child/fetus with an NTD.
- The woman is taking anti-epileptic drugs.
- The women has diabetes, coeliac disease, sickle cell disease, thalassaemia or a body mass index (BMI) over 20 kg/m²
  (NICE 2023).

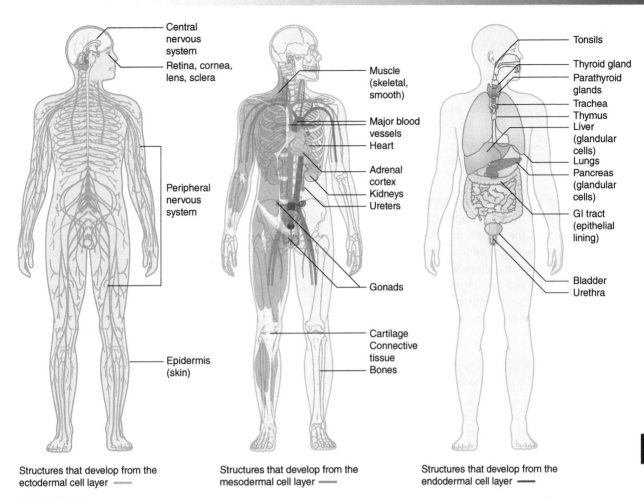

Structures that develop from the ectodermal cell layer ——

Structures that develop from the mesodermal cell layer ——

Structures that develop from the endodermal cell layer ——

49

FIGURE 3.7 The fate of the three germ layers. GI, gastrointestinal. Source: Reproduced with permission from Webster and de Wreede (2016) / Wiley.

Post-Implantation Development (Weeks 4–8): Organogenesis

By the beginning of the fourth week of gestation, the embryo's head develops primitive eyes and the inner ear canals. The heart has also begun to develop from a tube of mesoderm and has started beating. The arm and leg buds also arise from a combination of ectoderm and mesoderm. By week 5, the arm buds begin to flatten and become 'paddle-like'. The remainder of week 5 is largely characterised by rapid brain growth, where distinct brain areas and cranial nerves begin to develop. During this time the heart chambers have also begun to develop, and the primitive gonads form at the genital ridge. By the end of this week the embryo is has reached approximately 1 cm in length.

During week 6, the embryonic eyes gain pigment and the external ears form. The brain and the head expand, while the hand buds form finger rays. The heart continues to develop and establishes the first circulation as the liver begins to produce blood cells. In terms of the reproductive system, the primordial germ cells complete their migration from the hindgut to the gonads at the genital ridge.

Weeks 7 and 8 mark the final two-week period of embryonic development. This time is marked by distinct facial, organ system and neuromuscular development. The mouth, tongue and palate are completed during this time and the gonads differentiate into testes or ovaries based on the genetic sex of the embryo (the chromosomes it carries: XX for a genetically female individual and XY for a genetically male individual). Fetal movement is also now visible on ultrasound.

Examination Scenarios: Ultrasound

Ultrasound or sonography is an imaging method that uses sound waves to produce images of structures within a body. An ultrasound (transabdominal and/or transvaginal) is offered to all women during the first trimester of pregnancy to determine pregnancy viability, number of fetuses, location (i.e. intrauterine or ectopic) and to screen for major fetal malformations (i.e. acrania, absence of a fetal skull). Gestational age may also be calculated by measurement of the fetus's crown–rump length (CRL), which is electronically compared to a standard reference chart to offer an accurate estimated due date.

Source: Adapted from Knight et al. (2018).

It is also during this period of development, between implantation to around 60 days post-conception, that the embryo is most sensitive to developmental abnormalities, specifically teratogenesis. By definition, a human teratogen is an agent that alters the growth or structure of the developing embryo or fetus, causing birth defects (Alwan and Chambers 2015). However, in addition to birth defects, a teratogenic exposure may lead to death or manifest as growth retardation, or a functional disorder. The term functional disorder encompasses neurological impairments, including intellectual disability and long-term effects on cognition, learning, attention and/or behaviour that may appear later in childhood. It is important to note that outcome severity is influenced by the dose and duration of a teratogenic exposure as well as the timing of exposure, as some developmental stages are more susceptible than others.

Health Promotion: Teratogens

Numerous teratogenic agents have been identified, including physical agents (ionising radiation and hyperthermia), maternal health factors (obesity and diabetes), environmental chemicals (heavy metals and herbicides) and drugs (prescription, over the counter or recreational). Infectious agents have also been shown to have teratogenic effects (cytomegalovirus, rubella varicella, herpes simplex, toxoplasma, syphilis) on infants.

It is usually advised that during pregnancy known teratogens should be avoided. However, in the case of prescription medications, if the woman has a medical condition or becomes ill during her pregnancy, the health and welfare of both the mother and the unborn baby may also be at risk without treatment. In these situations, it is important that healthcare providers discuss with their patients the potential risks and benefits of continuing to use these medications during pregnancy.

It is also important to note that the risk of a birth defect for any baby is about 4%, regardless of the circumstances during pregnancy. This means that even those who strictly avoid known teratogens while pregnant may still bear children with a birth defect.

The Fetal Stage

The fetal stage describes the period of time from the ninth week of gestation until birth. At this point the embryo is now known as a fetus. This period of prenatal development is marked primarily by additional changes in the brain, maturation of the organ systems and overall physical growth (weight and length).

Late Gestation and Birth (Embryonic Weeks 11–38 and Gestational Weeks 13–40)

A human pregnancy is divided into three-month periods termed trimesters. The first trimester extends from conception to the 12th week of pregnancy (embryonic week 10). The second trimester extends from weeks 13 to 27, and the third trimester from 28 weeks until birth. A typical pregnancy should span a total of 40 weeks from the first day of the last menstrual period to the birth of the baby. Birth occurring earlier than 37 weeks is considered 'preterm' birth and carries considerable risk for the fetus. In this section we will primarily focus on the changes to the body of the pregnant woman, but will also touch on the major changes taking place in the fetus.

The First Trimester (Also See Post-Implantation Development)

During the first trimester, elevated progesterone levels and other hormonal changes affect almost every organ system in the pregnant body. Tender, swollen breasts, morning sickness (nausea with or without vomiting), increased urination, fatigue, food cravings or aversions, mood swings, heartburn and constipation are complaints regularly associated with pregnancy. In the fetus, by the end of the first trimester all major systems and organs have developed and are functioning, including the circulatory, nervous, digestive and urinary systems, but the fetus cannot yet survive independently.

Antenatal Care During the First Trimester
The first antenatal care appointment should be scheduled during the first trimester, usually before 10 weeks' gestation. In this first visit, the midwife should focus on assessing the pregnant woman's overall health and well-being. Detailed questions about the woman's health history (mental and physical), socioeconomic environment and previous pregnancies, if any, should also be collected to identify any risk factors that may affect the patient and the developing fetus. This appointment should also incorporate discussion surrounding the patient's health behaviours such as smoking and substance misuse, and sensitive enquiries about domestic violence and, if suspected, if female genital mutilation has occurred. At the conclusion of this visit, a plan for the remaining antenatal care appointments should be made; the schedule of appointments will depend on the woman's parity and the identification of any risk factors (NICE 2021b).

Case Study 3.1   Smoking During Pregnancy

Sophie, 30, is eight weeks' pregnant with her second baby and currently smokes 5–10 cigarettes a day. She has said that she does not want to stop smoking and asks her midwife what the risks are to the fetus. Her midwife explains that cigarette smoke contains >7000 substances, including nicotine and carbon monoxide. Both of these chemicals have been shown to cross the placenta and have teratogenic effects to the developing fetus. The midwife also explains that smoking during pregnancy has been shown to affect the formation of new blood vessels, which are needed for appropriate placental development, and is associated with an increased risk of miscarriage, perinatal death, premature birth, fetal growth restriction, and congenital malformations.

Source: Adapted from Royal College of Physicians (2010).

Learning Event

Reflect on your experiences of caring for pregnant women during the first trimester.

- What are the most common symptoms of pregnancy?
- Consider which hormone(s) cause these and the role in normal adaptation to pregnancy.

The Second Trimester (13–27 Weeks' Gestation)

During the second trimester of pregnancy, nausea and fatigue usually begin to ease due to a decrease in the levels of hCG and an adjustment to the levels of oestrogen and progesterone. Physical signs of pregnancy also begin to manifest. These include expansion of the uterus to house the growing fetus, commonly referred to as the 'baby bump', increases in breast size in preparation for milk production as well as hormone-related changes to skin (melasma and linea nigra), teeth (sensitivity and bleeding) and nose (bleeding, congestion), coupled with dizziness, leg cramps and Braxton Hicks contractions (mild, irregular contractions). Regarding the latter, if the woman begins to experience more regular contractions or a steady increase in their strength, a healthcare provider should be contacted as this could be a symptom of preterm labour.

In the fetus, since all the major organs and systems have developed, the remaining six months of gestation are largely spent growing. In fact, the weight of the fetus will increase by roughly seven times and will measure between ~33 and 40 cm by the end of this stage of development. During weeks 17–19, in the female (XX carrying) fetus the uterus and vaginal canal will form, while the testes begin to descend in males (XY carrying). The 20th week marks the halfway point of the pregnancy, but it is only after the end of 24 weeks that a fetus may survive in a neonatal intensive care unit if delivered. Chances of survival following preterm birth increase significantly during week 26, when the lungs develop. At week 27, the second trimester ends.

Antenatal Care During the Second Trimester

During the second trimester, all pregnant women are offered a routine ultrasound scan to screen for fetal anomalies. It is also possible at this stage to determine the sex of the fetus, should the parent(s) wish. Antenatal appointments focus on fetal growth by measurement of the symphysis–fundal height (SFH) and/or ultrasound scan and the detection of potential emerging physical and mental health problems. The woman will also be offered regular weight, blood (blood cell and iron levels), urine (examining albumin, a protein that may indicate pre-eclampsia) and blood pressure checks to monitor their health as the pregnancy progresses. Other blood tests offered to some pregnant women include screening for diabetes that can develop during pregnancy (gestational diabetes). The frequency and type of antenatal appointments may be increased from the usual schedule depending on the progress of the pregnancy (NICE 2021b).

Medicines Management: Vitamin D Deficiency

Vitamin D plays an essential role in calcium metabolism, bone growth and mineralisation. Around 90% of our vitamin D requirement comes from exposure of the skin to sunlight, with only 10% coming from our diet (from fish with a high fat content, red meat, milk and eggs). Babies of women with vitamin D insufficiency during pregnancy are at risk of infantile rickets, hypocalcaemia and seizures, myopathy, diabetes, asthma and reduced intra-uterine long-bone growth (Morley et al. 2006).

A patient with vitamin D insufficiency/deficiency is at risk of osteomalacia, accelerated osteoporosis due to secondary hyperparathyroidism and muscle weakness. During pregnancy, vitamin D insufficiency may be associated with poor placental function leading to hypertension, pre-eclampsia and increased primary caesarean section rates (Bodnar et al. 2007).

Vitamin D supplementation should be offered to all patients throughout pregnancy and is particularly important for those who have limited exposure to sunlight (i.e. night-shift or office workers), have darker skin, including women who are of Asian, African Caribbean or Black African descent, or cover their skin for cultural reasons ('veiled'). BMI has also been found to be inversely proportional to serum vitamin D levels, so women with higher BMIs should also receive vitamin D supplementation. Current recommendations are for women to take 10 mg a day of vitamin D throughout pregnancy.

Learning Event

Think about your experience of caring for smokers during pregnancy.

- How would you provide information about the risks of smoking in relation to the patient's health and the health of development of the fetus?
- What could you do to support the cessation of smoking and what resources are available?

Medicines Management: Iron-Deficiency Anaemia

Pregnant women are at increased risk of iron-deficiency anaemia. This is a condition in which the body does not have sufficient iron to produce haemoglobin. Haemoglobin is the protein found in red blood cells that carries oxygen to the organs and tissues of the body. Iron-deficiency anaemia during pregnancy can cause severe fatigue and can increase the risk of premature birth (birth prior to 37 weeks), low birth weight and postpartum depression.

Women are at increased risk of developing anaemia during pregnancy if they:

- Have a history of anaemia or heavy periods before pregnancy.
- Have closely spaced pregnancies.
- Have a twin or higher-order multiple pregnancy (multiparity).
- Do not consume enough iron-rich foods.
- Are under 20 years old when pregnant.

Often good nutrition and prenatal vitamins that contain iron can help prevent and/or treat iron-deficiency anaemia during pregnancy. During pregnancy, a dietary intake of 27 mg of iron per day is recommended.

Source: Adapted from Pavord et al. (2020).

Case Study 3.2 Combined Screening and Trisomy 21

At an antenatal ultrasound department, a patient consents to having the combined screening test for trisomy 21 (Down's syndrome). The result indicates that the chance of their fetus having trisomy 21 is 1 in 1000, meaning that the fetus is considered to have a low chance. The patient is also told that the level of pregnancy-associated plasma protein-A (PAPP-A) in the maternal blood is low (less than <0.4 MoM).

Role of the Midwife

- Explain that the screening test result indicates a low chance of the fetus having Down's syndrome.
- Explain that the detection of low PAPP-A can be associated with an increased risk of having a baby that is small for gestational age (SGA) and that additional ultrasound scans to monitor fetal growth should be offered later in pregnancy.

Points for Consideration

- New parents may not be aware of the implications of a low PAPP-A result.
- Information should be provided in a way that is easy to understand and tailored to the needs of the individual.
- New parents may need support from midwives when considering their options.

Clinical Investigation: Prenatal Combined Screening

Prenatal screening for trisomy 21 (Down's syndrome), trisomy 18 (Edwards' syndrome) and trisomy 13 (Patau's syndrome) is available during pregnancy in many countries including the United Kingdom. These tests estimate the chance of a fetus/baby having a chromosomal or physical abnormality and can be carried out when the fetal CRL measurement is between 45 and 84 mm.

The combined test is used to calculate the chance or risk of a fetus having either trisomy 21, 13 or 18 and is conducted by taking into consideration the following:

- Maternal age.
- Biochemical markers in a maternal blood sample (free β-hCG) and (PAPP-A).
- Ultrasound measurement of the fetal CRL and nuchal translucency, a fluid-filled space behind the baby's neck during the first trimester between 11 and 14 weeks of pregnancy.

While in most countries these tests are offered to all pregnant women, the decision to have this test remains with the individual. While for many, these scans can be reassuring and indicate that their baby is developing normally, for others they may not be and as such the healthcare professional should provide clear information prior to the test, which should supplement the information offered by the person who is performing the investigation. It is important that this information be given in such a way that the patient understands why the test is being carried out, what it involves and what might be discovered so that they are able to make an informed decision. It is also important that new parents understand that there are different types of tests available, which vary in how accurate they are and what information they can provide.

Case Study 3.3   Trisomy 13 – Patau's Syndrome

Following a discussion with her midwife, Hayley, who is pregnant for the first time, consented to have the combined test when she was 12 weeks' gestation. The result shows that there is a 1 in 65 chance of the fetus having Patau's syndrome, a serious rare genetic disorder caused by having an additional copy of chromosome 13. The ultrasound scan did not detect any major fetal abnormalities, however.

Role of the Midwife

- Provide an explanation of the meaning of the result and explore how Hayley and her partner feel about the findings.
- Discuss the accuracy of the combined test and other options available to the parents: non-invasive prenatal testing (NIPT), invasive testing, no further screening or testing.
- Provide information about the risks associated with an invasive test and the time frame for a result.

Points for Consideration

- The patient and their partner may be unsure whether to opt for further testing and need time to consider their options.
- Information should be provided in a way that is easy to understand and tailored to the individuals.
- Continued support from midwives should be provided to patients when considering their options.

The Third Trimester (27 Weeks Onwards) and Birth

Fetal development continues during the third trimester. The fetus begins to open their eyes, continues to gain weight, and prepares for delivery. At 28 weeks the eyelashes have formed. The central nervous system begins to direct rhythmic breathing movements and control body temperature. By the 30th week, the layer of lanugo that has covered the skin since the second trimester begins to fall off. After this, to prepare for birth the fetal head descends into the pelvis to facilitate delivery. By the end of the third trimester, the fetus is about 48–53 cm long and weighs, on average, 2.5–4 kg.

An expectant mother may experience significant discomfort in this trimester, as the quick growth of the fetus crowds the abdominal cavity and places more pressure on the internal organs. Upward pressure of the fetus on the diaphragm may make breathing difficult and create gastric reflux, especially when the woman is lying down, and downward pressure on the bladder reduces its capacity, making frequent urination a feature. Many women also begin to experience an increase in 'false labour' or Braxton Hicks contractions. Another hallmark of this stage of development is the secretion of colostrum (a fluid from the breasts that nourishes the baby until breast milk becomes available) from the expectant mother's nipples.

Antenatal Care During the Third Trimester, Birth, Delivery and Postpartum

Antenatal visits during the third trimester usually include blood pressure measurement, urine testing to continue examining for indicators of pre-eclampsia (late onset), hypoglycaemia, and blood work assessing full blood count, blood group and antibodies at 28 weeks' gestation. The position, growth and development of the fetus will also be monitored by measurement of the SFH (NICE 2021b). Notably, by week 37 the fetus is considered 'full term' and at this point the organs are fully functional.

Postnatal care is just as crucial as antenatal care. A new mother may experience a range of physical and psychological changes, including soreness due to perineal trauma, incontinence, haemorrhoids, tender breasts (due to engorgement), after-pains (contraction of the uterus as it returns to its pre-pregnant state) and mental health concerns ranging from low mood to postpartum psychosis. Important topics to consider during these appointments include an emotional and physical well-being assessment, contraception, birth spacing and the review information relating to infant care and feeding.

Complications of Pregnancy

Given the intricacy of biological events that drive conception, embryo development and pregnancy establishment and maintenance, it should not be surprising that an approximately two-thirds of all pregnancies end in loss prior to the completion of the first trimester, with as many as 15–20% lost prior to the woman being aware of the pregnancy (Wang et al. 2003; Wilcox et al. 1998; Zinaman et al. 1996).

Orange Flag: Pregnancy Loss

While the burden of every lost pregnancy or failed *in vitro* fertilisation cycle does not have a direct impact on maternal mortality, the psychological and emotional impact of a sudden and unexpected pregnancy loss leads to immediate and sustained distress. In fact, pregnancy loss is now documented as a leading cause of anxiety and depressive disorders in women of reproductive age (Carter et al. 2007; Fisher et al. 2012; Geller et al. 2001, 2004).

In addition to this psychological morbidity (Rai and Regan 2006), loss of a previous pregnancy dramatically increases the risk of an adverse outcome in a subsequent pregnancy, including preterm delivery, premature rupture of membranes and low birth weight (Jauniaux et al. 2006; Bhattacharya and Bhattacharya 2009).

It is important to note that pregnancy loss can occur any time during pregnancy and is categorised based on the timing of the loss. Implantation failure occurs when no quantifiable signs of implantation are evident following embryo transfer in an assisted reproduction context; spontaneous abortion/miscarriage occurs prior to and stillbirth after 20 weeks of pregnancy (23 weeks in the UK). The causes of pregnancy loss are multivariate and can be physical (trauma, morphological defects of the placenta/cervix/uterus, exposure to toxicants such as drugs or alcohol) or physiological (chromosomal abnormalities, shallow/incomplete placentation, maternal age or infection). In addition, the aetiology may also be idiopathic or a secondary consequence of a chronic disease (high blood pressure, diabetes, thyroid disease or polycystic ovary syndrome) or immunological disorder (autoimmune diseases). Regardless of the cause, pregnancy loss must be handled with extreme care and consideration for the family.

Red Flag: Ectopic Pregnancy

An ectopic pregnancy occurs when an embryo implants and grows outside of the uterus. An ectopic pregnancy most often occurs in a fallopian tube, which carries eggs from the ovaries to the uterus, and is called a tubal pregnancy. Signs of ectopic pregnancy can vary but can include:

- Abdominal pain/tenderness
- Absent periods (amenorrhoea)
- Vaginal bleeding
- Faintness
- Shoulder tip pain
- Urinary and gastrointestinal symptoms
- Breast tenderness
- Pain on defecation

On clinical examination, a woman may also show signs of tachycardia, hypotension, pallor or shock.

Source: Adapted from NICE (2021a).

Some other common pregnancy complications are discussed next.

Anembryonic Pregnancy (Formally a Blighted Ovum)

An anembryonic pregnancy is a pathological pregnancy characterised by the development of a gestational sac and the absence of an embryo (Chaudhry et al. 2022). Anembryonic pregnancy constitutes a significant but unknown proportion of miscarriages, but may constitute up to half of all first-trimester miscarriages. While the exact aetiology of anembryonic pregnancies is difficult to ascertain, some common features include morphological and chromosomal abnormalities, genetic defects and endocrinological disorders.

Expert Midwife

Common risk factors for anembryonic pregnancy include consanguineous marriages, obesity, maternal infection and immunological disorders, morphological abnormalities of the uterus, gestational drug use and advanced maternal age.

Source: Adapted from Cavalcante et al. (2019).

A molar pregnancy, also known as hydatidiform mole, is a specific form of an anembryonic pregnancy. There are two types of molar pregnancy: complete molar pregnancy and partial molar pregnancy. In a complete molar pregnancy, the placental tissue is abnormal and swollen and appears to form fluid-filled cysts. There is also no formation of fetal tissue. In a partial molar pregnancy, there may be both normal and abnormal placental tissue together with a non-viable fetus. These are usually miscarried early in the gestation.

A significant difference between an anembryonic pregnancy and a molar pregnancy is that the molar pregnancy can develop serious secondary complications, including a rare form of cancer called choriocarcinoma. If a choriocarcinoma was to develop it has the potential to metastasise to other organs and will need to be treated with combination chemotherapy. Additionally, persistent gestational trophoblastic neoplasia may also occur. Gestational trophoblastic neoplasia can be diagnosed with an abnormally high level of hCG after the molar pregnancy has been removed. Persistent gestational trophoblastic neoplasia can nearly always be successfully treated, most often with chemotherapy, but in some cases hysterectomy might also be necessary.

Red Flag: Molar Pregnancy

Approximately 1 in every 1000 pregnancies is diagnosed as a molar pregnancy. Various factors are associated with molar pregnancy, including:

- Maternal age: a molar pregnancy is more likely in women older than 35 or younger than 20 years.
- Previous molar pregnancy: recurrent molar pregnancies happen on average in 1 out of every 100 women.
- Children conceived within a consanguineous relationship.

Preterm Birth

Preterm birth is classified as birth prior to 37 completed weeks of gestation and is the second leading cause of perinatal morbidity and mortality (behind chromosomal abnormalities) (Lawn et al. 2006). Children who are born premature are at a higher risk of developing cerebral palsy, learning difficulties, respiratory diseases and sensory deficits than those who make it to term (Hack et al. 1995). Preterm labour and delivery may occur due to cervical insufficiency, intra-uterine infection, placental abruption and/or decidual haemorrhage, but may be due to other causes such as a history of a previous premature birth, pregnancy with multiples and maternal infection. Preterm babies typically need a longer hospital stay and may require admission to the neonatal intensive care unit.

Take-Home Points

- Conception, embryo development and pregnancy are complex biological phenomena.
- An entire pregnancy can be broken up into three stages: the germinal stage, which refers to the period from fertilisation through the development of the early embryo until implantation; the embryonic stage, which refers to the period encompassing the third through to the eighth week of gestation; and the fetal stage, which describes the time from the ninth week of gestation until birth.
- The causes of pregnancy complications are multivariate and can be physical, physiological, a secondary consequence of a chronic disease or idiopathic (unknown).
- The midwife has an extremely important role in the care of pregnant women.
- Prenatal, postnatal and postpartum care are incredibly important to the health and well-being of the mother, child and partner.

Conclusion

Health professionals have an extremely important role throughout conception, embryo development, pregnancy establishment and maintenance. For those wishing to specialise in this field, a robust knowledge of fertilisation, conception, embryo development, gestation and birth is an essential attribute.

References

Alwan, S. and Chambers, C.D. (2015). Identifying human teratogens: an update. *Journal of Pediatric Genetics* 4 (2): 39–41. https://doi.org/10.1055/s-0035-1556745.

Bhattacharya, S. and Bhattacharya, S. (2009). Effect of miscarriage on future pregnancies. *Women's Health* 5: 5–8.

Bischof, P. and Campana, A. (1997). Trophoblast differentiation and invasion: its significance for human embryo implantation. *Early Pregnancy* 3 (2): 81–95.

Bodnar, L.M., Simhan, H.N., Powers, R.W. et al. (2007). High prevalence of vitamin D insufficiency in black and white pregnant women residing in the northern United States and their neonates. *Journal of Nutrition* 137 (2): 447–452. https://doi.org/10.1093/jn/137.2.447.

Brosens, I., Robertson, W.B., and Dixon, H.G. (1967). The physiological response of the vessels of the placental bed to normal pregnancy. *Journal of Pathology and Bacteriology* 93: 569–579. https://doi.org/10.1002/path.1700930218.

Carter, D., Misri, S., and Tomfohr, L. (2007). Psychologic aspects of early pregnancy loss. *Clinical Obstetrics and Gynecology* 50: 154–165.

Cartwright, J.E., Fraser, R., Leslie, K. et al. (2010). Remodelling at the maternal–fetal interface: relevance to human pregnancy disorders. *Reproduction* 140 (6): 803–813.

Cavalcante, M.B., Sarno, M., Peixoto, A.B. et al. (2019). Obesity and recurrent miscarriage: a systematic review and meta-analysis. *Journal of Obstetrics and Gynaecology Research* 45 (1): 30–38.

Chaudhry, K., Tafti, D., and Siccardi, M.A. (2022). Anembryonic pregnancy. In: *StatPearls*. Treasure Island, FL: StatPearls Publishing https://www.ncbi.nlm.nih.gov/books/NBK499938.

Fisher, J., Cabral de Mello, M., Patel, V. et al. (2012). Prevalence and determinants of common perinatal mental disorders in women in low- and lower-middle-income countries: a systematic review. *Bulletin of the World Health Organization* 90: 139g–149g.

Geller, P.A., Klier, C.M., and Neugebauer, R. (2001). Anxiety disorders following miscarriage. *Journal of Clinical Psychiatry* 62: 432–438.

Geller, P.A., Kerns, D., and Klier, C.M. (2004). Anxiety following miscarriage and the subsequent pregnancy: a review of the literature and future directions. *Journal of Psychosomatic Research* 56: 35–45.

Gellersen, B., Brosens, I.A., and Brosens, J.J. (2007). Decidualization of the human endometrium: mechanisms, functions, and clinical perspectives. *Seminars in Reproductive Medicine* 25: 445–453.

Hack, M., Klein, N.K., Gerry, H., and Taylor. (1995). Long-term developmental outcomes of low birth weight infants. *Future of Children* 5 (1): 176–196.

Hunkapiller, N.M., Gasperowicz, M., Kapidzic, M. et al. (2011). A role for Notch signaling in trophoblast endovascular invasion and in the pathogenesis of pre-eclampsia. *Development* 138: 2987–2998. https://doi.org/10.1242/dev.066589.

Jauniaux, E., Farquharson, R.G., Christiansen, O.B., and Exalto, N. (2006). Evidence-based guidelines for the investigation and medical treatment of recurrent miscarriage. *Human Reproduction* 21: 2216–2222.

Knight, B., Brereton, A., Powell, R.J., and Liversedge, H. (2018). Assessing the accuracy of ultrasound estimation of gestational age during routine antenatal care in in vitro fertilization (IVF) pregnancies. *Ultrasound* 26 (1): 49–53. https://doi.org/10.1177/1742271X17751257.

Lawn, J.E., Wilczynska-Ketende, K., and Cousens, S.N. (2006). Estimating the causes of 4 million neonatal deaths in the year 2000. *International Journal of Epidemiology* 35: 706–718.

Lowe, J.S. and Anderson, P.G. (2015). Female reproductive system. In: *Stevens & Lowe's Human Histology*, 4e (ed. J.S. Lowe and P.G. Anderson). Philadelphia: Mosby, ch. 17.

Morley, R., Carlin, J.B., Pasco, J.A., and Wark, J.D. (2006). Maternal 25-hydroxyvitamin D and parathyroid hormone concentrations and offspring birth size. *Journal of Clinical Endocrinology and Metabolism* 91: 906–912.

National Institute for Health and Care Excellence (NICE) (2021a). Ectopic pregnancy and miscarriage: diagnosis and initial management. https://www.nice.org.uk/guidance/ng126 (accessed November 2023).

National Institute for Health and Care Excellence (NICE) (2021b). Antenatal care. https://www.nice.org.uk/guidance/ng201 (accessed November 2023).

National Institute for Health and Care Excellence (NICE) (2023). Antenatal care – uncomplicated pregnancy. https://cks.nice.org.uk/topics/antenatal-care-uncomplicated-pregnancy/management/antenatal-care-uncomplicated-pregnancy/#nutritional-supplements (accessed November 2023).

Navot, D., Scott, R.T., Droesch, K. et al. (1991). The window of embryo transfer and the efficiency of human conception in vitro. *Fertility and Sterility* 55: 114–118. https://doi.org/10.1016/S0015-0282(16)54069-2.

Pavord, S., Daru, J., Prasannan, N. et al. (2020). UK guidelines on the management of iron deficiency in pregnancy. *British Journal of Haematology* 188: 819–830. https://doi.org/10.1111/bjh.16221.

Pijnenborg, R., Vercruysse, L., and Hanssens, M. (2006). The uterine spiral arteries in human pregnancy: facts and controversies. *Placenta* 27 (9–10): 939–958. https://doi.org/10.1016/j.placenta.2005.12.006.

Rai, R. and Regan, L. (2006). Recurrent miscarriage. *Lancet* 368: 601–611.

Ramathal, C.Y., Bagchi, I.C., Taylor, R.N., and Bagchi, M.K. (2010). Endometrial decidualization: of mice and men. *Seminars in Reproductive Medicine* 28 (1): 17–26. https://doi.org/10.1055/s-0029-1242989.

Royal College of Physicians (2010). *Passive Smoking and Children. A Report by the Tobacco Advisory Group*. London: RCP.

Wang, X., Chen, C., Wang, L. et al. (2003). Conception, early pregnancy loss, and time to clinical pregnancy: a population-based prospective study. *Fertility and Sterility* 79: 577–584.

Webster, S. and de Wreede, R. (2016). *Embryology at a Glance*, 2e. Chichester: Wiley.

Wilcox, A.J., Weinberg, C.R., and Baird, D.D. (1998). Post-ovulatory ageing of the human oocyte and embryo failure. *Human Reproduction* 13: 394–397.

Zinaman, M.J., Clegg, E.D., Brown, C.C. et al. (1996). Estimates of human fertility and pregnancy loss. *Fertility and Sterility* 65: 503–509.

Further Resources

World Health Organization: Maternal health. www.who.int/health-topics/maternal-health (accessed November 2023).

World Health Organization: Stillbirth. www.who.int/health-topics/stillbirth (accessed November 2023).

World Health Organization: Abortion. www.who.int/health-topics/abortion (accessed November 2023).

World Health Organization: Newborn health. www.who.int/health-topics/newborn-health (accessed November 2023).

Glossary

Blastomeres	A type of cell produced by cell division of an embryo
Choriocarcinoma	A malignant, fast-growing tumour that develops from trophoblastic cells
Cilia	A microscopic hairlike structure found on the surface of certain cells
Consanguineous	Relating to or denoting people descended from the same ancestor
Corpus luteum	A temporary endocrine structure in ovaries that produces progesterone
Decidualisation	The functional and morphological changes that occur within the endometrium to form the decidual lining into which the blastocyst implants
Diploidy	The presence of two complete sets of chromosomes in an organism's cells
DNA	Deoxyribonucleic acid, the hereditary material in humans and almost all other organisms
Epiblast	The pluripotent primary lineage that will form the definitive germ layers in a complex process of differentiation and morphogenetic movements called gastrulation
Genital ridge	The somatic precursor of gonads in both sexes
Gestational trophoblastic neoplasia	A type of gestational trophoblastic disease
Gonads	The primary reproductive organs, the testes and the ovaries
Haploid	The presence of a single set of chromosomes in an organism's cells
Hypoblast	A thin monolayer of small cuboidal cells that make up the lower layer of the bilaminar embryonic disc
Lanugo	Thin, soft, usually unpigmented, downy hair found on the fetal body
Meconium	The first faeces, or stool, of the newborn
Proteases	Enzymes that break the peptide bonds of proteins
RNA	Ribonucleic acid, a single-stranded nucleic acid that converts the information stored in DNA into proteins
Toxaemia	Disease caused by the spread of bacteria and their toxins in the bloodstream
Trisomy	A chromosomal condition characterised by an additional chromosome

CHAPTER 4

Genetics and Genetic Conditions

Sarah Malone and James Castleman

Fetal Medicine Department, Birmingham Women's Hospital, Birmingham, UK

AIM

The aim of this chapter is to help the reader understand the principles of genetic screening, the screening tests available, their interpretation and options for diagnostic testing.

LEARNING OUTCOMES

On completion of this chapter the reader will be able to:

- Provide a fundamental description of the human genome.
- Understand sensitivity, specificity, and positive and negative predictive value.
- Know the options available in the context of a high-chance screening result.
- Ensure the woman is offered individual, non-judgemental support.

Test Your Prior Knowledge

1. What are sensitivity, specificity, and positive and negative predictive value?
2. What is aneuploidy?
3. What is reproductive carrier screening?
4. From what gestation can a chorionic villus sample (CVS) be performed?
5. What is the rate of cystic fibrosis carrier status in white European populations?

Midwives provide care throughout pregnancy, are often the sole providers of primary screening and triage risk for appropriate models of care. The midwife needs an understanding of genetics to provide safe and effective care for women and their families. This is essential when discussing and interpreting screening for common chromosomal conditions such as Down's, Edwards' and Patau's syndromes and assessing the risks of genetic conditions such as thalassaemia or sickle cell disease.

Fundamentals of Maternal Pathophysiology, First Edition. Edited by Claire Leader and Ian Peate.
© 2024 John Wiley & Sons Ltd. Published 2024 by John Wiley & Sons Ltd.
Companion website: www.wiley.com/go/leader/maternalpatho

Overview of Genetics

In order to get the most out of this chapter, it is important to have insight into the underlying principles of genetics. The following discussion provides a brief overview. A list of further resources is given at the end of the chapter.

Genetic information exists as deoxyribose nucleic acid (DNA). Most of the cell's DNA resides in the nucleus, but a small amount is in the mitochondria (structures that provide energy for the cell) (see Figure 4.1).

DNA is a double-stranded molecule. Each strand is made up of a string of nucleotides. A nucleotide is deoxyribose: a sugar phosphate backbone, with a nucleic acid (a nitrogenous base) attached. There are four types of nitrogenous base: adenine (A), guanine (G), cytosine (C) and thymine (T). The nitrogenous base will join only to a complementary base pair – A and T will form a bond and so will C and G. These two strands of DNA are held together by the bond between each complementary base pair (see Figure 4.2).

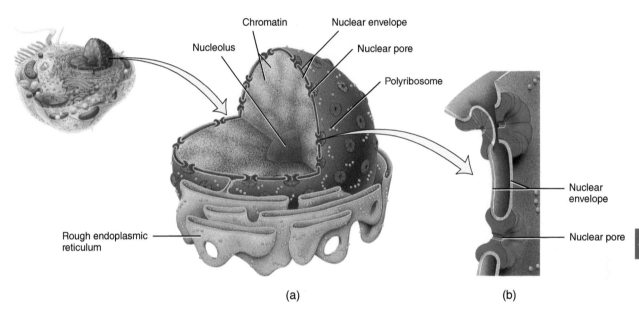

(a)

(b)

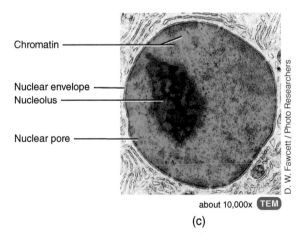

about 10,000x **TEM**

(c)

D. W. Fawcett / Photo Researchers

FIGURE 4.1 The nucleus houses genetic material. Within the nucleus, chromatin is stored, ribosomes are formed and substances are able to enter and exit the nucleus through the nuclear pore. The nucleolus is where ribosomes are made. Ribosomes produce proteins. (a) Details of the nucleus; (b) details of the nuclear envelope; (c) transverse section of the nucleus.

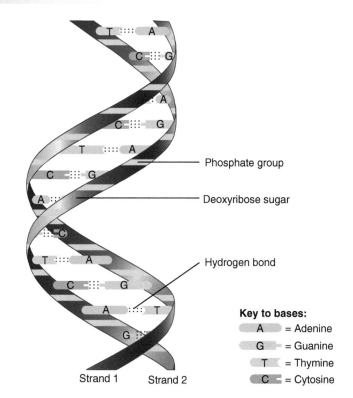

- DNA is made of two strands twisted in a spiral staircase-like structure called a double helix.
- Each strand consists of nucleotides bound together.
- Each nucleotide consists of a deoxyribose sugar bound to a phosphate group and one of 4 nitrogenous bases [adenine (A), thymine (T), guanine (G), cytosine (C)].
- The nitrogenous bases pair together through hydrogen bonding to form the 'steps' of the double helix.
- Adenine pairs with thymine and guanine pairs with cytosine.

Phosphate group

Deoxyribose sugar

Hydrogen bond

Key to bases:

A = Adenine
G = Guanine
T = Thymine
C = Cytosine

Strand 1   Strand 2

FIGURE 4.2   A pictorial representation of a portion of the double helix.

The double strand of DNA twists to form a double helix. That DNA double helix wraps itself around protein molecules called histones to form a densely packed structure called chromatin. Figure 4.3 depicts DNA from a double helix to the chromosome.

Chromosomes

In a human body cell there are 23 pairs of chromosomes, 22 of which are known as autosomes and the 23rd pair known as the sex chromosomes. In normal circumstances in humans, for female sex the 23rd pair is XX and for male sex it is XY. Overall, there are 46 chromosomes. This would be described for female sex as 46XX and for male sex 46XY. The word 'karyotype' describes an individual's complete set of chromosomes, which can be seen under a microscope. Figure 4.4 illustrates this.

The chromosomes are arranged in homologous pairs, which means that chromosome 1 inherited from the mother will match up with chromosome 1 from the father, chromosome 2 will do the same and so on.

Cells containing 46 chromosomes are known as diploid. Not all cells contain 23 pairs (46 in total) of chromosomes. The sex cells, known as gametes (sperm in males and oocytes in females), have 23 chromosomes only – they do not have pairs. These cells are known as haploid.

Genes

A gene is a section of DNA that contains the code to make a specific protein. Not all genes code for protein, however. The gene is an arrangement of nitrogenous base pairs (A, T, C, G) of a certain length. Genes can vary in size. Our genes determine everything that makes us who are we are. They code for everything down to our eye colour, our skin type and even our susceptibility to certain conditions.

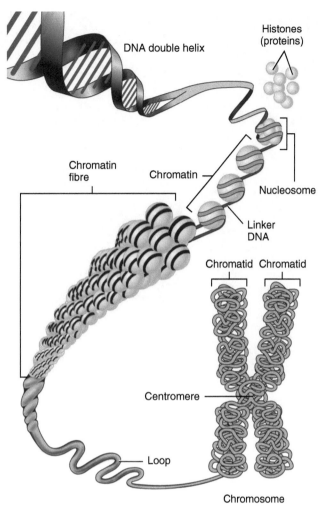

FIGURE 4.3 DNA for a double helix to chromosome.

What Can Go Wrong with Chromosomes

Triploidy

Triploidy describes a complete extra set of chromosomes. The karyotype here would be 69XXX, 69XXY or 69XYY. This results from a sperm or an egg cell that had a diploid number of chromosomes. This diploid sex cell fertilises with a haploid sex cell and the result is a triploid zygote. The effects in a baby depend on whether the diploid cell came from the maternal side (digynic) or from the paternal side (diandric).

Triploidy has a high chance of ending in miscarriage. Surviving to a later stage of pregnancy may reveal structural differences and severe fetal growth restriction. Most of these babies would pass away soon after birth with very few surviving to adulthood, and with significant health problems if they do.

Diandric triploidy is otherwise known as a partial molar pregnancy. An embryo forms but there is excessive placental tissue and usually ends in a miscarriage in the first trimester.

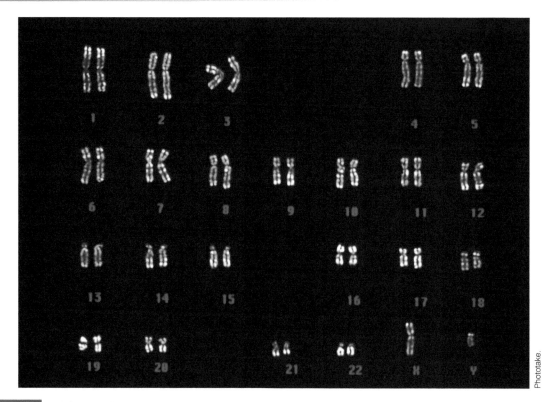

FIGURE 4.4   Male human chromosomes.

Loss or Gain of a Chromosome

This is otherwise known as aneuploidy. The most common aneuploidies in humans are when there is an additional chromosome on chromosome 13, 18 or 21, or if there is an extra or missing sex chromosome (X0, XXY, XXX, XYY). Other additional or missing chromosomes would most likely end in early miscarriage. When there is an extra copy of a chromosome this is called a trisomy – for example, trisomy 21, the condition also known as Down's syndrome.

Chromosomal Rearrangements

A segment of DNA may be inverted, deleted, duplicated or have undergone a translocation. This may or may not result in a change in the amount of genetic material in a cell. A translocation describes the swapping of genetic material from one chromosome to another. If this is an equal swap of genetic material then it is a balanced rearrangement. If the exchange has resulted in an incorrect amount of genetic material, then this is an unbalanced rearrangement.

Balanced rearrangements are unlikely to cause any problems for the individual but may cause problems for their children, as when their cells become haploid, an incorrect number of chromosomes may transferred to sex cells.

Unbalanced rearrangements can cause differences in the individual, which would depend on the size and genes involved. They are also a cause of miscarriage.

Mosaicism

Mosaicism is when there are two cell lines within an individual. For example, one group of cells may be 46XX and the second group of cells may be 45X0. The ratio of cells is variable. The effect on an individual will depend on the ratio of affected cells, but is generally milder than a full set of chromosomes affected with aneuploidy. This can still be difficult to predict based on the genotype alone.

Microduplications and Deletions

It is not only possible to have an abnormal number of chromosomes (as we see in aneuploidy and triploidy) or a different arrangement of the genetic material on the chromosome (rearrangements), it is also possible to have an incorrect amount of DNA within a chromosome. This is due to copy number variants (CNVs), which are submicroscopic deletions or duplications of segments of DNA that can vary in size. Not all microdeletions or duplications cause disease, but there are some well-recognised conditions that are a result of this process (Levy and Burnside 2019).

Mendelian Inheritance

There are two copies of each gene – one that has been passed down from the mother and one from the father. If there is a pathogenic mutation in one of the genes, whether it will cause a problem in that individual will depend on whether the gene is dominant or recessive. A faulty gene that is dominant means you only need one copy of the faulty gene to be affected by the condition. With a recessive inherited trait, both of the genes must be faulty before there is clinical disease. Being a carrier for a condition means that the individual is not affected but they carry a mutated gene, which they could pass on to their child.

Orange Flag

Be aware that the parents of children with thalassaemia may also have had health problems from thalassaemia, which can put them at higher risk of physical, emotional and social problems.

X-linked Conditions

These are conditions whereby the faulty gene is on the X chromosome. In females there are two X chromosomes, which means that if this was a dominant condition, they would have the disease, and if it was recessive, they would be a carrier. In a genetic male, since they only have one X chromosome, they would be affected regardless of whether this was a dominant or recessive trait.

Health Promotion

Pre-conception care is an important and often overlooked opportunity to improve the health of would-be mothers, their families and their babies. Finding out if the couple are at increased risk of having a baby with a genetic condition is important before a pregnancy, as it offers an opportunity to seek out more information and appropriate counselling.

Chromosomal or genetic conditions could happen to any of us, and this is not an exhaustive list, but they are more likely in those with:

- A personal or family history on the maternal or paternal side of a known genetic condition.
- A previous baby with structural differences (which may or may not have resulted in a live birth).
- A history of developmental delay in the family.
- Recurrent pregnancy loss.
- A consanguineous relationship with the baby's father.

Red Flag

There are some ethnic groups that are at higher risk of some genetic conditions:

- **Thalassaemia and sickle cell disease:** These are disorders of red blood cells affecting the haemoglobin and causing anaemia, more likely in those from South, East and South-East Asian, African, Middle Eastern, South American and Southern European countries. Treatments are available but these conditions can cause serious health problems and severe manifestations can be fatal.
- **Tay-Sachs disease:** This is a metabolic condition inherited in an autosomal recessive manner, which is 10 times more common in the Ashkenazi Jewish population. Ashkenazi Jews have a higher rate of several genetic conditions, so much so that routine screening is offered to check if they are carriers of gene mutations that may increase the risk of serious genetic diseases.
- **Cystic fibrosis:** This is seen more commonly in white European populations, with a carrier rate of 1 in 25 individuals. It causes sticky mucus to build up in the lungs and digestive system.

Testing for carrier status of some genetic conditions is increasingly being offered by some practitioners for anyone regardless of their history, if they are either planning pregnancy or pregnant. The Royal College of Australian and New Zealand Obstetricians and Gynaecologists (RANZCOG 2019) is the only college that has published guidelines stating that carrier screening should be discussed. This is an area of ongoing research and may become mainstream in the future.

Expert Midwife

When talking to patients about a 'mutated' or 'mutation' of a gene, the preferred terminology is 'pathogenic variant'. Midwives must always be conscious of the language they use.

Sally, Senior Midwife (screening)

Screening

Screening can identify which individuals in a population are at higher risk of a certain condition in comparison to the rest of the population. The aim is to focus resources on those at higher risk and minimise any harms – either physical or psychological – of further diagnostic investigations, which tend to be more invasive.

The perfect screening test would detect all truly positive cases and would be 100% accurate when a test result was negative. The performance of a screening test can be expressed mathematically by the following:

- **Sensitivity:** The ability of a test to correctly identify a 'positive' case in a population. If a test is 70% sensitive, it identifies 70% of the individuals who have the condition. It will miss 30% of those who have the condition.
- **Specificity:** The ability of a test to correctly identify a 'negative' case in a population. If a test is 90% specific, it identifies 90% of the individuals who truly do not have the condition. So 10% of the time, there will be a negative result but actually the individual has the condition.
- **Positive predictive value:** If the screening test comes back positive, the positive predictive value is the chance that this result is a true positive. For example, if a test has a positive predictive value of 80%, if you have a positive screening result there is an 80% chance you have the condition. There is a 20% chance that you do not have the condition and the test was a false positive.
- **Negative predictive value:** If the screening test comes back negative, the negative predictive value is the chance that you really do not have the condition. For example, if a test has a negative predictive value of 99%, then a negative result means you have a 99% chance that this is a true negative and a 1% chance that the result is a false negative.

Understanding that every screening test has a certain performance is important, particularly if you are providing people with options about what type of screening test they want to pursue and when interpreting results.

Aneuploidy Screening

Aneuploidy describes an abnormal number of chromosomes. In humans, we would expect to have 23 pairs of chromosomes – 22 autosomes and 1 pair of sex chromosomes. There are three aneuploidies that are most common in human reproduction, which make up the majority of chromosomal or genetic conditions in pregnancy. These are trisomy 13, 18 and 21 and are known as Patau's, Edwards' and Down's syndromes, respectively. To effectively counsel an individual as to whether they want to screen for a condition, it is important to explain the condition and what they may expect if they have an affected child.

Trisomy 13 (Patau's Syndrome)

This condition, which has an incidence of 2 in every 10 000 births (NHS England 2022), results from an extra copy of chromosome 13, and carries an increased risk of early miscarriage or stillbirth during pregnancy. On ultrasound scan there are often significant differences that can be noted, including thickened nuchal translucency (NT), smallness, holoprocencephaly (where the brain has not split into two sides), cleft lip and palate, micropthalmia (small eyes), polydactyly (extra digits), omphalocele, heart defects and differences in the kidneys, to name but a few (Kroes et al. 2014). This condition is traditionally recognised as one that is not compatible with life. There are in fact cases of babies that have survived to birth and beyond, but the average survival is between 7 and 10 days, with a minority surviving beyond 1 year of age (Meyer et al. 2015).

Trisomy 18 (Edwards' Syndrome)

This condition, with an incidence of 3 in every 10 000 births (NHS England 2022), is related to an extra copy of chromosome 18. As with Patau's syndrome, there is an increased risk of miscarriage and stillbirth in pregnancy. There are often significant differences seen on ultrasound, such as thickened NT, smallness, heart defects, brain differences, diaphragmatic hernia, omphalocele, kidney differences and rocker-bottom feet (Kroes et al. 2014). Again, as with Patau's syndrome, the prognosis is poor, with a median survival of eight days and a minority surviving into the first few years of life (Meyer et al. 2015).

Trisomy 21 (Down's Syndrome)

This condition, with an incidence of 10 in every 10 000 births (NHS England 2022), is related to an extra copy of chromosome 21. There can be features seen on ultrasound, yet one study found that ultrasound alone was responsible for detecting only 30% of cases (Offerdal et al. 2008). Ultrasound features can be varied: examples include a thickened NT or nuchal fold, ventriculomegaly, cardiac defects (a particular association with atrioventricular septal defect), hypoplastic nasal bone, short femurs and humeri, renal pelvis dilation, echogenic bowel, clinodactyly and growth restriction. As with all trisomies, there is an increased risk of miscarriage and stillbirth.

Children with Down's syndrome will likely have some degree of intellectual disability or behavioural difficulties. The physical effects are variable, depending on the presence or severity of other structural differences such as heart problems, which may have their own associated morbidity. These physical effects mean that about 5% of babies born with Down's syndrome do not live beyond their first birthday. There is a characteristic appearance of Down's syndrome with almond-shaped eyes, a larger tongue, a thick neck and short stature. Longer term, there is an increased risk of immune problems, thyroid issues and leukaemia. With no serious health problems, people with Down's syndrome have a life expectancy of 60 years or more (NHS England 2022). As adults there is variation in those who live independently and those who need more supportive care, but certainly those with Down's syndrome can live happy and fulfilling lives.

Sex Chromosome Aneuploidy

The sex chromosomes for genetic females are XX and for males XY. Aneuploidy can also occur in the sex chromosomes and cause recognised conditions:

- **Turner's syndrome** (X0, known as Monosomy X) is where there is one solitary X chromosome. As there is no Y chromosome this is a genetic female condition, associated with an increased risk of miscarriage, increased NT, cystic hygroma, heart defects and horseshoe kidney. Females have a characteristic appearance with short stature and webbed neck. Women with Turner's syndrome have problems with hypertension and hypothyroidism. The ovaries are underdeveloped, periods do not begin and therefore women with Turner's syndrome cannot have their own biological children.
- **Klinefelter syndrome** (XXY) is due to an additional X chromosome in a genetic male. This may not be obvious after the baby is born, but there may be some delays in meeting childhood milestones. Confidence may be low and the children may have dyslexia, dyspraxia or attention deficits. Men with Klinefelter's are usually tall and at puberty have only sparse facial hair, with a small penis and testicles and the development of breast tissue (gynaecomastia). Low libido and infertility are features in adulthood (NHS 2019). This condition may only be noted in later life.

Other sex chromosome aneuploidies include XXX and XYY, which tend to have associations with an increased chance of learning disabilities and behavioural problems.

Overall, screening for sex chromosome aneuploidy is not offered on a population level. Some countries reveal the sex chromosomes on non-invasive prenatal testing (see later in the chapter), which can identify a potential sex chromosome aneuploidy prenatally. The performance of these tests for that reason should be discussed in the pre-test consent.

Use of Ultrasound to Detect Genetic Differences

Prenatal ultrasound is a screening tool to attempt to identify babies with structural differences that may or may not be related to underlying chromosomal or genetic causes. Identifying these babies is helpful so, where appropriate, offer genetic testing and/or termination of pregnancy. Prenatal diagnosis allows for relevant specialists to be involved before and after birth and help parents psychologically prepare for the arrival of a baby with additional needs. In some circumstances, identifying a problem prenatally allows for treatment in utero, for example placing shunts, fetoscopic laser coagulation for complications of monochorionic multiple pregnancy and fetal tracheal occlusion in cases of diaphragmatic hernia. Prenatal ultrasound can also be used for screening for placenta praevia, preterm birth and fetal growth restriction.

Orange Flag

The role of a midwife is to provide maternity care and support for women and families during all stages of pregnancy, throughout labour and the early postnatal period. The care and support that women require have to be evidence based and tailored to meet their unique needs with respect to their unique circumstances. This includes the provision of information, in accessible formats, concerning screening programmes.

The initial recommended scan is the first-trimester ultrasound. This ensures that the pregnancy is intrauterine and viable, enables us to accurately calculate the gestation and can diagnose a multiple pregnancy. The first trimester is seen as an opportunity to diagnose many structural anomalies that may have previously been identified later in

TABLE 4.1 Nuchal translucency.

Nuchal translucency (NT) measurement (mm)	% Abnormal karyotype (T13/18/21/X0), other sex chromosome aneuploidies/triploidy/unbalanced translocations/mosaicism/duplications or deletions (%)
95th centile – 3.4	7.1
3.5–4.4	20.1
4.5–5.4	45.4
5.5–6.4	50.1
>6.5	Approximately 70

Source: Data from a large retrospective study of singleton pregnancies with a thickened NT undergoing invasive testing for karyotype. Adapted from Kagan et al. (2006).

pregnancy. Newer, high-frequency ultrasound machines, use of transvaginal scanning (which may produce superior images as the probe is closer to the fetus) and improving operator knowledge and expertise in this area have made this possible.

One component of the first-trimester scan is the nuchal translucency (NT), which is the thickness of the skin at the back of the fetal neck. It has been observed that the NT is thicker in babies affected by aneuploidy. The NT can only be measured between 11 and 13 + 6 weeks gestation, correlating to a crown–rump length (CRL) of 45–84 mm. In addition to aneuploidy, there are other causes of a thickened NT and the magnitude of NT thickness is directly related to a poor prognosis. Other causes of thickened NT are cardiac defects, major structural differences and specific syndromes (Table 4.1).

If a karyotype is normal, depending on the thickness of the NT and other ultrasound features, a microarray with or without prenatal exome may be offered. This depends on local practices and patient wishes. The cut-off in England (NHS) for further investigation is an NT ≥3.5 mm. In addition, a fetal echocardiogram would usually be organised due to the association with congenital heart defects.

Second-trimester ultrasound is performed for all pregnancies to detect differences in the structures of a fetus. This should be offered to all women and is generally performed from 18 to 22 weeks' gestation. It is not possible for ultrasound to pick up all differences and the detection rate will be variable dependent on maternal size, fetal position, operator expertise and quality of the ultrasound machine. It is also important to know that fetal development continues beyond this anatomy scan and therefore problems may still be identified later in pregnancy or after birth.

The principles of screening and the role of ultrasound have been discussed. In most high-income countries there are aneuploidy screening programmes for all pregnant women to access should they choose.

First-Trimester Combined Screening

First-trimester combined screening (FTCS) considers a pregnant woman's background risk of aneuploidy calculated by age and gestation. It has sensitivity of 85%, specificity of 95% and positive predictive value of approximately 7–10% (RANZCOG 2018).

The rate of aneuploidy is proportional to maternal age and we can estimate what that risk is at each age (Table 4.2). The background risk is adjusted by including the NT and measurements of two chemicals: pregnancy-associated plasma protein-A (PAPP-A) and beta-human chorionic gonadotropin (β-hCG). PAPP-A is a glycoprotein produced by the placenta. In low levels it has an association with Down's, Patau's and Edwards' syndromes. β-hCG is found in high levels in Down's syndrome, yet is low in Patau's and Edwards' syndromes.

Maternal ethnicity as well as smoking status can affect levels of chemical analytes.

TABLE 4.2   **The rate of aneuploidy is proportional to maternal age.**

	Maternal age at term					
	20	25	30	35	40	45
Risk of Down's syndrome live birth	1 in 1450	1 in 1350	1 in 940	1 in 350	1 in 85	1 in 35

Source: Adapted from Morris et al. (2003).

Learning Event

Much of the work in this area was pioneered by Professor Kypros Nicolaides, founder of the Fetal Medicine Foundation. Its website has a helpful online calculator where these parameters can be entered and the chance calculated: https://fetalmedicine.org/research/assess/trisomies.

The result is issued as a numerical risk, for example 1 in 1350 for Down's syndrome and 1 in 10 000 for Edwards' and Patau's. An arbitrary cut-off deems what is a high-risk result and will vary between countries. In the NHS, a high-risk result is higher than 1 in 150 (anywhere between 1 in 2 and 1 in 150) chance of Down's syndrome. A low-risk result does not mean no risk. The interpretation of risk is very personal and will differ depending on an individual's experiences and circumstances. In the context of a high-risk result (or a result that the family deems high risk), the options are to do nothing, perform non-invasive prenatal testing (NIPT) or undergo a diagnostic test. In contemporary practice the word 'chance' is preferred to 'risk' when discussing this with women and their families.

Non-invasive Prenatal Testing

For Down's syndrome the sensitivity of NIPT is 99%, specificity 99% and positive predictive value approximately 45% (RANZCOG 2018). For Edwards' and Patau's syndromes sensitivity is 97% and specificity 99.9% (Taylor-Phillips et al. 2016).

NIPT is otherwise known as cell free fetal DNA (cffDNA) testing. This test works on the premise that the fetus most often has the same genetic form as the placenta. In the maternal blood stream, fragments of the DNA from the placenta circulate from the first trimester. Maternal and fetal cell free DNA is sequenced, and this sequence reveals which chromosome it was derived from. If there is a comparatively increased or decreased amount of DNA proportionately from one of the chromosomes, this would indicate a trisomy or monosomy.

Case Study 4.1

Randeep and Joe have been referred to their local etal medicine unit. They have had a mid-trimester ultrasound showing that the baby is much smaller than expected, while the estimated date of delivery (EDD) is confirmed correct. They had not undergone any screening for aneuploidy, but they decide to undergo an amniocentesis. The quantitative fluorescence polymerase chain reaction (QF-PCR) result comes back as triploidy.

Randeep and Joe are counselled by the Fetal medicine specialist and the geneticist. They make the difficult decision not to continue with the pregnancy given the poor prognosis. They have a termination of pregnancy. They are offered a postmortem, but feel that they have enough information to process what has happened and have been informed that their risk of recurrence in the future is low.

This case illustrates a few points. The first is that even though the couple had not undergone aneuploidy screening, it should not be assumed that they would not want to have later invasive testing should a different problem present. Had they undergone FTCS they might have had a low PAPP-A, which could have given them a higher-chance result of aneuploidy and they would possibly have had testing at that point. Had they have performed NIPT, they would have been more likely to have a low fetal fraction. If a result had not been possible after two attempts, this is an indication for offering invasive testing. These problems are often seen with triploidy. The case also shows the nuanced decision about postmortem. It can be offered to everyone, but often there is greater value when there is not yet a diagnosis or genetic diagnosis. Not having a certain diagnosis means it can be challenging to quote a future chance of recurrence.

NIPT can be performed from 10 weeks of pregnancy with no upper gestational age limit. There are some situations where NIPT can have some shortcomings:

- **Low fetal fraction:** There has to be enough of the placental DNA to accurately analyse. This can be quantified using a term known as the 'fetal fraction'. Depending on the laboratory, this has to be at least 4% to test. At 10 weeks, there is approximately a 5% chance that the fraction will be low; of those who then repeat the test, 50–60% will have a result (Hui and Bianchi 2019). Higher maternal body mass index (BMI) can make this more likely, as can other factors such as treatment with low molecular weight heparin, maternal inflammation or vitamin B_{12} deficiency (Hui and Bianchi 2019). Sometimes a persistent low fetal fraction can be due to an aneuploidy or triploidy and after two failed attempts this is seen as an indication for invasive testing.
- **Maternal transplant:** This means that there are three sets of chromosomes: the mother, the organ donor and the placenta. It does not mean that NIPT cannot be performed, but it would need to be discussed with the genetics laboratory.
- **A multiple pregnancy with a co-twin demise:** It is not possible from the test to establish which twin's DNA would be contributing to the result.
- **Maternal malignancy:** There have been cases of abnormal results secondary to tumours contributing to the cell free DNA. This is very rare.

Expert Midwife

Aneuploidy screening can be offered in multiple pregnancies. FTCS can be used for twins. In triplet and higher-order multiples, NT with maternal age is used. NIPT can be used in ongoing twin pregnancies with comparable test performance (Benn and Rebarber 2021).

Jazmina, Midwife

Clinical Investigation: Non-invasive Prenatal Diagnosis

Non-invasive prenatal diagnosis (NIPD) is the same test as NIPT working on the same biological principle. The difference is that NIPD is considered diagnostic for certain conditions and a follow-up confirmatory invasive test is not needed. These are examples of conditions that can be diagnosed using NIPD:

- **Fetal sex:** Helpful for families at risk from X-linked conditions such as congenital adrenal hyperplasia, a genetic condition causing virilisation of a female fetus, where there is some evidence that steroids given to the mother in pregnancy reduce the morbidity associated with the condition.
- **Fetal rhesus status:** In all rhesus-negative mothers, anti-D was traditionally given to reduce sensitisation from a rhesus-positive fetus, which may cause haemolytic disease of the fetus or newborn in a subsequent pregnancy. In some countries the fetal rhesus status is genotyped using cffDNA and anti-D is given only to those mothers whose fetuses are rhesus positive. This avoids unnecessary anti-D administration.
- **Testing for certain specific gene changes:** Examples are fetal *FGFR3* mutations, which can cause the skeletal dysplasias achondroplasia and thanatotrophic dysplasia, and gene mutations for cystic fibrosis.

Quadruple Screening, 15–20 Weeks

This has sensitivity of 70–75%, specificity of 93% and positive predictive value of approximately 2–3% (RANZCOG 2018). A blood test is performed in the second trimester measuring the analytes oestradiol, inhibin A, alpha-fetoprotein and hCG to provide a risk for trisomy 21 and 18. Alpha-fetoprotein levels climb in spina bifida and abdominal wall defects and therefore an increased level can raise the suspicion of these conditions. A high-quality ultrasound can effectively diagnose such structural differences.

Genetic Testing

There are genetic tests available to examine each level of the genome. The test chosen must be relevant to the type of condition you are looking to diagnose. You could liken each test to zooming further and further in to see more detail of the genome.

We start with the overview of how many chromosomes are in a cell. That can be done by a karyotype. Cells from a patient are obtained and a medium is added to stimulate the cells to divide. The cells are arrested in metaphase, when the chromosomes appear very densely packed and are most easily visible. The chromosomes are fixed onto a slide and a dye (called Giemsa, which is why you may see the term G-banded karyotype) is used to stain the chromosomes, giving them an appearance of light and dark bands. A microscope is used to see these arranged chromosomes under magnification. The karyotype is able to identify aneuploidies, translocations (balanced or unbalanced) and inversions. What it cannot do is see to the level of microdeletions or duplications, so it cannot identify changes in DNA sequence. As cells need to be grown, a karyotype can take up to approximately two weeks.

Since a karyotype takes some time, particularly when trying to get rapid answers for parents, QF-PCR is a quicker way of finding out about a set number of chromosomes, which is used for chromosomes 13, 18, 21 and, depending on the laboratory and indication, the sex chromosomes. Chromosome-specific DNA is sequenced and read on a DNA scanner. You would expect to have two peaks for a normal number of each chromosome, so when there is a trisomy there will be an additional peak. This technique can have rapid a turnaround of 24–48 hours and can identify the common trisomies, sex chromosome aneuploidy and triploidy.

Fluorescent in situ hybridisation (FISH) is often used similarly to QF-PCR. This test involves tagging fluorescent DNA probes that will bind to a specific target – this could be a chromosome or a gene. The cells are looked at under the microscope and each fluorescent probe counted. For example, if there are three probes lighting up for chromosome 13, then we have trisomy 13. It can also be used to look for microdeletions (commonly used for DiGeorge syndrome, a microdeletion at location 22q11) or duplications, or the presence or absence of a specific DNA sequence. It can also detect chromosomal rearrangements. In short, FISH only looks at what we have asked it to. While it is a narrow test, the advantage is that the turnaround is rapid, at between 24 and 48 hours.

Chromosomal microarray is a test looking for problems relating to the amount of genetic material. It can work by two methods: comparative genomic hybridisation (CGH) and single-nucleotide polymorphisms (SNP). Both methods are able to detect gains and losses of DNA, but neither can detect if there are balanced chromosomal rearrangements – remember, this method is really looking to see if there is too much or too little DNA rather than where the DNA is located. CNVs are the submicroscopic deletions or duplications of segments of DNA that can vary in size. Not all microdeletions or duplications cause disease, but there are some well-recognised conditions that are a result of this process (Levy and Burnside 2019). CNVs are classified by their known pathogenic effect. This can sometimes cause some anxiety if a variant of uncertain significance is identified. It is important that this possibility is included in the consent process.

Next-Generation Sequencing: Exome and Genome Testing

Next-generation sequencing (NGS) refers to a group of high-throughput sequencing technologies developed over the last decade. It can be used to sequence single genes, gene panels (multiple genes), exomes or whole genomes (Muzzey et al. 2015). This is a further zoom-in closer than the level of the microarray, looking for changes at the level of the gene by sequencing the base pairs of DNA. This is helpful when we are looking for single-gene disorders.

Exomes are regions of coding DNA making up approximately 1–2% of the whole genome. The DNA in exomes is the source of 85% of disease-causing changes. Compared to the existing standard chromosomal/genetic testing, with prenatal exome sequencing (ES) there can be an additional diagnostic yield, greatest in fetuses with multiple anomalies. Exome testing can detect single-nucleotide variants (SNVs), small insertions and deletions, and some CNVs (Abou Tayoun et al. 2018).

Orange Flag

When the testing is performed for a microarray, exome or genome, a 'trio' may be performed. This means there is a sample from the mother, the father and the baby. This can help identify whether it is a de novo (new) gene change or if it has been passed down from one of the parents.

    The midwife will need to offer parental support.

Whole-genome sequencing is the sequencing of all the DNA in the genome, approximately 3 billion base pairs. This includes the exome, non-coding DNA and mitochondrial DNA. As there is more DNA to interrogate, it can be more costly and time consuming. As it can take so long, the pregnancy is often over before a result is available, which is why it is not helpful in the prenatal setting.

Learning Event

To summarise the tests available in a simple way and a way that can be easier for parents to understand, consider this.

    Think of a library where we have pairs of bookcases lined up from 1 to 23. When we check a karyotype/QF-PCR or FISH, we are seeing if there is an extra bookcase. The bookcases represent chromosomes.

    If we want to look more closely, we want to count how many pages are in the books on the bookcases and check if there are any missing or extra pages. This represents a chromosomal microarray.

    If we want to look closer still, we read the words and check for spelling mistakes in those books on the bookcase. This represents genetic tests at the level of the exome or genome.

Red Flag

Obtaining consent for any genetic test should be performed by an appropriately trained clinician.

Performing Diagnostic Testing

In order to acquire the DNA sample to perform the genetic tests during pregnancy, invasive testing is required. The sample can be a placental biopsy, amniotic fluid or sometimes fetal blood. Invasive testing should be offered to those who have high-risk screening results, some fetal structural differences or a history raising the chance of a chromosomal or genetic condition.

Chorionic Villous Sample

A placental biopsy is performed from 11 weeks' gestation by a specialist in fetal medicine. The woman is appropriately counselled and consent is taken. Local anaesthetic is used on the skin and a thin needle inserted into the placenta under ultrasound guidance. The needle is either aspirated directly or a specific chorionic villous sample (CVS) kit is used. It is usually performed transabdominally but can be performed transvaginally. The procedure takes a matter of minutes.

    Specific to CVS are the limitations by virtue of the fact that the sample is from the placenta. There is a small chance of placental mosaicism, meaning that the result of the placental chromosomes may not always be the same as those of the fetus. This occurs in 1–2% of women who undergo CVS. When this is suspected, an amniocentesis should be performed as the amniotic fluid is indicative of the fetal cells.

Amniocentesis

A thin needle is inserted into the uterus under ultrasound guidance and approximately 20 ml of amniotic fluid is aspirated. This can only be performed beyond 15 weeks' gestation. The needle is so fine that local anaesthetic may not be needed.

The main concern from performing invasive testing is the risk of procedure-related miscarriage, ruptured membranes or preterm birth. That risk has traditionally been quoted as 1 in 200, but a recent meta-analysis suggests it is likely to be much lower than that, with a loss rate from amniocentesis of 0.3% and no increased risk of loss following transabdominal CVS (Saloman et al. 2019).

Red Flag

Invasive testing is a sensitising event and anti-D will be required where appropriate.

Woman-Centred Care

There is no right or wrong for how a woman chooses to manage the diagnosis of a serious genetic diagnosis for their unborn baby. In some circumstances, families opt not to continue with a pregnancy when there are significant structural differences or a chromosomal or genetic diagnosis. The provision of termination and the lawful gestation at which it can be performed will vary based on the jurisdiction in which you practise. In the United Kingdom, the 1967 Abortion Act allows termination of pregnancy until the 24th week of pregnancy and beyond this it is only possible in certain circumstances. Those circumstances include the diagnosis of a fetal abnormality in which there is a substantial risk that the child, if born, would suffer physical or mental abnormalities that would result in serious handicap (Royal College of Obstetricians and Gynaecologists 2010).

After a termination of pregnancy, a postmortem can be helpful, particularly if a genetic diagnosis has not been reached. This can obtain more information about the phenotype, which can guide testing of the genotype. A diagnosis suspected prenatally may be confirmed or revised and there may be other findings noted that had not been identified on ultrasound. The postmortem procedure should be explained by an appropriately trained professional and, as with all decisions leading to this point, the couple's fully informed decision should be respected.

Future Pregnancies

Orange Flag

Knowing what the genetic change or chromosomal change is in the affected baby will aid counselling regarding risk in a future pregnancy.

The majority of the time, aneuploidy results from an isolated occurrence. Increasing maternal age increases the background risk. A recurrence risk is quoted as 1% or the maternal background age risk, whichever is higher. If a translocation is the cause of the extra chromosome material, rather than trisomy, the chance of recurrence is greater, there will be an increased risk of this repeating in the future.

For a chromosomal duplication or deletion, the recurrence risk depends on whether the duplication or deletion was de novo in the affected baby or if it was inherited from either parent. De novo mutations have a low chance of recurrence.

Woman-Centred Care

In conditions with a recognised recurrence rate, there are options for what a family may choose to do in a future pregnancy:

- Try for another pregnancy, accepting the risk of a future affected child. Genetic testing could be considered after birth or if symptoms develop.
- Try for another pregnancy and have invasive testing (or NIPD if available for the condition) to achieve a diagnosis prenatally. For some that information may mean opting for termination of pregnancy if the fetus is affected.
- Pre-implantation genetic diagnosis (PGD), which requires in vitro fertilisation (IVF) to create embryos. A small sample is taken from the embryo and tested. Only embryos that are euploid/without the gene change are suitable for transfer to the uterus. Only a small number of cells are tested, which leaves room for error due to mosaicism. Testing in pregnancy should still be offered as confirmation.
- Gamete donation.
- Choosing not to have a further pregnancy.

Case Study 4.2

Jasmine is pregnant with her first child. Her mid-trimester scan shows that her baby has a right aortic arch, confirmed by a paediatric cardiologist specialising in fetal echocardiography. The fetal medicine specialist cannot see any other structural differences. Jasmine is told there is an association with some genetic conditions, one of which is DiGeorge syndrome (a microdeletion of 22q11).

She decides to have an amniocentesis. A FISH and microarray are sent. The fetal medicine specialist has requested a probe for the FISH to check for 22q11 in addition to the common aneuploidies of chromosome 13, 18 and 21. The FISH result is ready after 48 hours, confirming DiGeorge syndrome. The final microarray also confirms the microdeletion at 22q11. Jasmine and her partner Tom have microarrays sent and it seems that this change for her baby is de novo.

Jasmine has counselling with the geneticist and the neonatal team and is told that this condition can cause some feeding, hearing and growth difficulties, immune issues and later behavioural and psychiatric problems. She is informed of the support available and that the extent of these issues is hard to predict. Jasmine feels comfortable continuing the pregnancy and is referred to the social work team for more support. She gives birth to a baby boy. Early support is arranged for feeding, and follow-up with the cardiologist, audiologist and developmental paediatric team is also arranged before she is discharged from hospital.

This case highlights that some parents may benefit from the opportunity to prepare for the birth of a baby with genetic differences. An early diagnosis can mobilise the appropriate team to offer the best care for the child, which may improve outcomes.

Conditions Associated with Genetics

The following are a list of conditions that are associated with genetics. Take some time and write notes about each of the conditions. Remember to include aspects of patient care. If you are making notes about people you have offered care and support to, you must ensure that you have adhered to the rules of confidentiality.

The condition	Your notes
DiGeorge syndrome	
Patau's syndrome	
Edwards' syndrome	
Down's syndrome	
Turner's syndrome	

Take-Home Points

- As midwives, it is important to be aware of those women who could benefit from further genetic counselling or investigation, either before or during pregnancy.
- Aneuploidy screening should be offered to all pregnant women in high-income countries.
- Understanding screening tests and their performance is essential in order to accurately counsel a woman prior to testing.
- Interpretation of genetic test results can be complex and in the context of high-risk results, it is important to recognise our own limitations and seek advice from the wider multidisciplinary team.
- All women should be offered the same standard of care and be treated with respect and compassion.

Conclusion

Prenatal genetics is a rapidly evolving field involving many complex situations, requiring the expertise of several specialists. Members of the multidisciplinary team include screening midwives, general practitioners, general obstetricians and gynaecologists, fetal medicine specialists, sonographers, genetic counsellors, geneticists, the genetic laboratory staff, neonatologists, relevant paediatric specialties, bereavement teams, social workers and psychologists. It is important to be aware of everyone's limitations and ensure that we work collaboratively to deliver the best care.

It is essential that all women and their families are offered the same options for investigation and management regardless of their background or the healthcare professionals' personal beliefs. Our responsibility is to offer up-to-date, evidence-based advice and our support. All women and their families should be treated with respect and compassion through what may be an unexpectedly challenging time.

References

Abou Tayoun, A., Spinner, N., Rehm, H. et al. (2018). Prenatal DNA sequencing: clinical, counselling and diagnostic laboratory considerations. *Prenatal Diagnosis* 38: 26–32.

Benn, P. and Rebarber, A. (2021). Non-invasive testing in the management of twin pregnancies. *Prenatal Diagnosis* 41: 1233–1240.

Hui, L. and Bianchi, D. (2019). Fetal fraction and noninvasive prenatal testing: what clinicians need to know. *Prenatal Diagnosis* 40: 155–163.

Kagan, K.O., Avgidou, K., Molina, F.S. et al. (2006). Relation between increased fetal nuchal translucency thickness and chromosomal defects. *Obstetrics and Gynecology* 107: 6–10.

Kroes, I., Janssens, S., and Defoort, P. (2014). Ultrasound features in trisomy 13 (Patau syndrome) and trisomy 18 (Edwards syndrome) in a consecutive series o 47 cases. *Facts, Views & Vision in ObGyn* 6: 245–249.

Levy, B. and Burnside, R. (2019). Are all chromosome microarrays the same? What clinicians need to know. *Prenatal Diagnosis* 39: 157–164.

Meyer, R., Liu, G., Gilboa, S. et al. (2015). Survival of children with trisomy 13 and trisomy 18: a multi state population based study. *American Journal of Medical Genetics* 170: 825–837.

Morris, J., Wald, D., Mutton, E., and Alberman, E. (2003). Comparison of models of maternal age-specific risk for Downs syndrome live births. *Prenatal Diagnosis* 23: 252–258.

Muzzey, D., Evans, E., and Lieber, C. (2015). Understanding the basics of NGS: from mechanism to variant calling. *Current Genetic Medicine Reports* 3: 158–165.

NHS (2019). Klinefelter syndrome. https://www.nhs.uk/conditions/klinefelters-syndrome (accessed November 2023).

NHS England (2022). Downs' syndrome, Edwards' syndrome and Patau's syndrome. https://www.gov.uk/government/publications/screening-tests-for-you-and-your-baby/downs-syndrome-edwards-syndrome-and-pataus-syndrome-combined-or-quadruple-test-taken-on-or-after-1-june-2021 (accessed November 2023).

Offerdal, K., Blaas, H.G.K., and Eik-Nes, S.-H. (2008). Prenatal detection of trisomy 21 by second trimester ultrasound examination and maternal age in a non selected population of 49,314 births in Norway. *Ultrasound in Obstetrics & Gynecology* 32: 493–500.

Royal Australian and New Zealand College of Obstetricians and Gynaecologists (RANZCOG) (2018). Prenatal screening and diagnostic testing for fetal chromosomal and genetic conditions. https://ranzcog.edu.au/wp-content/uploads/2022/05/Prenatal-Screening-and-Diagnostic-Testing-for-Fetal-Chromosomal-and-Genetic-Conditions.pdf (accessed November 2023).

Royal Australian and New Zealand College of Obstetricians and Gynaecologists (RANZCOG) (2019). Genetic carrier screening – C-obs 63. https://ranzcog.edu.au/wp-content/uploads/2022/05/Genetic-carrier-screeningC-Obs-63New-March-2019_1.pdf (accessed November 2023).

Royal College of Obstetricians and Gynaecologists (2010). Termination of pregnancy for fetal abnormality in England, Scotland and Wales. https://www.rcog.org.uk/guidance/browse-all-guidance/other-guidelines-and-reports/termination-of-pregnancy-for-fetal-abnormality-in-england-scotland-and-wales (accessed November 2023).

Saloman, L., Sotiriadis, C., Wulff, B. et al. (2019). Risk of miscarriage following amniocentesis or chorionic villus sampling: systematic review of literature and updated meta-analysis. *Ultrasound in Obstetrics & Gynecology* 54: 442–451.

Taylor-Phillips, S., Freeman, K., Geppert, J. et al. (2016). Accuracy of non-invasive prenatal testing using cell-free DNA for detection of Down, Edwards and Patau syndromes: a systematic review and meta-analysis. *BMJ Open* 6 (1): e010002.

Further Resources

Positive about Down syndrome. www.positiveaboutdownsyndrome.co.uk (www.youtube.com/channel/UCr3LqX6RKUb8d6jIt3UWqEA) (accessed November 2023).

Down Syndrome Association. www.downs-syndrome.org.uk (accessed November 2023).

SOFT UK, support organisation for trisomy 13/18. www.soft.org.uk (www.youtube.com/channel/UC4qwXysHkwfIXjDsRF9notA/videos) (accessed November 2023).

77

Glossary

Allele	A variation of a gene. For example, a gene for eye colour could have a blue or brown allele. We inherit one allele from our mother and one from our father
Aneuploidy	An abnormal number of chromosomes that is not an exact multiple of the haploid number
Diploid (2n)	Two complete sets of chromosomes (46 in humans – 23 pairs, present in somatic cells)
Euploid	A normal number of chromosomes in a cell
Exome	Makes up only 1–2% of all our genome yet accounts for 85% of disease-causing mutations
Expression	Conversion of the genotype to the phenotype
Gamete	A sex cell (contains a haploid number of chromosomes). Egg or sperm
Gene	A sequence of DNA that codes for a protein or function
Genome	All of our genetic material
Genotype	Describes the genetic material of an individual
Haploid (n)	One set of chromosomes (23 in humans – eggs and sperm)
Karyotype	Microscopic picture of the homologous chromosomes arranged in order from 1 to 23 after they have been stained (commonly with Giemsa)
Microarray	A test that can determine problems relating to the amount of genetic material in an individual

Monosomy   Only one copy of a chromosome
Mosaicism   More than one genetic cell line in an individual
Phenotype   Describes a feature, behaviour or appearance of an individual
Ploidy   Refers to the whole set of chromosomes
Triploid (3n)   A complete additional set of chromosomes (69 in humans)
Trisomy   Three copies of a chromosome

CHAPTER 5

The Reproductive System and Associated Disorders

Claire Ford

Department of Nursing, Midwifery and Health, Northumbria University, Newcastle upon Tyne, UK

AIM

This chapter aims to support midwifery practice, providing the reader with information about the pathophysiology of the reproductive system.

LEARNING OUTCOMES

On completion of this chapter the reader will be able to:

- Describe both the internal and external organs associated with the female reproductive system
- Understand the need to provide individualised woman-centred care
- Have an awareness of the pathophysiology associated with the female reproductive system
- Gain an appreciation of the role of the midwife in relation to managing and treating disorders affecting the reproductive organs

Test Your Prior Knowledge

1. Name two disorders of the reproductive system that can have negative impacts on female fertility.
2. What are the main symptoms associated with endometriosis?
3. What hormones are needed for an ovum to develop and be released from the ovary?
4. What treatments are available for managing dysmenorrhea?

The female reproductive system comprises both internal and external organs (see Figure 5.1) designed to adapt and change to produce female gametes, transport the ovum, assist fertilisation, protect the growing fetus, for birth and to feed a baby (Boore et al. 2021). Throughout this chapter the pathophysiology of the reproductive organs will be explored in greater depth. Reference will also be made to normal anatomy and physiology and the assessment and management strategies required to facilitate the reproductive process and improve physiological and psychological health.

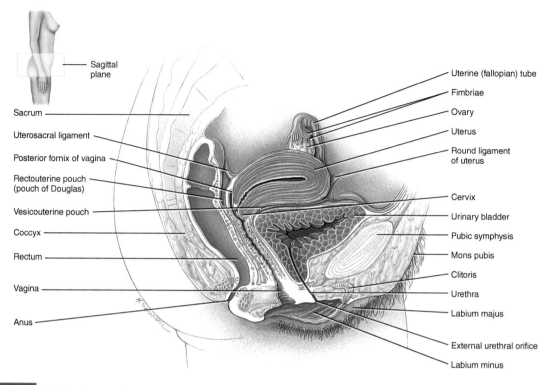

Sagittal plane

Sacrum

Uterosacral ligament

Posterior fornix of vagina

Rectouterine pouch (pouch of Douglas)

Vesicouterine pouch

Coccyx

Rectum

Vagina

Anus

Uterine (fallopian) tube

Fimbriae

Ovary

Uterus

Round ligament of uterus

Cervix

Urinary bladder

Pubic symphysis

Mons pubis

Clitoris

Urethra

Labium majus

External urethral orifice

Labium minus

FIGURE 5.1   The female reproductive organs (sagittal plane view).

Vulva (External Female Genitalia)

The vulva protects the urethra, lubricates the vagina and, due to an extensive nervous supply, also produces feelings of sensual intensity on stimulation. However, until recently the importance of the vulva in sexual pleasure has largely been underplayed and in some cultures female pleasure is not encouraged or even discussed.

Woman-Centred Care

For many women it is important that their identity is not only aligned to growing life but also as being sexual, with needs and desires. It is imperative that midwives encourage women to discuss their fears and concerns about the impacts pregnancy and birth may have on their sexual health, sexual identity and potential relationships with their partner(s). It is also important to consider the individual and unique needs of the woman herself. As such, midwives need to be open-minded, receptive to alternative lifestyles and practise in a non-discriminatory manner.

The vulva (see Figure 5.2) consists of the following structures:

- Vaginal orifice
- Clitoris
- Mons pubis
- Labia majora
- Labia minora
- Urethral orifice
- Vulval vestibule
- Vulval glands

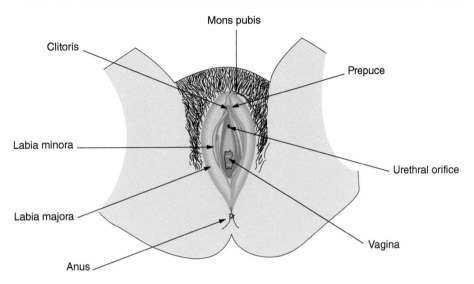

FIGURE 5.2 The vulva (external genitalia).

Mons Pubis

In females, this is a prominent mound of adipose tissue that is located directly anterior to the pubic bone. Its main functions are to ease and facilitate sexual intercourse, by cushioning and protecting the pubic bone and secreting pheromones, via the sebaceous glands, to induce sexual attraction. During puberty hair growth can be seen in this region, which also acts as a protective buffer, reducing friction and acting as a dry lubricant.

Labia Majora and Minora

The words 'labia majora' mean the larger lips and these two large prominences form the lateral longitudinal outer boundary of the vulva (Nguyen and Duong 2022). They are created from rounded folds of skin, adipose and fibrous tissue that join anteriorly and superiorly to the vaginal opening, forming the anterior labial commissure, and posteriorly to the vaginal opening to form the posterior labial commissure (Waugh and Grant 2018). They contain sebaceous and eccrine sweat glands and hair growth only occurs on the lateral surfaces, leaving the inner surfaces smooth. The hair acts as a protective barrier, reducing friction, and the inner smooth surface acts like a mucous membrane, preventing dryness.

The term 'labia minora' means smaller lips, which are also folds of skin with sebaceous and eccrine sweats glands but, as the name suggests, are smaller in size and completely hairless. They are found between the labia majora and their main function is the protection of the vestibule, urethra, vagina and clitoris. The anterior folds of the labia minora encircle the clitoris, which creates the clitoral hood and the frenulum of the clitoris (Nguyen and Duong 2022). These folds then descend obliquely and downwards to the posterior ends encompassing the vulva vestibule, before terminating as they are linked together by a skin fold called the frenulum.

Considerations for Pregnancy

It is not unusual for the labia minora and majora to appear swollen with or without sexual arousal, due to the increased blood flow experienced during pregnancy. They may also appear darker in colour to the rest of the woman's normal skin colour, because of the hormonal changes associated with pregnancy.

Considerations After Delivery

During birth and depending on the mode of delivery, the labia may be swollen due to the increased pressure from bearing down or trauma caused during delivery. Cold packs and non-steroidal anti-inflammatory drugs (NSAIDs) can be used to reduce the swelling and pain.

Vulva Varicosities

These are dilated veins in the labia majora and minora and are estimated to occur in around 20% of pregnant women due to an increase in pelvic blood flow and slow venous return (Gavrilov 2017; Lewis 2022). Women can often be asymptomatic or can experience feelings of pressure or fullness in the vulva along with discomfort, especially during sex, exercise or if standing for long periods. Most varicosities do not pose any significant problems for delivery and they usually reduce in size after delivery, but severe cases that persist postnatally may require surgery.

Health Promotion

Vulval varicosities are linked with venous stasis and venous thromboembolic events. It is therefore essential that any women presenting with this condition are advised of steps that can be taken to ease symptoms such as pain and swelling, and informed that an occupational health assessment may be required if their job involves long periods of standing. Additionally, strategies to reduce the risk of developing a venous thromboembolism may be required:

- To reduce venous stasis, encourage women to regularly change their position, from sitting to standing, and to sit with their legs elevated.
- To increase venous return, advise women that they can wear compression hosiery, take regular exercise and encourage calf muscle contraction even when their legs are elevated.
- To reduce the risk of hypercoagulability, stress the importance of drinking and hydration, stopping smoking and maintaining a healthy diet.

Vulval Cancer

Annually within the United Kingdom approximately 1300 women are diagnosed with cancer of the vulva. While any part of the vulva can be affected, such as the tip of the clitoris or the Bartholin's glands, the most common area is the labia (MacMillan 2022). Squamous cell carcinomas accounts for 90% of cases, which usually start with pre-cancerous changes to the outer layer of the skin cells of the vulva and can take years to develop (Isaac and Young 2011). Other vulval cancers include:

- Verrucous carcinoma, slow-growing wart-like growths.
- Malignant melanoma accounts for around 4% of vulval cancers and can be associated with pigment-producing cells.
- Lichen sclerosis, which appears as flat white moist patches.
- Basal cell carcinomas, cancer that develops in the basal deep layer and is associated with ultraviolet radiation damage.
- Paget's disease, a rare non-invasive cancer that originates from the epithelial cells and only affects women who are menopausal. Skin is often red or scaly and can cause itching and irritation.
- Merkel cell tumours, a very rare but aggressive cancer presenting as firm lumps of skin with a blue or red hue. They usually develop in women between the ages of 60 and 80 years.
- Sarcomas represent around 4% of vulval cancers and are associated with fast-growing lymphatic metastatic spread. They originate in connective tissue and can be felt as firm nodules.
- Adenocarcinoma develops from the vulval glands.

Health Promotion

Vulval cancers are not common, but early detection and treatment are vital for improving prognosis. It is therefore important that women are aware of the risk factors associated with the development of these cancers and what steps they can take to reduce these risks.

Risks

- Human papilloma virus (HPV): There is a clear link between HPV and squamous cell carcinoma.
- Smoking: Risks increase with number of years smoking and level of intensity.
- Age: Risk increases with age and is associated more with women over 50 years.
- Human immunodeficiency virus (HIV) and iatrogenic immunosuppression: Damaged immune systems can increase the risk of cancer development.

Screening
Women themselves can play a huge role in screening for potential cancer, as changes to the vulva are easily visible and can be palpated. Self-examination is therefore crucial, and midwives should encourage women to self-examine at least once a month and signpost them to self-examination guides.

Vaccination
Once of the most common preventative measure is to be vaccinated against HPV, particularly HPV 16, 18, 31, 33.

Source: Adapted from Isaac and Young (2011) and Olawaiye et al. (2021).

Vulval cancer symptoms include raised, thickened red, white or dark patches, itching, burning, vulvodynia, bleeding and ulceration. These cancers are graded based on the appearance of the cells under a microscope and provide a base for the anticipated speed of development, which is necessary to determine the most appropriate treatment. A low grade is used for cells closely resembling normal cells of the vulva, a moderate grade for more abnormal cells and a higher grade for cells that are extremely abnormal and more likely to spread (Olawaiye et al. 2021). As well as the grading of the cells, vulval cancer is also classified into stages, which help describe the size and spread (see Table 5.1).

Clitoris

The main function of this organ is for sexual pleasure; consequently, it is constructed largely of sensory nerve endings and erectile tissue. It is approximately 2 cm in diameter and consists of a shaft (body) and a glans (tips), which is the part of the clitoris that is visible. The glans clitoris is highly innervated by nerves and is estimated to contain over 8000 nerve endings. The underlying tissue that makes the clitoris is the corpus cavernous and erectile tissue, which is perfused by

TABLE 5.1   The stages of vulval cancer.

Stage 1	Stage 2	Stage 3	Stage 4
Growth isolated to the vulva and/or perineum Stage 1A: <2 cm and has grown 1 mm or less into the skin Stage 1B: >2 cm in size or has grown more than 1 mm into the skin	Any size of tumour that has spread to the lower part of the urethra, the vagina or the anus	Spread to the lymph nodes in the groin Stage 3A: 1 or 2 lymph node metastases <5 mm OR only 1 lymph node metastasis >5 mm Stage 3B: >3 lymph node metastases <5 mm OR >2 lymph node metastases >5 mm Stage 3C: Cancer has spread outside the capsule surround the lymph node	Stage 4A: Lymph node metastases that are ulcerated or fixed to nearby structures OR cancer has spread further to other structures, the bladder, rectum, pelvic bone Stage 4B: Lymph node metastases in the pelvis or other parts of the body

Source: Adapted from Isaac and Young (2011) and Olawaiye et al. (2021).

many blood vessels and responds to arousal by enlarging and becoming firm (Peate 2017). A fold of skin derived from an extension of the labia minora, known as the clitoral hood, protects this very sensitive organ.

Red Flag: Female Genital Mutilation

The World Health Organization (WHO 2022a) recognises female genital mutilation (FGM) as a violation of the human rights of women and girls and suggests that the practice reflects deep-rooted gender inequalities. Globally more than 200 million girls and women have been subjected to FGM. It is illegal in the United Kingdom and constitutes a form of child abuse. Therefore, it is imperative when caring for women that midwives and midwifery students observe for signs of FGM and ask women about any possible alterations to the external genitalia, as these may increase the risk of intrapartum complications and neonatal mortality. As it constitutes an extreme form of discrimination, it may also alert healthcare professionals to possible safeguarding concerns for the woman and female infants.

- FGM involves the partial or total removal of external female genitalia or other injury to the female genital organs for non-medical reasons (see Figure 5.3 and Table 5.2).
- It damages healthy genital tissue and interferes with the natural functions of girls' and women's bodies; it has no health benefits and can also result in loss of life.

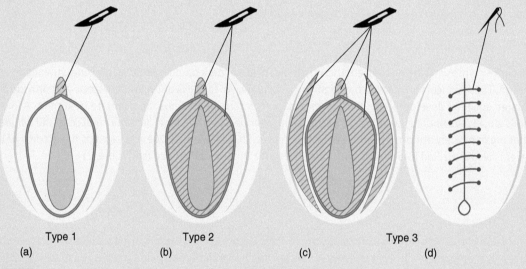

Type 1   Type 2   Type 3

(a)   (b)   (c)   (d)

FIGURE 5.3   (a–d) Types of female genital mutilation. Source: Adapted from WHO (2022a).

TABLE 5.2   **Types of female genital mutilation.**

Type 1	Type 2	Type 3	Type 4
Partial or total removal of the clitoral glans, the most external and visible part of the clitoris and also the most sensitive part of female genitalia	Partial or total removal of the clitoral glans and the labia minora, with or without removal of the labia majora	Narrowing of the vaginal opening by cutting and repositioning the labia minora and/or labia majora Also known as infibulation	All other harmful procedures to the female genitalia for non-medical purposes, including: • Pricking • Piercing • Incising • Scraping • Cauterising

Source: Adapted from WHO (2022a).

Orange Flag: FGM and Psychological Support

FGM can affect a woman's mental health long after the time of the physical trauma and can have significant impacts on all areas of her sexual, physiological and emotional well-being. It is often the case that the more extensive the physiological trauma, the higher the risk of developing mental health disorders.

Signs of long- and short-term psychological trauma include:

- Anxiety
- Shock
- Sadness
- Somatisation
- Depression
- Post-traumatic stress disorder
- Other mood disorders

Women can also report feelings of anger, particularly at family members who have violated their trust, and feelings of isolation as they do not feel they can confide in or talk to anyone about this. Midwives are in a prime position to recognise FGM and provide both an outlet for the women's concerns and a conduit for linking the woman to specialist support services.

Source: Adapted from Köbach et al. (2018) and WHO (2022a).

Considerations for Pregnancy

The clitoris may be more sensitive during pregnancy due to the increase in blood flow and some associated swelling. The colour of other areas of the skin may also darken due to the hormonal changes that occur, and women can often achieve orgasm more readily.

Consideration After Delivery

The clitoris may receive some tissue damage caused by trauma during delivery. Cold packs and NSAIDs can be used to reduce the swelling and pain, but if the clitoris became lacerated or torn sutures are not usually required, as it will usually heal via second intention.

Urethral Orifice

This is often referred to as the urinary meatus and is the exit point of urine out of the body, from the bladder through the urethra. It is located 2.5 cm inferior and posterior to the clitoris and superior and anterior to the vagina (Boore et al. 2021).

Vaginal Orifice

The introitus to the vagina is partially covered by the hymen, a thin protective layer that is made up of mucous membranes stretching across the vaginal lumen. It is usually incomplete to allow passage of menstrual loss, but can be broken further or completely removed by physical activity, the insertion of sanitary products, or sexual activities. It is therefore an unreliable indicator of the absence of sexual intercourse.

Vestibular Bulbs

The vestibular bulbs are structures formed from corpus spongiosum tissue, a type of erectile tissue (Nguyen and Duong 2022). These commence close to the inferior side of the body of the clitoris before extending, splitting and surrounding the lateral border of the urethra and vagina. During sexual arousal they become engorged with blood, which exerts pressure on the clitoris, inducing feelings of pleasure.

Vulval Vestibule and Vestibular Glands

The cleft between the labia minora is referred to as the vestibule. The change from the vulva vestibule to the labia minora is clearly defined by Hart's lines, which are formed when the skin transitions to the smoother skin of the vulva. There are two greater vestibular glands (Bartholin's glands) situated on either side of the inferior aspect of the vaginal orifice. They are approximately 1 cm in diameter and have ducts that open into the vestibule, laterally to the attachment of the hymen. These two glands secrete a mucus-like substance into the vagina that acts as a lubricant and helps to keep the vulva moist (Waugh and Grant 2018; Nguyen and Duong 2022). The two lesser or minor vestibular glands, also known as Skene's glands, are located around the inferior part of the urethral orifice and are believed to be the source of female ejaculation during sexual arousal. The substance is also believed to act as an antimicrobial, to prevent urinary tract infections.

Medicines Management: Bartholin's Cyst

If the ducts of the Bartholin's gland become blocked, usually due to bacterial infections such as *Escherichia coli* (*E. coli*), gonorrhoea or chlamydia, they can become engorged with fluid and expand to form a cyst. Some may be small and resolve on their own; however, others can become very large, causing significant pain and discomfort, and may become infected, resulting in an abscess.

Suspected infected cysts will need to be swabbed to identify the bacteria responsible and target the treatment more effectively. Antibiotic therapies for infected cysts include ceftriaxone, ciprofloxacin, doxycycline and azithromycin. Topical or local anaesthetics such as lidocaine and bupivacaine are also used to treat abscesses, and oral analgesics, such as paracetamol and ibuprofen, are recommended to manage the pain.

Ciprofloxacin adult dose by mouth: initially 500 mg twice daily; increased to 750 mg twice daily in severe or deep-seated infections.

Source: Adapted from Lee et al. (2015), BNF (2022a) and NHS (2022a).

Perineum

This is a triangular structure extending from the labia minora to the anal canal and its main function is the attachment to the muscles of the pelvic floor (see Figure 5.4). It consists of connective tissue, muscles and adipose tissue and tearing of these structures can often occur during childbirth. The Royal College of Obstetricians and Gynaecologists (RCOG 2022a) states that almost 9 out of 10 first-time mothers who have a vaginal birth will experience some trauma to the perineum. This trauma can occur inside the vagina or other parts of the vulva, including the labia, and for most women the tears are minor and heal on their own. However, for approximately 3.5 out of 100 women the tear may be deeper, resulting in significant damage to the anal sphincter, leading to complications such as anal incontinence, infections, fistulas and weakened pelvic floor (see Table 5.3 for the classification of perineal trauma).

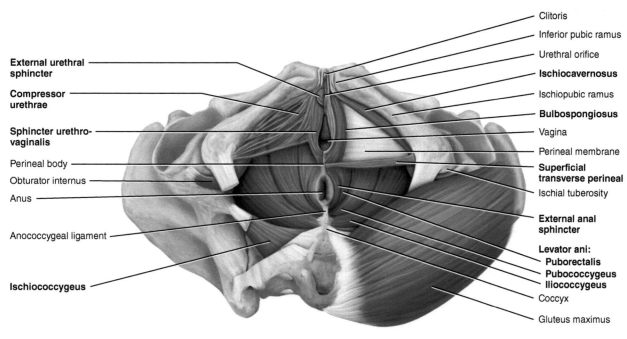

External urethral sphincter

Compressor urethrae

Sphincter urethro-vaginalis

Perineal body

Obturator internus

Anus

Anococcygeal ligament

Ischiococcygeus

Clitoris

Inferior pubic ramus

Urethral orifice

Ischiocavernosus

Ischiopubic ramus

Bulbospongiosus

Vagina

Perineal membrane

Superficial transverse perineal

Ischial tuberosity

External anal sphincter

Levator ani:
 Puborectalis
 Pubococcygeus
 Iliococcygeus
Coccyx

Gluteus maximus

Inferior superficial view of a female perineum

FIGURE 5.4 Muscles of the pelvic floor.

TABLE 5.3 **Classifications of perineal trauma.**

Classification	Description
First degree	Damage to the perineal skin and/or vaginal mucosa Will normally heal quickly Requires no intervention
Second degree	Damage to the perineal muscles and skin, but not anal sphincter Usually requires sutures to close the skin and muscle layers Repair can be performed by a competent midwife or medical professional with appropriate skill and knowledge
Third degree	Damage to the skin, muscles and anal sphincter Three subgroups of third-degree tears: 3a. Damage to external anal sphincter (EAS) <50% thickness 3b. Damage to EAS >50% thickness 3c. Internal sphincter also torn Surgical repair will be performed by obstetric medical staff in theatre
Fourth degree	Injury to both the external and internal anal sphincter as well as the anal epithelium Repair will be carried out in theatre, under local, regional or general anaesthetic by a member of the obstetric medical team

Source: Adapted from RCOG (2015, 2022a).

> ### Case Study 5.1   Perineal Trauma
>
> Melissa is a 27-year-old woman who has just given birth to her first child. During delivery she sustained a third-degree tear, which needed to be repaired and sutured by the medical team under local anaesthetic. She is ready for discharge but is anxious as she has not yet had a bowel movement and is experiencing pain and discomfort, especially when wearing clothing and sitting.
>
> - What advice can the midwife provide about easing bowel movements and reducing the risk of constipation?
> - What analgesic pharmacological and non-pharmacological strategies can be suggested?
> - What advice should be provided to Melissa before discharge about managing the wound and assessing for signs of infection?
> - To minimise ongoing complications, what additional advice do you think Melissa would benefit from?

Internal Reproductive Organs

The internal organs of the reproductive system sit within the pelvic cavity and consist of the vagina, the uterus, two ovaries and two uterine tubes (see Figures 5.1 and 5.5). Each organ has its own blood and nerve supplies (Waugh and Grant 2018).

Vagina

This is a fibromuscular tube that acts as a passageway for menstrual fluid and the birth of a baby and as such connects with the vestibule at one end and the uterine cervix at the other (Peate 2017). Both the arterial and venous blood supply to the vagina is via the internal iliac arteries and veins, and lymphatic draining is through the deep and superficial iliac glands (Boore et al. 2021). The vagina is also not completely vertical, but rather at an upward, inverted angle of about 45°, anterior to the rectum and posterior to the bladder and urethra. Hence, it has a longer posterior wall, around 9 cm, and a shorter anterior wall, approximately 7.5 cm. While the vagina itself has no secretory glands, it is kept moist by the cervical secretions and, with the assistance of oestrogen and lactic acid-secreting friendly bacteria, the vagina maintains an acidic bacteriostatic environment, inhibiting the growth of other microorganisms (Peate 2017).

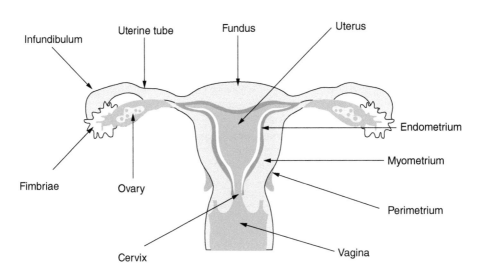

FIGURE 5.5   Vagina, uterus, ovaries and supporting structures.

TABLE 5.4 Types of vaginitis.

Type	Description
Candida infection	Caused by an increased balance of fungus *Candida*
	Symptoms include a thick, white vaginal discharge, itching, erythema and pain during sexual intercourse
	Treated with antifungal vaginal creams and suppositories, vaginal tablets and/or oral antifungals
Bacterial vaginosis	Caused by a bacterial imbalance
	Symptoms include 'fishy' malodour and thin discharge
	Treated with oral antibiotics
Non-infectious vaginitis	Caused by irritation from or allergy to vaginal sprays, douches, spermicidal products, or sensitivity to personal hygiene and laundry products
	Symptoms include itching, burning, increased discharge and pain
Viral vaginitis	Caused by viruses such as herpesvirus or human papillomavirus, usually sexually transmitted
	Symptoms include pain, lesions and sores
	Treatments such as antiviral medication can help alleviate the symptoms, but will not kill the virus, so immunisation against the virus is the best line of defence
Trichomoniasis vaginitis	Sexually transmitted infection caused by the parasite *Trichomonas vaginalis*
	Symptoms include frothy, malodorous greenish-yellow discharge, itching or burning, erythema, oedema, light bleeding, lower abdominal pain and pain during sexual intercourse
	Treatments include oral antibiotics and all sexual partners must also be treated

Source: Adapted from ACOG (2022) and NHS (2022b).

Vaginitis

Vaginitis refers to inflammation of the vagina, which can be infectious or non-infectious, transmitted through sexual contact or resulting from an imbalance in natural flora and fauna due to hormonal changes, personal hygiene or medications. It is one of the most common reasons for women seeking assistance from gynaecologists and there are many causes, including bacteria, yeast, viruses or even clothing, creams and soap (see Table 5.4) (ACOG 2022).

Vaginal Cancer

This type of cancer is very uncommon, accounting for less than 2% of all genital malignancies; thus, it is usually secondary to vulval or cervical cancer or from metastatic spread through the lymphatic system. Symptoms include pain and vaginal bleeding; however, some women are asymptomatic, and the cancer is only detected as part of regular cervical smears and vaginal examinations. As with vulvar cancers, vaginal cancer is graded using the International Federation of Gynecology and Obstetrics (FIGO) classification (see Figure 5.6) and survival rates for stages one are 70–80%, reducing to less than 20% for grade 4. Treatment and management will depend on the level of spread and if it is primary or secondary, but can include surgical excision, radiotherapy, chemotherapy, brachytherapy or a combination of all these approaches (Tinkler 2011).

Examination Scenario: Vaginal Examination

During undergraduate midwifery education, students will have the opportunity to undertake vaginal examination. However, this is an invasive procedure and therefore it is important to consider the following in relation to this clinical skill:

- Have you seen chaperones being used in practice?
- What is your understanding of informed consent regarding vaginal examination and what would you do if consent was not provided?
- How have you seen respect and dignity being maintained when observing this skill in practice?
- If you have undertaken this skill under supervision in practice, how did you feel?
- How did you articulate the findings to the woman?

CERVICAL CANCER

Normal

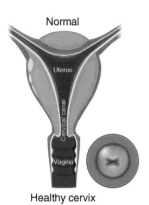

Healthy cervix

Early stage IB

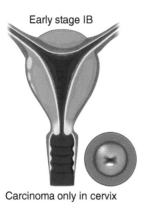

Carcinoma only in cervix

Late stage IB

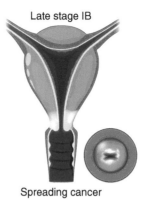

Spreading cancer

Stage IIB

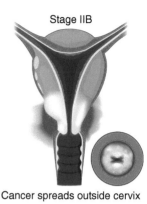

Cancer spreads outside cervix

FIGURE 5.6   Stages of vaginal cancer.

Orange Flag: Vaginismus

This is an uncontrolled physical reaction where the vaginal muscles tighten, which is initiated by an emotional reaction to the fear of some or all types of vaginal penetration (NHS 2022c). This can occur at any time in a woman's life and usually presents after an unpleasant medical examination, a bad first sexual experience, believing sex is shameful or a case of vaginitis. It is usually treated by attempting to find the cause and then treating the origin, therefore treatments might include psychosexual therapy, pelvic floor exercises, relaxation techniques or vaginal trainers.

The Uterus

The uterus is a pear-shaped organ, situated in the pelvic cavity posterior and superior to the bladder and anterior to the rectum. For most women it leans forward (anteverted), unlike the vagina, and is approximately 7.5 cm long, 5 cm wide and weighs between 30 and 40 g (Waugh and Grant 2018). It is divided into several sections, the largest of which is the body, occupying two-thirds of the uterus. The fundus is the rounded superior section commencing after the openings of the uterine tubes and the narrow inferior portion is referred to as the isthmus, which attaches to the cervix (see the separate section on the cervix). It is held in place within the pelvic cavity by the mesometrium ligaments, which attach to the pelvic floor, and the round ligaments anchor the anterior wall of the uterus to the pelvic cavity. The mesovarium (and the mesometrium), otherwise referred to as the broad ligaments, help preserve the position of the uterus within the pelvic cavity, but also maintain the relationship of the uterine tubes to the ovaries and the uterus.

The uterus is an extremely muscular organ, about 2.5 cm thick, with walls constructed from three varying muscle layers, the perimetrium, the myometrium and the endometrium:

- **Perimetrium:** This is the outer serous and protective layer of the uterus that merges with the peritoneum.
- **Myometrium:** This is the central and thickest part of the uterus, which contains several smooth muscle layers, running in various directions and interlaced with blood vessels and nerves. This structural design aids in contraction during labour and menstruation, and enables the uterus to grow and expand, up to 20 times its normal size, during pregnancy (Peate 2017).
- **Endometrium:** This is the inner layer of the uterus, constructed from a basal and functional layer of mucosa. The basal layer, which is permanent and closest to the myometrium, plays a role in the replication and regeneration of the uterine lining during the menstrual cycle. The functional layer is the section of the mucosa that sheds during menstruation if the ovum released by the ovaries is not fertilised or implanted.

The uterus is extremely vascular and significant amounts of blood can be delivered to it via two uterine arteries branching from the internal iliac arteries. There are two uterine arteries on either side of the uterus supplying the endometrium, splitting further into straight radial arteries that feed the basal layer and spiral radial arteries that supply the functional layer. The myometrium is fed via the arcuate arteries.

Menstrual Cycle

For most women, the menstrual cycle (consisting of menses, follicular/proliferation, ovulation and luteinising/secretion phases) occurs every 28 days (see Figure 5.7) and is associated with changes in the uterus, ovaries, breast and vagina, aligned with hormonal fluctuations (see Figure 5.8). Regulation and control of the menstrual cycle are highly dependent on the anterior pituitary gland and the release of follicular stimulating hormones (FSH) and luteinising hormones (LH). FHS, as the name suggests, simulates several immature ovarian follicles to grow and secrete oestrogen and LH causes at least one follicle to mature, rupture and eject an ovum, stimulating the development of the corpus luteum (Huether and McCance 2017). The role of hormones in the initiation of menses is discussed later in this chapter.

One of the most crucial periods of the menstrual cycle is ovulation. The fertilisation of the oocyte by sperm can only occur within a limited time frame, as most sperms' fertilising abilities diminish after 72 hours post-ejaculation and most ejected oocytes are no longer viable after 48 hours (Patton and Thibodeau 2018). The window of possible fertilisation is therefore very small and restricted to three to six days in every menstrual cycle.

Menstrual Disorders and Abnormal Bleeding

Menstrual disorders and abnormal bleeding can arise from hormonal imbalances, infections, diseases, trauma and certain medications. These can also occur at various stages of a woman's life, such as in puberty, during pregnancy, postnatally, through to menopause and beyond (see Table 5.5).

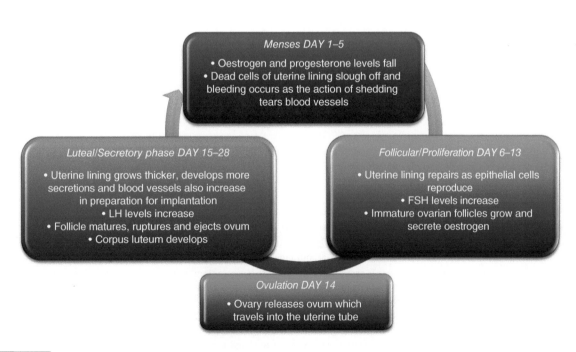

FIGURE 5.7 Phases of the menstrual cycle. Source: Adapted from Huether and McCance (2017) and Patton and Thibodeau (2018). FSH, follicular stimulating hormone; LH, luteinising hormone.

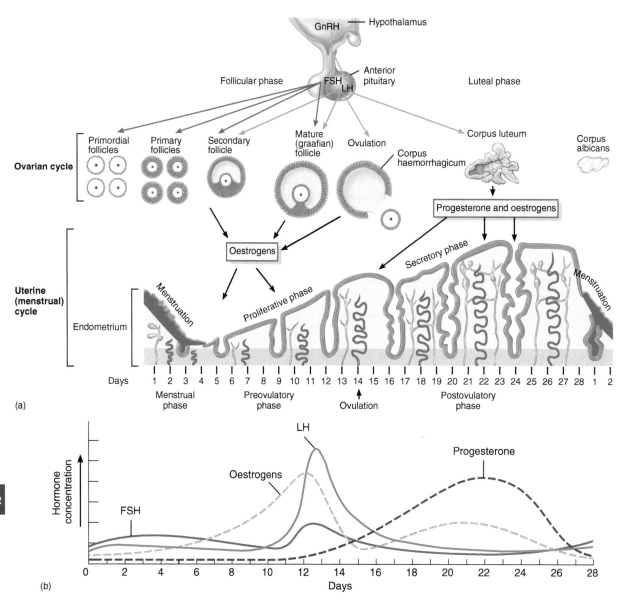

FIGURE 5.8   A typical 28-day menstrual cycle. (a) Hormonal regulation of changes in the ovary and uterus. (b) Changes in concentration of anterior pituitary and ovarian hormones.

TABLE 5.5   Menstrual disorders and abnormal bleeding.

Disorder	Description
Dysmenorrhoea	Pain and other negative symptoms accompanying menstruation
	Primary dysmenorrhoea is associated with excessive prostaglandin release in the endometrium that increases contractions in the myometrium, restricting blood vessels, causing pain and ischaemia. Usually occurs in women between 15 and 25 years old
	Secondary dysmenorrhoea occurs in later life and is linked with altered pelvic pathologies such as fibrosis, polyps, cancer and cysts
	Pain can be debilitating as it radiates to the groin and back and can also cause headaches, diarrhoea and vomiting
	Treatments include contraceptive medication, non-steroidal anti-inflammatory drugs, heat, massage, electrical nerve stimulation or radiofrequency endometrial ablation

TABLE 5.5 *(Continued)*

Disorder	Description
Amenorrhoea	Absence or cessation of menstruation
	Primary amenorrhoea is failure to establish menstruation by the age of 15 years in girls with normal breast development or by 13 years in girls with no secondary sexual characteristics
	Causes can include disorders of the uterus and the ovaries, genetic disorders such as Turner's syndrome, congenital abnormalities of the reproductive system or congenital disorders affecting hormone production and release
	Treatment is dependent on identifying the underlying pathology and usually involves extensive investigations, hormone therapy or surgery
	Secondary amenorrhoea is associated with cessation of menstruation for 5–6 months in women with previous normal menses, or for 6–12 months in women with previous oligomenorrhoea
	It can be caused by excessive weight loss and exercise and malnutrition, pregnancy, menopause and hormone imbalances
	Pregnancy is the main cause and therefore a pregnancy test is imperative before assessing for other causes
	Treatments can include hormone replacement and surgery
Other types of abnormal bleeding	Polymenorrhoea: Cycle shorter than 3 weeks, often associated with endocrine disorder resulting in increased ovulation
	Oligomenorrhoea: Cycles longer than 6–7 weeks, associated with imbalance in hormones and ovulation
	Metrorrhagia: Bleeding between cycles, usually occurring due to pelvic disease
	Hypermenorrhoea: Excessive loss usually associated with organic disease
	Menorrhoea and menorrhagia: Excessive loss that is also prolonged
	Menometrorrhagia: Excessive prolonged flow, with spotting between bleeding episodes

Source: Adapted from Huether and McCance (2017), Patton and Thibodeau (2018), NICE (2022b).

Medicines Management: Tranexamic Acid

Tranexamic acid is used as an antifibrinolytic and due to its clotting properties is often prescribed to treat menorrhoea.

Dose: Orally, 1 g three times a day for up to four days, to be initiated when menstruation has started. Maximum dose 4 g/day.
Contra-indications: Fibrinolytic conditions, history of convulsions and thromboembolic disease
Side effects: Common – diarrhoea, nausea, vomiting. Uncommon – allergic dermatitis. Rare – colour vision change, embolism and thrombosis.

Source: Adapted from BNF (2022c).

Examination Scenario: Discharge Examination

To help identify underlying pathologies or disorders and abnormal postnatal recovery, it may be necessary to discuss or visually examine vaginal discharge with women who present with symptoms. This includes the colour, consistency, amount, odour, onset, duration and other associated symptoms.

- How do you think subjectivity can be reduced when examining vaginal discharge?
- How do midwives ascertain amount of blood loss accurately, especially during delivery and postnatal recovery?

Medicines Management: Uterotonics

Globally, obstetric haemorrhage remains one of the major causes of maternal death. Primary postpartum haemorrhage (PPH), commonly defined as a blood loss of 500 ml or more within 24 hours after birth, affects about 6% of all women giving birth. To minimise the risk of bleeding, pharmacological intervention in the form of prophylactic uterotonics is often used in maternity and obstetric practice, to stimulate and encourage uterine contraction. Several uterotonics have been developed, including prostaglandin analogues (misoprostol, sulprostone, carboprost) and ergot alkaloids (ergometrine/methylergometrine). However, the most popular and widely used are the oxytocin receptor agonists (oxytocin or carbetocin), with 10 IU of oxytocin by intramuscular injection being recommended following the birth of the baby for the prevention of PPH for all births.

Source: Adapted from Mavrides et al. (2022), Vogel et al. (2019) and BNF (2022b).

Endometrial Polyps

These are individual masses of endometrial tissues that contain glands, blood vessels and stroma and usually originate in the fundus. They can also form in clusters in the lower uterine segment and can be classified as hyperplastic, atrophic or functional. They can develop at any stage of a woman's reproductive life cycle, but more often occur between the ages of 40 and 50 years, as the risk of incidence increases with hypertension, obesity and when oestrogen levels are at their highest (Huether and McCance 2017). They can cause menorrhoea and metrorrhagia, are diagnosed via hysteroscopy or ultrasound and treatment usually involves surgical removal.

Uterine Fibroids (Leiomyomas)

These are benign tumours that develop from the myometrium and affect between 70% and 80% of women, usually between the ages of 30 and 50 years. The cause is not yet fully understood, but it is believed that they are related to hormonal fluctuations aligned with oestrogen and progesterone. They are classified into three main types depending on their location within the layers of the uterine wall (see Figure 5.9).

While most small fibroids are uncomplicated, others can lead to significant symptoms including menorrhagia, dysmenorrhoea, anaemia, polyuria, constipation and back pain, and during pregnancy can increase the risk of miscarriage and premature labour (British Fibroid Trust 2022). They are confirmed via bimanual examination, pelvic sonography or magnetic resonance imaging (MRI) and treatment will depend on age, size, number and position of

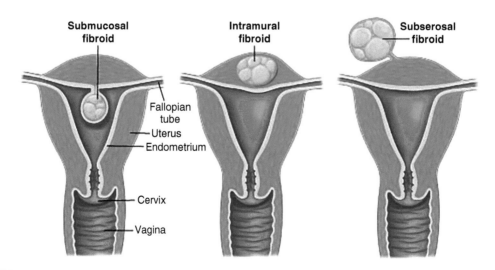

FIGURE 5.9   Types of uterine fibroids.

fibroids and whether the woman is wanting to have further pregnancies. In the latter case, the fibroids will be conservatively observed, but if they are causing significant symptoms, hormones may be prescribed to manage growth or a myomectomy may be undertaken. If the woman no longer wants to have children, a hysterectomy can be performed.

Endometriosis

This is a disorder associated with the presence of functioning endometrial tissue outside of the uterus that responds to hormonal changes, proliferates and sheds, bleeding into the surrounding area and causing inflammation and for some women significant pain. The most common sites are the ovaries, uterine ligaments and pelvic peritoneum; however, endometrial tissue has also been found in the bowel, bladder, vulva, extremities and lungs (Huether and McCance 2017). Globally endometriosis affects approximately 190 million women of reproductive age and is associated with severe dysmenorrhoea and chronic pelvic pain, which has negative impacts on sexual intercourse, bowel movements and/or urination and causes nausea, fatigue, bloating and infertility (WHO 2022b). What is extremely concerning is that there is currently no cure and treatments such as contraceptive steroids, NSAIDs, analgesics, hormone therapy and surgery largely attempt merely to control symptoms.

Woman-Centred Care

In many countries endometriosis is not taken seriously, as pelvic pain in women is frequently normalised in modern societies. Consequently, women's voices are often silenced, or their symptoms minimised and not prioritised. This can have a devastating impact on their sexual and reproductive health, quality of life and overall well-being as well as their psychological health and feelings of worth.

It is paramount that women's reports of pain are not dismissed but thoroughly investigated to find the origin. Due to the variety of symptoms, it may also be necessary to adopt a multidisciplinary and multimodal, tailored approach to manage their symptoms effectively. This can include referrals to gynaecologist, pain specialist, pelvis physiotherapist, psychologist and alternative therapies as adjuncts to pharmacological management.

Source: Adapted from WHO (2022b).

Cervix

The cervix, the narrowest part of the uterus, is a thickened ring of muscle and fibrous tissue that changes during pregnancy, and in particular in labour. The external os of the cervix can be found protruding into the fornix of the vagina and the internal os opens into the uterus. The endocervical canal between these openings is approximately 2.5 cm long and is the only pathway between the uterus and the vagina. It is held in place by the lateral cervical ligaments, which attach the cervix and the vagina to the lateral pelvic walls.

Cervical Cancer

This type of cancer accounts for 2% of all female cancers and 99% are associated with persistent infection from high-risk subtypes of HPV, particularly strands 16 and 18, with peak incidences in the UK among women between the age of 30 and 34 years (NICE 2022a). Other risk factors include immunosuppression, long-term use of the contraceptive pill and women who smoke, have multiple partners or have children before the age of 17 years (Metcalf and McCarthy 2011). Due to the worldwide screening programme, many cervical cancers are preceded by a pre-invasive stage referred to as cervical intraepithelial neoplasia (CIN), which can be mild, moderate or severe. Women with an abnormal routine smear may then require further investigations, normally a colposcopy and removal of the diseased tissue by a large loop excision of transformation zone (LLETZ).

Expert Midwife

It is not unusual for women who are pregnant and have previously had an LLETZ procedure to be concerned about the ability of the cervix to remain closed during pregnancy and then adapt during labour and delivery.

- The risk of miscarriage is associated with multiple treatments or when large areas of the cervix have been removed.
- Scans are often used to assess cervical length and health.
- If risk of miscarriage is high, a cerclage can be placed in situ to reduce the risk of premature birth.

Sally, Registered Midwife

As with all gynaecological cancers, cervical cancer is staged and the more severe the spread, the shorter the life expectancy (see Figure 5.10). Treatments also vary depending on the severity of the disease, but can include radiotherapy, radical hysterectomy, trachelectomy, pelvic lymphadenectomy, chemotherapy, bilateral salpingo-oophorectomy and lymphadenectomy.

Ovaries

Within females, gametes are produced in the ovaries, which are also responsible for the production of several sex hormones (see Table 5.6). There are usually two flat, almond-shaped ovaries, 2.5–3.5 cm long, 2 cm wide and

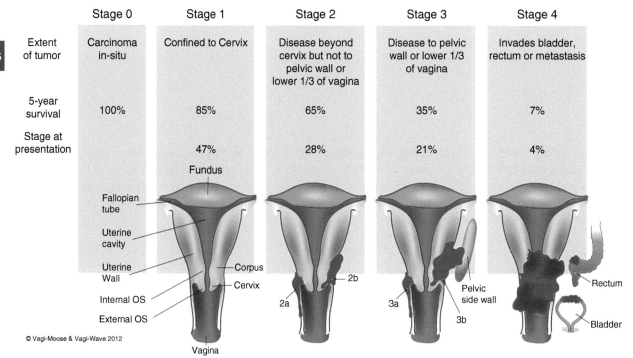

FIGURE 5.10   Staging of cervical cancer and life expectancy.

TABLE 5.6   Female reproductive hormones.

Oestrogen	Progesterone	Relaxin	Testosterone	Anti-Müllerian
Main function is to mature and maintain the reproductive system	Secreted by the corpus luteum	Secreted in the ovary by the corpus luteum	Produced in small amounts	Helps in the early development of follicles, which hold and support eggs before fertilisation
Responsible for maturation and release of the ovum	Triggers thickening of the uterine lining	Relaxes the wall of the uterus and prepares it for pregnancy	Essential for the development of new blood cells, enhancing libido and influencing follicle stimulating hormones	Measuring levels can indicate remaining egg supply
Aids in the thickening of the uterus lining	Prohibits uterine muscle contractions	Aids in implantation and placental growth	Low levels associated with fatigue, muscle weakness and mood changes	Levels are highest during puberty and decline after menopause
High levels linked to acne, constipation, reduced sex drive, depression, cancer and cardiovascular disease	Low levels can result in abnormal menstrual cycles or difficulties with conception	Prevents uterine contractions to prevent early delivery		
Reduced levels associated with osteoporosis and mood swings	High levels linked to anxiety and agitation, breast swelling and tenderness, depression, fatigue and weight gain	During labour, helps to relax the ligaments in the pelvis		

Source: Davidge-Pitts and Solorzano (2022).

1 cm thick, situated in a shallow fossa, flanking both the right and left sides of the uterus, inferior to the uterine tubes (Waugh and Grant 2018).

The ovaries are suspended in place within the peritoneal cavity by the suspensory ligaments that attach the ovary to the pelvic floor, the ovarian ligament that anchors the ovary to the uterus and the mesovarium, which acts as the main suspension ligament. Blood is supplied to the ovaries via the ovarian and uterine artery and the ovaries are supplied with parasympathetic and sympathetic nerves from the sacral and lumber outflow, respectively. Although the primordial ova are present within the ovaries at birth, these are held in stasis and are only activated at puberty, are then released during menstruation, and slowly reduce in number as the woman ages.

Polycystic Ovary Syndrome

As the name suggests, polycystic ovary syndrome (PCOS) is a disorder affecting the ovaries and is linked to one or more cysts and/or elevated levels of androgens and few or anovulatory menstrual cycles. This is the most common female endocrine disorder and is a leading cause of infertility (Patton and Thibodeau 2018). It is often diagnosed with other endocrine conditions such as congenital adrenal hyperplasia, Cushing's syndrome and thyroid disease. Symptoms are usually linked with obesity, as 41% of women with PCOS are obese, and range from acne to hirsutism, amenorrhoea, hypertension and dyslipidaemia. As such treatments and management strategies include promoting weight loss and healthy eating and oral contraceptives to help regulate menstrual cycles.

Ovarian Cysts

These should not be confused with cysts associated with PCOS and are common in women of reproductive age. These can be separated into two main categories, functional cysts (follicular and corpus luteum), which are the more common, and pathological ovarian cysts that arise due to abnormal cell growth, such as dermoid and endometrioid cysts (see Figure 5.11).

Cysts usually occur unilaterally and range from 5–6 cm to 8–10 cm. Most functional cysts resolve on their own and women may not experience symptoms, or even realise that they had a cyst. However, larger cysts that cause significant symptoms of pain within the pelvis, bloating and irregular menses or may be cancerous may need to be removed via surgery.

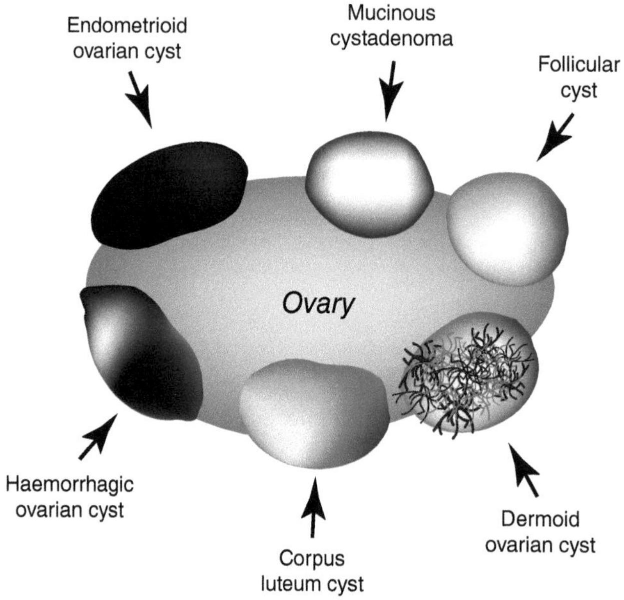

FIGURE 5.11 Types of ovarian cysts.

Red Flag: Ovarian Torsion

A painful and dangerous complication associated with the ovaries is ovarian torsion (or adnexal torsion). This can occur in women with ovarian cysts or tumours and is when the ovary and/or fallopian tube twists on its vascular and ligamentous supports. This blocks adequate blood flow to the ovary and causes acute and severe unilateral pain, often described as throbbing or pulsating.

Learning Event: Ovarian Cancer Screening

Within the United Kingdom ovarian cancer is the leading cause of death by a gynaecological cancer and the incidence rate has risen significantly in the last few decades. Due to extensive study within this area, a genetic link has been proven and carriers of the *BRCA1* and *BRCA2* (tumour suppressor) genes are at an increased risk of developing breast and ovarian cancer. Screening tests such as transvaginal ultrasound and serial Ca125 have gone some way to helping with the detection of this disease, but more still needs to be done to raise the awareness of the signs and symptoms to assist with early detection.

Source: Adapted from NICE (2011).

Uterine (Fallopian) Tubes

The ovum released from the ovaries is directed towards the uterine tubes (otherwise referred to as the fallopian tubes or salpinges) by the action of the fimbriae, which are tentacle-like ciliated protections situated at the funnel end (infundibulum) of the fallopian tube, the longest of which is the ovarian fimbria (Patton and Thibodeau 2018). Due to peristaltic and kinetic movement of the ciliated inner wall lining, the ovum moves towards the uterus for implantation, through the uterine tube, which is approximately 10 cm long (the largest part being the ampulla, and the narrowest and final section the isthmus) (Peate 2017). The uterine tubes are suspended and held in place by the mesosalpinx.

Red Flag: Ectopic Pregnancy

An ectopic pregnancy occurs when the fertilised ovum implants outside of the uterus. The RCOG (2022b) states that in the United Kingdom, 1 in 90 pregnancies results in an ectopic pregnancy and women are at higher risk if they have previously had an ectopic pregnancy. Most ectopic pregnancies develop in the fallopian tubes, but in 3–5% they can occur in the cervix, ovary and abdominal cavity. An ectopic pregnancy is life threatening and if suspected should be managed quickly via surgical, pharmacological or conservative interventions. As the fetus grows trauma can occur to the surrounding structures, causing pain and ruptured vessels, which can result in significant blood loss. As ectopic pregnancies can occur in a variety of positions, atypical presentation is common, but symptoms can include abdominal pain, amenorrhoea, vaginal bleeding, breast tenderness, gastrointestinal symptoms, dizziness, fainting or syncope and pallor, rectal pressure or pain on defecation, abdominal distension and enlarged uterus, tachycardia or hypotension, shock or collapse and orthostatic hypotension.

Source: Adapted from NICE (2021); RCOG (2016, 2022b).

Pelvic Organs Prolapse

If the muscles of the pelvic floor lose tone and strength due to the ageing process, surgery or childbirth, progressive descent of the pelvic organs may lead to urinary and faecal incontinence and uterine prolapse (see Figure 5.12). A cystocele occurs when the bladder and the anterior wall protrude into the vagina, a rectocele is when the rectum and the posterior wall bulge into the vagina, a urethrocele is associated with sagging of the urethra and an enterocele is when the rectouterine pouch has herniated into the rectovaginal septum. Uterine prolapse is staged depending on the severity of the descent. Around one in four women will suffer from one of these disorders during their lifetime and management strategies include pessaries, pelvic floor exercises, oestrogen therapy in postmenopausal women and surgery if all other strategies have failed.

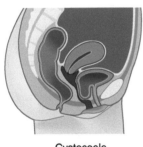
Cystocoele

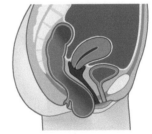
Rectocoele

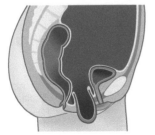
Vaginal vault prolapse with enterocoele

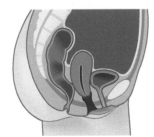
Uterine prolapse

FIGURE 5.12 Types of pelvic organ prolapse.

Breasts

These are often referred to as mammary glands and are considered external accessory sexual organs and part of the reproductive system, as they play a pivotal role in the nurturing and feeding of newborns (Peate 2017) (see Figure 5.13). They are not located within proximity to the other reproductive organs already mentioned in this chapter; instead, they are located on the upper chest, between the third and seventh ribs, and are supported in place by the pectoral muscles. The breasts are made of adipose tissue, fibrous connective tissue and glandular tissue that provides support and structure to the breast and is further divided into 15–25 lobes. These lobes comprise alveolar gland 'lobules', which produce milk and connect to the nipple via small lactiferous ducts. During the last two-thirds of pregnancy, the breasts enlarge due to the proliferation of additional glandular tissue and milk is also stored in the lactiferous sinuses.

Blood supply to the breasts is provided via the thoracic branches of the axillary arteries and the internal mammary and intercostal arteries (Waugh and Grant 2018). Lymphatic draining is carried out via the superficial axillary lymph vessel and nodes and the breast is supplied with many nerves branching from the fourth, fifth and sixth thoracic nerves. There are also several sensory nerve endings in the breast, especially around the nipple, which when stimulated by sucking pass impulses to the hypothalamus to increase the secretion of oxytocin, a hormone needed for milk production.

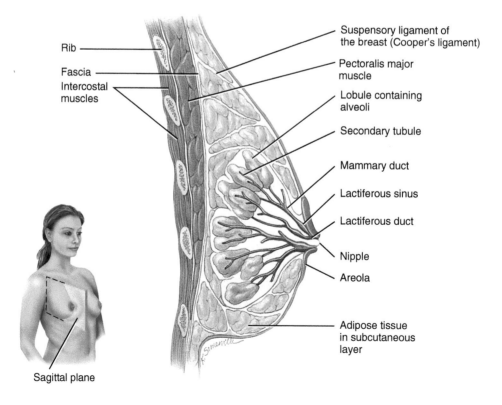

Rib

Fascia
Intercostal
muscles

Sagittal plane

Suspensory ligament of
the breast (Cooper's ligament)

Pectoralis major
muscle

Lobule containing
alveoli

Secondary tubule

Mammary duct

Lactiferous sinus

Lactiferous duct

Nipple

Areola

Adipose tissue
in subcutaneous
layer

Sagittal section

FIGURE 5.13   Sagittal view of the breast.

Case Study 5.2   Mastitis

Blessing is a 32-year-old mother of a newborn boy. With the support of her family and midwife, she is successfully breastfeeding her son, who is thriving. At the last visit before handing over care to the health visiting team, the midwife notices that Blessing is having some trouble holding the baby and seems to wince when her breasts are touched. Blessing admits when asked that her breasts have been very tender for the last two days and she found it difficult to feed her son this morning and needed to use some of her saved breast milk and bottles.

The midwife suspected mastitis and therefore needed to ask further questions to ascertain the severity of the condition and whether an immediate referral was needed.

- What questions will the midwife need to ask and what other assessment will she need to undertake?

Blessing's observations were within normal parameters, but she described the pain as throbbing and scored it 6 out of 10 using a numerical rating scale. There were no signs of an abscess, but both breasts were swollen and there were signs of erythema. The midwife did not think admission was required but did suspect that both breasts were inflamed and affected by mastitis.

- What can the midwife do to reassure Blessing and encourage her to continue breastfeeding?
- What advice and information can the midwife provide to manage Blessing's symptoms?

Conditions Associated with the Reproductive System

The following is a list of conditions that are associated with the reproductive system. Take some time and write notes about each of the conditions. Think about the altered pathophysiology involved. Remember to include aspects of patient care. If you are making notes about people you have offered care and support to, you must ensure that you adhere to the rules of confidentiality.

The condition	Your notes
Vulvodynia	
Turner's syndrome	
Pelvic inflammatory disease	
Ovarian cancer	
Uterine tubal abscess	

Take-Home Points

- When caring for any woman it is important to have a sound understanding of the anatomy and physiology of the reproductive system and how this may adapt and change during pregnancy and birth.
- This enables midwives to carry out procedures safely, but also to recognise disease and reproductive disorders that may have negative impacts on the perinatal journey.
- It is also essential to include women and their partners in their care and not to make a decision for women, but with women.
- Any decisions made must be tailored to the individual needs of the woman and need to take into consideration their holistic picture.

Conclusion

The reproductive organs play an essential role in the repopulation of the human race and as midwives' primary role is to 'be with women', before, during and after birth, midwifery students must understand alterations in normal anatomy and physiology to practise safely and effectively. The female body goes through a series of adaptations to develop and deliver life, but these processes do not always change in the way they should; thus, this chapter has provided additional information on some of the pathophysiological complications that can occur.

References

American College of Obstetricians and Gynecologists (ACOG) (2022). Vaginitis. https://www.acog.org/womens-health/faqs/vaginitis (accessed November 2023).

Boore, J., Cook, N., and Shepherd, A. (2021). *Essentials of Anatomy and Physiology for Nursing Practice*, 2e. London: Sage.

British Fibroid Trust (2022). Symptoms. https://www.britishfibroidtrust.org.uk/Fib_info/wif.php (accessed November 2023).

British National Formulary (BNF) (2022a). Ciprofloxacin. https://bnf.nice.org.uk/drugs/ciprofloxacin (accessed November 2023).

British National Formulary (BNF) (2022b). Oxytocin. https://bnf.nice.org.uk/drugs/oxytocin (accessed November 2023).

British National Formulary (BNF) (2022c). Tranexamic acid. https://bnf.nice.org.uk/drugs/tranexamic-acid (accessed November 2023).

Davidge-Pitts, C. and Solorzano, C.B. (2022). Reproductive hormones. Washington, DC: Endocrine Society. https://www.endocrine.org/patient-engagement/endocrine-library/hormones-and-endocrine-function/reproductive-hormones (accessed November 2023).

Gavrilov, S.G. (2017). Vulvar varicosities: diagnosis, treatment, and prevention. *International Journal of Women's Health* 28 (9): 463–475.

Huether, S.E. and McCance, K.L. (2017). *Understanding Pathophysiology*, 7e. London: Elsevier.

Isaac, B.H. and Young, L. (2011). Cancer of the vulva. In: *Women's Cancers* (ed. A. Keen and E. Lennan), 183–198. Chichester: Wiley.

Köbach, A., Ruf-Leuschner, M., and Elbert, T. (2018). Psychopathological sequelae of female genital mutilation and their neuroendocrinological associations. *BMC Psychiatry* 18: 187.

Lee, M.Y., Dalpiaz, A., Schwamb, R. et al. (2015). Clinical pathology of Bartholin's glands: a review of the literature. *Current Urology* 8 (1): 22–25.

Lewis, F.M. (2022). Vascular abnormalities and the vulva. In: *Ridley's The Vulva*, 4e (ed. F.M. Lewis), 240–242. Chichester: Wiley.

Macmillan (2022). Vulval cancer. www.macmillan.org.uk/cancer-information-and-support/vulval-cancer (accessed November 2023).

Mavrides, E., Allard, S., Chandraharan, E. et al. (2022). Prevention and management of postpartum haemorrhage. *BJOG* 24: e106–e149.

Metcalf, K. and McCarthy, K. (2011). Cancer of the cervix. In: *Women's Cancers* (ed. A. Keen and E. Lennan), 142–156. Chichester: Wiley.

National Health Service (NHS) (2022a). Bartholin's cyst. https://www.nhs.uk/conditions/bartholins-cyst/treatment (accessed November 2023).

National Health Service (NHS) (2022b). Vaginitis. https://www.nhs.uk/conditions/vaginitis (accessed November 2023).

National Health Service (NHS) (2022c). Vaginismus. https://www.nhs.uk/conditions/vaginismus (accessed November 2023).

National Institute for Health and Care Excellence (NICE) (2011). *Ovarian Cancer: Recognition and Initial Management*. London: NICE.

National Institute for Health and Care Excellence (NICE) (2021). Ectopic pregnancy and miscarriage: diagnosis and initial management. www.nice.org.uk/guidance/ng126/resources/ectopic-pregnancy-and-miscarriage-diagnosis-and-initial-management-pdf-66141662244037 (accessed November 2023).

National Institute for Health and Care Excellence (NICE) (2022a). Cervical cancer. https://cks.nice.org.uk/topics/cervical-cancer-hpv (accessed November 2023).

National Institute for Health and Care Excellence (NICE) (2022b). Amenorrhoea. https://cks.nice.org.uk/topics/amenorrhoea (accessed November 2023).

Nguyen, J.D. and Duong, H. (2022). Anatomy, abdomen and pelvis: female external genitalia. In: *StatPearls*. Treasure Island, FL: StatPearls Publishing https://www.ncbi.nlm.nih.gov/books/NBK547703.

Olawaiye, A.B., Cuello, M.A., and Rogers, L.J. (2021). Cancer of the vulva: 2021 update. *International Journal of Gynecology & Obstetrics* 155 (Suppl. 1): 7–18.

Patton, K. and Thibodeau, G. (2018). *The Human Body in Health and Disease*, 7e. London: Elsevier.

Peate, I. (2017). The reproductive system. In: *Fundamentals of Anatomy and Physiology for Nursing and Healthcare Students*, 2e (ed. I. Peate and M. Nair), 371–402. Chichester, UK: Wiley.

Royal College of Obstetricians and Gynaecologists (RCOG) (2015). *The Management of Third- and Fourth-Degree Perineal Tears*. Green-top Guideline No. 29. London: RCOG.

Royal College of Obstetricians and Gynaecologists (RCOG) (2016). *Diagnosis and Management of Ectopic Pregnancy*. Green-top Guideline No. 21. London: RCOG.

Royal College of Obstetricians and Gynaecologists (RCOG) (2022a). Perineal tears and episiotomies in childbirth. https://www.rcog.org.uk/for-the-public/perineal-tears-and-episiotomies-in-childbirth (accessed November 2023).

Royal College of Obstetricians and Gynaecologists (RCOG) (2022b). Ectopic pregnancy. www.rcog.org.uk/for-the-public/browse-all-patient-information-leaflets/ectopic-pregnancy-patient-information-leaflet (accessed November 2023).

Tinkler, S. (2011). Cancer of the vagina. In: *Women's Cancers* (ed. A. Keen and E. Lennan), 172–182. Chichester: Wiley.

Vogel, J.P., Williams, M., Gallos, I. et al. (2019). WHO recommendations on uterotonics for postpartum haemorrhage prevention: what works, and which one? *BMJ Global Health* 4 (2): e001466.

Waugh, A. and Grant, A. (2018). *Ross and Wilson Anatomy and Physiology in Health and Illness*, 13e. London: Elsevier.

World Health Organization (WHO) (2022b). Endometriosis. https://www.who.int/news-room/fact-sheets/detail/endometriosis (accessed November 2023).

World Health Organization (WHO) (2022a). Female genital mutilation. https://www.who.int/news-room/fact-sheets/detail/female-genital-mutilation (accessed November 2023).

Further Resources

FGM National Clinical Group. www.fgmnationalgroup.org (accessed November 2023).

The Ectopic Pregnancy Trust. www.ectopic.org.uk (accessed November 2023).

NCT. Breastfeeding support from NCT. www.nct.org.uk/baby-toddler/feeding/early-days/breastfeeding-support-nct (accessed November 2023).

British Fibrosis Trust. Fibroids: Causes - symptoms - types. www.britishfibroidtrust.org.uk/Fib_info/wif.php (accessed November 2023).

Endometriosis UK. www.endometriosis-uk.org (accessed November 2023).

Glossary

Adipose tissue	Connective tissue consisting mainly of fat cells
Amenorrhea	Absence of menstruation
Anterior	Near to the front
Anteverted	Tilted forward
Atrophic	Decrease in size of a body part or tissue
Benign	Not harmful in effect
Bilateral salpingo-oophorectomy	Surgery to remove both ovaries and both uterine tubes
Brachytherapy	A type of internal radiotherapy
Chemotherapy	Treatment of cancer by cytotoxic drugs
Cleft	A hollow between ridges or protuberances
Commissure	A point or line of union between two anatomical parts
Cushing's syndrome	A metabolic disorder caused by overproduction of corticosteroid hormones, often involving obesity and high blood pressure
Dermoid	Cyst filled with tissues normally found in the outer layers of the skin, including sweat and oil glands

Dyslipidaemia	Imbalance of lipids
Effacement	Thinning of the tissue of the cervix
Erythema	Reddening of the skin
Fistula	An abnormal passage that leads from one hollow organ or part to another
Frenulum	A connecting fold of membrane serving to support a part of the body
Fundus	The large upper end of the uterus
Gamete	Sex cell
Glans clitoris	The conical, highly innervated body forming the external extremity of the clitoris
Hirsutism	A condition in which women have a lot of hair growth in places usually associated with men
Hypercoagulability	Abnormally increased coagulability of the blood
Hyperplasia	Enlargement of an organ or tissue caused by an increase in the reproduction rate of its cells
Hypertension	High blood pressure
Inferior	Situated lower down
Infibulation	The complete excision of the clitoris, labia minora and most of the labia majora, followed by stitching to close most of the vagina
Introitus	The orifice of a body cavity
Isthmus	A narrow anatomical part or passage connecting two larger structures or cavities
Lateral	Of or relating to the side
Lumen	The cavity of a tubular organ or part
Malignant	Very virulent or infectious
Malodour	A very unpleasant smell
Metastasis	Secondary malignant growth found at a distance from a primary site
Osteoporosis	A condition that is characterised by a decrease in bone mass with decreased density and enlargement of bone spaces
Ovum	A female gamete
Pelvic lymphadenectomy	Surgery to remove the pelvic lymph nodes
Pessaries	An elastic or rigid device that is inserted into the vagina to support the uterus
Pheromones	A chemical substance produced to serve as a stimulus to other individuals of the same pecies
Posterior	Situated behind
Radical hysterectomy	Surgery that involves the removal of the uterus, cervix, ovaries, uterine tubes and other supporting tissues
Radiotherapy	Treatment that uses high doses of radiation to kill cancer cells and shrink tumours
Second intention (wound)	A wound remaining open and healing from the base up
Serial Ca125	A tumour marker used to indicate ovarian cancer
Squamous cell carcinoma	Second most common form of skin cancer
Superior	Situated higher up
Trachelectomy	Surgery to remove the cervix
Uterotonics	Stimulating muscular tone in the uterus
Venous thromboembolism	Blood clots in the veins
Vulvodynia	Chronic discomfort of the vulva

CHAPTER 6

Homeostasis

Deborah Gurney and Janet G. Migliozzi

School of Life & Medical Sciences, University of Hertfordshire, Hatfield, UK

AIM

This chapter introduces the concept of homeostasis and explores the body's regulatory mechanisms that ensure health is maintained. The second part of the chapter then explores the physiological changes that occur during pregnancy and discusses how the body's homeostatic mechanisms change and adapt to enable fetal development and growth.

LEARNING OUTCOMES

On completion of this chapter the reader will be able to:

- Define the concept of homeostasis
- Describe the body's regulatory mechanisms
- Describe the functions of the placenta and its role in maintaining homeostasis
- Describe the physiological adaptations the body undergoes during pregnancy
- Describe the physiological processes involved in the intrapartum period

Test Your Prior Knowledge
1. What does 'homeostasis' mean?
2. What are feedback mechanisms?
3. What does extracellular fluid consist of?
4. What are the main functions of the placenta?
5. Which hormone initiates and maintains uterine contractions?

The idea that a constant internal environment is critical to the healthy functioning of the human body and the maintenance of life is not a new concept and can be traced back to the work of the French physiologist Claude Bernard in the mid-nineteenth century. In 1857 Bernard wrote that 'the consistency of the internal environment is the condition for free life' (Roberts 1986) in which the idea of a constant internal environment of the organism led to the modern-day concept

Fundamentals of Maternal Pathophysiology, First Edition. Edited by Claire Leader and Ian Peate.
© 2024 John Wiley & Sons Ltd. Published 2024 by John Wiley & Sons Ltd.
Companion website: www.wiley.com/go/leader/maternalpatho

of homeostasis. The term 'homeostasis' is derived from two Greek words – *homeo* meaning staying the same and *stasis* meaning standing still. It is the regulation of homeostasis that maintains life.

An understanding of the concepts of the body's internal environment is fundamental to explaining homeostasis, as many characteristics of the internal environment are regulated but not controlled; that is, they can adapt to changing requirements. The internal environment refers to interstitial fluid and blood plasma, both of which make up extra-cellular fluid. The concentration of substances in the intercellular fluid directly affects the concentration of substances in cells and failure to regulate the internal environment can lead to the accumulation of toxins and destruction of cells and tissues, which can result in ill health and death. However, the body has many mechanisms to enable the cells of the body to remain in balance – this is critical to cell function as most operate within relatively narrow parameters. Therefore, the maintenance of a constant, stable internal environment of the body's cells, tissues and organ systems is crucial to maintaining health, as any disruption or imbalance in the internal environment may lead to ill health.

If an imbalance occurs, the body's regulatory/control systems become active to restore optimum conditions and these are dependent on the following three basic components:

- Receptor
- Control centre
- Effector

The initial disturbance in a physiological parameter is detected by receptors that are located throughout the body. These include chemoreceptors that monitor the concentration of chemicals, baroreceptors that monitor pressure, osmoreceptors that monitor the amount of water within the body, and thermoreceptors that monitor body temperature. Each receptor constantly monitors the parameter it is regulating and detects one specific variable. If a receptor detects any change in the parameters of the variable, it conveys this to the control centre for further action. The control centre is a part of the central nervous system (CNS); that is, it is predominantly within the brain but may also involve the spinal cord, where information is received and integrated with other messages arriving from other parts of the CNS, before an appropriate response is coordinated. Within the control centre are set points of acceptable physiological limits that ensure the body remains healthy. If a change is required, the control centre then sends an output or stimulus to effectors – muscles, organs and glands – in order to produce an appropriate response or change. Table 6.1 outlines common changes that receptors can instigate.

If the incoming signal indicates that an adjustment is needed, the control centre responds and its output to the effector is changed. Nearly all of these are controlled by two feedback mechanisms that continually report back to the control area.

Feedback Mechanisms

Negative Feedback Mechanisms

Most of the body's homeostatic control mechanisms operate on the principle of negative feedback – when a disturbance in homeostasis occurs the body's inbuilt, self-regulatory mechanisms come into play to reverse the disturbance. An example of this might be the regulation of blood glucose, where an increase or decrease in blood

TABLE 6.1 Changes that receptors can initiate.

Blood pressure
Blood glucose levels
Oxygen and carbon dioxide levels within tissues and blood
Body fluid pH levels
Concentration levels of water and electrolytes

glucose levels outside of the homeostatic range sets in motion processes that will either reduce or increase glucose levels so that blood glucose levels remain constant over time.

Positive Feedback Mechanisms

Positive feedback mechanisms play a much smaller role in the body's homeostatic control and there are only a few of these 'amplifier' systems in the body (Waugh and Grant 2018). In positive feedback mechanisms, the disturbance is allowed to increase in its direction and resultant loss of homeostasis. While this homeostatic disturbance can be detrimental and lead to ill health, positive feedback is desirable when rapid change is required. An example of this is lactation. A suckling action of the baby at its mother's breast leads to the production of prolactin, which leads to milk production. The more the baby suckles, the more prolactin and ultimately breast milk is produced. When the demand for breastfeeding stops, prolactin levels decrease and breast milk production stops.

The body's nervous and endocrine systems are the two main systems that are involved in the maintenance of homeostasis. While each of the body's individual systems works independently and is to a certain degree self-regulating, they are also reliant on one another to maintain homeostasis, as a disturbance in one body system can affect the functioning of another. Therefore, there is a need for systems to interrelate and work together to maintain a constant and balanced, stable internal environment that maintains health. Table 6.2 outlines the functions that individual body systems perform that maintain homeostasis.

TABLE 6.2 Body systems that play a major role in maintaining homeostasis.

System	Role in homeostasis
Nervous system	Nerve impulses from the central and peripheral nervous systems play a major role in the monitoring, control and regulation of the body to maintain homeostasis
Endocrine system	Endocrine organs regulate metabolism through the secretion of chemical messengers in the form of hormones and play a major role in maintaining homeostasis
Cardiac system	The heart pumps blood that contains the requisites for cell function around the body
Renal system	The renal system plays a key role in the elimination of toxic waste and fluid, electrolyte and acid–base balance
Respiratory system	The respiratory system enables oxygen to reach cells, removes carbon dioxide and plays an important role in the regulation of blood gases to ensure cellular homeostasis
Musculoskeletal system	The skeletal system is a reservoir for essential minerals. Bone marrow helps to form blood cells and maintain calcium levels in the blood
Digestive system	The digestive system enables nutrients required for the body's function to reach the cells through the process of digestion
Skin	The skin plays an important role in helping to maintain homeostasis through assisting with temperature regulation, providing protection and sensory perception, and the synthesis and absorption of chemicals
Senses	The senses play a part in helping to maintain homeostasis by measuring and detecting changes in the external environment of the body and relaying these to the central nervous system, where information is interpreted and adaptations made to ensure homeostasis is maintained

Source: Adapted from Peate 2021.

Homeostasis in Pregnancy

In this section, homeostasis during pregnancy will be outlined and adaptations to the cardiovascular and pulmonary systems will be discussed. Haematological and biochemical changes will also be explored as well as the impact of neuro-hormonal adaptations to pregnancy, with a discussion around the significance of the placenta in these physiological adaptations.

Homeostasis relates to the body's mechanisms for maintenance of the appropriate levels of salt, fats, water, glucose, proteins and oxygen. Disruption to homeostasis usually occurs in response to illness. Pregnancy, of course, is not an illness, but there are profound alterations to the maternal systems during pregnancy that change the normal parameters of vital signs, haematological and biochemical investigations. Midwives need to understand these alterations to enable them to recognise when there is a pathological cause and to make appropriate referrals and clinical decisions.

Pregnancy is defined as the period from conception through to birth (Ishida et al. 2011) and is usually considered a normal physiological event. It is divided into three parts, first, second and third trimesters. During pregnancy, adaptations occur in all organs and body systems to some degree, and following birth there should be few, if any, permanent effects. Blows (2018) highlighted that this almost complete reversal enables us to determine that pregnancy is not pathological but physiological, and these adaptations are necessary to create the pregnancy-specific processes in the mother and facilitate the development and growth of the fetus (Ishida et al. 2011). Although each system will be considered individually, all these physiological changes are complex, synchronised and have impacts on one another (McNabb 2017).

The Placenta

The placenta is a temporary organ of pregnancy and is critical to fetal survival as it regulates maternal and fetal metabolism. Disruption to placental homeostasis can lead to the development of conditions such as pre-eclampsia that may be detrimental to fetal growth and ultimately fetal well-being. The placenta has several functions but is entirely dependent on maternal blood for oxygen and nutrients and removal of waste products via the maternal circulation. It is derived from embryonic trophoblast cells. The trophoblastic cells divide into two layers, the inner cytotrophoblastic layer and the outer syncytiotrophoblast. Optimal diffusion gradients are established, but the structure of the placenta means that maternal and fetal blood never mix. The mechanisms by which substances are transferred are not clear for all substances, but include:

- Simple diffusion of lipid-soluble substances.
- Water pores transferring water-soluble substances.
- Facilitated diffusion of substances.
- Active transport mechanisms.

Transport across the placenta increases as the pregnancy progresses and the placenta increases in size. The rate of transfer is influenced by increased fetal demands, but also by maternal nutritional status, exercise and the presence of disease. For example, hypertension reduces nutrient transfer due to decreased placental blood flow and maternal hyperglycaemia present in diabetes mellitus increases glucose transfer to the fetus (Coad and Dunstall 2017)

Table 6.3 provides an overview of the function of the placenta and Table 6.4 considers the hormones of pregnancy (Chapter 7 discusses the placenta in more detail).

TABLE 6.3 The functions of the placenta.

Function	Description
Endocrine	In very early pregnancy, the trophoblast produces hCG, which maintains the corpus luteum and its production of progesterone and oestrogen, and the production of these hormones increases as the pregnancy enters the second trimester
	Other hormones produced by the placenta include prostaglandins, relaxin, endothelin, prolactin, thyroid stimulating hormone and adrenocorticotropic hormone (see Table 6.4)
Transport and transfer	The placenta transports glucose, iron, nutrients and vitamins. Lipids and fat-soluble vitamins (A, D and E) cross slowly, and these differ in their molecular structure
	Fluid levels are balanced by hydrostatic and colloid osmotic pressure
	Glucose is the carbohydrate necessary for fetal energy production and is transferred via a protein molecule
	A healthy placenta has capacity to transfer glucose that far exceeds fetal needs
Storage	Glycogen is stored in the placenta and when required this can be converted into glucose
Protection	The trophoblast has immunological properties that prevent rejection of the fetus as foreign tissue
	The placenta provides a protective barrier against most bacteria
	Some viruses, including varicella-zoster cytomegalovirus and human immunodeficiency virus (HIV) as well as some small bacterial organisms, such as syphilis, can cross the placenta to the fetus
	Some drugs, anaesthetics and carbon monoxide (CO) from maternal smoking can also cross the placenta.
Respiration	Oxygen (O_2) and carbon dioxide (CO_2) are transferred between maternal and fetal circulation by a partial pressure concentration gradient
	The diffusion gradient is enhanced by the higher fetal haemoglobin (HbF) as well as the increased affinity to O_2 of HbF
	The lipid solubility of CO_2 results in a more rapid transfer for gas across cell membranes
Excretion	In addition to CO_2, heat and other by-products of metabolism, including bilirubin, urea and uric acid, are transferred to the maternal circulation to be excreted

TABLE 6.4 Hormones of pregnancy and their functions.

Hormone name	Location produced or synthesised	Functions and effects
Human chorionic gonadotropin (heterodimer glycoprotein) type	Corpus luteum up to first 10 weeks then syncytiotrophoblast cells of the placenta Smaller amounts found in pituitary gland, liver and colon	Maintains corpus luteum to ensure progesterone secretion until placenta established and function adequate Stimulates fetal testosterone and corticosteroid production to enhance fetal growth and development Suppression of maternal immune system to prevent rejection of the placenta Detected in maternal urine/serum to confirm presence and viability of pregnancy Increases the number and size of myometrial cells Dominant in first and second trimesters
Human placental lactogen Also known as human chorionic somatomammotropin (hCS)	Corpus luteum up to 10 weeks then syncytiotrophoblast cells of the placenta	Regulating fetal glucose availability for the fetus, works as an insulin antagonist Promotes fetal growth by altering maternal protein, carbohydrate and fat metabolism Increases maternal metabolism and use of fat stores for energy Growth-promoting hormone – reduces glucose uptake by maternal cells, making more glucose available to the fetus

(Continued)

TABLE 6.4 (*Continued*)

Hormone name	Location produced or synthesised	Functions and effects
Progesterone Steroid hormone	Corpus luteum up to first 10 weeks then synthesised primarily by the placenta	Produced from cholesterol Maintains the uterus for pregnancy, enabling the fertilised ovum to be implanted and begin development, by preventing the endometrium from being shed (menstruation) Promotes blood vessel growth to the uterus Progesterone levels remain high throughout pregnancy to maintain myometrial quiescence, preventing premature contractions, and early lactation stimulates uterine growth, relaxing the smooth muscle of blood vessels and causing vasodilation
Relaxin polypeptide hormone	Corpus luteum up to 10 weeks then syncytiotrophoblast cells of the placenta	Levels increase rapidly until 20 weeks' gestation Causes rapid and sustained vasodilation of the vascular system Decreases systemic and renal vascular resistance Inhibits the response of numerous vasoconstrictors, such as vasopressin, angiotensin and catecholamines, by altering the molecular composition of small and medium arteries Prevents uterine contractions along with progesterone
Oestrogen Steroid hormone Three types Oestradiol – strongest type Oestriol – levels rise during pregnancy Oestrone – weakest type of oestrogen, more prevalent after menopause	Produced in the ovaries, and from the corpus luteum until the placenta takes over	Oestrogen levels steadily rise throughout pregnancy Required to promote progesterone production Stimulates synthesis of structural and contractile proteins and enzymes that supply energy for the process of contraction Influences molecules within the plasma membrane that control permeability for ions such as sodium, potassium, calcium and chloride, which determines the electrical excitability and resting potential of myometrial cells Oestrogens synchronise the formation of oxytocin receptors that promote uterine contractions
Oxytocin Octapeptide hormone	Produced in the hypothalamus and stored in the posterior lobe of pituitary gland	Produced in low levels during pregnancy Circulating levels increase gradually during pregnancy, reaching a peak at the onset of labour The key hormone in both initiating and maintaining labour Causes regular uterine contractions and has an important role in cervical ripening Induces feelings of love and bonding Continues to contract uterine muscles following birth to expel the placenta and control uterine bleeding Stimulates the milk ejection reflex postpartum

Source: Adapted from Stables and Rankin (2014).

Cardiovascular Adaptations

The cardiovascular system comprises both the heart and the circulatory system. The circulatory system functions in conjunction with other organs and body systems, as it is required to transport oxygen and nutrients to body cells that have been absorbed through the respiratory and gastrointestinal tracts. It also transports the waste products from metabolism, such as carbon dioxide to the lungs for elimination and other waste products to the kidneys to be excreted in urine (Blackburn 2016). The cardiovascular system is also essential for cell functioning as it distributes hormones and other substances and plays a vital role in temperature regulation. Blood pressure and cardiovascular volume and fluid balance fluctuate throughout the ovarian cycle and are influenced by oestrogen and progesterone. In pregnancy, significant changes occur in both cardiac function and haemodynamics to prepare to meet the increased demands of both the maternal and fetal tissues. The changes occur both indirectly, as a result of hormonal alterations, and directly, by mechanical forces resulting from an increased load on the system (Chapter 9 discusses the cardiovascular system). The formulation and growth of the placenta enable uteroplacental circulation, which allows the exchange of oxygen (O_2) and carbon dioxide (CO_2), nutrients and waste products between the mother and the fetus (Stables and Rankin 2014). The veins in the lower limbs become dilated under the influence of hormones as well as increased blood volume. This can result in decreased venous return.

The Heart

In early pregnancy the hormone-mediated decrease in vascular resistance initiates an increase in cardiac output of 40–50% (McNabb 2017). This rises significantly in the first trimester and peaks between 20 and 28 weeks (Blows 2018), with a plateau or small decrease closer to term (McNabb 2017). Stables and Rankin (2014) point out that this increase in cardiac output results in an increased requirement for oxygen within the myocardium (Coad and Dunstall 2017). The heart volume increases by 70–80 ml and its size by around 12% by the third trimester. In addition, the expanding uterus pushes the diaphragm upwards, consequently displacing the heart upwards and laterally (Stables and Rankin 2014), which may need to be considered if undertaking or interpreting an electrocardiogram (ECG).

Distribution and Effects of Increased Blood Flow

The majority of the increased blood flow is focused on the uterus and the placental site, but blood flow is also increased to other organ systems, including the kidneys, breasts and skin (Coad and Dunstall 2017), which is evident in some surprising ways. Renal blood flow increases by around 400 ml/min from early in the pregnancy, in response to reduced vascular resistance and increased cardiac output. This triggers an increase in glomerular filtration. Despite this, the kidneys retain both sodium and water, which expands plasma volume further (McNabb 2017). Increased blood flow in the breasts may be evident from early in the pregnancy, as there may be superficial veins that are dilated and visible, although these may be less visible in darker skin tones. The breasts and nipples in particular may feel tender or sensitive as they are engorged with blood, resulting from the increase in blood flow. In the skin, the effects of superficial capillary vasodilation and increased blood flow to the skin mean that pregnant women frequently have warm hands and feet, with accompanying palmar erythema, as well as stimulating growth of hair and nails. These changes will return to their pre-pregnancy state in the postnatal period (NHS 2022).

Blood Pressure

Blood pressure is the force exerted by circulating blood on the vessel walls and is controlled by the baroreflex system that provides a negative feedback loop controlling blood pressure in response to external stimuli, such as stress or exercise (Figure 6.1). Blood pressure is also affected by the volume of circulating blood and the resistance of peripheral blood vessels, which become more relaxed, leading to a significant decrease in blood pressure at around six to eight weeks' gestation (McNabb 2017). Increasing levels of progesterone in early pregnancy relax the smooth muscle walls of blood vessels, causing vasodilation. Additionally, the development of new vascular beds also contributes to a reduction in resistance in the blood vessels. Coad and Dunstall (2017) highlight that there is little change to the systolic blood pressure in pregnancy, but the diastolic blood pressure is lower in the first two trimesters and returns to values seen pre-pregnancy in the third trimester.

Dysregulation or dysfunction in the adaptation of cardiovascular regulatory mechanisms during pregnancy can lead to hypertension and pregnancy-specific conditions such as pre-eclampsia.

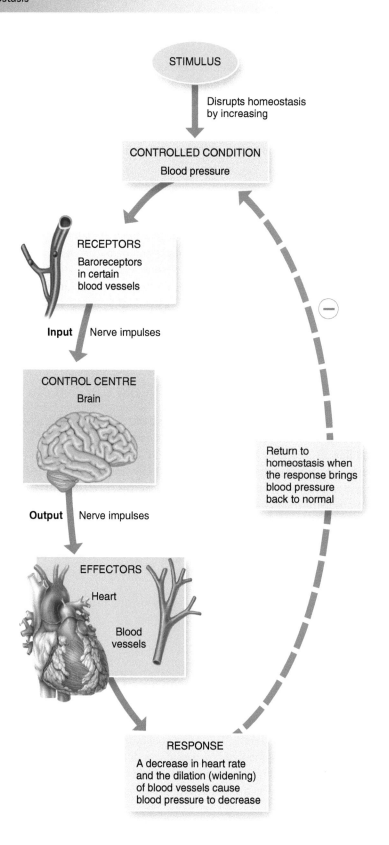

FIGURE 6.1   Homeostatic regulation of blood pressure by a negative feedback system. The broken return arrow with a negative sign represents negative feedback. Source: Reproduced with permission from Tortora and Derrickson (2017) / Wiley.

Red Flag: Hypertension

Hypertension

- Mild >140/90 mmHg
- Moderate >150/100 mmHg
- Severe >160/110 mmHg

Pre-eclampsia

New onset of hypertension (over 140 mmHg systolic or over 90 mmHg diastolic) after 20 weeks of pregnancy and the coexistence of one or more of the following new-onset conditions.

Proteinuria

- Urine protein: creatinine ratio of 30 mg/mmol or more
- OR albumin: creatinine ratio of 8 mg/mmol or more
- OR at least 1 g/l [2+] on dipstick testing

Other Maternal Organ Dysfunction

- Renal insufficiency (creatinine >90 μmol/l)
- Liver involvement (elevated transaminases, with or without right upper quadrant pain)
- Neurological complications such as eclampsia (seizures)
- Altered mental status
- Blindness
- Stroke
- Clonus
- Severe headaches
- Visual scotomata
- Haematological complications (thrombocytopenia – platelets <150 000/μl), haemolysis or disseminated intravascular coagulation (DIC)

Uteroplacental Dysfunction

Such as fetal growth restriction, abnormal umbilical artery waveform analysis or stillbirth.

Source: Adapted from NICE (2019).

113

White Blood Cells

White blood cells are part of the body's immune system. Types of white blood cells include granulocytes (neutrophils, eosinophils and basophils) as well as monocytes and lymphocytes, which are also known as T cells and B cells. There is an overall increase in the number of white blood cells in pregnancy, largely due to the rise in the number of neutrophils (Stables and Rankin 2014). The level peaks at around 30 weeks' gestation and this is maintained until birth. Higher circulating levels of oestrogen are thought to precipitate a further rise in labour before the levels return to normal by day 6 following birth. No change is seen in the number of circulating B cells and T cells, but there is a profound decline in cell-mediated immunity as human chorionic gonadotropin (hCG) and prolactin are known to supress the function of lymphocytes. This process is vital to the survival of the fetus, but increases the mother's susceptibility to viral infections including influenza and COVID-19.

Haemostasis

Haemostasis is defined as the body's normal physiological response to prevention or arrest of bleeding and this response occurs in several stages. Abnormalities in haemostasis can result in thrombosis formation or haemorrhage (Coad and Dunstall 2017). When there is active bleeding, the body's haemostatic mechanisms are initiated, there is localised vasoconstriction to reduce blood flow to the area, and the platelets then form a temporary plug in the vessel walls. Following this, a cascade of clotting factors is activated bringing fibrinogen to the damaged vessels, which provides a polymer fibrin plug to prevent further blood loss while the tissue beneath is being regenerated (LaPelusa and Dave 2022).

During pregnancy several adaptations occur within the blood to minimise the amount of blood that may be lost. As discussed previously, there is an increase to the volume of circulating red blood cells and plasma. There are also alterations to the cellular components of blood to protect maternal homeostasis. The mechanisms to protect maternal homeostasis are reliant on a complex interaction between platelets, blood vessel walls, fibrinolysis and coagulation factors. The normal non-pregnant negative feedback mechanisms are altered in preparation for anticipated blood loss at delivery as the blood changes to a hypercoagulable state and the following changes are seen:

- Plasma volume increases around 45–50% from 2600 to 3900.
- Plasma proteins decrease, reducing osmotic pressure, predisposing to oedema.
- Platelet count decreases slightly, in response to haemodilution, function unaffected.
- Red blood cell mass increases by around 18%, which can be up to 30% with iron supplementation.
- Neutrophil count increases in both number and activity in response to physiological stress.
- Clotting factors VIII, IX and X all increase and fibrinogen increases by up to 80%.
- Protein S and antithrombin are reduced.

Red Flag: Venous Thromboembolism

The normal physiological changes of pregnancy and the puerperium increase the risk of venous thromboembolism (VTE) including deep vein thrombosis (DVT) and pulmonary embolism (PE) due to:

- Venous stasis
- Endothelial damage
- Hypercoagulability

These normal adaptations represent a four- to sixfold increase overall compared to the non-pregnant state, but vary depending on the stage of pregnancy or postnatal period.

Source: Adapted from Singh et al. (2011).

Renal System Adaptations

Increased frequency of micturition, urinary leakage and nocturia are very common in pregnancy, and are considered normal physiological adaptations (Stables and Rankin 2014). The hormonal and haemodynamic changes that occur in pregnancy also lead to significant changes to renal function. In response to the extra demands of fetal metabolism, as well as the changes in maternal metabolism, the kidneys increase excretion of waste, and the cardiovascular adaptations previously discussed lead to retention of fluid and electrolytes (Coad and Dunstall 2017). Hormone-mediated vasodilation increases blood flow in the renal system, causing an upsurge in the glomerular filtration rate (GFR), and the kidneys are enlarged by around 1 cm and by around 30% in volume. A small amount of hydronephrosis is seen as the calyces (urine-collecting system) are also dilated and their peristaltic action is reduced. This results in some urine being retained in the kidney. In addition, the ureters become elongated to accommodate the increased volume of urine, but these alterations are associated with an increased risk of infection due to urine stasis.

Biochemical Adaptations

The increase in circulating blood volume and resulting haemodilution occur because the kidneys increase the reabsorption of sodium. This results from the activation of the vascular renin–angiotensin–aldosterone cycle. Sodium regulates osmotic forces along with chloride and bicarbonate. It also works alongside potassium to regulate acid–base balance and maintain neurotransmission. In the presence of an excess of sodium, a combination of hormonal (aldosterone) neural and renal mechanisms (renin–angiotensin system) work together to control the balance and maintain concentrations of sodium within the narrow range of 136–145 mEq/l. Renin is produced by the juxtaglomerular apparatus within the kidney. Levels remain stable in early pregnancy, with a small rise seen after 20 weeks' gestation. In the circulation, renin separates part of angiotensin, initiating an enzymatic cascade to form angiotensin I. In pregnancy there follows a downregulation of angiotensin-converting enzyme (ACE), a glycoprotein that divides angiotensin I and forms angiotensin II. It is angiotensin II that stimulates increased fluid and bicarbonate reabsorption and, although plasma concentrations of angiotensin II are double those seen pre-pregnancy by the second week of pregnancy, its effects on increasing blood pressure are mitigated by hCG and relaxin (Stables and Rankin 2014).

Vital Signs

Monitoring vital signs gives an objective measurement of homeostasis, by measuring the person's essential physiological functions (Sapra et al. 2022). The degree to which vital signs are outside of normal parameters may assist the midwife in assessing the severity of illness and the potential time frame for their subsequent actions. Work has been undertaken to standardise these parameters and escalation of concerns across the National Health Service (NHS) with the introduction of the National Early Warning Score (NEWS2) tool from the Royal College of Physicians (RCP 2017). The six physiological measurements assessed are:

- Systolic blood pressure
- Pulse rate
- Temperature
- Respiratory rate
- Oxygen saturation
- Level of consciousness

Findings are recorded on a colour- and score-coded chart. An aggregate score of these physiological measurements is calculated to enable early detection of deterioration of acutely ill patients and to identify trends, with a pathway of actions and escalation to follow depending on the score. The NEWS2 tool has been adapted to the MEOWS to account for differences in normal parameters in view of the physiological changes in pregnancy (Figure 6.2).

The use and value of early warning scores in maternity care are widely acknowledged, with benefits cited as reducing length of hospital stay, timely identification of deterioration and appropriate escalation. However, there remains a lack of consensus on the acceptable parameters and in their review of the literature, Smith et al. (2021) concluded that these scores do not have any impact on the number of maternal and neonatal deaths.

Red Flag: Sepsis

The physiological adaptations discussed in this chapter and the alterations to acceptable vital signs parameters may make the early diagnosis of sepsis more challenging. The classical signs and symptoms of sepsis in pregnant women may be absent, more subtle and not always reflective of the severity of disease compared to = the non-pregnant population. The Royal College of Obstetricians and Gynaecologists (RCOG 2012) recommends that healthcare professionals use a high index of suspicion and consider individual risk factors, gestation, medical history and clinical presentation along with any clinical observations undertaken.

Sepsis in pregnancy may present in an atypical way, such as constant abdominal pain, nausea and vomiting, and the disease progression may be much more rapid than in a non-pregnant state, so urgent referral to obstetric and anaesthetic colleagues is essential.

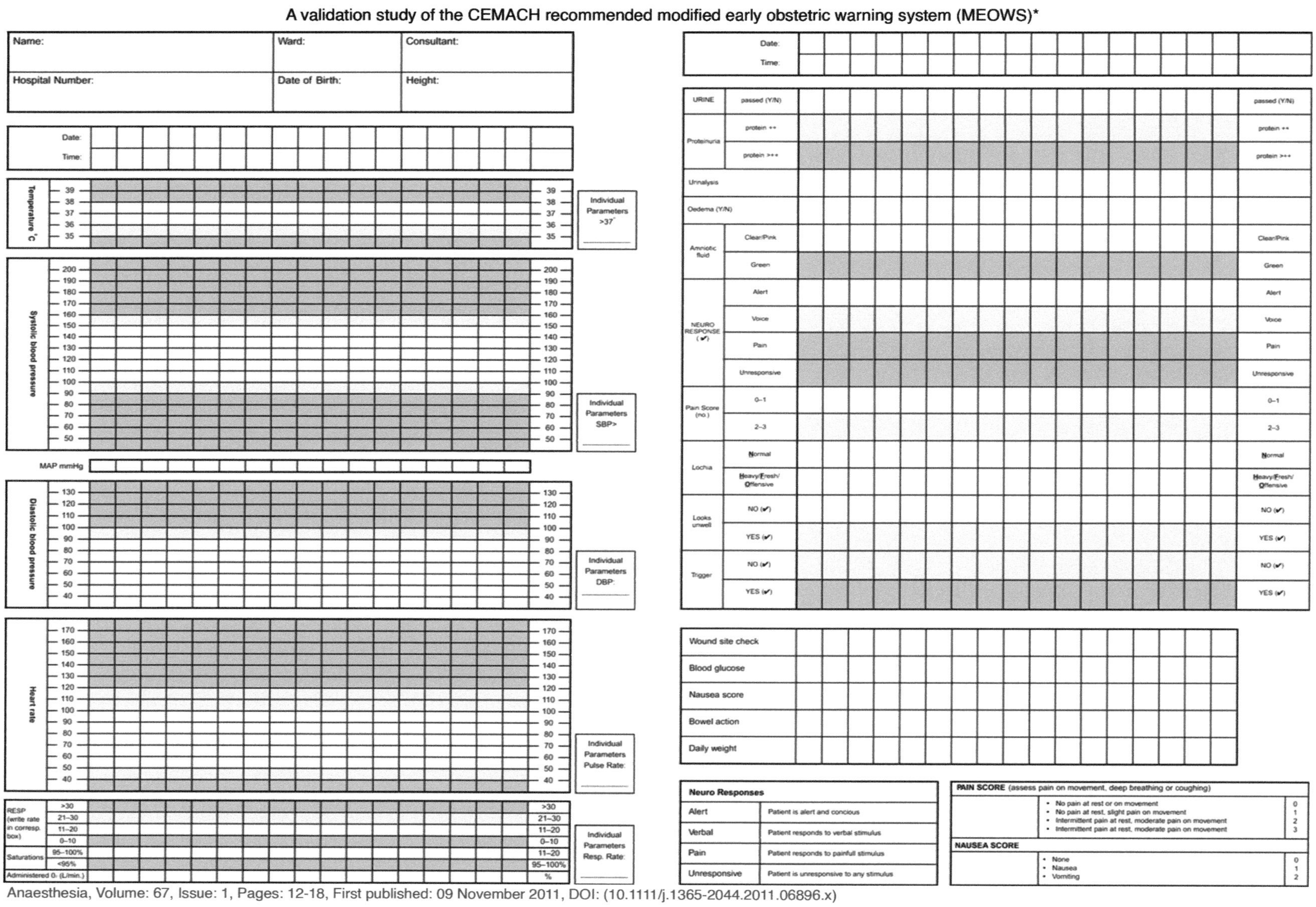

116

FIGURE 6.2   Modified Early Obstetric Warning Score (MEOWS) chart. Source: Reproduced by permission from Singh et al. (2011).

Anaesthesia, Volume: 67, Issue: 1, Pages: 12-18, First published: 09 November 2011, DOI: (10.1111/j.1365-2044.2011.06896.x)

Signs and Symptoms of Septic Shock

- Temperature: <36°C or >38°C
- Heart rate: <40 bpm or >100 bpm
- Systolic blood pressure: <90 mmHg
- Respiratory rate: >20/min
- Impaired mental or conscious state
- Significant oedema
- Oliguria <25 ml/h
- Oxygen saturation <95% on room air
- Hyperglycaemia 7.7 mmol/l (without diabetes)

Source: Adapted from RCOG (2012).

Psychological Stress and Homeostasis

Although the main focus of this chapter is on homeostasis and physiological adaptations that occur in pregnancy to facilitate and nurture the developing fetus, the impact of psychological stress on the body's homeostatic mechanisms should also be considered. Traylor et al. (2020) highlighted that disruptions in the maternal–placental–fetal immune and endocrine responses can result from both acute and chronic stress causing allostatic overload, where there is a long-term imbalance in mediators of homeostasis that may be associated with adverse pregnancy outcomes through a positive feedback loop. In pregnancy these disruptions increase the risk of preterm birth, low birth weight, neonatal death and pre-eclampsia. Maternal anxiety and depression are common in pregnancy, with rates reported by Filippetti et al. (2022) at 47% and 60%, respectively. In their study they highlight that this represents an increase in reported rates of perinatal mental health issues since the Covid-19 pandemic. Traylor et al. (2020) also pointed out that pregnancy can be a time when women are anxious about their financial stability and relationships as well as the stresses of everyday life.

Labour

In physiological pregnancy labour occurs naturally, but the mechanism that controls the onset of this is not well understood, and many of the preparatory actions occur a number of weeks before the onset of labour. In clinical terms labour is usually divided into three distinct phases. The first stage is characterised by regular, painful uterine contractions, progressive cervical effacement and dilation, ending when the cervix is fully dilated. The second stage begins when the cervix is fully dilated and ends with complete delivery of the baby. In the third stage of labour the placenta separates and is expelled along with the membranes. The physiology, however, is not divided into phases and the progression of each stage of labour relies on a continuous positive feedback mechanism, in which uterine contractions represent the stimulus, applying axial pressure, flexing the fetal head, which in turn applies pressure to the cervix. The stretch receptors in the cervix send messages to the brain, which instructs the pituitary gland to release oxytocin into the blood stream that intensifies contractions, applying additional pressure to the cervix. Thus the cycle repeats until a definite end point is reached (Figure 6.3). In this case, it is the birth of the baby and following this, delivery of the placenta and membranes.

The maintenance and continuation of this homeostatic, positive feedback loop aid progression through labour, but it can be affected by internal factors, such as cephalopelvic disproportion, fetal abnormalities, fetal malpresentation or malposition and a full bladder. All of these can interrupt the effectiveness of the feedback loop by a reduction in pressure on the cervix, reducing the degree to which stretch receptors are activated, or the oxytocin uptake being reduced in the myometrial muscle. There are also external factors, including a psychologically secure birthing environment, continuity of carer, as well as maternal mobility and upright positions (Goldkuhl et al. 2021), which have been shown to influence the sensitive progress of physiological labour. In physiological labour oxytocin

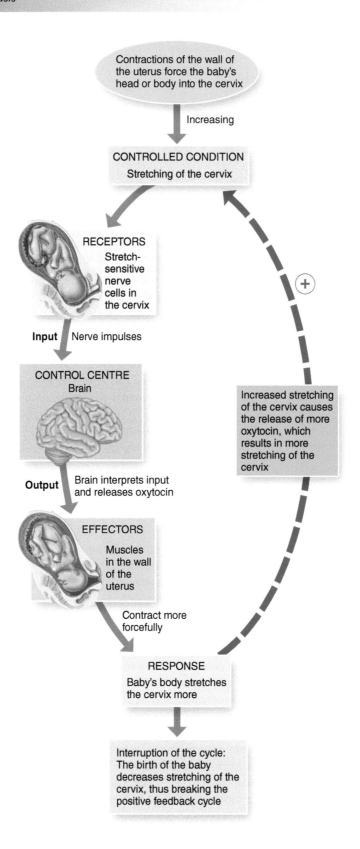

FIGURE 6.3   Positive feedback control of labour contractions during the birth of a baby. The broken return arrow with a positive sign represents positive feedback. Source: Reproduced with permission from Tortora and Derrickson (2017) / Wiley.

activates the parasympathetic nervous system, leading to an increase in uterine blood flow and dilation of uterine arteries, ensuring adequate fetal oxygen supply. However, in stress, rising levels of adrenaline and noradrenaline cause a shift in the autonomic nervous system, increasing to dominance of the sympathetic nervous system, activating beta-adrenoreceptors. The activation of these receptors inhibits uterine contractions, leading to a slowing of progress in labour (Walter et al. 2022).

The partogram may be electronic or paper based and gives an overall view of measures of both fetal and maternal well-being. If accurately completed, it allows for timely recognition of an arrest of progress in labour or a deviation from the normal parameters of the maternal vital signs or fetal heart rate monitoring. Identification of any deviation from normal should prompt a plan for action to resolve the issue, which could include bladder care, maternal position change or obstetric review.

Take-Home Points

- Homeostasis is the complex, internal, self-regulatory physical and chemical conditions that maintain stability within homeostatic ranges by controlling variables including fluid and electrolyte balance, body temperature, glucose levels and blood pressure.
- During pregnancy the body undergoes significant adaptations to facilitate the conditions necessary for the fetus to develop and grow.
- The placenta, via the maternal circulation, conducts the metabolism, respiration and excretion for the fetus. It also provides passive immunity to the fetus and creates a state of immunotolerance to ensure that the mother's immune system does not target the fetus as a foreign body.
- Accepted normal ranges for vital signs such as blood pressure, heart rate and respiratory rate are altered and modified obstetric warning score charts should always be used in the perinatal period.
- Physical and mental illness can disrupt mechanisms of homeostasis and management, and treatment should seek to support the body in returning to and maintaining stable internal conditions.
- Progress in labour is influenced by numerous internal and external factors. It is imperative that the midwife understands how to recognise these and optimise maternal and fetal conditions as well as the birthing environment.
- Any deviation from the acceptable parameters in clinical findings should be accurately recorded and appropriately escalated to multidisciplinary colleagues in a timely manner.

119

Conclusion

Homeostasis is the term used in reference to the stability of the internal environment within the body. It is a self-regulating process by which numerous biological systems maintain stability while adjusting to changing external conditions. This chapter has outlined and given examples of both negative and positive feedback mechanisms and how observation and documentation of vital signs, such as blood pressure, pulse rate, oxygen saturation, respiration rate, temperature and level of consciousness, give objective measures of any homeostatic imbalance. The profound physiological changes that the body undergoes during pregnancy have been highlighted with their impact on the normal ranges of vital signs. It is essential that those caring for pregnant women are aware of the underlying adaptations and are using appropriate early warning score charts that are adjusted to account for the altered parameters of pregnancy.

It should always be borne in mind that there can also be a pathophysiological reason for changes in vital signs. Midwives need to be aware that while there are changes to acceptable parameters for vital signs such as physiological hypotension, slight tachycardia or respiratory rate that may be increased in pregnancy, they should also consider clinical risk factors, presentation, medical and obstetric history in addition to subjective observations, such as colour and behaviour, to make a diagnosis, rather than exclude a diagnosis (Knight et al. 2022). Assumption of normal physiological causes and complacency around abnormal vital signs can lead, and has led, to a failure to recognise early, subtle changes to these measurements. Failure to recognise deterioration has featured in several maternal deaths from cardiac disease, sepsis and epilepsy among other causes. This highlights the importance of thorough assessment, prompt escalation and appropriate treatment.

References

Blackburn, S. (2016). *Maternal, Fetal and Neonatal Physiology: A Clinical Perspective*. Philadelphia: Elsevier.

Blows, W. (2018). *The Biological Basis of Clinical Observations*. Oxford: Taylor & Francis.

Coad, J. and Dunstall, M. (2017). *Anatomy & Physiology for Midwives*. Edinburgh: Churchill Livingstone.

Filippetti, M., Clarke, A., and Rigato, S. (2022). The mental health crisis of expectant women in the UK: Effects of the COVID-19 pandemic on prenatal maternal mental health, antenatal attachment and social support. *BMC Pregnancy and Childbirth* 22 (1): 68.

Goldkuhl, L., Dellenbourg, L., Berg, M. et al. (2021). The influence and meaning of the birth environment for nulliparous woman at a hospital-based labour ward in Sweden: an ethnographic study. *Women and Birth* 35 (4): e337–e347.

Ishida, J., Matsuoka, T., Saito-Fujita, T. et al. (2011). Pregnancy-associated homeostasis and dysregulation: lessons from genetically modified animal models. *Journal of Biochemistry* 150 (1): 5–14.

Knight, M., Bunch, K., Patel, R. et al. (ed.) (2022) (Eds.) on behalf of MBRRACE-UK). *Saving Lives, Improving Mothers' Care Core Report – Lessons Learned to Inform Maternity Care from the UK and Ireland Confidential Enquiries into Maternal Deaths and Morbidity 2018–20*. Oxford: National Perinatal Epidemiology Unit, University of Oxford.

LaPelusa, A. and Dave, H. (2022). Physiology, haemostasis. In: *StatPearls*. Treasure Island, FL: StatPearls Publishing https://www.ncbi.nlm.nih.gov/books/NBK545263.

McNabb, M. (2017). Maternal neurohormonal and systemic adaptations to feto-placental development. In: *Mayes' Midwifery* (ed. S. Macdonald and G. Johnson), 484–502. Oxford: Elsevier.

National Health Service (NHS) (2022). Common health problems in pregnancy. https://www.nhs.uk/pregnancy/related-conditions/common-symptoms/common-health-problems (accessed November 2023).

National Institute of Health and Care Excellence (NICE) (2019). Hypertension in pregnancy: diagnosis and management. https://www.nice.org.uk/guidance/ng133 (accessed November 2023).

Peate, I. (ed.) (2021). *Fundamentals of Applied Pathophysiology: An Essential Guide for Nursing and Healthcare Students*. Chichester, UK: Wiley.

Roberts, M.B.V. (1986). *Biology; a Functional Approach*, 4e. Nelson: Salisbury.

Royal College of Obstetricians & Gynaecologists (RCOG) (2012). Bacterial sepsis in pregnancy. https://www.rcog.org.uk/media/ea1p1r4h/gtg_64a.pdf (accessed November 2023).

Royal College of Physicians (RCP) (2017). National Early Warning Score (NEWS) 2. www.rcplondon.ac.uk/projects/outputs/national-early-warning-score-news-2 (accessed November 2023).

Sapra, A., Malik, A., and Bhandari, P. (2022). Vital sign assessment. In: *StatPearls*. Treasure Island, FL: StatPearls Publishing https://www.ncbi.nlm.nih.gov/books/NBK553213.

Singh, S., McGlennan, A., England, E., and Simons, R. (2011). A validation study of the CEMACH recommended modified early obstetric warning system (MEOWS). *Anaesthesia* 67 (1): 12–18. https://doi.org/10.1111/j.1365-2044.2011.06896.x.

Smith, V., Kenny, L.C., Sandall, J. et al. (2021). Physiological track-and-trigger/early warning systems for use in maternity care. *Cochrane Database of Systematic Reviews* (9): CD013276. https://doi.org/10.1002/14651858.CD013276.pub2.

Stables, D. and Rankin, J. (2014). *Physiology in Childbearing with Anatomy and Related Biosciences*, 3e. London: Balliere Tindall.

Tortora, G.J. and Derrickson, B.H. (2017). *Tortora's Principles of Anatomy and Physiology*. Hoboken, NJ: Wiley.

Traylor, C., Johnson, J., Kimmel, M., and Manuck, T. (2020). Effects of psychological stress on adverse pregnancy outcomes and non-pharmacologic approaches for reduction: An expert review. *American Journal of Obstetrics and Gynecology* 2 (4): 100229. https://doi.org/10.1016/j.ajogmf.2020.100229.

Walter, M., Abele, H., and Plappert, C. (2022). The role of oxytocin and the effect of stress during childbirth: Neurobiological basics and implications for mother and child. *Frontiers in Endocrinology* 12: https://doi.org/10.3389/fendo.2021.742236.

Waugh, A. and Grant, A. (2018). *Ross and Wilson: Anatomy and Physiology in Health and Illness*, 13e. Edinburgh: Elsevier-Churchill Livingstone.

Further Resources

Peate, I. and Hamilton, C. (2022). *Fundamentals of Pharmacology for Midwives*. Chichester, UK: Wiley.

Open Educational Resources.1.3 Homeostasis – Anatomy & Physiology. https://open.oregonstate.education/aandp/chapter/1-3-home-ostasis/ (oregonstate.education) (accessed January 2024).

Glossary

Antithrombin	A protein produced by the liver to help control blood clotting
Cephalic	Relating to the fetal head
Diaphragm	A dome-shaped muscular partition separating the thorax from the abdomen in mammals. It plays a key role in breathing, as its contraction increases the volume of the thorax and so inflates the lungs
Diastolic	The period of relaxation of the ventricles of the heart
Endothelium	The tissue that forms a single layer of cells lining various organs and cavities of the body, especially the blood vessels, heart and lymphatic vessels
Enzyme	A substance produced by a living organism that acts as a catalyst to bring about a specific biochemical reaction
Haematocrit	The ratio of the volume of red blood cells to the total volume of blood
Haemodynamic	Relating to the flow of blood within the organs and tissues of the body
Haemoglobin	A red protein responsible for transporting oxygen in the blood
Haemostasis	Stopping of a flow of blood
Lipid	Any of a class of organic compounds that are fatty acids or their derivatives and are insoluble in water
Myocardium	The muscular tissue of the heart
Platelets	A small, colourless disc-shaped cell fragment without a nucleus, found in large numbers in blood and involved in clotting
Protein S	A vitamin K-dependent, anticoagulant glycoprotein that acts chiefly in enhancing the ability of protein C to inactivate factor V and factor VIII
Systolic	The phase of the heartbeat when the heart muscle contracts and pumps blood from the chambers into the arteries

CHAPTER 7

The Placenta

Raya Vinogradov[1,2,3] and Vikki Smith[4]

[1] *Newcastle upon Tyne NHS Hospitals Foundation Trust*

[2] *Faculty of Medical Sciences, Newcastle University, Population Health Sciences Institute*

[3] *National Institute for Health and Care Research Applied Research Collaboration North East and North Cumbria*

[4] *Department of Nursing, Midwifery and Health, Northumbria University, Newcastle upon Tyne, UK*

Raya Vinogradov is funded by the National Institute for Health and Care Research (NIHR) Applied Research Collaboration (ARC) North East and North Cumbria (NENC) (in-practice fellow APF2209). The views expressed are those of the author(s) and not necessarily those of the NIHR or the Department of Health and Social Care.

AIM

This chapter provides an overview of commonly occurring placental pathophysiology and its impact on fetal and maternal well-being during pregnancy and postnatally. Screening, diagnosis and management are discussed in relation to the provision of midwifery care.

LEARNING OUTCOMES

On completion of this chapter the reader will be able to:

- Identify the variations of placental morphology and the most common disorders of the placenta and umbilical cord
- Explain the pathophysiology of human placental disorders and relate this to normal placental anatomy and physiology
- Describe the risks for the woman and fetus associated with placental pathophysiology
- Discuss the principles of management of care for women with complications of the placenta

Test Your Prior Knowledge

1. Describe the early development of the human placenta.
2. Describe the anatomy of the human placenta at full term.
3. List the functions of the human placenta.
4. List the functions of amniotic fluid.
5. Outline the structure of the umbilical cord.

Structure and Function of the Placenta

Prior to attempting this chapter, we recommend that readers review their knowledge of anatomy and physiology, as many major complications of pregnancy are consequences of defective placentation, therefore a good understanding of processes involved in placentation will aid comprehension. In this chapter we will focus on pathology and will offer only a brief recap of the development and anatomy of the placenta.

A developed placenta is a disc-shaped organ that grows in volume as pregnancy progresses. A mature placenta weighs approximately 500 g and is 22 cm in diameter and 2.5 cm in thickness.

Structurally, the placenta can be divided into three key areas:

- The chorionic plate is connective tissue containing amnion, umbilical vein and two arteries (umbilical cord) extending into chorion as chorionic veins and arteries, then to arterioles leading to main stem villi.
- The intervillous space supports exchange between fetal and maternal circulation.
- The basal plate is vascularised by endothelial vessels and consists of a mixture of decidua basalis (maternal cells) and trophoblast cells (fetal cells).

The placenta performs several key functions during pregnancy supporting the growth and development of the fetus: respiration, nutrition, endocrine regulation, excretion and protection.

Health Promotion

Alcohol consumed by a mother can easily pass through the placenta and reach the fetal blood stream. Due to an inability to metabolise alcohol in the same way as its mother, the fetus is exposed to a higher concentration of alcohol for longer.

Alcohol causes irreversible damage to the placental structure and developing fetus.

Alcohol exposure is associated with placental dysfunction, impaired blood flow and nutrient transport, endocrine changes, increased rates of stillbirth, placental abruption, umbilical cord vasoconstriction and low birth weight. Alcohol exposure in fetuses can lead to fetal alcohol syndrome (FAS) or a broader range of fetal alcohol spectrum disorders (FASD) that encompass an array of >400 coexisting conditions. There is no known safe level of alcohol consumption in pregnancy.

Source: Adapted from NICE (2021).

123

> ### Learning Event
>
> Reflect on your experiences of discussing alcohol use with women during pregnancy.
>
> - What approach do you take to make sure that women feel comfortable discussing their alcohol consumption?
> - Do you ask about the types and number of alcoholic drinks consumed?
> - What advice do you provide about the risks to the woman and her fetus?

Structural Pathology of the Placenta

Variations in Placenta and Umbilical Cord Morphology

Velamentous Cord Insertion

This occurs when the umbilical cord attaches to the membranes surrounding the placenta rather than being attached centrally to the placenta, meaning that the umbilical vessels run through the membranes to the placenta. This finding can be associated with vasa praevia (see later discussion). The appearance of a velamentous cord insertion is shown in Figure 7.1.

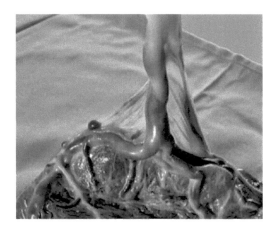

FIGURE 7.1   Velamentous cord insertion. Source: Reproduced by permission from Sepulveda (2006) / John Wiley & Sons.

Battledore Insertion of the Cord

This is also known as a marginal cord insertion and refers to a cord that inserts close to the placental margin (edge). In some cases this type of cord can detach from the placenta during active management of the third stage of labour.

Succenturiate Lobe

Although most placentas are uniform in appearance, in 0.6–1% of pregnancies a smaller accessory placental lobe that is separate from the main placental mass can be found; this is called a succenturiate lobe (Suzuki and Igarashi 2008) (Figure 7.2).

 The presence of a succenturiate lobe can be diagnosed during a routine antenatal ultrasound scan. Although this is a normal variant, there are a number of clinical considerations worth keeping in mind when looking after a woman with a known succenturiate lobe, because of the association with an increased incidence of vasa praevia and a higher risk of postpartum haemorrhage due to retained placental tissue.

Case Study 7.1

Laura is a 35-year-old woman who has given birth vaginally to her first baby at 40 weeks' gestation. The pregnancy was uncomplicated, Laura has no identified medical problems and went into labour spontaneously. During a routine ultrasound scan, it was suspected that there was a succenturiate lobe of the placenta. She had a physiological third stage of labour.

 Laura is experiencing heavy vaginal bleeding two hours after the birth of her baby.

- What should you consider in this case and what action should be taken?

Notes

- Identification of a succenturiate lobe of placenta is a risk factor for retained placental tissue after birth.
- A detailed examination of the placenta, cord and membranes should be performed soon after birth to determine whether the placenta is intact.
- If part of the placenta is retained in the uterus it cannot contract effectively, resulting in maternal haemorrhage.
- The cause of vaginal bleeding should be investigated as a matter of urgency and medical assistance should be sought.

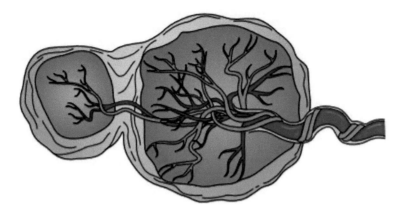

FIGURE 7.2   Succenturiate lobe of placenta.

Two-Vessel Cord/Single Umbilical Artery

Blood supply from the placenta to the fetus flows through a single vein. Due to the unique features of the fetal circulation, nutrient- and oxygen-rich blood enters the fetal circulation via the umbilical vein and reaches the right cardiac atrium through the ductus venosus and inferior vena cava. Blood carrying waste products leaves the fetal circulation via two umbilical arteries, which can be easily visualised during routine antenatal ultrasound examination. Therefore, most umbilical cords consist of one vein (with nutrient- and oxygen-rich blood) and two arteries (carrying fetal waste products to the placenta).

In some pregnancies the umbilical cord consists of one rather than two umbilical arteries. The incidence of single umbilical artery is reported as 0.5–6% (Vafaei et al. 2021). Although isolated cases are most likely to have a normal outcome, the presence of a single umbilical artery can be associated with several chromosomal conditions such as trisomy 13, 18 and triploidy; congenital anomalies most commonly in genitourinary, cardiovascular and musculoskeletal systems; fetal growth restriction (FGR); and fetal demise (Hua et al. 2010). Fetal karyotyping is not recommended in isolated cases of single umbilical artery.

Abnormal Localisation

Placenta Praevia

Placenta praevia refers to a condition where the placenta partially or completely covers the internal cervical os and it has an estimated incidence of 1 in 200 pregnancies (Silver 2015). The localisation of the placenta is determined by transabdominal or transvaginal ultrasonography, generally during the mid-trimester (anomaly) scan at 18–20 weeks' gestation. A low-lying placenta is defined as a placenta where the placental edge is within 2 cm of the internal cervical os, and a further ultrasound scan is recommended to determine whether the placenta has migrated or remains low-lying or placenta praevia (Jauniaux et al. 2018). Apparent migration of the placenta refers to the development of the lower segment of the uterus during the third trimester, resulting in a positional change in the placenta away from the internal cervical os.

Placenta praevia is associated with high rates of maternal and neonatal morbidity and mortality. Severe, usually unprovoked, haemorrhage may occur during pregnancy as a result of placenta praevia. The incidence of placenta praevia is higher in women who have had a caesarean birth, are older, have used assisted reproductive techniques and in women who smoke (Silver 2015). The definitions of bleeding, based on estimated volume of blood loss, are shown in Table 7.1.

125

Red Flag

Heavy vaginal bleeding during pregnancy (antepartum haemorrhage (APH)) is a risk factor for adverse outcomes including blood clotting disorders, shock and fetal hypoxia.

- What are the possible causes of APH?
- How would you assess a woman presenting with heavy vaginal bleeding?

TABLE 7.1   Definitions of vaginal bleeding.

Quantity of vaginal bleeding	Description
Spotting	Staining, streaking or blood spotting noted on underwear or sanitary protection
Minor haemorrhage	Blood loss less than 50 ml that has settled
Major haemorrhage	Blood loss of 50–1000 ml with no signs of clinical shock
Massive haemorrhage	Blood loss greater than 1000 ml and /or signs of clinical shock

Source: Adapted from RCOG (2011).

Placenta Accreta Spectrum

Placenta accreta spectrum (PAS) is a term used to describe a complication of pregnancy where the placenta is abnormally adhered to and/or invades the uterine wall. The reported prevalence of the condition is varies between 1 in 300 and 1 in 2000 pregnancies (Varlas et al. 2021). Recognised risk factors for PAS are previous caesarean section, other uterine surgery that involved breach of the myometrium (e.g. myomectomy), assisted reproduction techniques and placenta praevia, with increasing prevalence of all risk factors and incidence of PAS over the last decade (Collins et al. 2016).

PAS occurs when recovery of the endometrium (endometrial re-epithelialisation) is impaired in the area of uterine scarring, most commonly from caesarean section, resulting in deep invasion of the trophoblast and villous tissue (placenta) into the myometrium (smooth muscle of the uterus) and in some cases the pelvic organs (Jauniaux et al. 2018). Due to the worldwide increase in caesarean sections, the rate of PAS will continue to rise.

The spectrum encompasses placenta accreta, increta and percreta and represents degrees of placental invasion into and through the myometrium at the site of prior surgical scarring, with the degree of invasion being determined following histopathological examination of the placenta. In cases of placenta accreta, the villi adhere to the myometrium; placenta increta occurs when the villi invade into the uterine myometrium; and placenta percreta refers to the villi invading through the myometrium (Jauniaux et al. 2018). The range of placental adherence is shown in Figure 7.3.

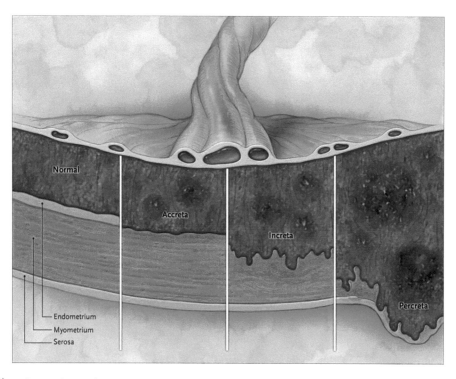

FIGURE 7.3   Placenta accreta spectrum.

In cases of PAS the placenta does not separate normally after birth and predisposes women to massive postpartum haemorrhage, resulting in a substantial increase in maternal morbidity and mortality. For some women PAS is a life-threatening complication, which can result in hysterectomy after birth. The risk of morbidity is dependent on the degree of placental invasion, with the deepest invasion, placenta percreta, having a fatality rate of up to 7%.

The risks associated with PAS are reduced when it is diagnosed antenatally and women give birth in a hospital with a specialist multidisciplinary care team (Collins et al. 2016). Antenatal ultrasound screening for PAS should be performed in all women who have had uterine surgery (with the most common being caesarean section) and have a low, anteriorly positioned placenta or placenta praevia. Screening involves an ultrasound scan (usually transabdominally) to screen for four signs of PAS and in some cases women will be offered magnetic resonance imaging (MRI) to assist with diagnosis of the condition.

Red Flag

A pregnant woman who has previously had a caesarean section and is known to have an anterior low-lying placenta or a placenta praevia covering the internal os should be referred for ultrasound screening for PAS.

Orange Flag

Women who have a diagnosis of PAS can experience significant adverse psychological outcomes, including relatively high rates of post-traumatic stress disorder (PTSD) (Tol et al. 2019).

Vasa Praevia

Vasa praevia is a condition where the placental blood vessels are unprotected by the umbilical cord or placental tissue and cross or are close the internal cervical os. It occurs in approximately 1 in 365 to 1 in 5000 pregnancies (Oyelese et al. 2023). Vasa praevia can be associated with either a velamentous umbilical cord or a succenturiate placental lobe (Figure 7.4).

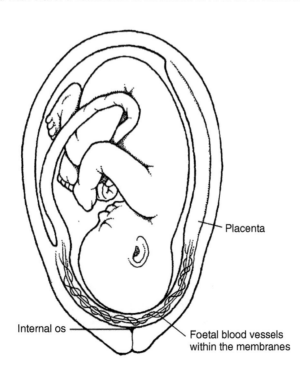

FIGURE 7.4 Vasa praevia.

When the fetal vessels run across the internal cervical os, there is the likelihood that the vessels will rupture during active labour or when amniotomy is performed. This is associated with a fetal mortality rate of around 60% due to exsanguination, although this rate is reduced with antenatal diagnosis and planned caesarean section (Oyelese et al. 2023; Silver 2015).

Pre-eclampsia

Definition and Prevalence
Pre-eclampsia is a pregnancy-related multisystem syndrome with disease onset after 20 weeks of gestation and up to 6 weeks postnatally. Pre-eclampsia affects up to 2–5% of all pregnancies (Abalos et al. 2013). Pre-eclampsia is diagnosed by new onset of hypertension (>140 mmHg systolic or >90 mmHg diastolic) with proteinuria or/and maternal organ dysfunction or/and uteroplacental dysfunction (NICE 2019).

Symptoms of Pre-eclampsia
Symptoms of pre-eclampsia include:

- Visual disturbances.
- Right upper quadrant abdominal (epigastric) pain.
- Oedema (swelling of the hands, face or feet).
- Oliguria (low urine output).

Short-Term Consequences of Pre-eclampsia
If not diagnosed and closely monitored, pre-eclampsia can lead to eclampsia, HELLP syndrome (haemolysis, elevated liver enzymes and low platelets), disseminated intravascular coagulation, stroke or organ dysfunction, and maternal and fetal death. Women suffering from hypertensive disease of pregnancy are at increased risk of placental abruption, and are more likely to have a small baby and give birth early.

Pathogenesis
Pre-eclampsia is believed to be a consequence of defective trophoblast invasion and subsequent poor remodelling of spiral arteries, resulting in reduced uteroplacental perfusion that leads to a systemic inflammatory response (failure of physiological transformation of the spiral arteries is illustrated in Figure 7.5). However, an alternative hypothesis suggests that pre-eclampsia has a cardiovascular origin (Thilaganathan and Kalafat 2019).

Screening and Prophylaxis
All pregnant women should be screened at the time of pregnancy booking for risk factors of pre-eclampsia. There are number of approaches to screening, however the most common approach is based on maternal characteristics (see Table 7.2). Women with one major or two or more moderate risk factors should be advised to take a daily prophylactic dose (75–150 mg) of aspirin (NICE 2019), if aspirin is not otherwise contra-indicated. Maternal risk factors for pre-eclampsia are shown in Table 7.2.

Medicines Management

Daily low-dose aspirin (75–150 mg) is recommended by NICE (2019) to women identified at increased risk of pre-eclampsia. This recommendation is based on decades of research and clear evidence demonstrating that 150 mg of daily aspirin started from 12 weeks of gestation can reduce the risk of early-onset pre-eclampsia (Rolnik et al. 2017; Henderson et al. 2014).

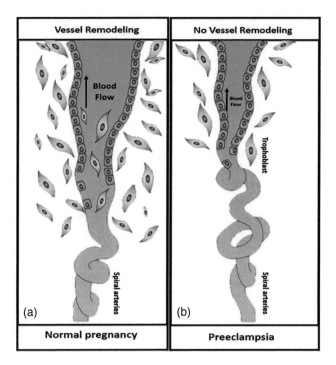

FIGURE 7.5 Failure of physiological transformation of the spiral arteries is implicated in pre-eclampsia. (a) In a normal pregnancy, physiological transformation of the myometrial segment of the spiral artery occurs. Trophoblast cells extend to both the decidual segment and one-third of the myometrial segment of the spiral artery. Both the arterial media and endothelium are destroyed by trophoblasts, converting the arteries into wide-calibre vessels and increasing the delivery of blood to the intervillous space. (b) In pregnancies affected by pre-eclampsia, a key feature associated with the failure of physiological transformation of the spiral arteries is lack of invasion of the trophoblasts into the myometrial segment of the spiral artery. The resulting lack of transformation of blood vessels results in narrow spiral arteries, a disturbed pattern of blood flow and reduced uteroplacental perfusion. Source: Reproduced from Shaikh et al. (2021) / CC BY 3.0 Deed.

TABLE 7.2 Risk factors for pre-eclampsia.

Major risk factors	Moderate risk factors
Hypertensive disease during a previous pregnancy	Nulliparity
Chronic kidney disease	Age 40 years or older
Autoimmune disease such as systemic lupus erythematosus or antiphospholipid syndrome	Pregnancy interval of more than 10 years
Type 1 or type 2 diabetes	Body mass index (BMI) of 35 kg/m² or more at first visit
Chronic hypertension	Family history of pre-eclampsia
	Multifetal pregnancy

Although widely used, aspirin is contra-indicated for women with known haemorrhagic disorders, hypersensitivity to aspirin, active peptic ulceration, under 16 years of age or severe cardiac failure (analgesic dose), and is advised to be used with caution in people with asthma, anaemia, dehydration, G6PD deficiency, history of gout, hypertension, previous peptic ulceration and thyrotoxicosis. The most up-to-date information about contra-indications can be found at the British National Formulary (BNF, https://bnf.nice.org.uk), which is updated regularly.

Examination Scenario

All women should have blood pressure assessment and urinalysis at every antenatal visit. Women at increased risk of pre-eclampsia should have more frequent antenatal visits and be aware of signs and symptoms of pre-eclampsia.

Biochemical tests such as the placental growth factor (PlGF) test or ratio of soluble fms-like tyrosine kinase 1 (sFlt-1)/PlGF could be used for women who have suspected pre-eclampsia between 20 weeks' and 34 weeks and 6 days' gestation (NICE 2019).

Management

While symptoms of pre-eclampsia can be managed by medication, there is no treatment for pre-eclampsia once it has developed, therefore close monitoring is required and may include hospitalisation. Monitoring includes blood pressure measurement, urine protein: creatinine ratio, blood tests to assess full blood count, liver function and renal function, and fetal monitoring. In the case of maternal or fetal concerns, early birth may be indicated.

Medicines Management: Pre-eclampsia

Antihypertensive drugs (such as labetalol, nifedipine or methyldopa) may be required to control blood pressure during pregnancy. Consideration should be given to existing medication, risks and the woman's preference (NICE 2019).

Orange Flag

Evidence suggests that pregnant women may not take aspirin as recommended (Abheiden et al. 2016). Women may worry about negative consequences or perceived side effects of taking aspirin that can affect themselves and their unborn child. When discussing low-dose aspirin with women, be aware that although it is widely used in obstetric practice, low-dose aspirin, like many other medicines, is used off-licence in pregnancy. This may cause confusion if women and healthcare professionals involved in women's care are not provided with up-to-date information about aspirin use for the prevention of pre-eclampsia.

Aim to provide an opportunity for women at risk of pre-eclampsia to ask questions and raise concerns about the use of aspirin.

Case Study 7.2

Bibi is a 35-year-old woman, pregnant with for the first time with twins. She attends the antenatal clinic for a routine appointment at 33 weeks' gestation.

On examination, Bibi's blood pressure is 154/100 mm/Hg and she has proteinuria.

- What would you ask Bibi to a gain greater understanding of the clinical situation?
- Does Bibi have other symptoms associated with pre-eclampsia?
- What would your plan of care be for Bibi?

Notes

- Bibi is pregnant for the first time and has a twin pregnancy, both of which are risk factors for developing pre-eclampsia.
- Bibi is hypertensive and has proteinuria, which are symptoms of pre-eclampsia.
- The midwife should ask Bibi whether she has experienced headaches, visual disturbance or other symptoms that she is concerned about.
- Explore Bibi's understanding of pre-eclampsia and explain what your concerns are in relation to her blood pressure and proteinuria.
- Refer Bibi for medical review the same day.

Fetal Growth Restriction

FGR is the term used to describe the growth of a fetus that does not reach its genetic growth potential. FGR is a leading cause of fetal and perinatal mortality and morbidity and is associated with premature birth (McIntyre et al. 1999). There is evidence to show that growth-restricted fetuses may be at higher risk of poorer long-term health outcomes as adults, including cardiovascular disease and diabetes. The Barker hypothesis of fetal programming states that the fetus adapts to a suboptimal intrauterine environment because of undernutrition, which causes disruption to metabolic controls and later-onset metabolic disease (Barker 1995).

Fetal growth is substantially influenced by the effectiveness of nutrient transfer from the maternal circulation to the fetus during pregnancy (see the earlier list of functions of the placenta), with growth being an important indicator of fetal health. Reduced placental blood flow results in impaired transport of oxygen and nutrients, which are required by the fetus to reach its optimum growth trajectory (growth potential). Less frequently, the ability of the fetus to utilise nutrients is affected by chromosomal or metabolic disorders, resulting in reduced fetal growth (Worton et al. 2014). Failure of trophoblastic invasion and spiral artery remodelling results in reduced uteroplacental blood flow (Lyall 2002); this is a factor in both FGR and the occurrence of pre-eclampsia.

Screening and Monitoring for Fetal Growth Restriction

Screening for FGR is undertaken by a thorough history taking and identification of risk factors during early pregnancy. Table 7.3 shows the classification of high and moderate risk factors relating to a woman's previous history and medical history.

Some factors that occur during pregnancy are also associated with an increased risk of FGR: fetal echogenic bowel identified by ultrasound scan, most commonly at the time of routine anomaly screening, significant maternal vaginal bleeding and a low level of pregnancy-associated plasma protein A (PAPP-A, <5th centile) detected through analysis of blood taken for the combined test for fetal trisomy screening. In the presence of one of more risk factors, fetal growth can be monitored by regular ultrasound scans performed every 2–4 weeks from 28 to 32 weeks' gestation to assess fetal growth trajectory and estimated fetal weight (NHS England 2023). Women who are not at increased risk of having a fetus that is growth restricted can be monitored during pregnancy by symphysis fundal height measurement, which should be plotted on a customised centile chart. This may be less accurate for women who are obese or have large fibroids.

131

Health Promotion

Mothers who smoke are more likely to deliver their babies early, have small for gestational age babies and have stillbirths. Babies of mothers who smoke are more likely to have respiratory issues and die from sudden infant death syndrome (SIDS). Specialised smoking cessation services are widely available, supporting referral of the mother and wider family members to encourage a smoke-free environment for pregnant women and families.

TABLE 7.3 Risk factors for fetal growth restriction (FGR).

High-risk factors	Moderate-risk factors
Chronic kidney disease	Previous small-for-gestational age (SGA) baby
Hypertension	Previous stillbirth (growth within normal parameters)
Autoimmune disease	Current smoker
Cyanotic congenital heart disease	Current drug misuse
Previous FGR baby	Maternal age >40 years
Hypertensive disease in a previous pregnancy	
Previous stillbirth (SGA)	

Learning Event

Reflect on your experience of discussing the effects of smoking with women and family.

- How can you introduce the use of carbon monoxide testing at booking and throughout pregnancy in a non-judgemental way?
- Are you confident in providing advice about smoking and referring women and family members to smoking cessation services?
- Do you have sufficient knowledge about ongoing care for women who smoke during pregnancy?

Placental Abruption

Placental abruption is a term used to describe the complete or partial separation of a normally situated placenta before birth. Placental abruption occurs in 0.4–1% of all pregnancies and it is a significant cause of maternal and perinatal morbidity and mortality (Tikkanen 2010). A woman with a placental abruption may present with vaginal bleeding, abdominal pain and uterine contractions or tenderness. Around 30% of cases of placenta abruption are described as 'concealed', where bleeding occurs but is contained behind the placenta (Tikkanen 2010). In this situation, women will show signs of hypovolaemic shock and abdominal pain without vaginal bleeding. A 'revealed' abruption will result in blood escaping from the placenta and draining through the cervix and out of the vagina. Figure 7.6 shows different sites for placental abruption.

Case Study 7.3

Sahra has attended the maternity assessment unit. She is pregnant with her third baby and is 37 weeks' gestation. She has had a straightforward pregnancy so far and the fetus is growing within the normal parameters. Sahra had a placental abruption during her first pregnancy.

Sahra is experiencing constant abdominal pain that appears to be severe. On palpation, her abdomen is tender, she is having tightenings and has fresh red vaginal bleeding.

- What should you consider in this case and what action should be taken?

Notes

- The symptoms that Sahra is exhibiting are indicative of placental abruption.
- Previous placental abruption is a risk factor for subsequent placental abruption.
- Measure Sahra's vital signs and be vigilant for signs of maternal shock.
- Ask Sahra about the presence of fetal movements and continuously monitor the fetal heart rate with a cardiotocograph (CTG) to identify fetal compromise.
- Seek urgent medical review.
- Explain the situation to Sahra and provide support.

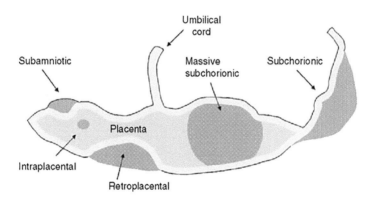

FIGURE 7.6 Sites of placental abruption.

Twin-to-Twin Transfusion Syndrome

Twin-to-twin transfusion syndrome (TTTS) results from rechannelling of the blood flow from one twin to another thorough abnormal vessel connections in the shared placenta. Therefore, TTTS only occurs in monochorionic twins, twins that share the placenta. This condition affects approximately 15% of all monochorionic twin pregnancies, with the most common onset between the 16th and 26th gestational weeks (Bamberg and Hecher 2019). As a result of abnormal shunting the twin with restricted blood supply, the donor twin, will become growth restricted and will attempt to spare vital organs such as the brain and heart by restricting flow to less important organs such as the kidneys, consequently developing oligohydramnios or anhydramnios. The recipient, the twin with an excess blood flow, develops circulatory overload, cardiac compromise and polyuria manifested as polyhydramnios.

If left untreated TTTS results in up to 80% mortality in both twins (Berghella and Kaufmann 2001). Long-term complications of TTTS include, but are not limited to, cardiac, renal and serious neurological morbidity. Women with TTTS may present with premature contractions, rapid increase in symphysis fundal height, rapid weight gain, breathlessness, abdominal tightness and a feeling of pressure in the abdomen due to polyhydramnios.

TTTS can be diagnosed during ultrasound examination by a discrepancy in the deepest vertical pocket (DVP) of amniotic fluid. Although variability due to gestational age should be considered, broadly speaking the diagnostic criteria for TTTS is met with a DVP in a donor's sac being ≤2 cm, while that in the recipient's sac is ≥8 cm (Khalil 2017).

Management options for TTTS include expectant management, amnioreduction (drainage of excess fluid), septostomy (rupture of the dividing membranes), laser ablation of abnormal vascular connections and selective fetal termination of one or termination of both twins (NICE 2006). Laser ablation is the technique of choice for the treatment of TTTS; it is performed under regional analgesia or local anaesthesia with maternal sedation by a trained fetal medicine specialist (see Figure 7.7). The survival rate post laser ablation is up to 65% for both twins and up to 88% for one of the twins (Miller 2021). The most common complications of the procedure are premature rupture of the membranes, placental abruption and fetal loss.

133

Red Flag

The development of TTTS should be considered in woman with a monochorionic twin pregnancy and symptoms of polyhydramnios. Signs include increased abdominal size, maternal breathlessness and discomfort.

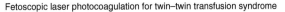

Fetoscopic laser photocoagulation for twin–twin transfusion syndrome

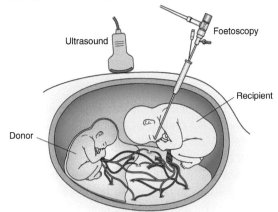

J of Obstet and Gynaecol, Volume: 44, Issue: 5, Pages: 831-839, First published: 13 February 2018, DOI: (10.1111/jog.13600)

FIGURE 7.7 A schematic representation of fetoscopic laser photocoagulation for twin-to-twin transfusion syndrome. A fetoscope is percutaneously inserted into the recipient sac through a cannula. Source: Reproduced by permission from Sago et al. (2018) / John Wiley & Sons.

Gestational Trophoblastic Disease

Gestational trophoblastic disease (GTD) represents a group of tumours formed by the trophoblastic cells. The most common type of tumour is a hydatidiform mole (molar pregnancy), an abnormal pregnancy due to the imbalance of chromosomal material. Molar pregnancies are rare (between 0.3% and 0.1%) and typically benign, but have a very small chance of becoming malignant (Makhseed et al. 1998). Risk factors for GTD include a history of molar pregnancy, spontaneous abortion, maternal age (<20 or >35 years) and ethnicity (Melamed et al. 2016).

There are two distinct types of molar pregnancy: partial and complete. Complete molar pregnancy is when the pregnancy lacks the maternal chromosomal component, with one or two sperm fertilising an egg lacking chromosomal material. Sperm cells then undergo mitosis and this results in a diploid set of cells (46XX or 46 XY). In the case of a complete molar pregnancy, an ultrasound examination will reveal grape-like clusters of tissue with no evidence of a developing fetus.

Fertilisation of a normal egg with two sperms result in a triploid (69, XXY) or tetraploid (92, XXXY) pregnancy – a partial mole. In the case of a partial molar pregnancy, an ultrasound examination can detect a fetus, but this condition results in early fetal demise.

Clinical presentation of a molar pregnancy can include abnormal vaginal bleeding in early pregnancy. Less common signs include a large-for-gestation uterus on palpation, hyperemesis, early-onset pre-eclampsia and hyperthyroidism. Due to an increased risk of malignancy, follow-up is required within a specialist unit (Tidy et al. 2021).

Preterm Prelabour Rupture of Membranes

Preterm prelabour rupture of membranes (PPROM) is defined as rupture of the fetal membranes before 37 completed weeks' gestation without signs of labour (Thomson et al. 2019). PPROM complicates up to 3% of pregnancies and is associated with 30–40% of preterm births (Thomson et al. 2019).

In women who present with PPROM, there is an increased risk of:

- Prematurity
- Sepsis
- Cord prolapse
- Pulmonary hypoplasia
- Chorioamnionitis
- Placental abruption

Diagnosis

PPROM is diagnosed by a woman's description of amniotic fluid loss vaginally and visualisation of amniotic fluid during sterile speculum examination. If amniotic fluid is not evident on speculum examination, the use of an insulin-like growth factor binding protein should be considered (IGFBP-1 or PAMG-1 if these tests are available) to determine whether the membranes have ruptured (Thomson et al. 2019).

Antibiotics are recommended for women who have PPROM until they are in established labour, to reduce the risk of chorioamnionitis. Corticosteroids and magnesium sulfate should be offered. Ongoing assessment should be implemented for women with PPROM, including clinical assessment for signs of infection, blood analysis to quantify white cell count and C-reactive protein and fetal heart rate monitoring. Expectant management until 37 weeks' gestation may be offered to women where this is not contra-indicated. Women and partners may require additional emotional support following PPROM due to the increased anxiety that can result.

Screening and Diagnostic Tests Relating to the Placenta

Chorionic Villus Sampling and Amniocentesis

Chorionic villus sampling (CVS), also referred to as chorionic villus biopsy (CVB), is a test where a small sample of the placenta is removed via a fine needle that is inserted into the uterus during pregnancy. This test is carried out from 11 weeks' gestation.

Amniocentesis is an invasive prenatal test that involves the removal of a small amount of amniotic fluid via a fine needle introduced through the uterus. This test can be performed from 15 weeks' gestation.

The chorion villus or amniotic fluid sample is taken for antenatal genetic testing, usually because of previous pregnancy outcome, family history or a suspicion of a fetal abnormality. The analysis of the sample provides information about the fetal chromosomes. Prenatal invasive tests are associated with an additional 1 in 200 chance of miscarriage (Navaratnam et al. 2022).

Imaging

In a context of placental pathology, ultrasound examinations are useful in the assessment of pregnancies when molar pregnancy is suspected, and for examination of placental localisation, cord insertion, fetal growth as well as maternal and fetal circulation (Doppler ultrasound). Although ultrasound examination is the imaging modality of choice in pregnancy, MRI examinations are extremely useful in assessment of invasive placentae and malignant neoplasms.

Human Chorionic Gonadotropin

Human chorionic gonadotropin (hCG) tests measure the beta subunit of the hCG specific to pregnancy. This is a hormone released by the trophoblastic cells and plays an important part in maternal recognition of the pregnancy. In normal pregnancy β-hCG level rise incrementally and reach the highest point at 9–12 weeks of gestation.

β-hCG tests can be done on urine or blood specimens and can be qualitative (positive or negative results) or quantitative (reporting number of international units within a given volume, e.g. 25 IU/l). Qualitative β-hCG tests are used to confirm pregnancy, while serial quantitative β-hCG tests could be used to help manage pregnancies of unknown locations, for management of molar pregnancies and for malignancies arising from the trophoblastic cells. Moreover, qualitative β-hCG is used in first- and second-trimester screening tests for Down's, Edwards' and Patau's syndromes, with higher levels of the hormone being associated with a higher chance of Down's syndrome, while lower levels of β-hCG are associated with a higher chance of Edwards' and Patau's syndromes. Possible reasons for false-positive results could include, but are not limited to, the use of hCG during fertility treatment and infections. False-negative results can be due to early testing or diluted samples.

Pregnancy-Associated Plasma Protein A

Pregnancy-associated plasma protein A (PAPP-A) is produced by the placenta, with its levels increasing rapidly during early pregnancy. Qualitative assessment of PAPP-A is performed as part of the first-trimester screening test for Down's, Edwards' and Patau's syndromes, also known as the combined test. Decreased levels of PAPP-A in the maternal blood in the first trimester in combination with high levels of β-hCG are associated with an increased chance of Down's, while decreased levels of PAPP-A in combination with reduced levels of β-hCG are associated with an increased chance of Edwards' and Patau's syndromes. Moreover, very low levels of PAPP-A could be associated with placental dysfunction and close surveillance of pregnancies with low PAPP-A may be recommended.

Placental Growth Factor

Placental growth factor (PlGF) is a key protein involved in angiogenesis, a process of remodelling and expansion of the vessels, which influences the feto-placental circulation and supports trophoblast growth. Low levels of PlGF are associated with abnormal placentation (Chau et al. 2017).

NICE recommends using PlGF-based testing alongside standard clinical assessment to rule or rule pre-eclampsia in or out in cases of suspected preterm (<37 weeks' gestation) pre-eclampsia (NICE 2022).

Conclusion

This chapter describes the most common placental pathologies that midwives may encounter during their clinical practice.

Take-Home Points

- Placental pathology results from various factors including underlying maternal conditions, iatrogenic factors and health behaviours.
- Placental pathology has an impact on the short- and long-term well-being of the woman, the fetus and the neonate, with increased risk of pregnancy loss and morbidity due to impaired fetal growth and premature birth.
- Effective maternity care involves early screening, application of preventative measures and monitoring during pregnancy.
- Multidisciplinary approaches to pregnancy care are key to achieving optimal pregnancy outcomes for pregnant women and their babies.

References

Abalos, E., Cuesta, C., Grosso, A.L. et al. (2013). Global and regional estimates of preeclampsia and eclampsia: a systematic review. *European Journal of Obstetrics, Gynecology, and Reproductive Biology* 170: 1–7.

Abheiden, C.N., Van Reuler, A.V., Fuijkschot, W.W. et al. (2016). Aspirin adherence during high-risk pregnancies, a questionnaire study. *Pregnancy Hypertension* 6: 350–355.

Bamberg, C. and Hecher, K. (2019). Update on twin-to-twin transfusion syndrome. *Best Practice and Research Clinical Obstetrics and Gynaecology* 58: 55–65.

Barker, D.J. (1995). Fetal origins of coronary heart disease. *BMJ* 311: 171–174.

Berghella, V. and Kaufmann, M. (2001). Natural history of twin-twin transfusion syndrome. *Journal of Reproductive Medicine* 46: 480–484.

Chau, K., Hennessy, A., and Makris, A. (2017). Placental growth factor and pre-eclampsia. *Journal of Human Hypertension* 31: 782–786.

Collins, S.L., Ashcroft, A., Braun, T. et al. (2016). Proposal for standardized ultrasound descriptors of abnormally invasive placenta (AIP). *Ultrasound in Obstetrics and Gynecology* 47: 271–275.

Henderson, J.T., Whitlock, E.P., O'Connor, E. et al. (2014). Low-dose aspirin for prevention of morbidity and mortality from preeclampsia: a systematic evidence review for the U.S. Preventive Services Task Force. *Annals of Internal Medicine* 160 (10): 695–703.

Hua, M., Odibo, A.O., Macones, G.A. et al. (2010). Single umbilical artery and its associated findings. *Obstetrics and Gynecology* 115: 930–934.

Jauniaux, E., Collins, S., and Burton, G.J. (2018). Placenta accreta spectrum: pathophysiology and evidence-based anatomy for prenatal ultrasound imaging. *American Journal of Obstetrics and Gynecology* 218: 75–87.

Khalil, A. (2017). Modified diagnostic criteria for twin-to-twin transfusion syndrome prior to 18 weeks' gestation: time to change? *Ultrasound in Obstetrics & Gynecology* 49: 804–805.

Lyall, F. (2002). The human placental bed revisited. *Placenta* 23: 555–562.

Makhseed, M., Al-Sharhan, M., Egbase, P. et al. (1998). Maternal and perinatal outcomes of multiple pregnancy following IVF-ET. *International Journal of Gynecology and Obstetrics* 61: 155–163.

McIntire, D.D., Bloom, S.L., Casey, B.M., and Leveno, K.J. (1999). Birth weight in relation to morbidity and mortality among newborn infants. *New England Journal of Medicine* 340: 1234–1238.

Melamed, A., Gockley, A., Joseph, N. et al. (2016). Effect of race/ethnicity on risk of complete and partial molar pregnancy after adjustment for age. *Gynecologic Oncology* 143: 73–76.

Miller, J.L. (2021). Twin to twin transfusion syndrome. *Translational Pediatrics* 10: 1518–1529.

National Institute for Health and Care Excellence (NICE) (2006). Intrauterine laser ablation of placental vessels for the treatment of twin-to-twin transfusion syndrome. Interventional procedures guidance IPG198. https://www.nice.org.uk/guidance/ipg198 (accessed November 2023).

National Institute for Health and Care Excellence (NICE) (2019). Hypertension in pregnancy: diagnosis and management. NICE guideline NG133. https://www.nice.org.uk/guidance/ng133 (accessed November 2023).

National Institute for Health and Care Excellence (NICE) (2021). *Antenatal Care*. NICE Guideline NG201. https://www.nice.org.uk/guidance/ng201/chapter/Recommendations (accessed November 2023).

National Institute for Health and Care Excellence (NICE) (2022). PLGF-based testing to help diagnose suspected preterm pre-eclampsia. Diagnostic guidance DG42. https://www.nice.org.uk/guidance/dg49 (accessed November 2023).

Navaratnam, K., Alfirevic, Z., and Royal College of Obstetricians and Gynaecologists (2022). Amniocentesis and chorionic villus sampling. *BJOG* 129: e1–e15.

NHS England (2023). Saving babies' lives version three. https://www.england.nhs.uk/publication/saving-babies-lives-version-three (accessed November 2023).

Oyelese, Y., Lees, C.C., and Jauniaux, E. (2023). The case for screening for vasa previa: time to implement a life-saving strategy. *Ultrasound in Obstetrics & Gynecology* 61: 7–11.

Rolnik, D.L., Wright, D., Poon, L.C. et al. (2017). Aspirin versus placebo in pregnancies at high risk for preterm preeclampsia. *New England Journal of Medicine* 377: 613–622.

Royal College of Obstetricians and Gynaecologists (RCOG) (2011). *Antepartum Haemorrhage*. Green-top Guideline No. 63. https://www.rcog.org.uk/guidance/browse-all-guidance/green-top-guidelines/antepartum-haemorrhage-green-top-guideline-no-63 (accessed November 2023).

Sago, H., Ishii, K., Sugibayashi, R. et al. (2018). Fetoscopic laser photocoagulation for twin–twin transfusion syndrome. *Journal of Obstetrics and Gynaecology Research* 44: 831–839.

Sepulveda, W. (2006). Velamentous insertion of the umbilical cord: a first-trimester sonographic screening study. *Journal of Ultrasound in Medicine* 25 (8): 963–968.

Shaikh, N., Nahid, S., Ummunnisa, F. et al. (2021). Preeclampsia: from etiopathology to organ dysfunction. In: *Preeclampsia* (ed. H. Abduljabbar). London: IntechOpen, ch. 4. https://doi.org/10.5772/intechopen.101240.

Silver, R.M. (2015). Abnormal placentation: placenta previa, vasa previa, and placenta accreta. *Obstetrics and Gynecology* 126: 654–668.

Suzuki, S. and Igarashi, M. (2008). Clinical significance of pregnancies with succenturiate lobes of placenta. *Archives of Gynecology and Obstetrics* 277: 299–301.

Thilaganathan, B. and Kalafat, E. (2019). Cardiovascular system in preeclampsia and beyond. *Hypertension* 73: 522–531.

Thomson, A. and Royal College of Obstetricians and Gynaecologists (2019). Care of women presenting with suspected preterm prelabour rupture of membranes from 24+0 weeks of gestation. *BJOG* 126: e152–e166.

Tidy, J., Seckl, M., Hancock, B.W., and On behalf of the Royal College of Obstetricians and Gynaecologists (2021). Management of Gestational Trophoblastic Disease. *BJOG* 128: e1–e27.

Tikkanen, M. (2010). Etiology, clinical manifestations, and prediction of placental abruption. *Acta Obstetricia et Gynecologica Scandinavica* 89: 732–740.

Tol, I.D., Yousif, M., and Collins, S.L. (2019). Post traumatic stress disorder (PTSD): the psychological sequelae of abnormally invasive placenta (AIP). *Placenta* 81: 42–45.

Vafaei, H., Rafeei, K., Dalili, M. et al. (2021). Prevalence of single umbilical artery, clinical outcomes and its risk factors: a cross-sectional study. *International Journal of Reproductive BioMedicine* 19: 441–448.

Varlas, V.N., Bors, R.G., Birsanu, S. et al. (2021). Maternal and fetal outcome in placenta accreta spectrum (PAS) associated with placenta previa: a retrospective analysis from a tertiary center. *Journal of Medicine and Life* 14: 367–375.

Worton, S.A., Sibley, C.P., and Heazell, A.E.P. (2014). Understanding placental aetiology of fetal growth restriction; could this lead to personalized management strategies? *Fetal and Maternal Medicine Review* 25: 95–116.

137

Further Resources

Royal College of Midwives: About Us. https://www.rcm.org.uk/about-us (accessed January 2024).
Royal College of Obstetricians and Gynaecologists: Home. https://www.rcog.org.uk/ (accessed January 2024).

Glossary

Amniocentesis	A medical procedure during pregnancy where a small amount of amniotic fluid is withdrawn from the amniotic sac surrounding the developing fetus. This fluid contains cells from the baby, and it can be analysed to detect certain genetic conditions or chromosomal abnormalities
Amnioreduction	A medical procedure in which the amount of amniotic fluid around a developing fetus in the womb is reduced. This is typically done to manage conditions such as polyhydramnios, where there is an excessive accumulation of amniotic fluid
Amniotic fluid	The fluid that surrounds and cushions the fetus within the amniotic sac, protecting it from external impacts
Amniotic sac	The membranous sac that encloses the fetus and contains amniotic fluid
Battledore Cord Insertion	The attachment of the umbilical cord to the edge or margin of the placenta, rather than at its centre
Chorioamnionitis	A condition where the protective layers around the baby during pregnancy become infected or inflamed
Chorion	The outermost membrane surrounding the embryo or fetus, which later forms part of the placenta
Chorionic Villus Sampling	A medical test during pregnancy where a small sample of tissue from the placenta (chorionic villi) is taken to check for certain genetic conditions in the developing baby
Cytotrophoblast	A layer of cells in the placental villi that supports the growth and maintenance of the syncytiotrophoblast
Decidua	The uterine lining that undergoes changes during pregnancy to support the placenta's development and function
Disseminated Intravascular Coagulation	A serious medical condition where there is widespread activation of blood clotting throughout the body
Down's Syndrome	A condition that happens when a person has an extra copy of chromosome 21
Echogenic	Terms, "echogenic" refers to the ability of a tissue to produce echoes in ultrasound imaging. If something is echogenic, it means it can reflect or bounce back ultrasound waves, making it visibly brighter on the ultrasound screen
Edwards Syndrome	Is a condition that happens when a person has an extra copy of chromosome 18
Embryo	The early stage of development after fertilisation, before the fetus is recognisable
Exsanguination	The process of bleeding to death
Fetal blood	Blood from the fetus that circulates within the placenta, allowing the exchange of nutrients, oxygen and waste products with maternal blood

Fibroid	A non-cancerous tumour that grows in the wall of the uterus (womb). It is made up of muscle and fibrous tissue and is also known as uterine fibroma or myoma
Haemolysis	A process of destruction of red blood cells, releasing their contents, including haemoglobin, into the surrounding fluid
Human chorionic gonadotrophin (hCG)	A hormone produced by the placenta shortly after implantation that is detected in pregnancy tests and helps maintain the uterine lining during early pregnancy
Hydatidiform Mole	An abnormal form of pregnancy. Instead of developing into a normal fetus, the cells form a mass or tumour
Hyperemesis	Severe and persistent vomiting during pregnancy
Hyperthyroidism	A medical condition where the thyroid gland produces too much thyroid hormone
Hypovolaemic shock	A serious condition when a person's body doesn't have enough blood volume to function properly. This can happen due to severe bleeding, dehydration, or fluid loss, leading to a drop in blood pressure and inadequate oxygen supply to the body's organs
Iatrogenic	Health issues or problems that are unintentionally caused by medical treatment or procedures
Karyotyping	A process of arranging and analysing the chromosomes to understand their overall pattern and identify any potential issues
Maternal blood	Blood from the mother that circulates through the placenta, allowing nutrient and gas exchange with fetal blood
Oliguria	A reduced amount of urine production
Patau's Syndrome	A condition that happens when a person has an extra copy of chromosome 13
Perfusion	A process of blood flowing through the tissues
Placenta accreta	A condition where the placenta attaches too deeply to the uterine wall, potentially causing difficulties during delivery and requiring special medical attention
Placenta increta	A more severe form of placenta accreta where the placenta grows even more deeply into the uterine wall
Placenta percreta	The most severe form of placenta accreta, where the placenta grows through the uterine wall and can even invade nearby organs
Placenta previa	A condition in which the placenta partially or fully covers the cervix, which can cause bleeding and complications during childbirth
Placental abruption	A serious condition in which the placenta separates from the uterine wall before delivery, potentially causing bleeding and endangering the fetus
Placental barrier	The protective barrier formed by the syncytiotrophoblast that separates maternal and fetal blood
Placental Growth Factor	A protein that plays a crucial role in the growth and development of blood vessels, particularly those in the placenta during pregnancy
Placental villi	Finger-like projections on the surface of the placenta that increase its surface area for nutrient exchange
Pregnancy-associated Protein A	Another protein that plays a role in the development of the placenta and is often used as a marker in prenatal screening tests to assess the health of the fetus
Pulmonary Hypoplasia	A condition where the lungs are underdeveloped or smaller than normal. This can lead to difficulties in breathing and other respiratory problems
Septostomy	A medical procedure that involves making an opening or hole in a structure called the septum
Stroke	A stroke occurs when the blood supply to part of the brain is cut off or reduced, usually due to a blood clot or a burst blood vessel

Succenturiate lobe	An addition lobe also called an accessory placental lobe
Syncytiotrophoblast	A layer of the placental villi responsible for hormone production and nutrient exchange between maternal and fetal blood
Vasa Praevia	A condition where the blood vessels from the umbilical cord or placenta cross the entrance to the birth canal, making them vulnerable to rupture if the water breaks or labour begins
Vasoconstriction	Narrowing of blood vessels
Velamentous Cord Insertion	A condition where the umbilical cord, which connects the baby to the placenta, is not attached directly to the centre of the placenta

CHAPTER 8

Inflammation and the Immune Response

Claire Ford and Claire Leader

Department of Nursing, Midwifery and Health, Northumbria University, Newcastle upon Tyne, UK

AIM

This chapter aims to support midwifery practice by providing the reader with information about the pathophysiology associated with inflammation and the immune response and how it changes and reacts during pregnancy, birth and the postnatal period.

LEARNING OUTCOMES

On completion of this chapter the reader will be able to:

- Have an awareness of the pathophysiology associated with inflammation and the immune response and how this can affect women during the perinatal journey.
- Appreciate the importance of understanding the underpinning evidence associated with the immune response, particularly during and after a traumatic delivery.
- Have a greater awareness of the importance of respecting individual choice and the need to provide individualised, woman-centred care.

Test Your Prior Knowledge

1. What do you already know about the physiology of the immune system?
2. What is the difference between innate and adaptive immunity?
3. How can inflammation be triggered in women during the perinatal journey?
4. Name as many autoimmune conditions as you can and indicate how these differ from one another.
5. What impacts can an altered immune response have on a women's well-being?

Fundamentals of Maternal Pathophysiology, First Edition. Edited by Claire Leader and Ian Peate.
© 2024 John Wiley & Sons Ltd. Published 2024 by John Wiley & Sons Ltd.
Companion website: www.wiley.com/go/leader/maternalpatho

Immunity is the ability of the body to mount a response to resist damage or disease from harmful agents found in internal or external environments. In pregnancy, some of these immune responses are reduced to prevent rejection of the placental and fetal tissue, which would otherwise be considered 'foreign'. This process can lead to an increased susceptibility to some invading antigens, such as viruses. However, the body during pregnancy also has the ability to enhance other defences to protect itself against antigens, such as bacteria, in order to ensure a safe environment for the growing fetus (Coad et al. 2020). In this chapter we explore how the immune system protects the body from disease and outline some of the potential disease processes that occur, with specific discussions on the impact of this in pregnancy when some of these immune responses are dysfunctional.

The Immune System

The immune system is formed by a collection of organs, cells, enzymes and proteins, and functions that provide external and internal physical and chemical barriers that protect the individual from invading microorganisms. Pathogenic microbes are disease-producing microbes that include viruses, bacteria and fungi (Delves et al. 2017). These are a constant source of invasion both internally and on the body's surface and are found in our environment in soil, water, air and food.

Due to the abundant presence of microorganisms in our daily lives, the intricate interplay of the many components of the immune system is thus constantly working to protect the body, making it resistant to these pathogens by mounting an immune response. This defence occurs in two ways, either innate or adaptive immunity. Innate refers to the immunity already present in the body, which acts as an early warning system, seeking to prevent harmful microbes from entering the body and eliminating those that do enter through physical and chemical barriers such as the skin and mucous membranes, natural killer cells, inflammation and fever (Coad et al. 2020). Adaptive immunity refers to how the body responds (or adapts) to a specific microbe through white blood cells, T cells and B cells (Tortora and Derrickson 2017).

Woman-Centred Care

During pregnancy, the immune response is altered to protect the fetus from being rejected as toxic or foreign tissue (antigen). While there are clear benefits to this process for the maintenance of the pregnancy, it can sometimes place the mother at greater risk of infection as well as potentially exacerbating pre-existing autoimmune disease. Consequently, midwives and other health professionals need to have an understanding of the key ways in which the immune system will be affected by pregnancy and the impacts this can have on existing co-morbidities and disease processes.

Types of Immunity

Innate (or Non-specific) Immunity

Innate immunity refers to the pre-existing defence mechanisms present from birth. Innate immunity does not target specific pathogens but provides an overall first line of defence in the form of physical and chemical barriers and a second line of defence through chemical and cellular defences (Tortora and Derrickson 2017; Patton and Thibodeau 2018). It is important to remember that there will be a high level of interdependence between these categories. See Table 8.1 for an outline of the first and second lines of defence.

TABLE 8.1 First and second lines of defence.

First line	Surface membrane barriers	Skin and mucous membranes In pregnancy: • Placenta • Placental membranes • Vernix
Second line	Cellular and chemical defences	Inflammation Pyrexia Compliment Phagocytosis Acidic secretions (vaginal, gastric, urine) Mucus Cilia Saliva Tears In pregnancy: • Amniotic fluid • Mucous plug • Accumulation of immune cells in the endometrium • Human chorionic gonadotrophin (hCG) stimulates neutrophil production • Cervical mucoid plug Postpartum: • Colostrum • Breast milk

143

Expert Midwife

Encouraging breastfeeding from birth will help prevent infections by transferring immunoglobulins that are passed on from the mother, coating the intestines and preventing pathogens from entering the circulation. Leucocytes found in human milk will also work to surround and destroy harmful bacteria through phagocytosis. Additional mechanisms involving lactoferrin provide bactericidal protection and bifidus factor promotes healthy gut flora. These defences protect the infant from a range of infections including prolonged diarrhoea, otitis media, urinary tract infections, neonatal necrotising enterocolitis and septicaemia (Hanson 1998) and inflammatory conditions such as asthma and allergies (El-Heneidy et al. 2018). There is also evidence that these benefits last for years after lactation (Hanson 1998).

Stacey, Midwife

First-Line Defence: Skin and Mucous Membranes

The skin is the largest organ in the human body with a surface area of approximately 1.5–2 m² in adults (Waugh and Grant 2018). The outer layer of the skin, the epidermis, prevents invasion by microorganisms by creating a physical barrier to the external environment, as well as producing sweat that provides an additional chemical barrier. The inner layer of the skin (the dermis) contains cells such as mast cells that serve as immune protection in collaboration with blood vessels, lymphatic vessels, sweat glands and nerves to prevent the colonisation of bacteria.

There are weaknesses within this mechanism created by the potential portals of entry, which include the orifices (mouth, nose, ears, vagina, anus and eyes). Here the mucous membranes provide an extra layer of protection by coating these passageways between the organs and the outside world. Additionally, mechanisms such as nose hair and cilia in the respiratory system move any foreign material through coughing or sneezing. The risk of ascending infections in the bladder and uterus is minimised by ensuring a one-way flow of urine and the presence of acidic secretions in the vagina, discouraging microbial growth (Boore et al. 2021).

In pregnancy, the placental barrier keeps the maternal and fetal circulatory systems separate and only certain antibodies can cross the placenta to provide passive immunity to the fetus. Intact placental membranes also directly protect the fetus from bacterial and viral pathogens; however, if these membranes are ruptured, the physical barrier is disrupted, making the fetus (and the woman) susceptible to infection (Macdonald and Johnson 2017). Liquor (amniotic fluid) contains properties that additionally protect the fetus from bacterial growth and the skin of the fetus is also coated in a protective layer of a thick, greasy substance called vernix caseosa. This substance is made up of fatty acids, water and proteins and, as it is slightly acidic, prevents bacterial colonisation. The fetus is also protected from ascending infection from the vaginal passage by the thick mucoid plug in the cervix containing antimicrobial proteins.

Examination Scenario

When performing vaginal examinations (VEs) to assess the progress of labour, midwives must ensure that rigorous hand hygiene practices are followed, including hand washing and the use of sterile gloves (Ford and Park 2018). As the frequency of VEs increases, so do the risks associated with infection such as chorioamnionitis, intrapartum fever, puerperal infection, neonatal sepsis and a longer stay in hospital (Downe et al. 2013; Başgöl and Beji 2015; Christopher et al. 2019). Midwives must therefore follow local and national guidance, limiting invasive VEs where possible to prevent infections from occurring.

Second-Line Defence

When microbes manage to penetrate the physical and chemical barriers that make up the first line of defence, the body has an innate second line of defence in the form of cells, inflammation and fever.

Cells of the Immune System

The innate system, the immunity that is present from birth, includes certain blood cells, namely leucocytes (white blood cells) and thrombocytes (platelets) (Vickers 2017). The white cells involved are the following:

- **Neutrophils:** These are the most common type of leucocyte, accounting for 50% of all white cells (Rankin 2017). They are chemically attracted to inflammation and will destroy bacteria and some fungi.
- **Eosinophils:** These make up between 1% and 4% of white cells and primarily attack parasitic worms, as well as assisting with the allergic response and tissue inflammation (Boore et al. 2021).
- **Basophils:** These are the rarest, accounting for less than 0.5% of white blood cells, and have a pale nucleus (Tortora and Derrickson 2017). They provide histamine as part of the inflammatory response and draw other white blood cells to the site of inflammation.
- **Mast cells:** These produce histamine, cytokine and chemotactic factors and are present in connective tissue (Devles et al. 2017).

During pregnancy, the white cell count will increase by 36% between 8 and 40 weeks' gestation. This is mainly due to an increased neutrophil count, which rises during ovulation and continues to rise if fertilisation occurs. There will be another significant elevation immediately post delivery (similar levels are found whether vaginal or operative delivery), which then drops to pre-labour levels within 7 days and returns to pre-pregnancy levels at around 21 days (Dockree et al. 2021). This increase is a physiological adaptation to pregnancy and birth, ensuring that the immune system is prepared to resist any antigens and to aid in repair.

Natural Killer Cells and Phagocytes

Natural killer (NK) cells are lymphocytes that are found in the blood, spleen, lymph nodes and red bone marrow. They are cytotoxic, which means they are able to kill a wide variety of infected cells as well as some tumour cells. They do so by identifying any plasma membrane proteins that they recognise as abnormal; consequently, these cells play a key role in immunity by mediating anti-tumour and anti-viral responses. During pregnancy, the number of NK cells is lowered, in order to reduce the risk of rejection of the developing embryo (Coad et al. 2020).

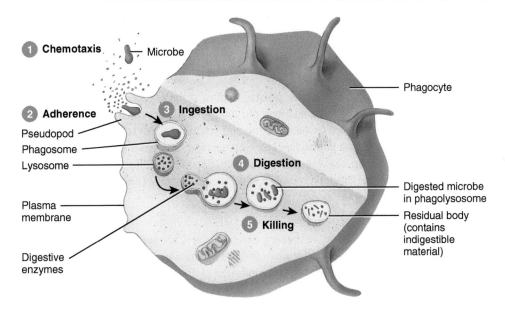

FIGURE 8.1 Phases of phagocytosis. Source: Reproduced by permission from Tortora and Derrickson (2017) / John Wiley & Sons.

Phagocytes are specialised cells that perform a process known as phagocytosis, the main phagocytes being macrophages (giant eaters) and neutrophils. Within an hour of the inflammatory process commencing, wandering macrophages form from monocytes that migrate through tissue spaces to the infected area, enlarging to ingest unwanted microorganisms such as bacteria, some viruses and dead or dying cells (Patton and Thibodeau 2018). They in turn stimulate other phagocytic cells, neutrophils and eosinophils to release enzymes that support the breakdown of the ingested microorganism. Fixed macrophages protect the organs by ingesting microbes or other cellular debris and these are found in connective tissue (histiocytes), the liver (Kupffer cells), the lungs (alveolar macrophages), the nervous system (microglial cells), the spleen, lymph nodes and red bone marrow (tissue macrophages). Figure 8.1 illustrates the process of phagocytosis.

Cell-mediated immunity in pregnancy is depressed by the production of oestrogen, human chorionic gonadotropin (hCG) from the placenta and the hormone prolactin. There is also a range of other complex cellular and hormonal processes occurring more widely within the uterus and placenta that are essential for ensuring that the fetus is not rejected. However, there is also a complex interplay between these mechanisms that adapt to the pregnant state and provide some continued immunity for the woman and the fetus.

Learning Event

While it is important to consider the risks to both the mother and the fetus from possible microorganisms, it is imperative that women are actively encouraged to engage in normal life. Controversy currently exists around claims that pregnancy leaves women immunocompromised, as the body naturally increases some of the first and second lines of defence to higher levels than would be found pre-pregnancy to protect both woman and fetus. As such, the term immunomodification or immunomodulation should be used when discussing immunity, to ensure that women are not restricted or prevented from socialising, working and taking part in some activities and events. Any advice provided should therefore be tailored to the individual woman's needs and take into account aspects of her life that may increase potential risk, while minimising the restrictions to her normal daily activities.

The Inflammatory Response

Inflammation is one of the body's second lines of defence. It emerges as a result of tissue injury caused by trauma or invasion by microorganisms and, while symptoms are unpleasant, aims to prevent the spread of harmful agents, dispose of the killed pathogens and cell debris and prepare the body for repair. Inflammation is characterised by four classic signs (Vickers 2017):

145

- Swelling (oedema)
- Pain
- Heat
- Redness (erythema)

A number of chemicals such as histamine, kinins, prostaglandins, complement and lymphokines are released by injured cells, phagocytes, lymphocytes, mast cells and blood proteins. This process causes vasodilation of localised small blood vessels, which accounts for the heat and redness (Patton and Thibodeau 2018). Capillary walls become more permeable, allowing a fluid exudate containing antibodies and clotting factors to enter the tissues, causing swelling and oedema. Pus is formed where the infection is severe, to create a collection of dead cells, microbes and phagocytes as well as fibrin and inflammation exudate at the site. Pain is caused when the localised swelling compresses the sensory nerves.

Pyrexia

Pyrexia is commonly defined as a body temperature that is greater than 38°C and is a response to the release of chemicals called pyrogens, which are secreted by macrophages when there is an invasion by microorganisms (Boore et al. 2021). The raised body temperature is thought to increase the metabolic rate of tissue, increasing the speed of defensive actions to aid repair. Mild to moderate fevers are helpful to this process; however, extremely high temperatures have a disrupting effect on these cellular and metabolic processes. Additionally, high temperatures can be extremely uncomfortable and anti-pyretics should always be considered. Table 8.2 outlines the grades of pyrexia.

The Complement System

The complement system consists of more than 30 proteins produced by the liver that circulate in the blood plasma and body tissues. When activated they destroy microbes by causing phagocytosis and increasing the inflammatory response (Tortora and Derrickson 2017). These steps, known as the complement cascade, facilitate the search and removal of antigens through the following steps:

- Binding to the blood vessels to increase permeability.
- Tagging pathogens for elimination by phagocytes (opsonisation).
- Attacking the pathogen's cell membrane, creating holes and causing its degeneration.
- Promoting inflammation.

Specific or Adaptive Immunity

Adaptive immunity is the body's defence against specific antigens that have leaked through the body's first lines of defence. It does this using two different mechanisms and lymphocytes referred to as B and T cells:

TABLE 8.2   Grades of pyrexia.

Low-grade pyrexia	Moderate- to high-grade pyrexia	Hyperpyrexia
Temperature normal–38°C	Temperature 38–40°C	Temperature: 40°C and above
This is indicative of an inflammatory response most likely caused by a mild infection, allergic reaction, minor trauma or surgery	Most likely caused by a wound, urinary tract or respiratory infection	This can occur with excessive environmental temperatures, damage to the hypothalamus or bacteraemia

Source: Reproduced by permission from Lister et al. (2020) / John Wiley & Sons.

TABLE 8.3 Types of antibodies.

Antibody	Function
IgG	The most common and the one that lives the longest It provides the majority of antibody-mediated immunity due to the wide range of pathogens it attacks IgG crosses the placenta to give temporary passive immunity to the fetus
IgA	Prevents antigens from crossing the epithelium Found in mucosal areas such as the gut, respiratory and urogenital tract and bodily secretions such as saliva, tears and breast milk and colostrum Important in preventing neonatal gut infections in babies who are breastfed
IgE	Found on the cell membrane of mast cells and basophils, often binds to antigens that can trigger allergic reactions by releasing histamine
IgM	The principal antibody is produced in an initial response to an antigen and activates the complement system
IgD	Little is known about this antibody except that it is found on the cell surface of B cells and acts as an antigen receptor

Source: Reproduced by permission from Coad et al. (2020) / Elsevier.

TABLE 8.4 Types of acquired immunity.

	Natural	Artificial
Active	Having a disease or infection stimulates the body to make antibodies	Short- or long-term immunity in response to having a dead or live vaccine
Passive	Short-term immunity acquired from the mother via the placenta or breast milk	Immunity from ready-made antibodies in donor human or animal serum

- **Cell-mediated immunity**, which involves cytotoxic T cells attacking antigens. This form of immunity is particularly effective against intracellular pathogens such as bacteria, viruses and fungi, as well as cancer cells and foreign tissue transplants. As well as cytotoxic T cells, there are also helper T cells, which are also known as CD4 cells as their plasma membrane contains a protein called CD4, and these are effectors of antiviral immunity.
- **Antibody-mediated immunity**, which involves B cells transforming into plasma cells, which then secrete proteins called antibodies. These work mainly against extracellular pathogens such as viruses, bacteria and fungi that are found in body fluids outside the cells. There are five main types of antibodies (see Table 8.3).

These two types of immunity work very well together as many pathogens are found in both intracellular and extracellular spaces. Further, the body adapts by memorising the antigen for future attacks and a healthy immune system can memorise millions of different antigens, producing both short- and long-term protection (Delves et al. 2017). Acquired immunity can be either **passive** or **active** as well as **naturally** or **artificially** acquired (see Table 8.4).

The Lymphatic System

The lymphatic system is the section of the body where the immune response takes place. It consists of organs and cells that serve to protect the body from invading pathogens and can be divided into the primary and the peripheral lymphoid organs. The primary system is where T cells and B cells mature, and this consists of the bone marrow and the thymus gland. The peripheral (or secondary) system includes the spleen, tonsils and lymph nodes (Vickers 2017). While the lymphatic system has other functions within the body, we will focus here on its role in the immune response.

- **The thymus** is situated between the sternum and the aorta, anterior to the top of the heart (Tortora and Derrickson 2017) (see Figure 8.2). Immature T cells migrate from the red bone marrow to the thymus to mature. A proportion of these mature T cells continually migrate from the thymus into the blood, spleen and lymph nodes, where they play a major role in the body's adaptive immune response. The size of the thymus reduces with age, changing into fatty tissue post adolescence when most of the body's T cells have matured.
- **The spleen** is an oval-shaped, highly vascular organ situated in the upper left side of the abdomen, behind the ribs and next to the stomach (see Figure 8.3). The primary function of the spleen is to act as a filter for the blood, bringing it into close contact with scavenging phagocytes and lymphocytes to remove unwanted pathogens.
- **Lymph nodes** are found in clusters around the body. They vary in size and shape, but are typically small, bean-shaped structures (see Figure 8.4). Antigens entering the body are swept along the lymphatic vessels and enter the lymph nodes along with any bacteria, dead or worn-out cells and inhaled particles. The nodes contain fixed macrophages, which detect and destroy pathogens and have a role in the adaptive immune system.

There are some instances when the immune system overreacts, resulting in allergic or hypersensitive reactions and autoimmune disorders, or fails in its primary functions, leading to immunodeficiency and increased susceptibility to microorganism-related illnesses (Norris et al. 2022) (see Table 8.5). Delves et al. (2017) claim that for autoimmune diseases a direct relationship exists between sex and hormones as more than 75% of these disorders occur in women, particularly during the childbearing years. When caring for women during the perinatal care continuum, it is therefore essential that midwifery students understand both primary and secondary immunodeficiency disorders as well as conditions that arise from an overactive immune system, since women with existing disorders may find that their condition improves or deteriorates, or they may develop new immune system dysfunctions or pass these to their unborn child (Coad et al. 2020).

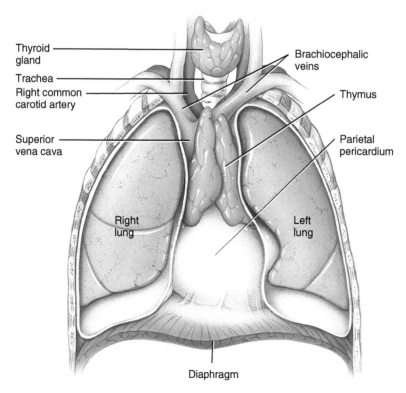

Thymus of adolescent

FIGURE 8.2   Anatomical position of the thymus.

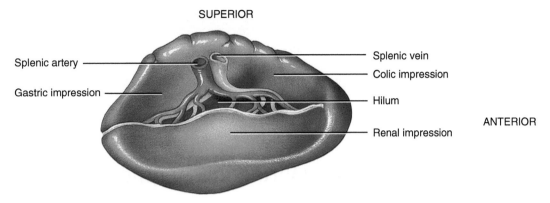

SUPERIOR

Splenic artery

Gastric impression

Splenic vein
Colic impression

Hilum

ANTERIOR

Renal impression

FIGURE 8.3 Structure of the spleen. Source: Reproduced by permission from Tortora and Derrickson (2017) / John Wiley & Sons.

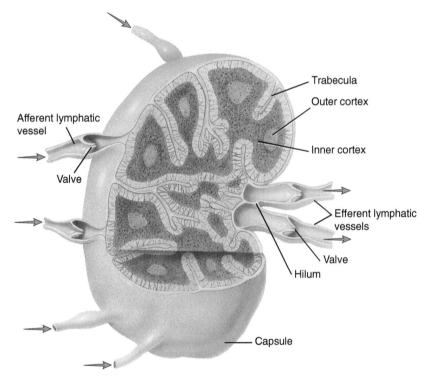

Trabecula
Outer cortex

Afferent lymphatic
vessel

Inner cortex

Valve

Efferent lymphatic
vessels

Valve
Hilum

Capsule

FIGURE 8.4 Structure of lymph nodes.

TABLE 8.5 Disorders of the immune system.

Hypersensitivity	Autoimmunity	Immunodeficiency
Levels vary based on the delay between exposure and the reaction	Antibodies attack self-antigens resulting in trauma to tissue and cells	This results in an impaired ability to react to microbes and increases risk of infection and death
Ranges from the most severe type I to type IV	Examples include rheumatoid arthritis, diabetes, Graves' disease, Addison's disease, coeliac disease, pernicious anaemia, Hashimoto's thyroiditis	Two types: primary (congenital) and secondary (acquired)
Examples include anaphylaxis, hay fever, asthma, dermatitis, rhinitis, Goodpasture's syndrome and haemolytic disease of the newborn		Examples include acquired immune deficiency syndrome (AIDS) and leucocyte adhesion deficiency

Learning Event

While endometriosis is not classified as an autoimmune condition, it is a chronic inflammatory condition and may increase the risk of developing an autoimmune disease. Therefore, it is paramount that women's reports of this condition are thoroughly investigated to find the origin. Due to the variety of symptoms, it may also be necessary to adopt a multidisciplinary and multimodal-tailored approach to manage their symptoms effectively.

Source: Adapted from WHO (2022).

Human Immunodeficiency Virus and Acquired Immunodeficiency Syndrome

Acquired immunodeficiency syndrome (AIDS) is a disease caused by the human immunodeficiency virus (HIV), which is a retrovirus that has the ability to infect body cells that have a protein CD4 receptor in their membrane (i.e. helper T cells). It is transmitted through bodily fluids such as blood, semen, vaginal fluids and breast milk (Waugh and Grant 2018). Globally, by the end of 2021, 38.4 million people were found to be living with HIV and 650 000 individuals had lost their lives to HIV-related causes (WHO 2023). The most common means of transmission in women in the United Kingdom are through sexual intercourse and contaminated blood via the sharing of intravenous drug needles or blood products; however, due to the implementation of screening programmes, there has been a significant decrease in the incidence of contaminated medical blood products in wealthier countries (Delves et al. 2017).

Symptoms in the early stages of contracting HIV include those associated with acute viremias such as sore throat, fever, headache and swollen lymph glands and these symptoms will normally last one to four weeks. During this period the levels of CD4 cells in the stomach rapidly reduce before the rate of loss slows. Most individuals then experience a period of latency lasting between 2 and 15 years, where the reduction of CD4 cells continues to decline; however, in pregnancy the progression to symptom development can be accelerated (Coad et al. 2020). Eventually, the levels become so low, and the immune system so compromised, that the individual begins to suffer from a variety of infections such as pneumonia, meningitis, cellulitis and so on due to the inability to fight invading pathogens. AIDS is officially diagnosed when the CD4 cell count falls below 200 cells/ml.

Orange Flag: HIV, Stigma and Discrimination

Unfortunately, despite an abundance of information about the disease and how it is transmitted and treated, individuals' well-being and lives are still being negatively impacted by stigma and discrimination. Social rejection, loss of employment and verbal abuse continue to be prevalent in today's society. Globally it is reported that 21% of people living with HIV were denied healthcare services and 47 countries maintain strict travel restrictions for individuals with HIV.

Source: Adapted from UNAIDS (2021)

Health Promotion

What is important to state at this juncture is that while HIV is a well-known disease, there is no known cure and individuals with the virus are infectious even when asymptomatic. In addition, pregnancy can mask some symptoms of HIV, such as fatigue and anaemia; therefore, women may not know they have HIV until they undergo routine blood screening during the antenatal period and they can transmit the virus to their unborn fetus in utero, or to the baby during birth or breastfeeding. However, treatment with antiretroviral therapy during pregnancy, for the mother and the newborn infant, can decrease perinatal transmission. Antivirals such as azidothymidine and ritonavir block HIV's ability to reproduce and reduce the number of viral particles in the blood.

Source: Adapted from Patton and Thibodeau (2018), Norris et al. (2022).

Case Study 8.1

Emily, a 25-year-old woman (approximately 16 weeks' gestation), is presenting to the midwife for the first time. She has just moved into the area and is receiving treatment for drug addiction. Her friend has recently died of an intravenous drug overdose after being diagnosed with AIDS and Emily is depressed, feeling tired and breathless. The pregnancy was not planned.

- Would you feel confident managing her care going forward?
- What considerations would you need to have in relation to the risk of HIV transmission?
- What referrals would you make and what additional advice would you give her?

Systemic Lupus Erythematosus

Systemic lupus erythematosus (SLE) is a multisystem autoimmune disease that is multifactorial and therefore the way in which it manifests itself can vary between individuals affected due to individual genetic characteristics and environmental factors such as ultraviolet light, hormones, chemicals and drugs, which can increase susceptibility to SLE or initiate relapses in disease remission (Rao et al. 2018). SLE is most commonly found in women, especially those from ethnic backgrounds, and is associated with B- and T-cell dysfunction, which results in multiple manifestations of symptoms involving several bodily systems including renal, musculoskeletal, haematological, gastrointestinal, pulmonary and cardiovascular (see Table 8.6). Due to the disease's varied nature, women with SLE must be monitored closely during the perinatal journey, and their care should involve the wider multidisciplinary team as their condition could worsen during this period (Delves et al. 2017).

Medicines Management: Hydroxychloroquine

Hydroxychloroquine is the first-line treatment for SLE and is used to decrease the pain and discomfort associated with joint and muscle inflammation and reduce the development of renal disease. It has steroid-sparing properties and if already prescribed can continue to be taken during pregnancy, as the inflammatory conditions associated with SLE are known to be more damaging to the mother and baby than the drug itself. It is also safe to take when breastfeeding, as long as the mother and baby are well.

　　　Dose: 200–400 mg daily.

Source: Adapted from BNF (2022b).

TABLE 8.6 Manifestations of SLE.

Mucocutaneous	Musculoskeletal	Haematological
Mouth ulcers	Arthralgia	Leucopenia
Alopecia	Arthritis	Lymphopenia
Malar rash	Joint swelling	Neutropenia
Photosensitivity	Myalgia	Thrombocytopenia
Renal	**Nervous system**	**Pulmonary**
Nephritis	Headaches	Pleurisy
Renal shutdown	Seizures	Pneumonitis
Accelerated hypertension	Meningitis	Pulmonary hypertension
	Cerebrovascular accidents	Pulmonary haemorrhage

(Continued)

TABLE 8.6 *(Continued)*

Cardiovascular	Gastrointestinal
Pericarditis	Nausea and vomiting
Myocarditis	Abdominal pain
Endocarditis	Diarrhoea
Pericardial tamponade	Peritonitis
	Pancreatitis

Source: Adapted from Rao et al. (2018).

Antiphospholipid Syndrome

Antiphospholipid syndrome (APS) can develop when the body produces abnormal antibodies known as antiphospholipids. It can be present as either a primary condition or a secondary condition associated with other autoimmune diseases, such as SLE. Women who are pregnant are at risk of developing venous thromboembolism (VTE) and pulmonary embolism (PE), and this is greatly increased if the woman also has APS. These can occur more than once and often in the arms as well as the legs; however, they can also occur in the arteries of the brain, presenting as strokes or transient ischaemia attacks. Pregnant women with APS are also at greater risk of miscarriage, especially during the second trimester, as the fetus is five times more likely to be stillborn and around 30% of pregnancies are unsuccessful (Arslan and Branch 2020). Other symptoms include hypertension, pre-eclampsia, preterm delivery and infants with low birth weight. Therefore, perinatal care should incorporate a multidisciplinary approach involving rheumatology and haematology expertise. Close monitoring of intrauterine growth is essential and planned early delivery may be necessary. To prevent APS-related pregnancy complications and reduce the risk of thrombosis, unfractionated heparin or low molecular weight heparin may need to be prescribed.

Learning Event

Catastrophic APS is caused by multiple vascular occlusions that occur simultaneously, resulting in catastrophic and devastating organ failure and most often death. It usually occurs primarily in the kidneys followed by the lungs, central nervous system, skin and heart.

Source: Adapted from Rao et al. (2018).

Health Promotion

Due to the risk of thrombosis, women must be made aware of the additional steps that can be taken to reduce the risk of developing VTE. These include the following:

- To reduce venous stasis, encourage women to regularly change their position, from sitting to standing, and to sit with their legs elevated.
- To increase venous return, advise women that they can wear compression hosiery, take regular exercise and encourage calf muscle contraction even when their legs are elevated.
- To reduce the risk of hypercoagulability, stress the importance of drinking and hydration, stopping smoking and maintaining a healthy diet.

Red Flag: Signs and Symptoms of a Venous Thromboembolism

It is important to advise woman with APS what the signs and symptoms of PE and deep vein thrombosis (DVT) are and that they must seek medical assistance if any of the following occur:

DVT
- Redness or darkened skin
- Swelling in the arm or leg
- Swollen, distended and tender veins
- Localised pain and tenderness/or throbbing or cramping pain
- Localised warmth and heat around the painful area

PE
- Sudden-onset shortness of breath
- Chest pain
- Anxiety
- Dizziness/fainting.
- Palpitations
- Haemoptysis
- Diaphoresis
- Tachycardia

Source: Adapted from NICE (2022a).

Rheumatoid Arthritis

Rheumatoid arthritis is an autoimmune disease, more common in females, usually affecting joints, which can become swollen, stiff and painful due to erosion of the cartilage and the associated inflammation. Up to 90% of affected women have rheumatoid factor autoantibodies and high levels are associated with more severe symptoms and disease progression (Waugh and Grant 2018). For some women the pain and swelling improve throughout pregnancy, but for others the symptoms worsen. Additionally, some of the medications used to control the symptoms can potentially affect fetal development (NRAS 2022). In order to manage this lifelong condition, it is important to commence treatment as soon as the condition is diagnosed and use combination therapy rather than monotherapy, including non-steroidal anti-inflammatory drugs (NSAIDs), disease-modifying anti-rheumatic drugs (DMARDs), steroids, immunosuppressant drugs and anti-cytokines (Chan et al. 2018).

Medicines Management: Ibuprofen

Among the most frequently used medications for the treatment of pain from rheumatoid arthritis are NSAIDs such as ibuprofen. Ibuprofen is a propionic acid derivative and can be given orally or topically, 600 mg four to six times a day, up to a daily maximum of 1.8 g.

Consequences for Pregnancy

Use of ibuprofen should be avoided unless the benefits outweigh the risks. The risk to the fetus increases after week 32 as ibuprofen can potentially cause closure of fetal ductus arteriosus in utero, resulting in persistent pulmonary hypertension of the newborn and lung and kidney damage. It can also delay the onset and progression of labour.

Consequences Postnatally

Many women find NSAIDs beneficial to treat pain after childbirth.

Source: Adapted from BNF (2022a).

Inflammatory Bowel Disease

Inflammatory bowel disease (IBD) is used as an umbrella term to describe conditions that cause chronic inflammation (including periods of relapse and remission) of the gastrointestinal (GI) tract, the two most common of which are Crohn's disease and ulcerative colitis (McErlean 2019) (see Table 8.7). IBD can often be confused with irritable bowel syndrome (IBS); while these are both gastrointestinal disorders and have similar symptoms, there are differences between the two conditions. IBS is a syndrome that is classified as a functional GI disorder, caused by interactions between the brain and gut, whereas IBD is categorised as an immune-mediated inflammatory disease (Crohn's and Colitis UK 2021a,b) that has the potential to permanently harm the intestines and increase individuals' risk of developing colon cancer (Crohn's and Colitis Foundation 2019).

While the exact cause of IBD remains unanswered, several factors have been found to contribute to the risk of IBD development, including genetics, environmental risk factors (i.e. virus, medication, smoking), imbalance or changes in the intestinal bacteria and abnormal immune system response. The most common symptoms associated with IBD are abdominal pain, frequent diarrhoea and faecal urgency, bleeding and mucus in stool, anaemia, weight loss, mouth ulcers, nausea and vomiting. IBD is associated with periods of relapse (flare-ups) and remission; as such, individuals are continuously transitioning from periods of having no symptoms to periods of managing mild to severe symptoms. For this reason, management of the symptoms can often be problematic and complex. However, while there is no known cure for IBD, there are several effective medications and treatments to help manage symptoms, such as steroids, immunosuppressants, antispasmodics, surgery and modified diets.

Orange Flag: Supporting Mental Health

Living with IBD can trigger several emotions such as feelings of stress, fear, anxiety and anger. Almost half of people with Crohn's stated that their condition had affected their mental health. Referrals to specialised services may therefore be required to support their overall health and well-being.

Myasthenia Gravis

This disease usually appears in women between the ages of 20–40 years and is associated with chronic muscle weakness, as the immune system attacks and blocks acetylcholine receptors on muscle cells at neuromuscular junctions, so nerve impulses to muscle fibres are blocked (Waugh and Grant 2018). The symptoms are normally isolated to the face (eyelids) and neck, resulting in speech, chewing and swallowing difficulties; however, they can become more chronic involving wider muscles and relapses are often associated with pregnancy. A myasthenia crisis occurs when all four limbs are affected, as such individuals are at greater risk of respiratory failure (Patton and Thibodeau 2018).

TABLE 8.7   Features of Crohn's disease and ulcerative colitis.

	Crohn's disease	Ulcerative colitis
Tissue and sites	From mouth to anus and involves the entire thickness of the wall of the digestive tract	Affects the mucosa of the rectum and colon
Lesions	Skip lesions are often found alongside ulcers and fistulae	Lesions are continuous and the mucosa is red and inflamed
Incidence	Affects both men and women between the ages of 20–40, the mean age is 26	Affects both men and women between the ages of 20–40, the mean age is 34
Prognosis	Surgery may be required but relapse is high	Surgery may be required to remove the entire colon, which cures the condition

Source: Reproduced by permission from Waugh and Grant (2018) / Elsevier.

Multiple Sclerosis

Multiple sclerosis (MS) is an autoimmune disorder where large sections of the myelin sheath that surrounds and protects nerve fibres are attacked and damaged by the body's natural immune system. For individuals affected by MS, areas of demyelinated white matter (plaques) replace myelin and grey matter in the spinal cord and brain. This leaves the nerves unprotected and thus susceptible to damage and can affect any nerves within the body. Symptoms are therefore varied but usually include vision, balance, loss of bladder and bowel control, swallowing difficulties and memory and cognition impairment. While it is not a complication of pregnancy, some women can display MS symptoms for the first time during pregnancy. The cause for this is unknown, but most people develop MS between the ages of 20–40 years and women are twice as likely to experience the condition than men (Waugh and Grant 2018); therefore, it is often discovered when women of childbearing age interact with healthcare professionals. While MS does not prevent women from becoming pregnant, it can sometimes result in babies with smaller birth weights. It can also make delivery more difficult, due to symptoms of reduced sensation and feeling; thus, there is an increased need for forceps or vacuum assistance during delivery (NICE 2022b).

Case Study 8.2

Sarah is a 32-year-old woman expecting her first child and within her first trimester. She contacted her midwife as she was experiencing some pain in the soles of her feet with some episodes of loss of balance and dizziness. She was also worried as she had been losing weight throughout the pregnancy, always seemed tired and was becoming very forgetful.

- What additional assessments and investigations would you undertake based on her symptoms?
- Who else would you need to be involved in Sarah's care, if you suspect multiple sclerosis?

Medicines Management: Corticosteroids

Steroids (also known as corticosteroids) may be used to treat relapses or acute exacerbations of MS, as they can reduce inflammation in the central nervous system. Methylprednisolone is the steroid most often prescribed and is considered safe to administer during pregnancy. However, it is only to be prescribed for short periods of time due to the side effects and associated complications of long-term use.

Dose: 500 mg once daily for five days.

Source: Adapted from BNF (2022c); NICE (2022b).

Conditions Associated with the Immune Response

The following is a list of some of the perinatal conditions that are associated with alterations in the inflammatory and immune response. Take some time and write notes about each of the conditions. Think about the altered pathophysiology involved. Remember to include aspects of women's care. If you are making notes about people to whom you have offered care and support, you must ensure that you have adhered to the rules of confidentiality.

The condition	Your notes
Neonatal lupus syndrome	
Polymyositis	
Dermatomyositis	
Haemolytic anaemia	
Livedo reticularis	

> ## Take-Home Points
>
> - When caring for any woman, it is important to have a sound understanding of the anatomy and physiology of the immune system and inflammatory processes.
> - This enables midwives to look for signs of abnormal immune function and assist women to manage pre-existing autoimmune disorders that may have an impact on the perinatal journey.
> - Any decisions made must be tailored to the individual needs of the woman and take into consideration her holistic picture.
> - It is also essential to practise in a non-discriminatory manner and include women and their partners in decisions made about their care.

Conclusion

Inflammatory processes and the immune system play essential roles in protecting the woman and her unborn baby from attacking and invading microorganisms during pregnancy and delivery. However, when these mechanisms fail or are inadequate, this can result in a variety of autoimmune conditions and immune deficiencies, which can increase risks for the mother and the baby. As such, midwives and midwifery students must understand normal and maladaptive functioning associated with the immune system and the process of inflammation in order to practise safely and minimise the risks, while also ensuring that their care is woman centred, individualised and holistically tailored to enable daily functioning and maintain physical and mental wellbeing.

References

Arslan, E. and Branch, D.W. (2020). Antiphospholipid syndrome: diagnosis and management in the obstetric patient. *Best Practice and Research Clinical Obstetrics and Gynaecology* 61: 31–40.

Basgol, S. and Beji, N. (2015). Common practices and evidence-based approach in first stage of labour. *Journal of the Health Sciences Institute* 5: 32–39.

Boore, J., Cook, N., and Shepherd, A. (2021). *Essentials of Anatomy and Physiology for Nursing Practice*, 2e. London: Sage.

British National Formulary (BNF) (2022a). Ibuprofen. https://bnf.nice.org.uk/drugs/ibuprofen (accessed November 2023).

British National Formulary (BNF) (2022b). Hydroxychloroquine sulfate. https://bnf.nice.org.uk/drugs/hydroxychloroquine-sulfate (accessed November 2023).

British National Formulary (BNF) (2022c). Methylprednisolone. https://bnf.nice.org.uk/drugs/methylprednisolone (accessed November 2023).

Chan, E.,.S.,.L, Wilson, A.G., and Cronstein, B.N. (2018). Treatment of rheumatoid arthritis. In: *ABC of Rheumatology*, 5e (ed. A. Adebajo and L. Dunkley), 77–80. Chichester: Wiley.

Christopher, U., Goldy, S., Bewin, O.J., and Adlin, R.C. (2019). Multiple vaginal examinations and early neonatal sepsis. *International Journal of Reproduction, Contraception, Obstetrics and Gynaecology* 8: 876–882.

Coad, J., Pedley, K., and Dunstall, M. (2020). *Anatomy and Physiology for Midwives*. London: Elsevier.

Crohn's and Colitis Foundation (2019). Inflammatory bowel disease vs. irritable bowel syndrome. https://www.crohnscolitisfoundation.org/sites/default/files/2019-10/ibd-and-IBS-brochure-final.pdf (accessed November 2023).

Crohn's and Colitis UK (2021a). Chron's disease. https://crohnsandcolitis.org.uk/media/pcsn5zoo/crohns-ed-8-with-links.pdf (accessed November 2023).

Crohn's and Colitis UK (2021b). Ulcerative colitis. https://crohnsandcolitis.org.uk/media/oogbwnym/uc-ed-10-with-links-2.pdf (accessed November 2023).

Delves, P.J., Martin, S.J., Burton, D.R., and Roitt, I.M. (2017). *Roitt's Essential Immunology*, 13e. Chichester: Wiley.

Dockree, A., Shine, B., Pavord, S. et al. (2021). White blood cells in pregnancy: reference intervals for before and after delivery. *eBioMedicine* 74: 103715.

Downe, S., Gyte, G.M., Dahlen, H.G., and Singata, M. (2013). Routine vaginal examinations for assessing progress of labour to improve outcomes for women and babies at term. *Cochrane Database of Systematic Reviews* 7: (Art. ID: CD010088). https://doi.org/10.1002/14651858.CD010088.pub2.

El-Heneidy, A., Abdel-Rahman, M.E., Mihala, G. et al. (2018). Milk other than breast milk and the development of asthma in children 3 years of age: a birth cohort study (2006–2011). *Nutrients* 10: 1798.

Ford, C. and Park, L.J. (2018). Hand hygiene and handwashing: key to preventing the transfer of pathogens. *British Journal of Nursing* 27: 1164–1166.

Hanson, L.A. (1998). Breastfeeding provides passive and likely long-lasting active immunity. *Annals of Allergy, Asthma and Immunology* 81: 523–533; quiz 533–534, 537.

Lister, S., Hofland, J., and Grafton, H. (2020). *The Royal Marsden Mannual of Clinical Nursing Procedures*, 10e. Chichester: Wiley.

Macdonald, S. and Johnson, G. (2017). *'ayes' Midwifery*, 15e. London: Elsevier.

McErlean, L. (2019). Gastrointestinal disorder. In: *Learning to Care: The Nurse Associate* (ed. I. Peate), 398–414. Edinburgh: Elsevier.

National Institute for Health and Care Excellence (NICE) (2022a). Antenatal care. https://www.nice.org.uk/guidance/qs22 (accessed November 2023).

National Institute for Health and Care Excellence (NICE) (2022b). Multiple sclerosis. https://www.nice.org.uk/guidance/conditions-and-diseases/neurological-conditions/multiple-sclerosis (accessed November 2023).

National Rheumatoid Arthritis Society (NRAS) (2022). Rheumatoid arthritis and pregnancy. https://nras.org.uk/resource/rheumatoid-arthritis-pregnancy (accessed November 2023).

Norris, T.L., Tuan, R.L., and Porth, C. (2022). *Porth's Essentials of Pathophysiology*, 5e. Philadelphia: Wolters Kluwer.

Patton, K. and Thibodeau, G. (2018). *The Human Body in Health and Disease*, 7e. London: Elsevier.

Rankin, J. (2017). *Physiology in Childbearing E-Book: With Anatomy and Related Biosciences*. London: Elsevier Health Sciences.

Rao, V., Ramsey-Goldman, R., and Gordon, C. (2018). Systemic lupus erythematosus and lupus-like syndromes. In: *ABC of Rheumatology*, 5e (ed. A. Adebajo and L. Dunkley), 119–127. Chichester: Wiley.

Tortora, G. and Derrickson, B. (2017). *Tortora's Principles of Anatomy and Physiology*. Singapore: Wiley.

UNAIDS (2021). HIV and stigma and discrimination: human rights fact sheet series 2021. https://www.unaids.org/en/resources/documents/2021/07-hiv-human-rights-factsheet-stigma-discrmination (accessed November 2023).

Vickers, P.S. (2017). The immune system. In: *Fundamentals of Anatomy and Physiology for Nursing and Healthcare Students*, 2e (ed. I. Peate and M. Nair), 371–402. Chichester, UK: Wiley.

Waugh, A. and Grant, A. (2018). *Ross and Wilson Anatomy and Physiology in Health and Illness*, 13e. London: Elsevier.

World Health Organization (WHO) (2022). Endometriosis. https://www.who.int/news-room/fact-sheets/detail/endometriosis (accessed November 2023).

World Health Organization (WHO) (2023). HIV. https://www.who.int/data/gho/data/themes/hiv-aids (accessed November 2023).

Further Resources

National Rheumatoid Arthritis Society. www.nras.org.uk/resource/rheumatoid-arthritis-pregnancy/ (accessed November 2023).
Multiple Sclerosis Society. www.mssociety.org.uk/about-ms/what-is-ms/women-and-ms/pregnancy-and-birth (accessed November 2023).
Multiple Sclerosis Trust. www.mstrust.org.uk/a-z/pregnancy (accessed November 2023).
Endometriosis Society. www.endometriosis-uk.org (accessed November 2023).
Lupus UK. www.lupusuk.org.uk/lupus-and-pregnancy (accessed November 2023).

Glossary

Alopecia	Partial or complete loss of body hair
Antigen	Derived from the word 'antibody generator', an antigen is a substance or molecule that provokes an immune response
Aorta	The main artery supplying oxygenated blood from the heart to the body
Arthralgia	Painful joints
Bifidus factor	A compound that enhances the growth of bifidobacteria
Chorioamnionitis	Inflammation, due to a bacterial infection of the amnion and chorion

Chemotactic factor	Molecules that stimulate the movement of cells
Cilia	A short hairlike structure
Colostrum	The first mammary gland secretion, which is rich in antibodies
Cytotoxic	Poisonous to living cells
Diaphoresis	Excessive perspiration/sweating due to a secondary condition
Endocarditis	Infection of the endocardium (the inner lining of the heart)
Erythema	Redness of the skin
Extracellular	Situated or occurring outside the cells of the body
Exudate	A fluid that leaks out of blood vessels into nearby tissues
Fibrin	A protein involved in the formation of blood clots
Haemoptysis	Expectoration of sputum containing blood
Histamine	A chemical found in the body that causes blood vessels to dilate and leak
Human chorionic gonadotrophin	A hormone made by chorionic cells in the placenta that stimulates the corpus luteum to produce progesterone, which maintains pregnancy
Intracellular	Situated or occurring inside the cells of the body
Kinins	Plasma proteins that increase vascular permeability
Lactoferrin	An iron-binding protein hindering the growth of bacteria and fungi
Leucopenia	Low levels of leucocytes
Lymphokines	A polypeptide generated by activated lymphocytes
Lymphopenia	Low levels of lymphocytes
Malar rash	Facial rash often red or purplish and usually presented in a butterfly pattern
Monotherapy	Treatment involving one drug
Mucus membranes	The moist inner lining of some organs and body cavities
Myalgia	Muscle pain
Myocarditis	Inflammation of the myocardium (heart muscle)
Neonatal necrotising enterocolitis	Inflammation of the bowel affecting newborn babies, which is a serious condition as the bowel also becomes ischaemic and necrotic
Nephritis	Inflammation of the kidneys
Neutropenia	Low levels of neutrophils
Oedema	Increased fluid causing the tissue to become swollen
Otitis media	Inflammation of the inner ear
Pancreatitis	Inflammation of the pancreas
Pathogen	A disease-producing microbe
Pericardial tamponade	Increased fluid/blood between the heart and pericardium
Pericarditis	Inflammation/infection of the pericardium (protective fluid-filled sac around the heart)
Peritonitis	Inflammation/infection of the peritoneal cavity (inner lining of the abdomen)
Permeability	The ability of a substance to allow the passage of gas or liquid
Pleurisy	Inflammation of the pleura
Pneumonitis	Inflammation of the lungs
Prolactin	Hormone that stimulates milk production
Puerperal infection	Caused by bacteria entering the genital tract and infecting the uterus and surrounding areas after birth
Pyrogens	Substance released by bacteria producing fever
Remission	A decrease or disappearance of signs and symptoms
Sternum	The long flat bone found in the centre of the chest wall, otherwise referred to as the breastbone
Thrombocytopenia	A condition associated with low levels of platelets in the blood
Vasodilation	The dilation (relaxing and widening) of blood vessels
Vernix	A covering found on the skin of a baby at birth, which is waxy and greasy

CHAPTER 9

Cardiovascular System and Associated Disorders

Komal Bhatt and Leo Gurney

Birmingham Women's Hospital, Birmingham Women's and Children's NHS Foundation Trust, Birmingham, UK

AIM

This chapter aims to provide an overview of changes in cardiovascular physiology in pregnancy, with examples of both common and rare pathology that may be encountered when working with women.

LEARNING OUTCOMES

On completion of this chapter the reader will be able to:

- Describe the physiological changes that occur to the cardiovascular system in pregnancy
- Recognise symptoms of cardiac disease
- Describe cardiac conditions that may arise in pregnancy
- Understand the impact of pre-existing cardiac conditions in pregnancy

Test Your Prior Knowledge

1. What changes occur to resting heart rate in pregnancy?
2. How would you investigate a patient presenting with chest pain?
3. What is cardiomyopathy?
4. Can patients with heart disease undergo labour?

The MBRRACE-UK (Mothers and Babies: Reducing Risk through Audit and Confidential Enquiries) report highlights the importance of a good understanding of cardiovascular presentations in pregnancy, as cardiac disease remains the largest single cause of indirect maternal deaths in the United Kingdom (Knight et al. 2021). The report highlighted the need for good postnatal contraceptive advice and the vital role of pre-pregnancy counselling for high-risk women with pre-existing cardiac disease, which is discussed in this chapter.

The chapter will consider cardiovascular physiology in the antenatal, intrapartum and postnatal periods and how the body during pregnancy must adapt to evolving physiology resulting in an altered heart rate and blood pressure, increased strength of cardiac muscle and increases in circulating blood volume.

Maternal Medicine Network

As of 2022 in the UK, services for maternal medicine are delivered via a maternal medicine network that operates using a 'hub-and-spoke' mechanism. Conditions are categorised into low, medium and high risk and then referred appropriately. Table 9.1 gives a local example, taken from the West Midlands Maternal Medicine Network arrangement of how different cardiac conditions may be categorised, but these referral pathways may vary locally.

Table 9.2 shows the main components of the maternal medicine multidisciplinary team (MDT). Midwives are vital to this MDT approach.

TABLE 9.1   **Managing cardiac conditions as part of a maternal medicine network.**

Category A (low risk)	Category B (medium risk)	Category C (highest risk)
Local expertise	**Shared care**	**Maternal medicine centre**
Seen at local unit but multidisciplinary team support and discussion available	Seen at maternal medicine centre for clinical review, advice and guidance	Booking and all care at maternal medicine centre
Mild pulmonary stenosis	Mild reduced left ventricular ejection fraction	Left ventricular ejection fraction <45%
Small/repaired patent ductus arteriosus	Hypertrophic cardiomyopathy with no high-risk features	Severe mitral stenosis
Mitral valve prolapse	Repaired aortic coarctation	Severe aortic stenosis
Repaired atrial septal defect	Mild mitral stenosis	Systematic right ventricle
Repaired ventricular septal defect	Other valve lesions not listed in category A or C	Fontan
Isolated atrial or ventricular ectopic beats	Atrioventricular septal defect	Previous peripartum cardiomyopathy
Treated cardiac electrophysiology conditions	Repaired tetralogy of Fallot	Ventricular arrhythmia
	Marfan (maternal medicine centre if not aortic centre)	Moderate aortic stenosis
	Bicuspid aortic valve (if aorta <45 mm)	Moderate mitral stenosis
	Unrepaired simple shunt lesions	Mechanical valve
	Treated ischaemic heart disease	Turner syndrome without aortic dilation
	Myocarditis	Turner syndrome with aortic dilation
	Ongoing supraventricular arrhythmia	Aortic dilation
		Unrepaired cyanotic disease
		Vascular Ehlers-Danlos
		Re-coarctation
		Heart transplant
		New ischaemic heart disease

TABLE 9.2   **Components of maternal medicine network core multidisciplinary team.**

Obstetrician	Specialist midwives	Obstetric physician or equivalent physician
Subspecialist in fetal-maternal medicine or equivalent	With expertise in antenatal, intrapartum and postpartum management of women with medical problems	In this instance, cardiologist with experience of running a joint obstetric clinic

Cardiovascular Physiology

Pregnancy is associated with significant changes in the cardiovascular system in order to meet the increased demands of the mother and fetus and to ensure adequate uteroplacental circulation for fetal development. If these adaptations do not occur, then the result can lead to morbidity for both mother and fetus. The changes that occur are summarised.

Cardiac Output

Cardiac output (CO) is the volume of blood pumped by the heart in a minute. Stroke volume is the volume of blood pumped by the heart with each beat and so the CO can be calculated by multiplying stroke volume by heart rate in beats per minute.

$$\textit{Cardiac Output (CO)} = \begin{array}{c} \textit{Stroke Volume (SV)} \\ \textit{X} \\ \textit{Heart Rate (HR)} \end{array}$$

CO increases throughout pregnancy, with the sharpest rise occurring at the start of the first trimester. By 24 weeks the increase in CO can be up to 45% compared to a non-pregnant woman (Sanghavi and John 2014). Early in pregnancy it is thought to be mediated by an increase in stroke volume (the volume of blood pumped out by the left ventricle after each systolic contraction). During labour, CO increases by an additional 30%, but by six weeks postpartum output will have returned to normal levels (Artal-Mittelmark 2021). The increased stroke volume is a consequence of various adaptations in pregnancy: the left ventricular wall muscle mass gets bigger, leading to increased blood volume in the ventricles prior to systole (end-diastolic volume) and increased myocardial contractility; and the heart rate gradually increases by approximately 10–20 beats/min, reaching higher levels in the third trimester (Nelson-Piercy 2020). Together, an increased stroke volume and a higher heart rate lead to an increase in the volume of blood pumped by the heart (i.e. CO).

The pregnant uterus compresses the inferior vena cava (IVC) in a supine (lying back) position, which reduces venous return to the heart. This will lead to reduced CO and so it is important that in emergency situations, or in situations where women may lie flat for prolonged periods (e.g. during an ultrasound scan), women are cared for on a lateral tilt.

161

Blood Pressure

There is a decrease in blood pressure (BP) occurring in the first trimester, usually around the time a patient may attend for their antenatal booking appointment. Hence BP recorded at booking may be lower than pre-conception values. Arterial pressures begin to increase during the third trimester and return to pre-conception levels postpartum. BP is the force exerted by circulating blood on the vessel walls. It is affected by CO, circulating blood volume, the elasticity of the vessel walls and systemic vascular resistance (SVR). The pressure that the peripheral circulation exerts against the blood pumping from the left ventricle is SVR. A decrease in SVR will lead to increased perfusion of peripheral tissues and increased venous flow back to the right ventricle.

During pregnancy there is an increase in peripheral vasodilation (relaxation of the blood vessel walls). This is because oestradiol is higher and this has an impact on chemicals that act on the blood vessel walls. This vasodilation leads to a drop in SVR and as a result there is a reduction in peripheral BP (Soma-Pillay et al. 2016).

Renin–Angiotensin–Aldosterone System

The renin–angiotensin–aldosterone system (RAAS) is a multiorgan pathway that involves regulation of BP, electrolytes, vascular resistance and tone. In pregnancy this pathway is activated, which results in an increase in plasma volume in early pregnancy. As a result of the higher oestrogen in pregnancy, angiotensinogen production increases, therefore increasing angiotensin production. This leads to salt and water retention, which balances against the peripheral vasodilation discussed earlier to maintain an adequate BP (Soma-Pillay et al. 2016).

Physiology in Labour

In labour, contraction of the uterus releases blood back into the maternal circulation leading to increased cardiac pre-load. Pre-load is the amount of blood that has filled in the ventricles when they are relaxed. The autonomic response to pain with contractions result in an increased heart rate and BP. The CO is therefore increased during labour (Nelson-Piercy 2020). Following delivery, compression of the IVC is reduced and the uterus remains contracted, releasing blood into the circulation. This increases CO by up to 80%. Patients are therefore most at risk of cardiovascular compromise during delivery and immediately postpartum. Postnatally CO will return to normal at around two weeks, but overall cardiovascular function may take up to six to eight weeks to return to normal.

Approach to Heart Disease in Pregnancy

History Taking

In order to assess for signs of cardiac disease, a thorough history should be taken from the woman. Symptoms to ask about include chest pain, palpitations, breathlessness, light-headedness or fainting (often called pre-syncope and syncope). Orthopnoea is worsening shortness of breath on lying flat and paroxysmal nocturnal dyspnoea (PND) describes acute shortness of breath that awakens the patient from sleep; often such women will describe waking and gasping for breath.

Woman-Centred Care

Remember to ask about the woman's past medical history including previous procedures and enquire about a family history of cardiac conditions or sudden cardiac death and their baseline exercise tolerance.

Assessment

Initial observations should be taken. The pulse rate should be measured. A pulse oximeter can be used to monitor the pulse rate and oxygen saturations, but if cardiac disease is suspected then a peripheral pulse should be palpated manually. Tachycardic or bradycardic patients may prompt further investigation. Oxygen saturation is the percentage of oxygenated haemoglobin and you would expect a healthy patient to have an oxygen saturation of more than 95% in air.

Learning Event

Some patients with known congenital cardiac disease may chronically have much lower oxygen saturations that may be normal for them. This should be checked with the cardiac team that knows the patient well, and the patient should be asked about any new symptoms.

Measured BP is necessary at each antenatal visit and also in labour. BP should be recorded in the sitting or left lateral recumbent position (Kinsella 2006) and the cuff size should be correctly fitted to the patient's upper arm. Respiratory rate is measured ideally when the patient is at rest and is the number of breaths taken per minute. Table 9.3 summarises normal ranges for basic observations and changes expected in pregnancy. A maternity early warning score (MEWS) tool will often be used to plot observations in order to identify deteriorating patients in pregnancy or the postnatal period.

Investigations

Those with suspected cardiac conditions or known cardiac conditions will likely need further investigation. A 12-lead electrocardiogram (ECG) is usually an initial baseline investigation and can be done at the patient's bedside. The electrical activity of the heart is recorded and it can pick up any abnormal rhythms, conduction problems, signs of ischaemia or strain on the heart muscle. In cases where an arrhythmia is suspected but not detected on the 12-lead ECG, a Holter monitor may be requested in order to monitor the electrical activity of the heart for a longer period.

Echocardiography is requested to investigate for structural abnormalities with the heart. It is an ultrasound scan and has to be performed by a trained professional, usually a cardiologist, cardiac physiologist or sonographer.

Acute Presentations in Pregnancy

Palpitations

Patients may describe a sensation of the heart fluttering or pounding. This can be a common symptom and if self-limiting and short lasting in a healthy patient may not be of any concern. It could, however, be a symptom of an arrhythmia, heart failure or structural heart disease. Non-cardiac differential diagnoses for palpitations include anaemia, hyperthyroidism, electrolyte disturbance, hypovolaemia or a panic attack.

TABLE 9.3 Normal observation ranges and how they may differ in pregnancy.

Observations	Normal ranges	Changes in pregnancy
Heart rate	60–90 beats/min	↑ by 10–20 beats/min
Blood pressure	90/60–140/90 mmHg	↓ by 15–20 mmHg in first and second trimesters
Respiratory rate	12–20 breaths/min	↔ unchanged The volume of air delivered to the lungs in each breath (tidal volume) increases to meet the increased oxygen demand
Oxygen saturation	95–100% on room air	↔ unchanged

Examination Scenario

A patient at 35 weeks' pregnant attends maternity triage with an unusual fluttering sensation in her chest.

- How can you initially assess the patient?

The woman's manual pulse should be palpated peripherally (radial pulse) for irregularities. Consider using a manual sphygmomanometer to measure BP. Check for peripheral signs of decompensation like pedal oedema and see if the jugular venous pulse is raised. The lung fields and heart beat should be auscultated with a stethoscope. A 12-lead ECG and blood tests may be requested to further investigate for arrhythmias.

Chest Pain

When any patient describes chest pain it is important to gain a thorough history of the onset, character and radiation of the pain.

Case Study 9.1

A 32-year-old woman admitted to the postnatal ward is 16 hours post normal vaginal delivery. She complains of chest pain. A set of routine observations are taken by her midwife and show a heart rate of 86 bpm, BP of 115/70, respiratory rate of 16 and saturations of 98% on air. She appears sweaty and reports central crushing chest pain.

- What are the possible differential diagnoses of chest pain?
  - Musculoskeletal: costochondritis, fractures.
  - Respiratory: pulmonary embolism, pneumothorax, pneumonia.
  - Cardiac causes: acute coronary syndrome (ACS), pericarditis.
  - Other: gastro-oesophageal reflux disease (GORD), aortic dissection.
- What is the appropriate next step to take?

The midwife should assess the patient through an A–E approach and request an urgent medical review.

- How would can we investigate cardiac causes for chest pain?
  - To investigate cardiac causes for chest pain the patient needs a 12-lead ECG.
  - A blood test may be taken to measure serum troponin levels (often two serial samples needed).
  - The patient may be discussed with cardiology if there are concerns.

Breathlessness

Breathlessness could be a symptom of a range of a serious conditions, but in pregnancy it also may be benign. Pregnancy results in an increase in oxygen demand, increased tidal volume (the volume of air moved in or out of the lungs in each breath) and diaphragmatic elevation, all contributing to this symptom (Soma-Pillay et al. 2016). Pulmonary oedema occurs due to accumulation of fluid in the lung spaces due to ineffective pumping of the heart and will typically lead to pink frothy sputum, orthopnoea, PND and exertional dyspnoea.

Case Study 9.2

A woman who is 34 weeks pregnant in her first pregnancy attends maternity triage with complaints of breathlessness, which has been getting worse and now stops her from walking short distances and lying flat.

- What initial assessments does this patient require?

She requires routine observations. If these are abnormal then she needs immediate medical review.

- What are some causes of breathlessness in pregnancy?
  - Asthma.
  - Pneumonia.
  - Influenza or Covid-19.
  - Pulmonary embolism (PE).
  - Pulmonary oedema due to pre-eclampsia or heart failure.
  - Physiological.
- How can we investigate and diagnose causes of breathlessness in pregnancy?
  - Auscultation of the thorax at the bedside and further clinical assessment (the patient may have ankle oedema or a raised jugular venous pressure).
  - Chest X-ray.
  - Viral throat swabs.
  - Full blood count, renal function and pro-BNP.
  - Arterial blood gas (ABG) could be considered if unwell.
  - Further imaging may be needed to investigate for a PE.

Pre-existing Cardiac Disease

Pre-existing medical conditions and conditions arising in pregnancy result in higher-risk pregnancies, therefore higher morbidity and mortality. The cardiac disease, symptoms and severity may all determine how the patient will tolerate pregnancy. Some conditions would be classified as low risk and so may need minimal specialist input, in contrast to higher-risk conditions that require more specialised and closer monitoring.

Mitral Stenosis

Mitral stenosis occurs when the mitral valve becomes narrowed, obstructing the blood flowing out of the left atrium into the left ventricle. Patients with mitral stenosis may have symptoms relating to pulmonary oedema, including orthopnoea, dyspnoea, postural nocturnal dyspnoea or cough.

Aortic Stenosis

Aortic stenosis is most commonly caused by congenital bicuspid valve disease; in addition, rheumatic heart disease is also a contributing cause (Regitz-Zagrosek et al. 2018). Symptoms of aortic stenosis are classically angina, breathlessness and syncope. Pre-pregnancy assessment of symptoms and exercise tolerance will help to guide pre-pregnancy counselling (Regitz-Zagrosek et al. 2018).

Aortic and Mitral Valve Regurgitation

Both aortic and mitral regurgitation are generally well tolerated in pregnancy. Aortic regurgitation occurs when the aortic valve does not shut completely, leading to backflow of blood into the left ventricle. In mitral regurgitation there is backflow of blood from the left ventricle to the atrium due to incomplete closure of the mitral valve. This can be caused by mitral valve prolapse, which occurs more commonly in young women, but is often mild.

Valve Replacement

There are two types of valve replacements: mechanical heart valves and tissue heart valves (usually from pig or human donors). Those with mechanical heart valves require lifelong anticoagulation due to the risk of blood clots forming at the valve, which can result in clotting events in the brain or other organs that may be fatal.

Medicines Management

Women taking anticoagulation due to a mechanical heart valve must continue during pregnancy. Pre-pregnancy they will usually be prescribed warfarin or oral vitamin K agonists, but these can be teratogenic and can lead to stillbirth. Any patient who becomes pregnant while taking these medications should continue but requires urgent referral to their local specialist pregnancy or haematology/cardiology team. They will often be prescribed an alternative blood thinner like a low molecular weight heparin (LMWH, such as enoxaparin) during the pregnancy (Regitz-Zagrosek et al. 2018).

Congenital Heart Disease

Congenital heart disease refers to heart disease that is present from birth. For mothers, it can encompass a spectrum of diseases of varying severity. Recently mortality rates from such conditions have declined owing to improvements in paediatric care, and increasing proportions of patients with congenital cardiac conditions are now becoming pregnant. With appropriate care, these pregnancies can be managed safely and with good outcomes for mothers and babies; however, it is vital that such conditions are picked up prior to pregnancy or early in pregnancy and the woman directed to the appropriate care team. There are a very wide variety of congenital heart conditions and therefore this section focuses on commoner lesions (Nelson-Piercy 2020).

Atrial Septal Defect

An atrial septal defect (ASD) is a communication between the two atria of the heart from a hole in the dividing septum. It is the most prevalent congenital cardiac defect in the adult population and is usually unproblematic in pregnancy.

Red Flag

There is a risk of paradoxical embolism with larger ASDs particularly, where a clot will cross the defect and enter the systemic circulation, causing potential blockage of systemic vessels (Nelson-Piercy 2020). In an ASD patient postpartum haemorrhage also poses a potential risk for cardiac decompensation due to the rapid loss of blood volume. These patients should be resuscitated early with fluid and blood product replacement.

Ventricular Septal Defect

A ventricular septal defect (VSD) is an opening in the interventricular septum that separates the ventricles. It allows the blood to pass from the left to the right ventricle and so allows for mixing of oxygenated blood back into the right side of the heart. The heart may have to work harder to pump blood into the systemic circulation. The majority of VSDs are surgically repaired at birth and so are usually well tolerated in pregnancy.

Patent Ductus Arteriosus

A patent ductus arteriosus (PDA) in most cases would either close soon after birth or be surgically corrected in childhood. The defect involves the communication between the aorta and pulmonary artery that was present in utero remaining open after birth. In most cases a persisting PDA would be well tolerated (Nelson-Piercy 2020), but if it is large then there is a potential for congestive cardiac failure due to flow of blood from the left side to the right side of the heart (Zhang et al. 2021).

Atrioventricular Septal Defect

In an atrioventricular septal defect (AVSD) there are holes between the right and left sides of the heart. In the case of a complete AVSD, there is one big hole in the middle of the heart allowing for mixing of blood between all four chambers. AVSD has a significant association with trisomy 21. The defect is usually repaired in childhood along with valve repairs.

Aortic Coarctation

Some people may be born with a narrowing of the aorta called aortic coarctation. This would usually be surgically corrected at birth, but if the narrowing is mild it may not be detected in childhood. They may present with shortness of breath or raised BP and would typically have higher BP readings in the arms compared to the legs.

Cyanotic Congenital Cardiac Disease

Cyanotic congenital heart disease results from deoxygenated blood entering the systemic circulation due to a congenital anomaly. It can cause significant problems in pregnancy due to an increase in shunting of the deoxygenated blood to the left side of the heart. The low oxygen levels in the systemic circulation can lead to polycythaemia (concentrated haemoglobin), which can predispose to thromboembolic events (like PE). There are risks of developing pulmonary hypertension and of fetal growth restriction (Nelson-Piercy 2020). The main causes of cyanotic cardiac disease that may be encountered in women of childbearing age are pulmonary atresia and tetralogy of Fallot (TOF).

TOF is usually corrected by adulthood and patients with resting oxygen saturations above 85% may tolerate pregnancy well and have a better outcome.

In transposition of the great arteries (TGA), the pulmonary artery is connected to the left ventricle and the aorta is connected to the right ventricle. This means that the oxygenated blood is pumped back to the lungs and the oxygen-depleted blood returning from the systemic circulation is recirculated around the body. This will be surgically corrected in infancy.

Children who are born with congenital anomalies that result in a single functioning ventricle should have surgical correction in childhood (Nelson-Piercy 2020). Following the procedure, a single ventricle pumps oxygenated blood to the body and this is termed a Fontan circulation. Due to the circulation, physiologically these patients are unable to sufficiently increase CO if required (Gewillig and Brown 2016) and there is a risk of decompensation in the third trimester. Patients with a Fontan circulation are considered high risk and should be managed in specialist centres (Zentner et al. 2016).

Cardiomyopathy

Cardiomyopathies describe illnesses involving the heart muscle, often leading to serious problems with the heart's pumping action and potentially heart failure. Examples of cardiomyopathy include hypertrophic cardiomyopathy (HCM), dilated cardiomyopathy (DCM) and peripartum cardiomyopathy (PPCM).

HCM is defined by a non-dilated left ventricular hypertrophy characteristically involving the septum (de Oliveira Antunes and Scudeler 2020). It has a strong genetic association and 70% of cases are autosomal dominant (Nelson-Piercy 2020).

Red Flag

These patients are at risk of tachyarrhythmias and sudden death. For this reason, they may be fitted with an implantable cardioverter defibrillator (ICD) that will deliver an electric shock if an arrhythmia is detected. A family history of sudden cardiac death should prompt further enquiry.

DCM groups together conditions that result in left ventricular dilation and dysfunction. Causes of DCM range from infection, drug-induced, secondary to ischaemic injury or idiopathic. Idiopathic causes can be hereditary in 20–35% of cases and so establishing diagnosis can be important for familial screening (Ware et al. 2016).

PPCM relates to heart failure towards the end of pregnancy or postnatally where other causes have been excluded (Nelson-Piercy 2020). The true cause is unknown but the condition will present with left ventricular systolic dysfunction. The maternal mortality rate is 9–15%, with PPCM accounting for 20% of cardiac maternal deaths in the United Kingdom (Nelson-Piercy 2020). Patients with multiple pregnancy, advanced maternal age, Afro-Caribbean race or multiparity may have a slight predisposition to the condition.

Orange Flag

The prognosis of PPCM is linked to the return to normal left ventricular size and function at six months postnatally and those with persisting cardiac dysfunction have a significant mortality risk in future pregnancies due to risk of recurrence and heart failure.

Disease Arising in Pregnancy

The changing physiology in pregnancy may reveal de novo cardiac disease in some patients. Although heart attacks are more common in an older population, cardiac ischaemia can still occur in pregnancy. Cardiac ischaemia occurs when there is restricted blood flow through the blood vessels that supply the heart (coronary arteries), which results in poor oxygen supply and injury to the heart muscle (myocardium). Some patients will present for the first time in pregnancy with an arrhythmia.

Acute Coronary Syndrome

Expert Midwife

ACS commonly presents with chest pain or discomfort, breathlessness, nausea or diaphoresis (excessive perspiration). If a myocardial infarction is suspected then the patient should have an urgent medical review, routine observations and, if appropriate, an ECG and serum troponin levels to make the diagnosis.

ACS relates to a group of conditions resulting in cardiac ischaemia or infarction due to reduced perfusion of the coronary arteries. The diagnostic criteria outside of pregnancy apply to pregnant women and include presence of chest pain, ECG changes and dynamic changes in cardiac enzymes (troponin I). Accumulation of plaque on the coronary artery walls (atherosclerosis) is the most common cause for ACS outside of pregnancy. In pregnancy other causes may be seen more frequently, including coronary artery dissection (tear in the vessel wall) (Nelson-Piercy 2020).

Health Promotion

Risk factors for atherosclerosis and subsequently ACS include smoking, diabetes, obesity, hypertension and hypercholesterolaemia. Some of these are modifiable risk factors.

The commonest disease process that causes ACS in pregnancy is spontaneous coronary artery dissection (SCAD) followed by atherosclerosis (James et al. 2006). With increasing maternal age, ACS in pregnancy is becoming more common (Ganz and Friedman 1995) and usually occurs in the third trimester, surrounding delivery or postnatally.

SCAD is reported more commonly in the postnatal period.

Aortic Dissection

Aortic dissection can be life threatening. A tear occurs in the medial layer of the aortic vessel wall and blood leaks between the layers. The presentation can vary, but there is typically severe chest pain, tearing in character, with radiation to the upper back. There may be raised systolic BP and the BP in both arms may be different. The dissection more commonly occurs in the ascending aorta but symptoms may depend on the blood supply affected. It occurs more commonly in the third trimester and postnatal period (Regitz-Zagrosek et al. 2018). Pregnancy is a predisposing factor in itself (Nelson-Piercy 2020).

Arrhythmias

Abnormal heart rhythms are detected by ECG and are caused by an issue with the cardiac conduction system. In normal physiology the electrical impulses that result in coordinated contraction of the myocardium originate from the sinoatrial (SA) node, and go on to activate the atrioventricular (AV) node that lies in the interventricular septum. The AV node allows some of the impulses to pass down the ventricles to generate ventricular contractions. If this pathway does not work in a synchronised way, the cardiac muscle contraction will not be coordinated, resulting in arrhythmia.

Common types of arrhythmias include atrial fibrillation, atrial flutter, supraventricular tachycardia (SVT) and heart blocks. These abnormal rhythms can be fast (tachyarrhythmia) or slow (bradyarrhythmia). These rhythms may be physiological for some patients, but they should still prompt investigation as they can on occasion be triggered by other pathology. Arrhythmias may present with palpitations, light-headedness, shortness of breath or fatigue and are diagnosed on ECG monitoring. Table 9.1 shows cardiac conditions stratified according to risk.

Paroxysmal SVT may be exacerbated in pregnancy (Regitz-Zagrosek et al. 2018). It is a narrow complex SVT resulting in a heart rate above 120 beats/min (Lehtoranta et al. 2016). The increased blood volume in pregnancy can increase the risk of SVT (Thorne et al. 2006).

Atrial flutter is a tachyarrhythmia with an atrial rate of around 300 beats/min. The resultant abnormal movement of the atria is coordinated (Faculty of Sexual and Reproductive Healthcare 2016), but the atria are unable to effectively pump blood into the ventricles.

Care of Women with Cardiac Conditions

Pre-pregnancy Care

Women can be referred for pre-pregnancy counselling through local maternal medicine networks. Pre-pregnancy counselling has the goal of defining the risks of the mother's condition for a pregnancy and detailing the risks of a pregnancy for the heart condition (as in severe cases a pregnancy may worsen the heart condition in an irreversible fashion).

Woman-Centred Care

Working with the woman and her partner, clinicians in the MDT (including specialist obstetric medical physicians, cardiologists, specialist cardiology nurses and midwives) will discuss planning for pregnancy with a view to optimising the mother's condition and minimising any risks. It is important to discuss the risks of pregnancy for their condition and any maternal and fetal mortality risks so that they are fully informed of the impact that pregnancy may have.

Medicines Management

When considering birth control, the options available may be guided by the risks outlined in the World Health Organization guidance on medical eligibility criteria for contraceptive use (Ruys et al. 2015). Patients should be advised to remain on their contraception until they have had appropriate pre-pregnancy assessments and counselling by their cardiology team.

Some medications may not be safe for the mother to stop and so the impact of continuing treatments that could affect fetal outcome needs to be discussed.

It is vital to take into account the woman's hopes and wishes and to ensure a joint plan is made going forward if she wishes to plan a pregnancy. It would be prudent to ensure there are reasonably up-to-date investigations to help stratify any risk that an upcoming pregnancy may pose.

Orange Flag

If a patient in early pregnancy has an increased risk of maternal death from pregnancy, then termination of pregnancy should be discussed in a sensitive manner, outlining the risks of the pregnancy to the mother and fetus while continuing to offer support should the mother wish to continue (Faculty of Sexual and Reproductive Healthcare 2016).

Antenatally, women should book their pregnancy through their local primary care service and if they have a cardiac history they should be referred within the maternal medicine network to establish an antenatal plan for care in the most appropriate setting. The woman may need monitoring or investigations in the first trimester. It is also an opportunity to counsel on the impact of pregnancy on their and the baby's health. Observations should be monitored at each antenatal appointment and escalated to the medical team if abnormal. Depending on their condition the woman should be seen at least in every trimester in a consultant clinic and some cardiac conditions will require much more regular input. Some may require regular echocardiograms in pregnancy to monitor their heart function. If there is risk of cardiac decompensation, then third-trimester growth scans will be arranged to monitor for signs of fetal growth restriction due to a potential risk of compromised uteroplacental perfusion.

In some cases more urgent referral to secondary care and maternal medicine services may be required. Patients with significant symptoms, for example poor exercise tolerance or signs of cardiac decompensation (like worsening symptoms or hypoxia), should be referred urgently and may need to be admitted to hospital to stabilise their condition. In cases of significant cardiac decompensation, hospital admission may be required to ensure rest until delivery, and a plan for early delivery (taking into account the risks of prematurity for the baby) will be made.

It may be prudent to discuss the impact that a cardiac condition may have on the delivery and prognosis for the baby. Pre-existing cardiac disease is a risk factor for other obstetric complications including postpartum haemorrhage, pre-eclampsia and preterm labour.

Labour and Delivery Management

Timing of delivery will depend on a number of other factors including maternal morbidity, fetal well-being and maturity and cervical assessment. In patients taking medications like beta-blockers, or at risk of cardiac decompensation in later pregnancy, induction of labour may be discussed (Zhang et al. 2021; Cauldwell et al. 2017). The method of induction of labour does not routinely need to be modified.

Medicines Management: Induction of Labour

High doses of misoprostol should be avoided in cardiac patients due to a potential risk of cardiac vasospasm and arrhythmia.

Propess® and Prostin® prostaglandins can be safely used vaginally for induction of labour.

Additional care may be given to speed titration of oxytocin infusions when augmenting labour in high-risk women who physiologically may have difficulty managing large fluid loads.

The mode of delivery must be individualised for each patient to take into account the underlying cardiac disease, gestation of delivery, any background obstetric factors and maternal wishes. In general, a vaginal delivery is considered safe for women due to a reduced risk of bleeding, venous thromboembolism (VTE) and infection and a quicker recovery. An elective caesarean may still be recommended for some, particularly those with severe aortic pathology, pulmonary hypertension or severe heart failure.

Some patients may be on a therapeutic dose of anticoagulation and so an unplanned delivery would increase the risk of maternal haemorrhage. If the anticoagulation is administered orally then caesarean is recommended to reduce the risk of fetal intracranial haemorrhage. In patients on therapeutic LMWH, the dose would have to be omitted 24 hours prior to surgery (Regitz-Zagrosek et al. 2018).

Examination Scenarios

A patient with a known cardiac condition is on the labour ward for induction of labour. She is currently on an antenatal oxytocin infusion. You are her midwife on the labour ward.

- What observations do you need to monitor?
  - Heart rate.
  - BP.
  - Oxygen saturations.
- What additional monitoring may be required intrapartum?
  - High-risk patients may require an arterial line for accurate BP monitoring.
  - Cardiac monitoring can be done with a continuous ECG to detect signs of strain on the heart.
  - The patient will require continuous electronic fetal monitoring.

Epidurals can be used but may cause systemic hypotension lowering the BP, and so in patients with reduced ventricular output should be titrated cautiously (Regitz-Zagrosek et al. 2018). Intravenous fluid must also be used with care depending on the cardiac lesion to ensure adequate pre-load or to avoid cardiovascular overload. In some cardiac cases, the Valsalva manoeuvre may cause a reduction in venous return to the heart and for this reason the active second (pushing) stage may need to be limited to less than one hour. In such cases, an allowance of two hours would be recommended for passive descent of the fetal head. Elective instrumental delivery may be indicated to shorten the active phase and limit maternal effort (Regitz-Zagrosek et al. 2018).

Care should be taken to avoid hypovolaemia through postpartum haemorrhage and so active management of the third stage should be considered. Oxytocin could theoretically cause peripheral vasodilation, but there is evidence of no significant impact on cardiovascular markers and observations (Cauldwell et al. 2017). In the event of bleeding, ergometrine should be only used with caution and avoided in severe cardiac disease, as ergot can cause coronary artery vasospasm that could lead to ischaemic injury to the heart. Prostaglandin F analogues like carboprost should also be avoided in cardiovascular disease (Regitz-Zagrosek et al. 2018).

Postnatal Management

Following delivery, a VTE risk assessment should be done and prophylaxis should be supplied to the patient.

Health Promotion

A discussion regarding postnatal contraception should be prioritised and if possible a suitable option offered in hospital. The patient should be advised to avoid pregnancy for at least one year and discuss with her medical team prior to trying to conceive again.

Appropriate follow-up with the cardiology team should be arranged. Breastfeeding is not contra-indicated, but it is important to consider any medications that may be passed via breast milk and their safety profile.

Take-Home Points

- As the body adapts to pregnancy, the increase in cardiac output can trigger arrhythmias and decompensation of the heart.
- The method of categorising heart conditions into low-risk, medium-risk and high-risk groups in order to optimally manage them is related to the morbidity and mortality risk associated with pregnancy.
- A thorough history and appropriate assessment can help to identify cardiac disease in pregnancy.

Conclusion

Midwives need to be aware of ways in which the risk of serous morbidity and mortality that can occur in pregnancy due to cardiac pathology can be reduced. This is particularly pertinent as cardiac disease remains the leading indirect cause of death in pregnancy. This chapter has described the basic concepts of the changes that occur in cardiac physiology during pregnancy and how cardiac conditions may be investigated and managed. Pre-existing cardiac conditions can significantly affect pregnancy and conversely pregnancy can have an impact on the cardiovascular function in heart disease. A holistic and multidisciplinary approach, taking into account the mother's wishes, providing psychosocial support and clearly outlining the risks and plan with the mother, will result in the best outcomes for mothers and babies.

References

Artal-Mittelmark, R. (2021). Physiology of pregnancy. In: *MSD Manual*. Rahwah, NJ: Merck https://www.msdmanuals.com/professional/gynecology-and-obstetrics/approach-to-the-pregnant-woman-and-prenatal-care/physiology-of-pregnancy.

Cauldwell, M., Steer, P.J., Swan, L. et al. (2017). The management of the third stage of labour in women with heart disease. *Heart* 103: 945–951.

Faculty of Sexual & Reproductive Healthcare (2016). UK medical eligibility criteria for contraceptive use. https://www.fsrh.org/documents/ukmec-2016 (accessed November 2023).

Ganz, L.I. and Friedman, P.L. (1995). Supraventricular Tachycardia. *New England Journal of Medicine* 332 (3): 162–173.

Gewillig, M. and Brown, S.C. (2016). The Fontan circulation after 45 years: update in physiology. *Heart* 102: 1081–1086. https://doi.org/10.1136/heartjnl-2015-307467.

James, A.H., Jamison, M.G., Biswas, M.S. et al. (2006). Acute myocardial infarction in pregnancy. *Circulation* 113 (12): 1564–1571.

Kinsella, S.M. (2006). Effect of blood pressure instrument and cuff side on blood pressure reading in pregnant women in the lateral recumbent position. *International Journal of Obstetric Anesthesia* 15 (4): 290–293.

Knight, M., Bunch, K., Tuffnell, D. et al. (ed.), on Behalf of MBRRACE-UK(2021). *Saving Lives, Improving Mothers' Care – Lessons Learned to Inform Maternity Care from the UK and Ireland Confidential Enquiries into Maternal Deaths and Morbidity 2017–19*. Oxford: National Perinatal Epidemiology Unit, University of Oxford.

Lehtoranta, L., Valta, M., Aantaa, R., and Perheentupa, A. (2016). Raskaudenaikainen supraventrikulaarinen takykardia [Supraventricular tachycardia during pregnancy]. *Duodecim* 132 (2): 173–175.

Nelson-Piercy, C. (2020). *Handbook of Obstetric Medicine*, 6e. London: Routledge.

de Oliveira Antunes, M. and Scudeler, T.L. (2020). Hypertrophic cardiomyopathy. *IJC Heart & Vasculature* 27: 100503.

Regitz-Zagrosek, V., Roos-Hesselink, J.W., Bauersachs, J. et al. (2018). ESC guidelines for the management of cardiovascular diseases during pregnancy: the Task Force for the Management of Cardiovascular Diseases during Pregnancy of the European Society of Cardiology (ESC). *European Heart Journal* 39 (34): 3165–3241.

Ruys, T.P., Roos-Hesselink, J.W., Pijuan-Domenech, A. et al. (2015). Is a planned caesarean section in women with cardiac disease beneficial? *Heart* 101: 530–536.

Sanghavi, M. and John, D. (2014). Rutherford cardiovascular physiology of pregnancy. *Circulation* 130 (12): 1003–10081.

Soma-Pillay, P., Nelson-Piercy, C., Tolppanen, H., and Mebazaa, A. (2016). Physiological changes in pregnancy. *Cardiovascular Journal of Africa* 27 (2): 89–94.

Thorne, S., Nelson-Piercy, C., MacGregor, A. et al. (2006). Pregnancy and contraception in heart disease and pulmonary arterial hypertension. *Journal of Family Planning and Reproductive Health Care* 32 (2): 75–81.

Ware, J.S., Li, J., Mazaika, E. et al. (2016). Shared genetic predisposition in peripartum and dilated cardiomyopathies. *New England Journal of Medicine* 374: 233–241.

Zentner, D., Kotevski, A., King, I. et al. (2016). Fertility and pregnancy in the Fontan population. *International Journal of Cardiology* 208: 97–101.

Zhang, Z., Wengrofsky, A., Wolfe, D.S. et al. (2021). Patent ductus arteriosus in pregnancy: cardio-obstetrics management in a late presentation. *CASE* 5 (2): 119–122.

Further Resources

BUMPS best use of medicines in pregnancy. www.medicinesinpregnancy.org (accessed November 2023).

MMBRACE-UK (2023). Lessons learned to inform maternity care from the UK and Ireland Confidential Enquiries into Maternal Deaths and Morbidity 2019-21. https://www.npeu.ox.ac.uk/mbrrace-uk/reports (accessed November 2023).

Glossary

Anticoagulation	Blood thinning medication to prevent blood from clotting
Arrhythmia	Abnormal heart rhythm
Bradycardia	A slow heart rate, less than 60 bpm
Cardiac output	Can be calculated by multiplying stroke volume by heart rate in beats per minute
Diastole	Relaxation of the heart
Hypovolaemia	A reduction in circulating blood volume
Stroke volume	The volume of blood pumped by the heart with each beat
Systole	Contraction of the heart
Tachycardia	A fast heart rate, over 100 bpm

CHAPTER 10

Shock

Claire Leader

Department of Nursing, Midwifery and Health, Northumbria University, Newcastle upon Tyne, UK

AIM

The aim of this chapter is to introduce the reader to the acute deterioration of a pregnant woman's condition and the recognition and management of shock.

LEARNING OUTCOMES

On completion of this chapter the reader will be able to:

- Develop an understanding of the pathophysiology of shock.
- Become familiar with stages of shock and the compensatory mechanisms involved, specifically relating to pregnancy.
- Have an understanding of the types of shock.
- Possess a fundamental knowledge of Airway, Breathing, Circulation, Disability, Exposure (ABCDE) assessment and treatment and the key considerations for pregnancy.

Test Your Prior Knowledge
1. What is the first stage of shock?
2. What is the last stage of shock?
3. What are the four types of shock?
4. What type of shock is sepsis?

The chapter provides an outline of the pathophysiology of the body systems and compensatory mechanisms. The key types of shock will be discussed to support the provision of gold-standard safe and effective treatment.

It is essential that midwives and other health professionals working in maternity services are competent and confident in providing first-line emergency care to the compromised or critically ill pregnant woman in the community as well as hospital settings. Early recognition of deterioration is fundamental to the provision of safe and effective care and the avoidance of further tragedies such as those reported following the Morecambe Bay (Kirkup 2015) and Shrewsbury and Telford (Ockenden 2022) inquiries. Midwives must be alert to early warning signs in order to keep the woman and fetus safe, to address the symptoms of clinical deterioration and improve the woman's condition. The Mothers and Babies: Reducing Risk through Audits and Confidential Enquiries across the UK (MBRRACE-UK) reports (Knight et al. 2022) highlight that failure to recognise critically ill pregnant women contributes to maternal mortality. The World Health Organization (WHO 2017) emphasises: 'The survival of a woman experiencing an obstetric emergency is determined by the amount of time it takes for care to be delivered and by the level and quality of care provided.' Midwives must ensure that comprehensive assessments are carried out and escalation is expedited where there are concerns.

Pathophysiology of Shock

The cardiovascular system maintains homeostasis through a complex and complementary interplay of four essential functions:

- Maintenance of adequate blood volume
- Continued blood flow
- Vascular resistance
- Contractility of the heart

If any of these mechanisms fail, the others will compensate to ensure that oxygen is delivered and utilised effectively by cells and tissues. Shock results where there is a failure to compensate or when more than one component is affected, leading to an inability of cells to obtain or utilise adequate oxygen and nutrients (Haseer-Koya and Paul 2021).

There exists a hierarchy among different organs and the body will prioritise perfusion of vital organs where there is impairment to normal functioning. This is a protective adaptation that has significant implications for the fetus in pregnancy as uterine and placental functioning are non-essential when the life of the mother is threatened. Additionally, a range of physiological and anatomical changes occur throughout pregnancy that reduce the woman's reserves and may expedite deterioration. Early recognition and management of shock are imperative to minimise the impact on the woman and fetus. The Modified Early Obstetric Warning Score (MEOWS) should be used for all women over 20 weeks' gestation undergoing observation to allow early recognition. The standard National Early Warning Score 2 (NEWS 2) may be used for women under 20 weeks' gestation (Chu et al. 2020).

175

Woman-Centred Care

It is important to remember that a woman in the early stages of shock will be aware that something is not right. Midwives and other health professionals must ensure that any concerns expressed by the woman are listened to and acted on. This is crucial for all women, but a particular focus should be given to women where communication may be additionally challenging, such as women with learning disabilities, women for whom English is not a first language or women with speech or hearing impairment. A key theme of the most recent MBRRACE-UK report is that women from ethnic minority backgrounds often have their concerns dismissed by health professionals and this may be a contributory factor to a disproportionate rate of morbidity and mortality (Knight et al. 2022).

Stages of Shock

Although the initial response to shock can vary depending on age, gestation and general state of health prior to the event leading to the shocked state, there are three distinct stages of shock.

Stage 1: Compensatory (Non-progressive) Stage of Shock

When the blood pressure is insufficient to adequately perfuse cells, a range of neural, hormonal and chemical compensatory mechanisms will be triggered to maintain homeostasis and restore blood flow to vital organs. At this early stage the individual may be experiencing symptoms of shock (e.g. increased heart rate, low blood pressure [BP], thirst), but these are reversible with appropriate interventions.

> ### Red Flag
>
> Fetal distress can be an early indicator of maternal shock and where there are pathological changes to fetal heart rate, maternal assessment should always be performed.

Neural Compensatory Mechanisms

The sympathetic nervous system regulates blood flow and pressure through its ability to increase heart rate and total peripheral resistance. In the shocked state, the baroreceptors and chemoreceptors located in the carotid sinus and aortic arch detect the reduction in blood pressure, and impulses are relayed to the vasomotor centre and medulla oblongata (Migliozzi 2021).

Hormonal Compensatory Mechanisms

When the sympathetic nervous system is stimulated this causes the release of catecholamines (epinephrine and norepinephrine) from the adrenal medullae. This increases the heart rate and the force of cardiac contractions to improve cardiac output. Blood flow to the heart increases as the coronary arteries vasodilate, supplying oxygen to the cells and tissue. Rate and depth of respiration will also increase to support gaseous exchange and oxygen levels in the blood (Sole et al. 2016).

Compensatory mechanisms work on a negative feedback loop. One example of this is when the drop in cardiac output affects the renal system. This causes the kidneys to release renin, which converts angiotensin into angiotensin I, which is then metabolised as a powerful vasoconstrictor angiotensin II. This triggers the adrenal gland to release aldosterone, which causes the reabsorption of sodium from the renal tubule. This results in retention of water as the body attempts to increase circulating blood volume. Furthermore, stimulation of the posterior pituitary gland releases anti-diuretic hormone (ADH), which increases the amount of water reabsorbed by the kidney tubules. This can result in reduced urine output (Migliozzi 2021).

Chemical Compensatory Mechanisms

There is decreased blood flow to the lungs that results from a lowered cardiac output, which the chemoreceptors located in the aorta and carotid arteries detect. The rate and depth of respiration increase to compensate, but this hyperventilation has a negative impact on gaseous exchange and results in a reduction in carbon dioxide. This, in turn, leads to reduced blood flow and oxygen delivery to the brain and can cause confusion or agitation.

When the compensatory mechanisms begin to fail, or if they are left untreated, the individual will move into the next stage of shock (Migliozzi 2021).

Stage 2: Progressive (Decompensated) Stage of Shock

Unless the cause of shock is corrected, tissue damage leading to organ failure will occur due to prolonged reduction of cardiac output, reduced circulating blood volume and inadequate perfusion. Vasoconstriction will continue with the aim of shunting blood to the vital organs at the expense of the extremities, leading to ischaemia. The inadequate oxygen and nutrient supply causes the metabolism to switch from aerobic to anaerobic, increasing the production of lactic acid, leading to metabolic acidosis.

Where anaerobic metabolism is prolonged, the production of adenosine triphosphate (ATP) is reduced and the sodium–potassium pump begins to fail, leading to an accumulation of sodium ions in the cell causing the cell to swell and malfunction. As shock progresses, histamine and bradykinin are released that have vasodilating properties, causing a further reduction in blood flow and a consequent decrease in cardiac output and blood pressure. This causes hypoxia, which leads to depression of the vasomotor centre in the medulla and the sympathetic nervous system. Levels of consciousness decrease and restlessness, agitation and confusion may ensue (Migliozzi 2021).

Stage 3: Irreversible (Refractory) Stage of Shock

The continued reduction in blood pressure, circulating blood volume and cardiac output will lead to irreversible damage to the cells and tissues of the organs. The body will fail to respond to any corrective treatment and multiorgan failure and death will occur.

Types of Shock

There are broadly four types of shock that can be classified as follows:

- Hypovolaemic shock
- Cardiogenic shock
- Distributive shock
- Obstructive shock

Red Flag

- The leading single cause of indirect maternal death in the United Kingdom is cardiac disease.
- Thrombosis and thromboembolism remains the leading cause of direct maternal death during or up to six weeks after the end of pregnancy.

Source: Adapted from Knight et al. (2022).

The identification of which organs are deprived can assist in identifying the type and degree of shock. Additionally, because of the compensatory adaptation, fetal distress can be an early signal and, taken in the context of other clinical indicators, can support midwives in the recognition and early escalation of deterioration. Through an effective multidisciplinary approach, it is possible to differentiate between the types of shock from the history, examination, focused investigations and response to treatment (Sarah Paterson-Brown and Howell 2016). Table 10.1 outlines the key actions and considerations to support rapid initial assessment (World Health Organization 2017).

Hypovolaemic Shock

Hypovolaemia is the form of shock that is due to blood/fluid loss. This can be caused by haemorrhage, diabetic ketoacidosis or from a relative loss of fluid following vasodilation, for example after spinal/epidural anaesthesia. Maternal deaths from hypovolaemia following haemorrhage are fortunately uncommon and account for 0.48 per 100 000 maternities; the rate of these deaths has halved since the reporting period 2013–2015 (Knight et al. 2022). This is due in part to improved recognition and early escalation of deterioration. However, haemorrhage emerges as the major cause of maternal morbidity in both developed and developing countries (WHO 2017).

TABLE 10.1   Key considerations for rapid assessment.

Assess	Danger signs	Consider
Airway and breathing	Cyanosis Respiratory distress	Severe anaemia Heart failure Pneumonia Asthma
Circulation	Skin: cool and clammy Pulse: fast (>110 bpm) and weak Blood pressure: low (systolic <90 mmHg)	Shock
Vaginal bleeding (early or late pregnancy or following childbirth)	Pregnancy (ascertain gestation) Recently given birth Placenta not delivered following childbirth	**Early pregnancy (first trimester)** Spontaneous abortion (miscarriage) Ectopic pregnancy Molar pregnancy **Late pregnancy and labour (second trimester onwards)** Placental abruption Placenta praevia Uterine rupture **Postpartum** Atonic uterus Tears to perineum, vagina, cervix Retained placenta Inverted uterus
Unconscious or convulsing	Blood pressure: low (diastolic >90 mmHg) Temperature: high (38°C or more)	Eclampsia Epilepsy (malaria or tetanus depending on country)
Dangerous fever	Weak, lethargic Frequent or painful urination Temperature: high (38°C or more) Unconscious Neck stiffness Shallow breathing Abdomen tender Vaginal discharge Tender breasts	**Pregnancy and labour** Urinary tract infection Chorio/amnionitis Group B streptococcal infection **Postpartum** Endometritis Retained placenta Pelvic abscesses Peritonitis Mastitis
Abdominal pain	Pregnancy – ascertain gestation Blood pressure: low (systolic <90 mmHg) Pulse: fast (>110 bpm) Temperature: high (38°C or more)	**Early pregnancy** Ectopic pregnancy Spontaneous abortion Ovarian cyst Appendicitis **Later pregnancy and labour** Labour (term or preterm) Chorio/amnionitis Placental abruption Uterine rupture

Source: Adapted from WHO (2017).

Historically assessment of blood loss has been underestimated. Guidance states that it is important to assess for signs of shock and that fetal compromise is an important indicator of volume depletion. Shock is associated with blood loss greater than 1000 ml. The drop in circulating blood volume results in a decrease in venous return, triggering the compensatory mechanisms discussed earlier. There is an increase in plasma volume during pregnancy of around 40%, which allows the woman to lose 1200–1500 ml of blood before any signs of hypovolaemia may be evident (Chu et al. 2020). Management and treatment should involve calling for help and following the Airway, Breathing, Circulation, Disability, Exposure (ABCDE) framework later in the chapter, with particular focus on replacing lost fluids and addressing the source of blood or fluid loss.

There can be a variety of causes of hypovolaemia, but in pregnancy the most common causes are:

- Ectopic pregnancy (first trimester)
- Antepartum haemorrhage (second and third trimester)
- Postpartum haemorrhage

Ectopic Pregnancy

An ectopic pregnancy occurs when the fertilised ovum implants outside the uterine cavity. In 93–98% of cases, the site of implantation is the uterine tube; however, it can occur within the ovary, the cervical canal or elsewhere in the abdominal cavity. The incidence in the United Kingdom is approximately 11 in 1000 pregnancies (National Institute for Health and Care Excellence 2021).

Ectopic pregnancy is a serious and life-threatening condition and the major cause of maternal death before 20 weeks' gestation. Risk factors include higher maternal age, smoking and damage to the uterine tube(s).

The major complication that leads to hypovolaemia is tubal rupture, which is most likely to occur between weeks 5 and 7 of gestation. This can make diagnosis more difficult as the woman may not be aware she is pregnant. However, symptoms may include:

- Abdominal tenderness and/or distension
- Cervical motion tenderness
- Shoulder tip pain
- Vomiting
- Dysuria
- Amenorrhea

Women with a suspected ectopic pregnancy should be transferred as an emergency to an appropriate acute care setting. An intravenous cannula should be inserted to treat hypovolaemia and bloods taken for cross-matching. Analgesia should be given and the woman should be transferred to the operating theatre where a salpingectomy may be performed.

Health Promotion

An avoidable cause of damage to the uterine tubes derives from sexually transmitted infections (STIs) such as chlamydia. If left untreated, STIs can lead to pelvic inflammatory disease (PID), which causes tubal scarring and loss of cilia that, under normal circumstances, would assist the fertilised ovum in its passage through the tubes to the uterine cavity. Health professionals can raise awareness of the impact of PID on subsequent fertility and increased risk of ectopic pregnancy by using a Making Every Contact Count (MECC) approach when seeing women in primary care contexts.

Antepartum Haemorrhage

Antepartum haemorrhage (APH) is defined as bleeding after the 24th week of pregnancy and before the birth of the baby (RCOG 2012). The bleeding occurs from the placental site and can be caused by placenta praevia, where the placenta is situated in the lower uterine segment, or placental abruption, where the placenta begins to separate prematurely from the uterine wall (see Chapter 7).

A woman with any active bleeding in pregnancy should be assessed in an appropriate acute care setting and management will depend on the amount of bleeding and the condition of the mother and fetus.

Woman-Centred Care

Healthcare professionals should be aware that APH can be caused by domestic violence. Women with repeated presentations of APH should be asked about domestic violence and supported as per local safeguarding policies.

Postpartum Haemorrhage

A primary postpartum haemorrhage (PPH) is defined as a blood loss of more than 500 ml within 24 hours of birth. This may occur as a sudden loss of >500 ml or may occur more slowly at around 150 ml/h over a few hours. However, any bleeding that leads to haemodynamic instability can be classified as a PPH (Coad 2018).

Secondary PPH is any blood loss occurring 24 hours after birth and can be caused by infection or retained placental tissue. The cause needs to be ascertained and treated before the blood loss ceases.

The causes of PPH can be broken down to the four Ts (Mavrides et al. 2017):

- **Tone:** The most common cause of PPH is poor uterine tone, accounting for 70% of incidences. Encourage the woman to try to pass urine and empty the bladder and consider massaging the fundus to stimulate the uterus to contract to prevent further blood loss.
- **Trauma:** This may involve any part of the perineum, vulva, vagina or cervix and will require repair to stem the blood loss. However, pressure may be applied directly to the area to maintain haemostasis until repair can be performed.
- **Tissue:** Tissue could mean retention of the placenta or a small part of the placenta, which should be removed by a trained professional to stop the bleeding. This accounts for 10% of incidences.
- **Thrombin:** This refers to the development of a condition called disseminated intravascular coagulopathy (DIC). This occurs where clotting factors are deranged and normal clotting is impeded (see Chapter 13). This accounts for 1% of incidences of PPH.

Medicines Management: Active Management of Third-Stage Labour

Evidence from Cochrane Reviews has established that an actively managed third stage of labour that includes prophylactic uterotonics, early cord clamping and controlled cord traction reduces the risk of PPH. McDonald et al. (2004) concluded that ergometrine-oxytocin (e.g. syntometrine), oxytocin 10 IU and oxytocin 5 IU all had similar efficacy in preventing PPH over 1000 ml. However, compared with oxytocin, ergometrine-oxytocin was associated with a fivefold increase in adverse effects such as raised blood pressure, nausea and vomiting. A shared decision-making conversation, including the risks and benefits of each of these drugs, needs to be conducted with the woman to support her to balance the risks of PPH with the potential adverse effects, which can interfere with maternal–infant bonding and breastfeeding.

It is imperative for the effective care and treatment of women experiencing a PPH to commence the ABCDE framework and involve the multidisciplinary team (MDT) in the early stages. This should include senior midwifery, anaesthetic and obstetric staff, with the haematologist and blood laboratory being informed.

Learning Event

Visit RCOG green top guideline no. 52 and review the major haemorrhage protocol for PPH: https://obgyn.onlinelibrary.wiley.com/doi/full/10.1111/1471-0528.14178.

Cardiogenic Shock

Cardiogenic shock occurs as a result of reduced cardiac contractility (see Chapter 9). The causes of cardiogenic shock include ischaemic heart disease, cardiomyopathy and arrythmias. The woman may present with chest pains, shortness of breath and orthopnoea. Reviews of maternal deaths due to cardiac disease found that when women present with classical symptoms they are attributed to the pregnancy and there is a failure to recognise and appropriately treat cardiovascular disease (Knight and Kurinczuk 2018).

While cardiogenic shock may present with symptoms similar to hypovolaemic shock, differentiating features include orthopnoea and extreme air hunger. Chest auscultation will help identify pulmonary congestion caused by an increased pressure in the pulmonary circulation. As with other forms of shock, early recognition is imperative and an assessment of the woman's condition utilising the ABCDE framework is indicated.

Health Promotion

With cardiac disease being reported as the leading cause of maternal death, there is a need for healthcare professionals to consider moving the focus from managing cardiac disease once the woman is pregnant and instead considering ways to support women with serious cardiac conditions in the prevention of pregnancies as a way of addressing morbidity and mortality (Knight and Kurinczuk 2018).

Distributive Shock

Distributive shock is characterised by widespread vasodilation and decreased vascular resistance. In distributive shock circulating blood volume remains normal, but cardiac output and blood pressure are impaired. The decreased vascular resistance results in the blood and fluid in large veins causing circulating blood volume to be abnormally displaced or, as the name suggests, 'distributed'. Blood pressure in the systemic circulation falls, causing a decrease in venous return and reduced cardiac output. Perfusion becomes impaired and shock ensues.

There are three types of distributive shock: anaphylactic, septic and neurogenic.

Anaphylaxis

The onset of anaphylactic shock is rapid and can progress to death in minutes if corrective treatment is not given. The incidence of severe obstetric anaphylaxis is approximately 1 in 30 000 pregnancies (Mulla et al. 2010). It is a severe generalised or systemic hypersensitivity (allergic) reaction to a proteinous substance such as peanuts, shellfish or foreign serum. However, the most common cause in an obstetric setting will be anaesthetic muscle relaxants and antibiotics (Sarah Paterson-Brown and Howell 2016). Intravenous drugs are more likely to cause a reaction than oral preparations. Latex sensitivity is also more predominant in the pregnant population and any latex sensitivity should be documented on the woman's notes so that all staff are aware. Anaphylactic reactions are usually triggered within 5–10 minutes of exposure to the allergen.

This type of shock involves a number of systems, which makes deterioration rapid. The redistribution of fluid into the tissues will cause oedema and swelling that can be observed externally, particularly in the face. Internally, this swelling will lead to bronchoconstriction causing upper airway obstruction and pulmonary oedema, resulting in respiratory distress. Ultimately, there will be reduced cardiac output and, as shock advances, acute ventricular failure and myocardial ischaemia may occur. Common signs will also include anxiety, gastrointestinal (GI) cramps, urticaria with severe itching and burning to the skin (Tortora and Derrickson 2017).

Rapid initial assessment and early multidisciplinary treatment are fundamental to dealing with anaphylaxis. ABCDE assessment should be performed and life-threatening features treated. Ensuring that the potential cause of the anaphylaxis has been removed/discontinued is the first priority (e.g. blood product/medication). First-line treatment for anaphylaxis is adrenaline. Additionally, a sudden change in posture should be avoided; a supine position is indicated with the pregnant woman being moved to the left lateral position.

181

Medicines Management

Adrenaline should be given early as an intramuscular (IM) injection into the anterolateral thigh to correct issues causing Airway, Breathing and Circulatory problems. UK resuscitation guidelines state that adrenaline is well tolerated and poses minimal risk to anyone having an allergic reaction. Essentially, if in doubt give IM adrenaline. If problems persist, repeat adrenaline after five minutes.

   Dose: Use adrenaline at 1 mg/ml (1 : 100) concentration.

   Adult and child >12 years old: 500 μg IM (0.5 ml)

   Where these measures are ineffective, as is the case for refractory anaphylaxis, intravenous (IV) adrenaline and fluids will be indicated. These should only be given by an experienced professional and urgent transfer to an acute unit should be initiated where incidences occur in the community setting.

Source: Adapted from Resuscitation Council UK (2021b).

Septic Shock

The most recent MBRRACE report identified that sepsis is the third most common direct cause of maternal death (Knight et al. 2022). The World Health Organization (2017) defines sepsis as 'a life threatening condition defined as organ dysfunction resulting from infection during pregnancy, childbirth, post-abortion or post-partum period'. Infections can be bacterial, viral, fungal or parasitic. However, the causes of sepsis in pregnancy may be indirect, such as influenza, pneumonia, GI infections, urinary tract infections and others. Causes directly related to pregnancy include systemic infections such as chorioamnionitis following prolonged rupture of membranes, or infections from perineal tears, caesarean section wounds or mastitis. Some authors have highlighted that the indirect causes of sepsis will be exacerbated by the pregnancy and that this way of categorising maternal morbidity and mortality due to sepsis may provide a misleading picture (Mohamed-Ahmed et al. 2015).

   The most common causes of sepsis identified in the most recent literature were genital tract infection (31%) and the presence of *Escherichia coli* (*E. coli*) (21%) (Amaan and Lamont 2019). There are a number of risk factors for sepsis (see Table 10.2) and it is incumbent on the midwife to ensure that guidelines are followed and, where sepsis is suspected, early escalation and assessment are offered. However, many of the signs related to sepsis are also normal physiological adaptations of pregnancy, which can render assessment challenging. For example, a drop in blood pressure is often associated with the vasodilation that occurs in trimesters 2 and 3 to accommodate the increase in circulating blood volume, along with compensatory tachycardia and tachypnoea. Amaan and Lamont (2019) state that all physiological

TABLE 10.2   Risk factors for maternal sepsis in pregnancy.

Obesity
Caesarean section
Impaired glucose tolerance/diabetes
Impaired immunity/immunosuppressant medication
Anaemia
Vaginal discharge
History of pelvic infection
History of group A, B or D streptococcal infection (group B more of a concern for neonate than mother)
Amniocentesis and other invasive procedures
Cervical cerclage
Prolonged spontaneous rupture of membranes
Black or other minority ethnic group origin
History of domestic violence
Higher maternal age
History of *Escherichia coli* (*E. coli*) infection

Source: Adapted from RCOG (2012); Bothamley and Boyle (2015); Paterson-Brown and Howell (2016).

changes associated with systemic inflammatory response syndrome (SIRS) would be expected in pregnancy except for a raised temperature (which is not present), and emphasise the importance of an adapted Modified Early Obstetric Warning System (MEOWS) for pregnant patients.

The incidence is decreasing thanks to the UK Sepsis Trust's raising of awareness of this issue, but even where aggressive management has been implemented for septic shock the mortality rate is approximately 40% (Paterson-Brown and Howell 2016). There is emphasis throughout guidance in pregnancy on early escalation and IV antibiotic administration.

Case Study 10.1   Maternal Sepsis

Marianna attended her local maternity assessment unit at 38 weeks' gestation with a history of painful contractions and diarrhoea and a pale, clammy appearance. A full set of maternal observations were recorded using a MEOWS chart. Tachycardia of 105 bpm and a temperature of 37.9°C were noted. The midwife was concerned and recognised this could be sepsis. This triggered the use of the maternal sepsis care bundle, which included the 'Sepsis Six'. The consultant obstetrician and consultant anaesthetist were alerted. Fetal monitoring was commenced and communication was sent out to the relevant MDT (obstetric, anaesthetic, paediatric medical team as well as theatre staff, haematology staff and so forth) to prepare for potential emergency caesarean section. Within 40 minutes, Marianna had been fully assessed, blood cultures taken, and IV fluids and antibiotics administered as per local protocol. Her lactate was raised and the fetal heart rate was showing an abnormal pattern, indicating distress. The baby was delivered via emergency caesarean section and required treatment for sepsis in the neonatal unit. Following swift and effective care and treatment, Marianna and her baby were well.

Consider the following:

- What are the key elements of good practice highlighted in this case study?
- Are you aware of your local policy in relation to managing sepsis?
- What are the implications for women and their babies where recognition of sepsis is delayed?

As with other forms of shock, sepsis assessment and treatment should follow the ABCDE approach. An additional mnemonic known as the Sepsis Six (Nutbeam and Daniels 2021) outlines key actions to be taken for the early and most appropriate treatment. Figure 10.1 outlines the Sepsis Six specific to pregnancy.

Learning Event

The UK Sepsis Trust has worked to raise awareness of sepsis in recent years using a composite approach to provide education to clinicians as well as the public. It advocates for six actions to be taken where sepsis is suspected (the Sepsis Six). Toolkits are available, including a toolkit for the management of sepsis in pregnancy:
https://sepsistrust.org/wp-content/uploads/2020/08/Sepsis-Acute-Pregnant-Version-1.4.pdf.

Neurogenic Shock

Neurogenic shock is a form of distributive shock caused by an imbalance between the sympathetic and parasympathetic stimulation of vascular smooth muscle. When the sympathetic stimulus is interrupted in its role in maintaining vascular resistance, shock will result. It is often referred to as vasogenic shock due to the resulting vasodilation that occurs, increasing the vascular compartments and creating a state of relative hypovolaemia (Tortora and Derrickson 2017).

There are a range of causes of neurogenic shock, including trauma (such as with inversion of the uterus), cerebral hypoxia, hypoglycaemia, anaesthetics and other drugs, pain and severe emotional distress.

The body compensates by increasing sympathetic activity leading to increased force of muscle contractions, increasing stroke volume and peripheral vasoconstriction to maintain blood pressure. Additionally, fainting may occur, which equalises blood pressure by preventing the woman from being in an upright position.

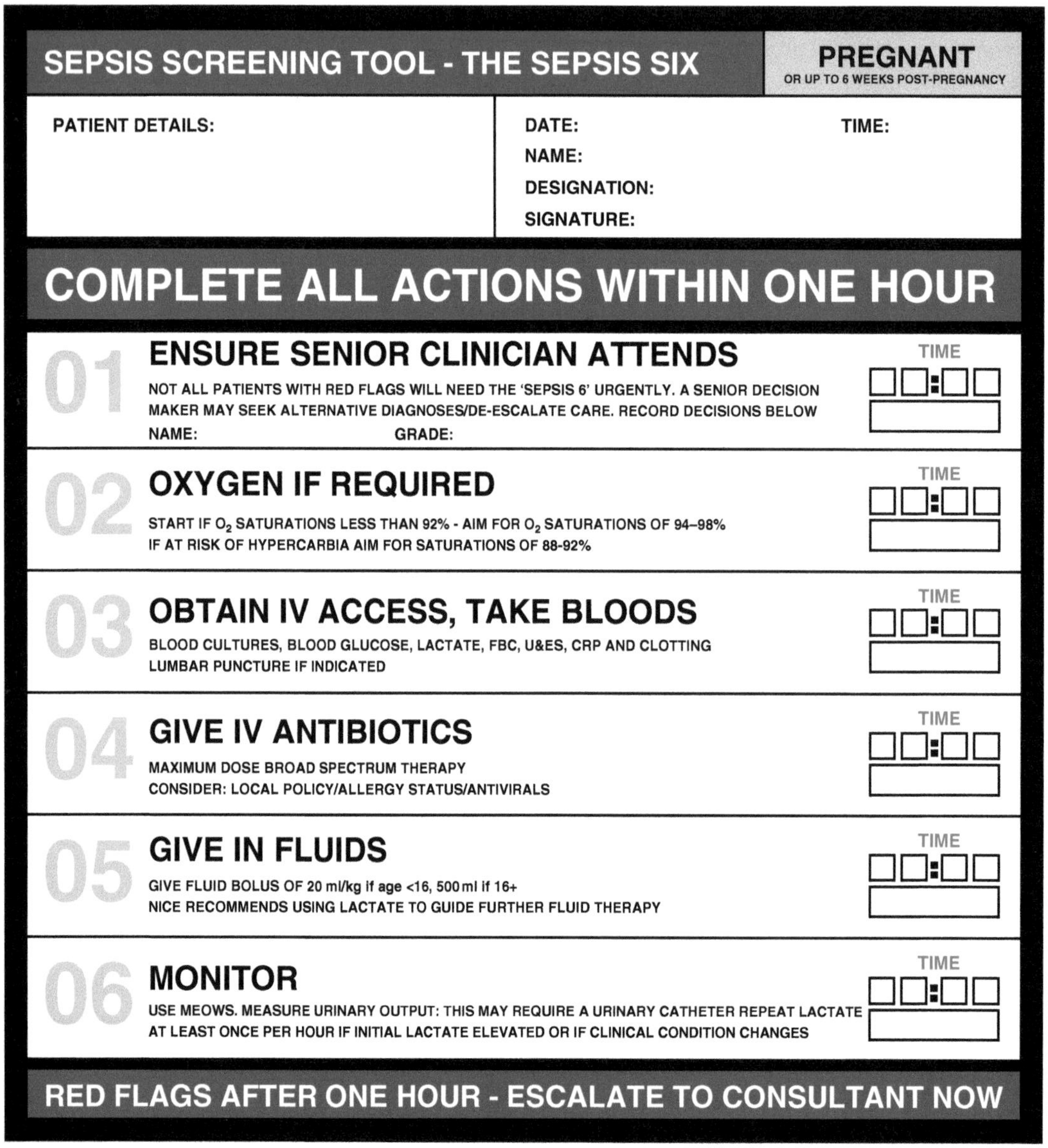

| SEPSIS SCREENING TOOL - THE SEPSIS SIX | PREGNANT OR UP TO 6 WEEKS POST-PREGNANCY |

PATIENT DETAILS:

DATE:
NAME:
DESIGNATION:
SIGNATURE:

TIME:

COMPLETE ALL ACTIONS WITHIN ONE HOUR

01 ENSURE SENIOR CLINICIAN ATTENDS
NOT ALL PATIENTS WITH RED FLAGS WILL NEED THE 'SEPSIS 6' URGENTLY. A SENIOR DECISION MAKER MAY SEEK ALTERNATIVE DIAGNOSES/DE-ESCALATE CARE. RECORD DECISIONS BELOW
NAME: GRADE:
TIME

02 OXYGEN IF REQUIRED
START IF O_2 SATURATIONS LESS THAN 92% - AIM FOR O_2 SATURATIONS OF 94–98%
IF AT RISK OF HYPERCARBIA AIM FOR SATURATIONS OF 88-92%
TIME

03 OBTAIN IV ACCESS, TAKE BLOODS
BLOOD CULTURES, BLOOD GLUCOSE, LACTATE, FBC, U&ES, CRP AND CLOTTING
LUMBAR PUNCTURE IF INDICATED
TIME

04 GIVE IV ANTIBIOTICS
MAXIMUM DOSE BROAD SPECTRUM THERAPY
CONSIDER: LOCAL POLICY/ALLERGY STATUS/ANTIVIRALS
TIME

05 GIVE IN FLUIDS
GIVE FLUID BOLUS OF 20 ml/kg if age <16, 500 ml if 16+
NICE RECOMMENDS USING LACTATE TO GUIDE FURTHER FLUID THERAPY
TIME

06 MONITOR
USE MEOWS. MEASURE URINARY OUTPUT: THIS MAY REQUIRE A URINARY CATHETER REPEAT LACTATE
AT LEAST ONCE PER HOUR IF INITIAL LACTATE ELEVATED OR IF CLINICAL CONDITION CHANGES
TIME

RED FLAGS AFTER ONE HOUR - ESCALATE TO CONSULTANT NOW

FIGURE 10.1 The Sepsis Six.

Obstructive Shock

Obstructive shock occurs when there is impaired perfusion and oxygen delivery to the tissues caused by a physical obstruction. Cardiac output is reduced because of the obstruction, which prevents blood from entering or leaving the heart. The most common cause of obstruction in pregnancy is pulmonary embolism (PE) (Tortora and Derrickson 2017). The normal physiological processes involved in pregnancy create a hypercoagulable state, which predisposes pregnant women to a greater risk of venous thromboembolism (VTE) that, if left untreated, can enter the blood stream and lodge in the lungs, causing a PE. Thrombosis and thromboembolism form the leading cause of direct maternal death, and 31 out of 32 women who died due to VTE died as a result of PE. Although there has been a marked decrease in the rate of VTE due to improved assessment, monitoring and treatment, it continues to be a risk that can be prevented through improvements in care, with obesity in particular highlighted as a key risk factor (Knight et al. 2022).

Obstructive shock can also occur as a result of tension pneumothorax, amniotic air embolism, pericarditis or high positive end-expiratory pressure (PEEP) during artificial ventilation, for example. Treatment of obstructive shock will involve identifying and treating the underlying cause. Ensuring that fast and effective assessment and care are offered will be the determining factor for morbidity and mortality.

Primary Assessment

The Airway, Breathing, Circulation, Disability, Exposure/Environment (ABCDE) framework is useful for assessing critically ill women (Resuscitation Council UK 2021a).

Airway

Airway assessment begins with assessing whether the woman can speak, by asking if she is OK. An appropriate response indicates that the airway is patent and brain perfusion adequate. Agitation, slurred speech or confusion can be an indication of hypoxia.

Inspect the airway for any obstructions and listen for abnormal sounds such as snoring or gurgling, which can indicate partial obstruction of the pharynx. Check for cyanosis around the mouth (this will appear as a bluish tint to the skin and mucous membranes in women with lighter skin tones, but will present as a greyish or white colour in darker skin tones; Raynor et al. 2021). Feel for the trachea to assess whether it is midline (an indication of pneumothorax is a deviated trachea most likely suspected in the incidence of trauma).

To maintain the airway manually, perform a head tilt and chin lift, or jaw thrust manoeuvre (where C-spine trauma is suspected). Where blood and secretions are present in the oropharynx, consider suction if available. Ultimately, if the woman is unable to maintain her own airway, a definitive airway is required. This will depend on the location and the resources available; oropharyngeal (such as Guedel, see Figure 10.2) or nasopharyngeal airways may be used, but endotracheal intubation (Figure 10.3) by a trained professional is gold standard in an unconscious patient (Paterson-Brown and Howell 2016).

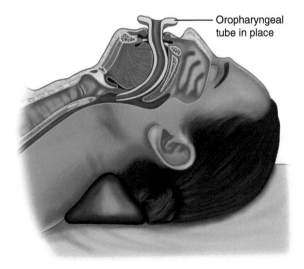

Oropharyngeal tube in place

FIGURE 10.2 Guedel airway position.

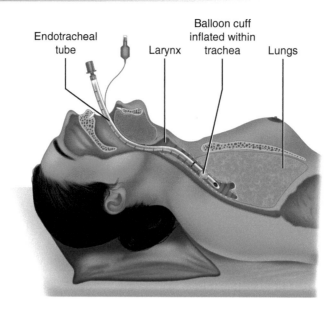

FIGURE 10.3   Endotracheal tube placement.

Considerations in Pregnancy

Obesity is associated with many of the causes of maternal death and is a cause of significant morbidity and mortality in the general population. When assessing the airway in a deteriorating or collapsed pregnant woman, the neck may be short and surrounded by excess adipose tissue, causing issues with airway management.

Additionally, women in later pregnancy may have engorged breasts or may have oedema related to pre-eclampsia, which can encroach on the airway and cause difficulties.

As the pregnancy advances there may be issues with the GI system that can increase the risk of gastric reflux, aspiration or regurgitation, which can make airway patency problematic. GI pressure may be increased as the uterus grows and presses on or displaces the organs within the GI system.

Breathing

Breathing may be compromised by an airway that is obstructed, but this can also be a result of altered ventilatory mechanics (such as respiratory disease) or central nervous system depression (for example with epilepsy or following opioid administration). Support with breathing is required to ensure adequate ventilation, gaseous exchange and sufficient perfusion are maintained.

An assessment of breathing should be undertaken using the Inspect, Palpate, Percuss, Auscultate (IPPA) framework:

- **Inspect:** Observe for chest movement and check for injuries.
- **Palpate:** Palpate for chest movement.
- **Percuss:** Percussion note should be resonant and equal bilaterally.
- **Auscultate:** Air entry should be equal and bilateral.

If breathing is compromised following appropriate airway management, then assistance will be required to improve the gaseous exchange in the lungs for the patient. Again, the way this is done will depend on the context and resources available (see Chapter 15 for a discussion of respiratory disorders).

In the unconscious patient ventilatory support can be achieved using the following techniques:

- Mouth to mouth (less likely in a hospital setting).
- Mouth to pocket mask.
- Self-inflating (resuscitator) bag and mask.
- Self-inflating bag and endotracheal tube (or other definitive airway).
- Automatic ventilation.

Considerations in Pregnancy

As the pregnancy progresses tidal volume continues to increase, from 20% in early pregnancy to 40% in later pregnancy (see Chapter 15 for a discussion of tidal volume).

Remember that the woman's lung capacity remains unchanged, meaning that she will have very few reserves if illness or injury occurs.

In a normal pregnancy the respiratory rate will increase and as the uterus grows, the rib cage will splay as the diaphragm plays a larger part in supporting respiration.

Circulation

The circulation throughout the body will be compromised where shock has progressed. Assessment of circulation will involve measuring the woman's pulse, blood pressure and capillary refill time (CRT), and observing colouration, temperature, urine output and sources of potential haemorrhage (consider hypovolaemia as the primary cause of shock until proven otherwise).

- Observe the appearance of the hands and digits: they may be blue, pink or pale in lighter skin tones and in women with darker skin tones may appear greyish or white in colour. Mottling may also be evident.
- Are the limbs cool or warm?
- CRT should be assessed by applying pressure for five seconds on a fingertip. The amount of time it takes for the skin to return to the colour of the surrounding skin after the pressure is released is the CRT. This should be less than two seconds.
- Are the veins underfilled or collapsed?
- Monitor blood pressure: although a decreased blood pressure can be a more advanced sign of shock due to compensatory mechanisms, the systolic should be above 90 mmHg.
- Assess central pulse for presence, rate (a fast pulse above 110 bpm is an indication of shock), quality, regularity and equality.
- Other signs of poor cardiac output may include reduced conscious level, reduced urine output (less than 0.5 ml/kg of weight per hour indicates reduced urine output).
- Fetal distress or compromise can also be indicative of maternal deterioration.
- Observe for haemorrhage.

Management of circulation will involve a multidisciplinary effort to gain intravenous access, commence fluids, take bloods and other investigations to identify and treat the underlying cause of shock.

Red Flag

Later in pregnancy the 'resistance' to the pumping action of the heart rises because the pregnant uterus begins to partially impede the return of blood flow in the vena cava to the heart. This means that the stroke volume increases to increase the circulating pressure to improve the return flow. For this reason, a pregnant woman must avoid lying flat on her back and should be moved to a left lateral position. Where there is suspected C-spine trauma, the health professional should ensure that the uterus is displaced to the left side manually (see Figure 10.4).

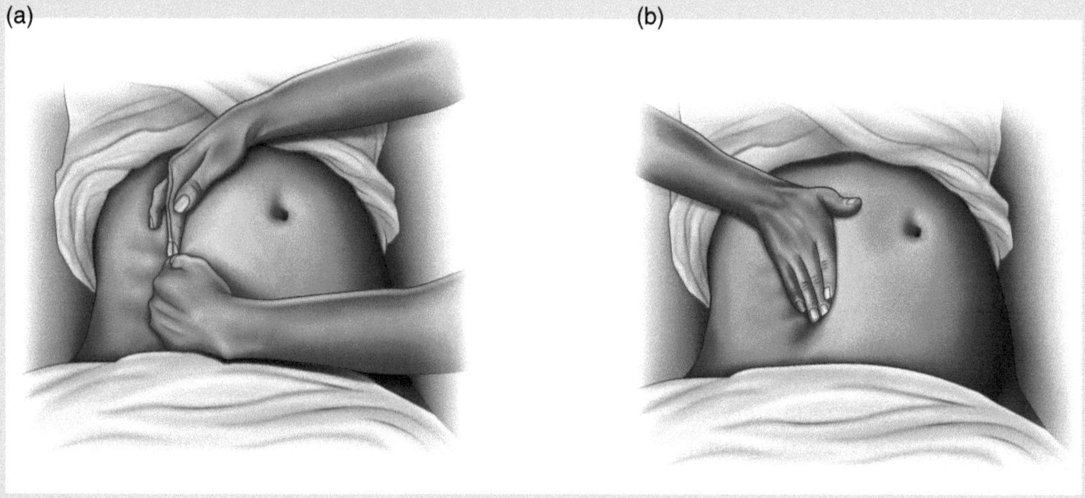

FIGURE 10.4   Uterine displacement. (a) Left uterine displacement using two-handed technique. (b) Left uterine displacement using one-handed technique.

Considerations in Pregnancy

To ensure that the placenta functions optimally, the woman's blood volume needs to increase dramatically, leading to an increase in the cardiac stroke volume and arterial pressure. Central venous pressure remains unchanged. Compared to non-pregnant women, a pregnant woman has a slightly lower haemoglobin concentration, because there is a larger plasma volume.

The fetal circulation and the mother's circulation are separate, and blood does not mix. The placenta belongs to the fetus and is filled with fetal blood. The oxygen tension in the fetal circulation is lower than that in the mother, so the fetus will always obtain oxygen from the mother. Fetal compromise can be an early sign of maternal deterioration and should always be recognised.

Disability .

Unconsciousness can be caused by a range of systemic failures as identified earlier. The assessment of disability will include the following:

- Checking the patient's drug charts for any reversible drug-induced causes (for example opioids).
- Perform neurological observations, including assessment of pupil size, equality and reactivity as well as assessment of whether she is alert, responds to vocal stimuli, responds to painful stimuli or is unresponsive (AVPU). Alternatively, a Glasgow Coma Scale score may be used to assess the patient's level of consciousness.
- Blood glucose measurement may be performed to check for hypoglycaemia as a potential reversible cause of unconsciousness (follow local protocols for management).

Considerations in Pregnancy

A woman who is experiencing seizures may be epileptic, septic or having an eclamptic seizure as a result of high blood pressure and proteinuria.

Exposure/Environment

Examining the woman by fully exposing the body will be necessary. Ensure that dignity and respect are maintained at all times.

Considerations in Pregnancy

Examine the introitus for any evidence of a presenting part, cord, membranes or bleeding (depending on stage of pregnancy).

Observe for evidence of blood loss in soaked clothes, sheets, sanitary pads and so forth.

Ensure that the room temperature is optimal for the woman and the baby and that the surroundings are clean and prepared for delivery of the baby or any emergency procedures that may be required.

Consider whether the woman is in the most appropriate setting. Transfer to theatre or intensive care as soon as possible when indicated.

Woman-Centred Care

When providing emergency care and treatment for women, it is imperative that the midwife and the wider MDT maintain the dignity of the woman throughout. This may include placement of sheets and screens as well as ensuring that only the essential personnel are in the room.

Take-Home Points

- **Competence in emergency care:** Midwives and health professionals in maternity services must be competent and confident in providing first-line emergency care for compromised or critically ill pregnant women, in both community and hospital settings.
- **Early recognition is key:** Early recognition of deterioration is crucial for the safe and effective care of pregnant women. Timely identification of warning signs is fundamental to preventing adverse outcomes.
- **Understanding shock:** Shock results from the body's failure to compensate, leading to cells' inability to obtain or utilise sufficient oxygen and nutrients. Awareness of the three distinct stages of shock is vital for appropriate response.
- **Women's awareness in early shock**: A woman in the early stages of shock will be aware that something is wrong. It is imperative for midwives and health professionals to listen to and act on any concerns expressed by the woman.
- **Disparities in care:** Women from ethnic minority backgrounds may face dismissal of their concerns by health professionals, contributing to disproportionate rates of morbidity and mortality. Cultural sensitivity is crucial for equitable care.
- **Tailored response to shock stages**: Health professionals need to tailor their response to the specific stage of shock, considering factors such as gestation, age and general health of the woman.
- **Understanding types of shock**: A fundamental understanding of the different types of shock is essential for midwives and health professionals in maternity services to provide appropriate treatment.
- **ABCDE approach for assessment**: Implementing the ABCDE approach (Airway, Breathing, Circulation, Disability, Exposure) is a structured framework for the primary assessment, addressing the care and treatment needs of women during shock.
- **Woman-centred care:** Adopting a woman-centred approach is crucial for timely identification and treatment of shock. Ensuring that care is tailored to the individual needs of the woman enhances the overall effectiveness of interventions.

Conclusion

This chapter has offered an outline of the fundamentals of shock. The stages of shock have been discussed together with the pathophysiology involved where compensatory mechanisms are impaired. An outline of the types of shock has been offered with an insight into the most effective care and treatment for women. The chapter has emphasised the importance of rapid initial assessment and the use of the ABCDE framework in the context of pregnancy. While midwives deal predominantly with healthy women and babies, it is imperative that we recognise early signs of deterioration and act on these swiftly for the best possible safe and effective care for women and their babies.

References

Amaan, A. and Lamont, R.F. (2019). Recent advances in the diagnosis and management of sepsis in pregnancy. *F1000Research* 8: F1000 Faculty Rev-1546.

Bothamley, J. and Boyle, M. (2015). *Infections Affecting Pregnancy and Birth*. London: CRC Press.

Chu, J., Johnston, T., Geoghegan, J., and Royal College of Obstetricians and Gynaecologists (2020). Maternal collapse in pregnancy and the puerperium. *BJOG* 127: e14–e52.

Coad, J. (2018). *Anatomy and Physiology for Midwives*. London: Elsevier.

Haseer-Koya, H. and Paul, M. (2021). Shock. In: *StatPearls*. Treasure Island, FL: StatPearls Publishing https://www.ncbi.nlm.nih.gov/books/NBK531492.

Kirkup, B. (2015). Morecambe Bay investigation: report. https://www.gov.uk/government/publications/morecambe-bay-investigation-report (accessed November 2023).

Knight, M. and Kurinczuk, J.J. (2018). Spotlight on . . . MBRRACE-UK. *Obstetrician & Gynaecologist* 20: 5–6.

Knight, M., Bunch, K., Tuffnell, D. et al. (2022). Saving lives, improving mother's care: lessons learned to inform maternity care from the UK and Ireland Confidential Enquiries into Maternal Deaths and Morbidity 2017–19. https://www.npeu.ox.ac.uk/assets/downloads/mbrrace-uk/reports/maternal-report-2021/MBRRACE-UK_Maternal_Report_2021_-_FINAL_-_WEB_VERSION.pdf (accessed November 2023).

Mavrides, E., Allard, S., Chandrahan, E. et al. (2017). Prevention and management of postpartum haemorrhage. *BJOG* 124: e106–e149.

Mcdonald, S., Abbott, J., and Higgins, S. (2004). Prophylactic ergometrine-oxytocin versus oxytocin for the third stage of labour. *Cochrane Database of Systematic Reviews* 1: CD000201. https://doi.org/10.1002/14651858.CD000201.pub2.

Migliozzi, J. (2021). Shock. In: *Fundamentals of Applied Pathophysiology*, 4e (ed. I. Peate), 130–152. Chichester, UK: Wiley.

Mohamed-Ahmed, O., Nair, M., Acosta, C. et al. (2015). Progression from severe sepsis in pregnancy to death: a UK population-based case-control analysis. *BJOG* 122: 1506–1515.

Mulla, Z., Ebrahim, M., and Gonzalez, J. (2010). Anaphylaxis in the obstetric patient: analysis of a state wide hospital discharge database. *Annals of Allergy, Asthma & Immunology* 104: 55.

National Institute for Health and Care Excellence (2021). Ectopic pregnancy. https://cks.nice.org.uk/topics/ectopic-pregnancy (accessed November 2023).

Nutbeam, T. and Daniels, R. (2021). Clinical tools: screening and action tools for community midwives. https://sepsistrust.org/professional-resources/community-services-nice (accessed November 2023).

Ockenden, D. (2022). Ockenden review: summary of findings, conclusions and essential actions. https://www.gov.uk/government/publications/final-report-of-the-ockenden-review/ockenden-review-summary-of-findings-conclusions-and-essential-actions (accessed November 2023).

Paterson-Brown, S. and Howell, C. (2016). Shock. In: *Managing Obstetric Emergencies and Trauma: The MOET Course Manual* (ed. S. Paterson-Brown and C. Howell), 39–51. Cambridge: Cambridge University Press.

Raynor, M., Essat, Z., Menage, D. et al. (2021). Decolonising midwifery education part 1: how colour aware are you when assessing women with darker skin tones in midwifery practice? https://www.all4maternity.com/decolonising-midwifery-education-part-1-how-colour-aware-are-you-when-assessing-women-with-darker-skin-tones-in-midwifery-practice (accessed November 2023).

Resuscitation Council UK (2021a). The ABCDE approach. https://www.resus.org.uk/library/abcde-approach (accessed November 2023).

Resuscitation Council UK (2021b). Emergency treatment of anaphylaxis. https://www.resus.org.uk/sites/default/files/2021-05/Emergency%20Treatment%20of%20Anaphylaxis%20May%202021_0.pdf (accessed November 2023).

Royal College of Obstetricians and Gynaecologists (2012). Sepsis in pregnancy. Green-top guideline no. 64a. https://www.rcog.org.uk/guidance/browse-all-guidance/green-top-guidelines/sepsis-in-pregnancy-bacterial-green-top-guideline-no-64a (accessed November 2023).

Sole, M., Klein, D., and Moseley, M. (2016). *Introduction to Critical Care Nursing*. St Louis: Saunders.

Tortora, G. and Derrickson, B. (2017). *Tortora's Principles of Anatomy and Physiology*. Singapore: Wiley.

World Health Organization (2017). Managing complications in pregnancy and childbirth: a guide for midwives and doctors. https://apps.who.int/iris/bitstream/handle/10665/255760/9789241565493-eng.pdf (accessed November 2023).

Further Resources

Blumlein, D. and Griffiths, I. (2022) Shock: Aetiology, Pathophysiology and Management. *British Journal of Nursing* 31: 8.

British Medical Journal (2022) Shock - Symptoms, diagnosis and treatment. *BMJ Best Practice* https://bestpractice.bmj.com/topics/en-gb/3000121 (accessed January 2024).

Glossary

ABCDE assessment	Airway, Breathing, Circulation, Disability, Exposure – a framework to conduct a primary assessment
Antepartum haemorrhage (APH)	A bleed that occurs after 24 weeks of pregnancy and prior to the birth of the baby
Domestic violence (DV)	Characterised as an incident or pattern of incidents involving controlling, coercive, threatening, degrading and violent behaviour. This behaviour extends to include sexual violence. While perpetrators are commonly partners or ex-partners, domestic abuse can also be perpetrated by family members or caregivers
IPPA	Inspect, Palpate, Percuss, Auscultate – a systematic tool for conducting a respiratory assessment
MBRRACE-UK	Mothers and Babies: Reducing Risk through Audits and Confidential enquiries across the UK. A national collaborative programme of work involving surveillance and investigation of maternal deaths, stillbirths and neonatal deaths
Modified Early Obstetric Warning Score (MEOWS)	A tool to allow early recognition of physical deterioration in pregnant and postnatal women
National Early Warning Score 2 (NEWS2)	A tool to allow early recognition of physical deterioration in adult patients
National Institute for Health and Care Excellence (NICE)	Provides national guidance and advice to improve health and outcomes for patients
Positive end-expiratory pressure (PEEP)	The pressure that will remain in the airways at the end of the respiratory cycle
Postpartum haemorrhage (PPH)	Heavy bleeding from the vagina after birth and up to 6 weeks following
Pulmonary embolism (PE)	A blockage in the pulmonary arteries
Sexually transmitted infection (STI)	An infection that is contracted during sexual intercourse
Systemic inflammatory response syndrome (SIRS)	An exaggerated defence response of the body to a stressor

CHAPTER 11

The Nervous System and Associated Disorders

Abbie Tomson[1] and Kristian Tomson[2]

[1] *Midwife Maternity, Women's and Children's Services, University Hospitals Plymouth NHS Trust, Plymouth, UK*

[2] *Paramedic Acute care Team, Bosvena Health, Bodmin, UK*

AIM

To understand the pathophysiology of the nervous system and its associated disorders in relation to the pre-conception, pregnancy and postnatal periods.

LEARNING OUTCOMES

On completion of this chapter the reader will be able to:

- Describe the gross anatomy and physiology of the central nervous system, including the structure of a neurone
- Understand the pathophysiological process underpinning some of the common neurological conditions encountered during pregnancy
- Understand the medicines management involved in pregnancy care and disorders of the nervous system
- Develop an awareness of some of the red flags of common neurological conditions in pregnancy, as well as the appropriate examinations for those conditions

Test Your Prior Knowledge

1. Describe the structure of a nervous cell.
2. Describe the structure of the central nervous system and peripheral nervous system.
3. What is the difference between the somatic and autonomic nervous systems?
4. Explain the role of the sympathetic and parasympathetic nervous systems.
5. What are the adjustments to the nervous system in pregnancy?

Anatomy and Physiology of the Nervous System

The nervous system is one of the smallest (accounting for approximately 3% of total body mass) but most vital and complicated of all the body systems. It is responsible for all voluntary and involuntary actions and plays a very influential part in coordinating homeostasis within all body systems as well as playing an influential role in the endocrine system (Tortora and Derrickson 2014). It achieves this through a complicated structure of specialised cells (neurons) that can transmit signals throughout the body. This is achieved by the nervous system through its three functions:

- **Sensory function:** to detect stimuli (either external or internal) and transmit these to the appropriate processing centre.
- **Processing or integrative function:** to process sensory stimuli to analyse and decide about the stimuli.
- **Motor function:** if the integrated sensory stimuli are deemed to need an effect, a motor function will be activated, i.e. muscle movement or secretion from a gland. This will only occur if the sensory information needs an appropriate motor response.

Structure of the Nervous System

The nervous system has two components: the central nervous system (CNS) and the peripheral nervous system (PNS):

- The CNS consists of the brain and spinal cord.
- The PNS consists of all other nervous tissue outside of the brain and spinal cord. This includes the cranial nerves, sensory and motor neurons as well as the enteric plexuses. These nerves carry impulses to and from the spinal cord.

193

Nerve Cells

There are many different nervous cells, which can be broadly divided into neurons and neuroglia. The neurons are the highly specialised cells that can span great lengths of the body and form complicated connections and interactions with other cells. Because of their specialist function and size, they are unable to undergo mitosis. Neuroglia, on the other hand, are much smaller and play a supportive role to protect, nourish and hydrate neurons in interstitial fluid. Due to their less specialist role, they can undergo mitosis throughout a person's life span, similar to most other cells in the body.

Dependent on their role there are many different shapes and structures of neurons and neuroglia. However, neurons generally share similar base components. See Figure 11.1 for an illustration of the general neuronal cell structure. The components are:

- **Dendrites:** the receiving aspect of a neuron, with the cell membrane having multiple neurotransmitter receptors. They also play a role in the integrative/processing function.
- **Cell body:** typical of most cells, contains the nucleus and other organelles such as lysosomes, mitochondria and Golgi apparatus. Due to their inability to undergo mitosis, neurons contain extra ribosomes and rough endoplasmic reticula to allow for increased protein synthesis, permitting the cell to replace and repair damaged components.
- **Axons:** long, protruding structures that are responsible for sending 'impulses' or carrying messages from one neuron to another neuron, muscle fibres or gland/secretory cells. The axons are often covered in a Schwann cell, which consists of a myelinated sheath allowing more efficient transport of impulses to the axon terminal and subsequently synapses.

Action Potential and Synaptic Transmission

The impulses that travel along an axon are called an action potential and these are also often referred to as electrical impulses. This is due to the change in overall ionic charge within the cytoplasm due to leaking of potassium ions and an influx of sodium ions, leading to a positively charged cell membrane. This occurs primarily at the nodes of Ranvier

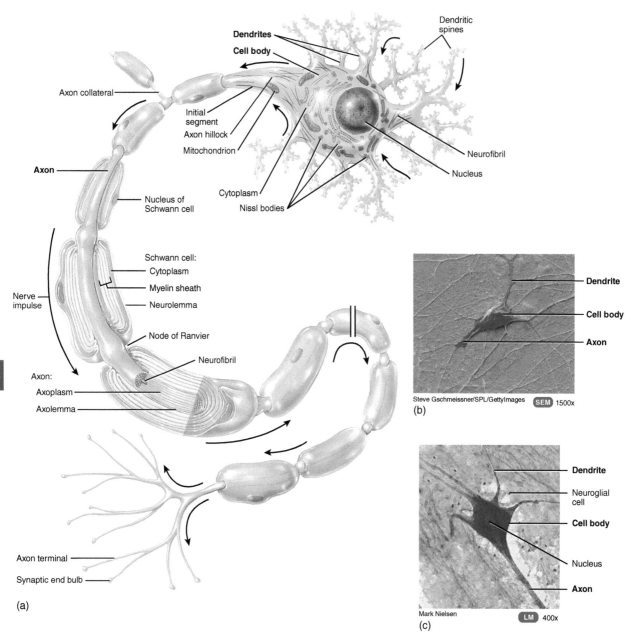

Steve Gschmeissner/SPL/GettyImages   SEM 1500x
(b)

Mark Nielsen   LM 400x
(c)

194

(a)

FIGURE 11.1   Structure of neuron. (a) Parts of a neuron. (b, c) Motor neurons. Source: Reproduced by permission from Tortora and Derrickson (2014) / John Wiley & Sons.

(located between Schwann cells), so it allows for big jumps of alternating charge along the axon, to quickly propagate a 'message'.

When the action potential reaches the synaptic bulbs at the axonal terminals, this subsequently activates voltage-gated calcium channels. These allow an influx of calcium, which triggers the vesicles containing neurotransmitter chemicals to exit (exocytosis). Once at the cell membrane, the vesicles release the neurotransmitter that binds with receptors at the receiving dendrite, triggering an effector response. In the case of dendrites, it triggers an influx of ions and a further action potential within the next neuron.

Central Nervous System

The CNS consists of the brain and spinal cord. The brain is an organ made up of approximately 85 billion neurons, located in the skull. The major components of the brain are brainstem, diencephalon, cerebellum and cerebrum. See Table 11.1 and Figure 11.2 for the functions and structure of the brain within the CNS.

The other component, the spinal cord, is responsible for relaying messages from sensory nerves to the brain, and from the brain to motor nerves. It also plays a role in integration, through facilitating reflexes. The spinal cord is in the spinal column, made up of spinal vertebrae. There are 33 vertebrae: 7 cervical spine, 12 thoracic, 5 lumbar, 5 sacral and 4 coccyges (as illustrated in Figure 11.3). At each level the vertebrae have openings allowing for the CNS to connect with the PNS.

The CNS's complex structure and diverse functions predispose it to a multitude of pathologies, each capable of causing varying types and degrees of dysfunction.

Peripheral Nervous System

The PNS consists of all tissue that is not part of the brain or spinal cord. This system is responsible for receiving or detecting sensory stimuli and sending the information about the stimuli to the CNS, as well as enacting the motor response decided by the CNS based on the integration of the stimuli.

The PNS can be broken down into two subgroups: the somatic nervous system and the autonomic nervous system.

The somatic nervous system is responsible for detecting external stimuli within its sensory capacity (of the five senses: sight, smell, hearing, taste and touch) and its motor function is that of controlling skeletal muscle only. This means that the action/motor function of the somatic PNS is voluntary only.

TABLE 11.1 Components of the brain and their function.

Component	Function
Cerebrum	The largest structure in the brain. It houses both sensory and motor areas within the cerebral cortex. These motor areas are responsible for voluntary motion. The cerebral cortex houses associated areas responsible for more complex functions such as memory, personality and intelligence. The cerebrum houses the limbic system that controls emotions.
Cerebellum	The second largest structure in the brain. It is responsible for unconscious control of skeletal muscle, through smoothing and correcting any complicated muscular components. It regulates balance and posture and is believed to play a role in cognition and integration of sensory stimuli.
Diencephalon	Consists of: • Thalamus: responsible for relaying sensory stimuli, as well as motor information from the cerebellum to the cerebral cortex. Believed to play a role in maintaining consciousness. • Hypothalamus: responsible for controlling and processing autonomic nervous system activities, as well as producing homeostatic hormones playing an endocrine role. It also works in partnership with the limbic system to regulate behaviour and emotions. Additionally, it controls the body's circadian rhythm, as well as its temperature control. • Epithalamus: plays a role in producing melatonin and processing smell (olfactory) stimuli.
Brainstem	Consists of: • Medulla oblongata: responsible for cardiovascular and respiratory control centres as well as being one of the primary structures where cranial nerves attach. • Pons: another site with many cranial nerve nuclei sited within it. The pons also has another respiratory centre that works in conjunction with the medullary respiratory centre. • Mid-brain: contains the nuclei of the cranial nerves responsible for ocular motor function. Collectively these structures also contain many tracts for both sensory and motor neurons to convey stimuli and effector messages throughout the body.

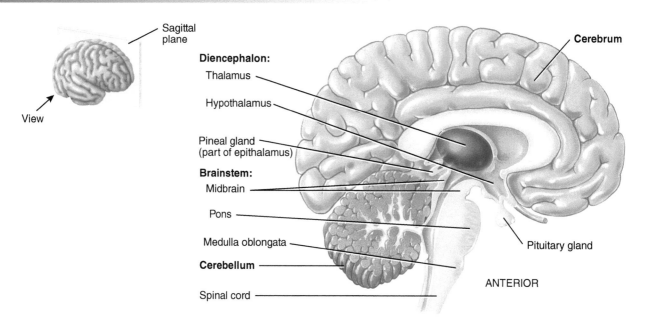

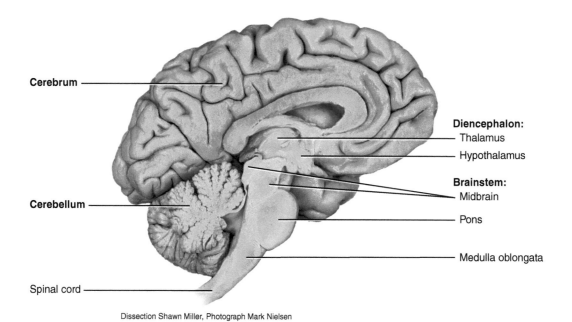

Dissection Shawn Miller, Photograph Mark Nielsen

FIGURE 11.2   Structure of the brain. Source: Reproduced by permission from Tortora and Derrickson (2014) / John Wiley & Sons.

The autonomic nervous system is responsible for the sensory stimuli from within the body's visceral organs such lungs and abdominal organs and the motor function affects that of smooth muscle, the heart and secretory glands. These functions reflect the origins of its name, *auto* being Greek for 'self' and *nomic* meaning 'law', thus self-law, or governing oneself. However, the autonomic nervous system is considered to act involuntarily due to no conscious decision being made about its actions.

The motor functions of the autonomic nervous system are further subdivided into the sympathetic and parasympathetic nervous systems. These are the nervous systems that are responsible for the 'fight or flight' and 'rest and digest'

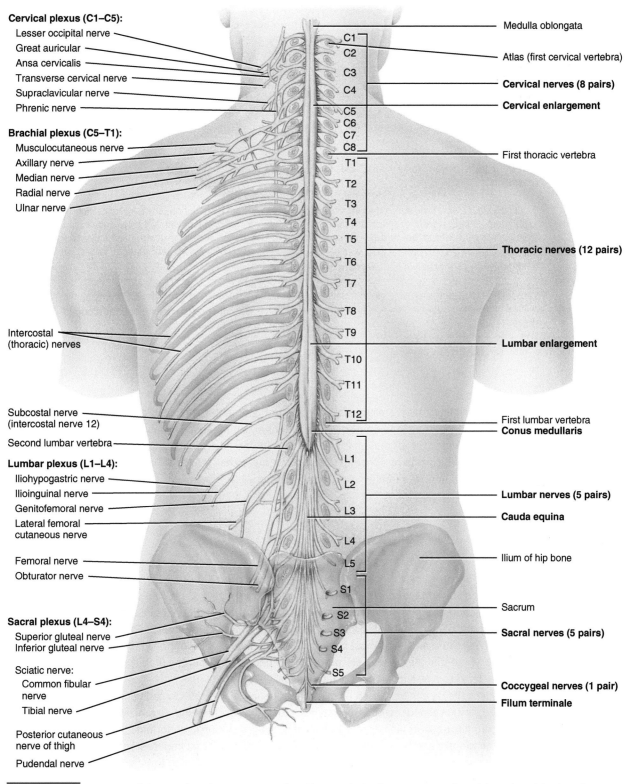

Cervical plexus (C1–C5):
- Lesser occipital nerve
- Great auricular
- Ansa cervicalis
- Transverse cervical nerve
- Supraclavicular nerve
- Phrenic nerve

Brachial plexus (C5–T1):
- Musculocutaneous nerve
- Axillary nerve
- Median nerve
- Radial nerve
- Ulnar nerve

Intercostal (thoracic) nerves

Subcostal nerve (intercostal nerve 12)

Second lumbar vertebra

Lumbar plexus (L1–L4):
- Iliohypogastric nerve
- Ilioinguinal nerve
- Genitofemoral nerve
- Lateral femoral cutaneous nerve

Femoral nerve
Obturator nerve

Sacral plexus (L4–S4):
- Superior gluteal nerve
- Inferior gluteal nerve

Sciatic nerve:
- Common fibular nerve
- Tibial nerve

Posterior cutaneous nerve of thigh

Pudendal nerve

C1
C2
C3
C4
C5
C6
C7
C8
T1
T2
T3
T4
T5
T6
T7
T8
T9
T10
T11
T12
L1
L2
L3
L4
L5
S1
S2
S3
S4
S5

Medulla oblongata

Atlas (first cervical vertebra)

Cervical nerves (8 pairs)

Cervical enlargement

First thoracic vertebra

Thoracic nerves (12 pairs)

Lumbar enlargement

197

First lumbar vertebra
Conus medullaris

Lumbar nerves (5 pairs)

Cauda equina

Ilium of hip bone

Sacrum

Sacral nerves (5 pairs)

Coccygeal nerves (1 pair)
Filum terminale

FIGURE 11.3 Structure of the spinal cord. Source: Reproduced by permission from Tortora and Derrickson (2014) / John Wiley & Sons.

TABLE 11.2   **Effects of sympathetic and parasympathetic nervous systems.**

Effector	Sympathetic nervous motor function	Parasympathetic nervous motor function
Glands	Secretion of adrenaline, glucagon, antidiuretic hormone, melatonin and renin Increases lipolysis, glycogenolysis and gluconeogenesis Inhibits digestive enzymes, bile and insulin release, while also increasing release of sweat from glands all over the body	Secretion of digestive enzymes, bile and insulin Stimulation of glycogen synthesis
Cardiac muscle	Increase in heart rate and force of atrial and ventricular contractions	Decrease in heart rate and force of atrial and ventricular contractions
Smooth muscle	Pupil dilation, airway (bronchial) dilation, relaxes gallbladder (to help store bile), decreases tone of stomach but contracts gastrointestinal sphincters Innovates uterine contractions in pregnant women, yet inhibits uterine contraction in non-pregnant women	Pupil constriction, bronchial constriction, constriction of gallbladder to increase bile release, increased gastrointestinal motility and tone with associated sphincter relaxation
Vascular smooth muscle	Vasodilation to vessels supplying blood to skeletal muscle and heart, with vasoconstriction to other organs	Vasoconstriction to vessels supplying the heart Vasodilation to vessels suppling blood to digestive and secretory glands

Source: Adapted from Tortora and Derrickson (2014).

responses. The sympathetic nervous system is responsible for fight or flight actions while the parasympathetic nervous system is responsible for rest and digest actions. Some of these actions are summarised in Table 11.2.

Within pregnancy the autonomic nervous system is affected with increased sympathetic stimulation and reduction in parasympathetic stimulation, which is in response to the cardiovascular changes (Yousif et al. 2019). This increased sympathetic stimulation returns to normal baseline homeostasis postnatally.

Epilepsy

Epilepsy is a relatively common neurological condition affecting around 1 in 200 pregnant women (Thangaratinam et al. 2016). It refers to a sudden abnormal discharge of electrical energy from cerebral neurones, which disrupts normal function and causes a seizure, and is a group of disorders rather than a signal condition. Epilepsy affects each woman differently, with varying symptoms and degrees of severity. The causes of epilepsy are complex. Primary (idiopathic) epilepsy has no obvious underlying cause and is the most common form of epilepsy, accounting for 60% of people with the condition. Although there is no identifiable cause of seizures in many people, an inherited predisposition to hypersensitivity of the neurons is considered to play a role (Thangaratinam et al. 2016).

Secondary (sympathetic) epilepsy can be caused by prenatal or perinatal injuries, congenital abnormalities, severe head injury, stroke, infection, certain genetic syndromes and brain tumours (World Health Organization 2023).

A seizure is caused by sudden, uncontrolled depolarisation of neurons resulting in abnormal motor or sensory activity with or without loss of consciousness (Thangaratinam et al. 2016). The activities that initiate seizures are not clear, but there are theories such as altered permeability of the neuronal membrane, reduced inhibitory neuronal control and an imbalance of neurotransmitters (Thangaratinam et al. 2016).

Factors that may trigger epilepsy in some people include physical stimuli such as loud noise and/or bright light, or biochemical stimuli such as excessive fluid retention, hypoglycaemia, change in medication, alkalosis, sudden withdrawal from sedatives and alcohol (Thangaratinam et al. 2016).

Expert Midwife

As a registered midwife, I must ensure that the care and support I offer women and their families is up to date and evidence based. It is essential that we use and apply any robust guidelines to care provision, such as Royal College of Obstetricians and Gynaecologists' Green-top guideline no. 68, Epilepsy in pregnancy. The second edition is currently under development (Thangaratinam et al. 2016).

Li Yi, Senior Midwife

Case Study 11.1   Epilepsy

Emma is a 24-year-old-woman who is attending her booking appointment with the community midwife. This is Emma's first pregnancy, and she has epilepsy diagnosed when a teenager. This was an unplanned pregnancy, and Emma has not had any preconception counselling.

On questioning, Emma mostly has focal type of seizures, but did experience tonic–clonic seizures as a teenager. She has been seizure free for the past three months and typically has five to six seizures a year, more if going through a particularly stressful time. Emma is medicated currently with Keppra®.

- What else would you like to know about Emma's medication?
- What advice would you be providing regarding folic acid?
- What would your plan of care be for Emma?

199

Pre-conception Care in Epilepsy

Between 55% and 80% of women with epilepsy reported unintended pregnancies, compared to 45% in the general population (Stephen et al. 2019). The following are the main aims of pre-conception care in epilepsy:

- Anti-epileptic drug (AED) therapy on the lowest possible dose to maintain seizure control.
- AED adherence to reduce risk of sudden unexpected death in epilepsy (SUDEP) and status epilepticus.
- Prescription of 5 mg folic acid tablets.
- Discussion of genetic factors.
- Smoking cessation – higher risk of preterm labour compared with women with epilepsy who do not smoke.

Red Flag

An 'aura' is a term that some people use to describe the warning they feel before they have a tonic–clonic seizure. An epilepsy aura is in fact a focal aware seizure (FAS). This can be described as:

- A rising feeling in the stomach.
- Unusual smell or taste.
- Stiffness or twitching in part of the body.
- Visual disturbances.

Source: Adapted from Epilepsy Society (2017).

First-Trimester Care in Epilepsy

Most women with epilepsy will meet their midwife for the first time at around 8–10 weeks' gestation (Thangaratinam et al. 2016) at the pregnancy booking appointment. The midwife must:

- Explore adherence to medication and ensure medication adjustments are made with the GP under the direction of an epilepsy specialist
- Discover what type of seizures the woman experiences and their current frequency. Uncontrolled tonic–clonic seizures are the strongest risk factor for SUDEP, which is the main cause of death in pregnancy women with epilepsy.
- Ensure the woman is taking 5 mg folic acid as prescribed.
- Discuss early pregnancy side effects, and ensure the woman is referred to her GP if there are any effects caused by nausea and vomiting on the absorption of medication.
- Provide information about the UK Epilepsy and Pregnancy Register and invite the woman to register.

The Royal College of Obstetricians and Gynaecologists (Thangaratinam et al. 2016) advises that women with a history of epilepsy who are not considered to have a high risk of unprovoked seizures can be managed as low risk in pregnancy. However, they should be referred to a specialist epilepsy team.

A discussion should be held around the woman bathing herself in shallow water and with assistance to minimise risk.

Labour/Birth Care in Epilepsy

- Women at risk of peripartum seizures should be giving birth in a consultant-led unit with facilities for one-to-one midwifery care and maternal and neonatal resuscitation facilities.
- Water birth is fine if the woman is not taking AEDs and has been seizure free for a significant period. She may be offered a water birth after discussion with an epilepsy specialist (Thangaratinam et al. 2016).
- There is a 4% increased risk above average of seizures during labour and the 24 hours following (Carhuapoma et al. 2017).
- Adequate analgesia and appropriate care in labour should be provided to minimise risk factors for seizures such as insomnia, stress and dehydration.
- Analgesia should be prioritised – pethidine should be used with caution, with diamorphine. Pethidine is metabolised to norpethidine, which is known to be an epileptogenic when administered in high doses to patients with normal renal function.
- Early epidural can be considered to minimise precipitating factors for seizures during labour, such as over-breathing, sleep deprivation, pain and emotional stress.
- The midwife should encourage the woman to take her usual AEDs at her regular time, and if not tolerated orally, a suitable alternative given by intravenous (IV) or rectal route. .
- Long-acting benzodiazepines such as clobazam can be considered if there is a very high risk of seizures in the peripartum period.

Postnatal Care in Epilepsy

- AED levels need to be assessed with blood levels in the postnatal period. There is a danger that lack of sleep will trigger seizures.
- AEDs should be reviewed within 10 days of delivery to avoid postpartum toxicity.
- Care for women in single rooms only with continuous observation.
- Breastfeeding is still encouraged.
- Babies born to mothers taking AEDs may have adverse effects such as lethargy, difficulty in feeding, excessive sedation and withdrawal symptoms with inconsolable crying. Individualised assessments should be conducted for the

level of postdelivery monitoring required for withdrawal symptoms, and for any signs of toxicity. This is especially important in premature babies.

- Safety strategies with babies include nursing the baby on the floor, using very shallow baby baths, laying the baby down if there is a warning aura, not bathing the baby unaccompanied, and avoiding sleep deprivation and alcohol if prone to myoclonic jerks.

Orange Flag: Psychological Considerations in Epilepsy

In a study of adults aged 18 years and older, it was found that adults with epilepsy were twice as likely to report feelings of depression compared to adults without epilepsy. This is thought to be related to certain areas of the brain responsible for some types of seizures, and can affect mood and lead to depression.

Source: Adapted from Kobau et al. (2006).

Medicines Management: Epilepsy

- Sodium valproate taken in pregnancy is associated with neural tube defects, facial cleft and hypospadias.
- Phenobarbital and phenytoin are associated with cardiac malformations.
- Phenytoin and carbamazepine are associated with cleft palate.
- The aim is no sodium valproate or AED polytherapy, whereby multiple AEDs are used.

   A Medicines and Healthcare products Regulatory Agency report (MHRA 2021) found that lamotrigine (Lamictal®) and levetiracetam (Keppra) are safer to use in pregnancy than other epilepsy medicines. This is because they are not linked with an increased risk of birth defects compared with the general population.

Multiple Sclerosis

Multiple sclerosis (MS) is mostly diagnosed in young women, many of whom will still wish to have children. It is therefore important that family planning is proactively discussed, particularly when considering disease-modifying treatments.

   MS is an autoimmune neurological condition, thought to affect 0.1–0.6% of people in the United Kingdom (Naryan 2015). In MS there is activation of the immune cells, CD4 T cells, which attack a protein component of the myelin sheath. Scarring and oedema occur at the site as part of the inflammatory response. Hardened areas or plaques known as sclerosis develop. Multiple lesions form in various locations seemingly randomly, hence the name multiple sclerosis. The process of demyelination, as seen in Figure 11.4, involves the breakdown of the myelin occurring because of the repeated and progressive inflammatory damage. Without this protective covering the nerves do not function as efficiently, leading to the neurological symptoms that characterise MS. The cause of the autoimmune response is unknown, but it is thought to be an interaction of a genetic tendency with environmental factors. Proposed environmental triggers are inadequate vitamin D, Epstein–Barr viral infection, smoking and obesity during adolescence.

Expert Midwife

The UK consensus on pregnancy in multiple sclerosis is outlined in the Association of British Neurologists' guidelines (Dobson et al. 2019).

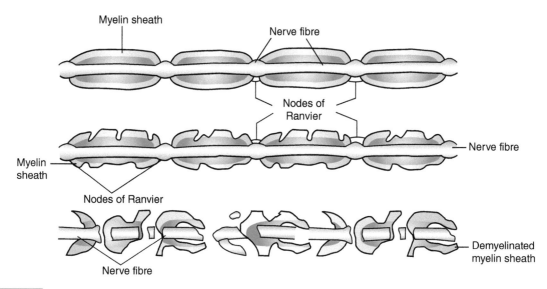

FIGURE 11.4   The process of demyelination.

Pre-conception Care in Multiple Sclerosis

At or soon after diagnosis, all women with MS of childbearing age should have pre-pregnancy counselling. This should be repeated at regular intervals, particularly for those who are on or considering starting medication.

Pregnancy Care in Multiple Sclerosis

- The MS team should be notified as soon as possible if a woman with MS becomes pregnant so that they can provide appropriate support and liaise with her obstetric team.
- Antenatal care can still be led by a midwife.
- No additional scans are required.
- Urinary tract infections (UTIs) are more frequent in pregnancy and are a common relapse trigger in epilepsy.
- Relapses are less common during pregnancy. Any woman with MS suffering from a disabling relapse should be offered IV methylprednisolone at the recommended dose in MS, regardless of trimester, once an underlying infection such as a UTI has been excluded.
- If a woman has problems with spasticity or severe weakness of the pelvis and/or legs, she should be referred to a neuro-physiotherapist early in pregnancy to work collaboratively with her and her obstetric team to optimise labour and delivery.
- The multidisciplinary team – midwife, obstetrician, neurologist, specialist nurse, occupational therapists, physiotherapists, incontinence nurses – all should be woman centred.

Woman-Centred Care

The midwife should ensure that a detailed, honest dialogue takes place concerning the woman's needs and ability, so that the midwife can offer appropriate help or suggest resources. Continuity of care with the same midwife should be ensured where possible, so that the woman and midwife can develop a trusting relationship. The possibility should be considered of the midwife and woman attending the hospital together to try to predict any problems and ensure a plan is made and resources are accessed before delivery.

Labour/Birth and Postnatal Care in Multiple Sclerosis

- Increased spasticity during labour may be controlled using benzodiazepines and/or an epidural anaesthetic.
- Women with spinal cord involvement or loss of sensation below T11 may not be aware of the onset of labour. They should be advised about other symptoms, including increase in spasticity, gastrointestinal upset, flushing and back pain.
- For women with MS who have severe spinal cord disease, autonomic dysreflexia should be considered in the differential diagnosis for pre-eclampsia.
- Distension of the bladder must be avoided, as urinary retention is very common.

Postnatal Care in Multiple Sclerosis

- Support breastfeeding alongside treatment considerations. Methylprednisolone is not contra-indicated in breastfeeding.
- There is an increased risk of postnatal depression.

Case Study 11.2   Multiple Sclerosis

You are working in the community, and are due to see Louise, who is 36 weeks' pregnant. You will be discussing her birth preferences and providing information regarding onset of labour. This is Louise's first pregnancy and she has MS that has spinal cord involvement.

- How else would you describe the onset of labour to Louise, besides the sensations of contractions?
- Regarding bladder care, what will be important to Louise during labour?
- Louise is concerned about the risk of relapse and increased spasticity during labour, but wants to try to avoid an epidural. What alternatives could you discuss with her?

Eclampsia

Eclampsia is considered a complication of severe pre-eclampsia, commonly defined as new onset of grand mal seizure activity and/or unexplained coma during pregnancy or postpartum in a woman with signs or symptoms of pre-eclampsia. It typically occurs during or after the 20th week of gestation or in the postpartum period. Eclampsia in the absence of hypertension with proteinuria has been demonstrated to occur in 38% of cases reported in the United Kingdom (Siddiqi and Platt 2017). It accounts for a third of maternal mortality in developing countries.

The neurological manifestations of eclampsia consist of seizures and alteration of sensorium or coma on a background of pre-eclampsia (Thomas 1998). Occasionally there can be focal neurological deficits too. Computed tomography (CT) scan and magnetic resonance imaging (MRI) demonstrate the presence of cerebral oedema and/or cerebral haemorrhage in eclampsia. The electroencephalogram (EEG) graph in patients with eclampsia has revealed evidence of diffuse cerebral dysfunction (delta waves) and epileptiform transients (spikes or sharp waves). There is also evidence of extensive vasculopathy within the brain parenchyma. A variety of mechanisms have been suggested to explain these changes, the most important being failure of autoregulation of cerebral blood flow that leads to cerebral oedema and haemorrhage.

Pre-conception Advice for Women at Risk of Pre-eclampsia

- Most pre-conception advice related to reducing the risk of pre-eclampsia will focus on those who already have chronic hypertension (NICE 2019).

- Offer women with chronic hypertension referral to a specialist in hypertensive disorders of pregnancy to discuss risks and benefits of treatment.
- Advise women who take angiotensin-converting enzyme (ACE) inhibitors or angiotensin II receptor blockers (ARBs) to discuss alternative treatments.
- Offer them advice on weight management, exercise, healthy eating and lowering the amount of salt in their diet.

First-Trimester Care for Women at Risk of Pre-eclampsia

Risk assess the care, including using the table in Medicines Management: Low-Dose Aspirin.

- Ensure aspirin 75–150 mg daily is prescribed from 12 weeks' gestation until birth based on the risk factors (National Institute for Health and Care Excellence [NICE] 2022).
- Offer healthy lifestyle advice.
- Consider referral for consultant-led care.

Medicines Management: Low-Dose Aspirin

Treatment with low-dose aspirin in women at high risk for pre-eclampsia resulted in a lower incidence of pre-eclampsia when compared to a placebo (Rolnik et al. 2017) in a randomised control trial. The women were treated from 14 weeks' gestation until birth.

One of the following high-risk factors	Two of the following moderate-risk factors
A history of hypertensive disease during a previous pregnancy	First pregnancy
Chronic kidney disease	Aged 40 years or older
Autoimmune disease, such as systemic lupus erythematosus or antiphospholipid syndrome	Pregnancy interval of more than 10 years
Type 1 or type 2 diabetes	Body mass index (BMI) of 35 or higher at first visit
Chronic hypertension	Family history of pre-eclampsia
	Multiple pregnancy

Second- and Third-Trimester Care for Women at Risk of Pre-eclampsia/with Pre-eclampsia

- This is for all pregnant women, but particularly important for those at risk of pre-eclampsia or with a history of pre-eclampsia. Dipstick the urine for protein and measure blood pressure at each visit.
- NICE guidance advises that a urine dipstick screening that is positive of 1+ or more for protein should have a protein: creatinine ratio to quantify the amount of protein in the urine.
- Discuss the signs and symptoms of pre-eclampsia.
- Continue aspirin for those with risk factors.

Labour Care for Women with Pre-eclampsia

Birth may be expedited if any of the following known features of severe pre-eclampsia are present, and the woman is therefore at greater risk of eclampsia:

- Inability to control maternal blood pressure despite three or more classes of antihypertensives being administered.
- Maternal pulse oximetry less than 90%.
- Progressive deterioration in liver function, renal function, haemolysis or platelet count.
- Ongoing neurological features, such as severe intractable headache, repeated visual disturbances, eclampsia, placental abruption, reversed end-diastolic flow, abnormal cardiotocography (CTG) or stillbirth.

Postnatal Care for Women with Pre-eclampsia

- Women with pre-eclampsia should be considered at high risk of eclampsia for at least three days postnatally and should have their clinical observations taken every four hours while awake for this duration.
- Antenatal antihypertensives should be continued, and consideration should be given to treating any hypertension before day 6 postnatally with antihypertensive therapy.
- Eclamptic seizures may develop for the first time in the early postpartum period.
- Avoid non-steroidal anti-inflammatory drugs for postnatal analgesia.

Red Flag

An eclamptic seizure is often preceded by changes in mental status, frontal and/or occipital headaches, nausea and/or visual changes (Wallace et al. 2019).

Medicines Management: Magnesium Sulfate

Magnesium sulfate is the only medication that should be used to manage eclampsia (Winter et al. 2017).

Magnesium sulfate appears to act primarily by reducing cerebral vasospasm. The Magpie Trial (Altman et al. 2002) demonstrated that magnesium sulfate can also prevent eclampsia, although it found that the number of women needing treatment with magnesium sulfate to prevent one woman having an eclamptic seizure is high, particularly where the pre-existing risk of eclampsia is low.

Always adhere to local policy and procedure.

Loading Dose: 4 g Magnesium Sulfate over Five Minutes

- Draw up 8 ml of 50% magnesium sulfate solution (4 g) followed by 12 ml of 0.9% normal saline into a 20 ml syringe. Give as an IV bolus over 5 min.

Maintenance Dose: 1 g/h

- Draw up 20 ml of 50% magnesium sulfate solution (10 g) followed by 30 ml of 0.9% normal saline into a 50 ml syringe.
- Place into a syringe driver and set the pump to run IV at 5 ml/h.
- Continue maintenance infusion for 24 hours following birth or the last seizure, whichever is the more recent.

Recurrent Seizures While on Magnesium Sulfate

- Draw up 4 ml of 50% magnesium sulfate (2 g) followed by 6 ml of 0.9% normal saline into a 10 ml syringe.
- Give as an IV bolus over 5 min.

Magnesium Toxicity Can Occur, Observations Required

- Blood pressure, respiration rate and urinary output closely observed.
- Regular patellar reflex.

Source: Adapted from Winter et al. (2017).

Examination Scenario: Eclampsia

You are caring for Sally on the postnatal ward. She is staying in hospital for blood pressure monitoring, due to concerns she may have pre-eclampsia. Sally has been reporting a headache that has been getting worse and has started seeing 'floaters' in her vision. As you are about to offer her support, her limbs start jerking and there are head movements.

Call for help, activating the emergency buzzer and ask for the senior midwife, experienced obstetrician and anaesthetist, additional midwives and maternity support workers. This may be via the emergency number in the hospital. Note the time the seizure occurred, and request that someone takes on the role of note taker.

Move the mother into a left lateral position, protecting her from injury, and provide high-flow facial oxygen via a non-rebreathe mask with a reservoir bag.

Magnesium sulfate should then be given as per the regimen cited in the earlier Medicines Management box.

Eclamptic seizures are usually self-limiting.

Sally's care should now be escalated to a one-to-one basis, ideally on a high dependency unit within a labour ward setting. A debrief should be provided to the team and also to Sally and anyone present with her at this time.

Source: Adapted from Winter et al. (2017).

Stroke

A stroke is a neurovascular condition, but a universal definition does not exist (Coupland et al. 2017). The term 'stroke' has only recently been adopted within the medical lexicon, but its symptoms have been recognised since the time of Hippocrates through the term 'apoplexy'. This was used to define any condition that rendered a person's neurological function reduced in the absence of respiratory or circulatory disturbance (Coupland et al. 2017).

The most modern definition of a stroke is that of the American Heart and Stroke Associations (Sacco et al. 2013). It broadly defines a stroke as ischaemia (lack of oxygen or other essential nutrients) of central nervous tissue, which results in cell death, and is detectable through pathological (i.e. autopsy), radiological (imaging) and other objective or clinical evidence. The significance of this definition is that it recognises pathological processes that cause central nervous tissue death in the absence of clinical signs and symptoms, but detectable through imaging or other processes (Coupland et al. 2017).

The term stroke is commonly used both medically and also by the public. It can also be termed a cerebrovascular accident (CVA) or cerebral vascular event (CVE). Similarly, you may come across mini-strokes or 'transient ischaemic attacks' (TIAs), which are defined as temporary ischaemia that results in clinical signs and symptoms but does not result in cellular death or permanent symptoms.

Orange Flag: Stroke

Strokes are known to have a psychological impact on those who experience them, due to neurological damage, but also coming to terms with the potential long-term effects, such as residual weakness (Welch 2008). Evidence suggests that women are more severely affected following an ischaemic stroke than men, including by psychological distress (Moatti et al. 2014). This tends to come in the form of depression and anxiety, and may be exaggerated in pregnant women, owing to the additional worries a mother may have about caring for and bonding with a new baby.

The woman should be offered care in conjunction with a multidisciplinary team including the perinatal mental health team to assist with bonding with the baby, managing emotional distress and tailored rehabilitation to meet the needs of the mother, baby and family.

Source: Adapted from Moatti et al. (2014).

Pathophysiology of Strokes

Strokes are broadly separated into two primary causes: ischaemia and haemorrhage.

Ischaemic Strokes

Ischaemic stroke is a term used to describe any stroke that results in ischaemia to the brain, but excludes haemorrhage or bleeding as the primary cause of the ischaemia. This can be for a range of reasons, from venous thrombus secondary to atheromatic plaque (similar to myocardial infarctions), to arterial embolus, to dissecting blood vessels (a tearing in the walls allowing layers to separate) (Kuriakose and Xiao 2020).

The primary end point for this type of stroke is the ischaemia of nervous tissue, where ischaemia is due to lack of blood flow and oxygen supply, which can result in cellular death.

Within pregnancy the primary aetiologies of ischaemic stroke are venous hypostasis, coagulation and thrombo-embolus formation in cerebral vessels (Yger et al. 2021). Atrial fibrillation (AF) is one of the most common causes or risk factors for stroke regardless of pregnancy, where there is dysfunctional atrial electrical conduction resulting in the atria fibrillating rather than contracting, causing stagnant blood flow and thrombus formation, which can lead to cerebral thrombo-embolus (Essa et al. 2021). However, some pregnancy-specific aetiologies of ischaemic stroke exist, including peripartum cardiomyopathy, a form of dilated cardiomyopathy that results in stagnant flow and thrombus formation, increasing stroke risk (Yger et al. 2021).

An amniotic fluid embolus is where an embolus of amniotic fluid causes cerebral ischaemia, however the mechanism is poorly understood, due to its extremely rare occurrence, and it is a diagnosis of exclusion (Yger et al. 2021). It is associated with increased risk from trauma such as instrumental and surgical deliveries, multiparity and increased age (Yger et al. 2021).

The final pregnancy-related cause of ischaemic and haemorrhagic stroke is choriocarcinoma. This is a malignant (cancerous) mass of cells developed from placental trophoblasts and is a particularly aggressive form of cancer, metastasising early on to vagina, liver, lungs and brain. If it metastases to the cerebral vessels it can results in vessel occlusion causing ischaemic stroke, or rupture causing haemorrhagic stroke (Yger et al. 2021).

Haemorrhagic Strokes

Haemorrhagic strokes are caused by haemorrhages or bleeds, leading to neural cell death within the CNS. They account for 10–15% of strokes and are generally subdivided into intercranial haemorrhage (ICH) and subarachnoid haemorrhage (Chen et al. 2014). The primary difference is that in ICH the bleed occurs into the cerebral tissue itself – that is, within the brain – while a subarachnoid haemorrhage occurs within the subarachnoid space, part of the meninges covering the CNS (Tortora and Derrickson 2014).

The accumulation of blood within the skull increases the pressure on cerebral tissue, causing injuries leading to hypoperfusion and death. In the case of herniation, this is often referred to as 'coning', where the brainstem is forced into and through the foramen magnum and leads to brainstem injury and death due to the key functions supporting respiration and cardiac function being within the brainstem, and thus is often fatal. Prior to herniation, cerebral haemorrhages increase intercranial pressure (ICP), which decreases cerebral profusion pressure (the pressure needed to supply the brain with oxygen-rich blood), compounding the complex picture of injury to cerebral tissues by causing further ischaemic damage and cellular death.

Red Flag

The following are red flag signs and symptoms indicating urgent intervention and investigation:

- Reduction in consciousness (anything that is not Alert on the AVPU scale, including acute confusion).
- Dysphasia, including expressive dysphasia.
- Unilateral weakness or paraesthesia.

- Facial asymmetry (or droop).
- Cranial nerve abnormalities.
- Acute visual impairments.
- Vertigo and dizziness.
- Ataxia and balance issues.
- Dyspraxia and coordination impairment.
- Alterations in cognition.
- Sudden onset of worst headache ever, often described as similar to a thunderclap (potentially a sign of a subarachnoid haemorrhage).

Pre-conception Care for Women at Risk of Stroke

As with all pre-conception care, the aims are to promote general health and stabilise any co-morbidities, to optimise the chance of a healthy successful pregnancy with minimal complications. This section focuses on women who have had a prior stroke attempting to become pregnant rather than the prevention of stroke (see the Health Promotion box).

Women with prior stroke should receive appropriate pre-conception counselling, which focuses specifically on the aetiology of their stroke (Khalid et al. 2020). This means optimising their medications, stopping any teratogenic medications, and swapping to safe alternatives to use within pregnancy. This often includes stopping clopidogrel and vitamin K antagonists for aspirin, and if thrombotic risk is high beginning prophylaxis of enoxaparin or low molecular weight heparin (Khalid et al. 2020).

Evidence suggests that when well managed and controlled, further stroke risk during pregnancy is up to 2%, but can rise to 20% if poorly controlled or where there are significant hypertensive co-morbidities (Khalid et al. 2020).

Health Promotion

Stroke is a preventable disease when modifiable risk factors are considered and reduced. These can include factors such as alcohol and drug abuse, smoking and obesity. Weight loss and a healthy diet can reduce the risk of diabetes, which can help prevent secondary kidney injuries and other complications that may give rise to a risk of pre-eclampsia/eclampsia, as this is one of the largest risk factors for pregnancy-related stroke.

Additionally, good blood pressure control through exercise and healthy diet is suggested, but if chronic hypertension is present ensure that it is adequately managed to normotensive levels.

Care During Pregnancy for Women at Risk of Stroke

The inherent risk of having a stroke as a female is higher at a younger age. Evidence suggests that this is linked primarily to pregnancy itself and that the risk of having a stroke as a young female is higher when pregnant versus non-pregnant (Kuriakose and Xiao 2020). This is mainly due to complications of pregnancy, but also to the increased risk of coagulation associated with the hormones of pregnancy (Kuriakose and Xiao 2020).

Despite this increased risk, evidence suggests that strokes in the antenatal period are uncommon, and the most common occurrence of a stroke is during intrapartum care (Liu et al. 2019). The current consensus statement/guideline from the European Stroke Organisation is that these patients can be treated by either thrombolysis or thrombectomy for ischaemic strokes (Kremer et al. 2022), yet they neglect to suggest what the treatment of haemorrhagic stroke should be.

A study regarding thrombolysis in pregnancy suggests that rates of complication among the pregnant population are like those for non-pregnant women, but that pregnancy-specific complications include fetal death (1.4%), neonatal death (0.7%), miscarriage (6.4%) and pre-term deliveries (9.9%) (Khalid et al. 2020).

One study on thrombectomy of four pregnant women showed good neurological outcome and no fetal complications in all cases, although this is only indicated in 10% of ischaemic strokes and has to be conducted at a specialised stroke centre (Khalid et al. 2020).

Haemorrhagic strokes can be treated conservatively through targeting maintenance of homeostasis and aggressive blood pressure control, although severe haemorrhage and those at risk of brainstem compression may need surgical intervention (Khalid et al. 2020).

The risks associated with stroke occurrence in pregnancy are as follows:

- Increased maternal age
- Multiparity
- Multifetal gestation
- Chronic hypertension
- Pre-eclampsia
- Eclampsia
- Connective tissue disorders
- HIV infection
- Migraines
- Congenital heart defects

Source: Adapted from Liu et al. (2019).

Postnatal Care for Women at Risk of Stroke

The postnatal period is the most common period for the occurrence of pregnancy-related stroke (Liu et al. 2019). The risk factors and management are much the same as outlined previously for the entire peripartum period, including postnatally.

Examination Scenario: Stroke

You are working in the maternity triage department. You have recently advised a woman called Jessica with some vague-sounding symptoms to come into triage for an assessment.

While waiting for her arrival you look at her medical notes and see that she is 36 years old, this is her first pregnancy, and she is currently at 38+2 weeks' gestation. Prior to booking her body mass index (BMI) was 27.0, and she previously smoked and was mildly hypertensive but not on medication. She has attended triage once before at gestation of 24 weeks for a headache and swollen feet, but there are no notes on the outcome of this encounter.

Jessica arrives 20 minutes later and is shown into the waiting area by the reception team.

You gather your notes and call her into an assessment room. She walks over to the room and appears to be acting drunk and is potentially dragging or limping with her left leg.

Once in the assessment room, you ask what has brought her into triage today.

She replies, 'I have a headache in my postcard.' Her facial expression appears anxious but frustrated when trying to speak. You spoke to her on the telephone 20 minutes ago and recall her complaining of a headache and general weakness, but she was speaking in complete, easy-to-understand sentences.

The next step is to carry out a FAST test. This looks for facial droop or asymmetry due to unilateral facial weakness, any speech difficulties and unilateral limb weakness.

You are concerned this may be a neurological presentation, so ask Jessica to raise her arms in front of her to 90° from her body and keep them there for 10 seconds. Jessica is only able to keep her right arm raised completely for the whole 10 seconds, as after approximately 4 seconds of a lot of straining, effort and wobbling, her left arm drifted back down to her side. You then ask her to smile and show her teeth. She can raise her right eyebrow and crease the corner of the right side of her mouth, but there is no movement in the left side of her face at all.

Jessica is FAST positive for all aspects of the test. She is displaying expressive dysphasia, has a unilateral limb weakness and facial droop. Any single aspect being positive is considered FAST positive, which yields an 85% sensitivity for an acute stroke (Purrucker et al. 2015).

The next step is to test capillary blood glucose levels, to rule out hypoglycaemia as a mimic of an acute stroke. Jessica's capillary glucose was 9.8 mmol/l, thus not hypoglycaemic.

You must suspect a stroke and if in a hospital contact the on-call stroke team and obstetrician. If not in a hospital, call for an emergency ambulance. To enhance care, you should then gather a full set of observations, including blood pressure. If you are competent to do so, insert an intravenous cannula.

Take-Home Points

- The nervous system is very complex and interrelated to multiple other body systems, so is susceptible to changes within other systems.
- In order to offer women and their family safe, effective, evidence-based care, an understanding of the pathophysiological changes that may occur in the nervous system is a prerequisite.
- Neurons are high specialised cells and do not undergo mitosis, thus once damaged nerve tissues do not 'regenerate'.
- Pregnancy has the potential to deterioration within the nervous system, such as increasing the stroke risk of women compared to non-pregnant women.

Conclusion

This chapter has delved into the intricate web of nervous system physiology, offering midwives a comprehensive understanding of the challenges and considerations associated with pre-conception, pregnancy and postnatal care in the context of neurological disorders.

Navigating the delicate balance between the physiological adaptations of pregnancy and the potential exacerbation of neurological conditions requires vigilance and a collaborative, multidisciplinary approach. Midwives play a pivotal role in ensuring optimal outcomes for both mother and baby by integrating their knowledge of neurophysiology with the principles of obstetric care. The complexities surrounding epilepsy management, the heightened risk of stroke, the unique challenges posed by multiple sclerosis, and the potential life-threatening implications of pre-eclampsia and eclampsia underscore the critical need for midwives to be well versed in the intricacies of the nervous system.

References

Altman, D., Carroli, G., Duley, L. et al. (2002). Do women with pre-eclampsia, and their babies, benefit from magnesium sulphate? The magpie trial: a randomised placebo-controlled trial. *Lancet* 359 (9321): 1877–1890. https://doi.org/10.1016/s0140-6736(02)08778-0.

Carhuapoma, J.R., Varner, M.W., and Levine, S.R. (2017). Neurological complications in pregnancy. In: *High-Risk Pregnancy: Management Opinions*, 5e (ed. D.K. James, P.J. Steer, C.P. Weiner, et al.), 1273–1321. Cambridge: Cambridge University Press.

Chen, S., Zeng, L., and Hu, Z. (2014). Progressing haemorrhagic stroke: categories, causes, mechanisms and managements. *Journal of Neurology* 261 (11): 2061–2078. https://doi.org/10.1007/s00415-014-7291-1.

Coupland, A.P., Thapar, A., Qureshi, M.I. et al. (2017). Definition of stroke. *Journal of the Royal Society of Medicine* 110 (1): 9–12. https://doi.org/10.1177/0141076816680121.

Dobson, R., Dassan, P., Roberts, M. et al. (2019). UK consensus on pregnancy in multiple sclerosis: Association of British Neurologists' guidelines. *Practical Neurology* 19 (2): 106–114. https://doi.org/10.1136/practneurol-2018-002060.

Epilepsy Society (2017). Epilepsy auras. https://epilepsysociety.org.uk/about-epilepsy/what-epilepsy/epilepsy-auras (accessed November 2023).

Essa, H., Hill, A.M., and Lip, G.Y.H. (2021). Atrial fibrillation and stroke. *Cardiac Electrophysiology Clinics* 13 (1): 243–255. https://doi.org/10.1016/j.ccep.2020.11.003.

Khalid, A.S., Hadbavna, A., Williams, D., and Byrne, B. (2020). A review of stroke in pregnancy: incidence, investigations and management. *Obstetrician and Gynaecologist* 22: 21–33. https://doi.org/10.1111/tog.12624.

Kobau, R., Gilliam, F., and Thurman, D.J. (2006). Prevalence of self-reported epilepsy or seizure disorder and its associations with self-reported depression and anxiety: results from the 2004 Health Styles Survey. *Epilepsia* 47 (11): 1915–1921. https://doi.org/10.1111/j.1528-1167.2006.00612.x.

Kremer, C., Gdovinova, Z., Bejot, Y. et al. (2022). European Stroke Organisation guidelines on stroke in women: management of menopause, pregnancy and postpartum. *European Stroke Journal* 7 (2): 1–19. https://doi.org/10.1177/23969873221078696.

Kuriakose, D. and Xiao, Z. (2020). Pathophysiology and treatment of stroke: present status and future perspectives. *International Journal of Molecular Sciences* 21 (20): 1–24. https://doi.org/10.3390/ijms21207609.

Liu, S., Chan, W.S., Ray, J.G. et al. (2019). Stroke and cerebrovascular disease in pregnancy incidence, temporal trends, and risk factors. *Stroke* 50: 13–20. https://doi.org/10.1161/STROKEAHA.118.023118.

Medicines and Healthcare products Regulatory Agency (MHRA) (2021). Antiepileptic drugs in pregnancy: updated advice following comprehensive safety review. https://www.gov.uk/drug-safety-update/antiepileptic-drugs-in-pregnancy-updated-advice-following-comprehensive-safety-review (accessed November 2023).

Moatti, Z., Gupta, M., Yadava, R., and Thamban, S. (2014). A review of stroke and pregnancy: incidence, management and prevention. *European Journal of Obstetrics & Gynecology and Reproductive Biology* 181: 20–27. https://doi.org/10.1016/j.ejogrb.2014.07.024.

Naryan, H. (2015). *Compendium for the Antenatal Care of High-Risk Pregnancies*. Oxford: Oxford University Press.

National Institute for Health and Care Excellence (NICE) (2019). Hypertension in pregnancy: diagnosis and management. NG 133. https://www.nice.org.uk/guidance/ng133 (accessed November 2023).

National Institute for Health and Care Excellence (NICE) (2022). Hypertension in pregnancy: Scenario: pre-eclampsia. https://cks.nice.org.uk/topics/hypertension-in-pregnancy/management/pre-eclampsia (accessed November 2023).

Purrucker, J.C., Hametner, C., Engelbrecht, A. et al. (2015). Comparison of stroke recognition and stroke severity scores for stroke detection in a single cohort. *Journal of Neurology, Neurosurgery, and Psychiatry* 86 (9): 1021–1028. https://doi.org/10.1136/jnnp-2014-309260.

Rolnik, D.L., Wright, D., Poon, L.C. et al. (2017). Aspirin versus placebo in pregnancies at high risk for preterm preeclampsia. *New England Journal of Medicine* 377: 613–622. https://doi.org/10.1056/NEJMoa1704559.

Sacco, R.L., Kasner, S.E., Broderick, J.P. et al. (2013). An updated definition of stroke for the 21st century a statement for healthcare professionals from the American Heart Association/American Stroke Association. *Stroke* 44: 2064–2089. https://doi.org/10.1161/STR.0b013e318296aecaStroke.

Siddiqi, U. and Platt, F. (2017). The treatment of hypertension in pregnancy. *Anaesthesia and Intensive Care Medicine* 18 (2): 106–109. https://doi.org/10.1016/j.mpaic.2016.11.005.

Stephen, L.J., Harden, C., Tomson, T., and Brodie, M.J. (2019). Management of epilepsy in women. *Lancet Neurological* 18 (5): 481–491. https://doi.org/10.1016/S1474-442(18)30495-2.

Thangaratinam, S., Fong, F., McCorry, D. et al. on Behalf of the Royal College of Obstetricians & Gynaecologists (2016). Epilepsy in pregnancy. Green-top guideline no. 68. https://www.rcog.org.uk/guidance/browse-all-guidance/green-top-guidelines/epilepsy-in-pregnancy-green-top-guideline-no-68 (accessed November 2023).

Thomas, S.V. (1998). Neurological aspects of eclampsia. *Journal of Neurological Sciences* 155 (1): 37–43. https://doi.org/10.1016/S0022-510X(97)00274-8.

Tortora, G.J. and Derrickson, B.H. (2014). *Principals of Anatomy and Physiology EMEA Edition*, 14e. Hoboken, NJ: Wiley.

Wallace, K., Harris, S., and Bean, C. (2019). The cerebral circulation during pregnancy and preeclampsia. In: *Sex Differences in Cardiovascular Physiology and Pathophysiology* (ed. B. LaMacra and B.T. Alexander), 149–163. London: Elsevier https://doi.org/10.1016/B978-0-12-813197-8.00010-5.

Welch, R. (2008). Considering the psychological effects of stroke. *British Journal of Healthcare Assistants* 2 (7): 335–338.

Winter, C., Crofts, J., Draycott, T., and Muchatuta, N. (ed.) (2017). *Practical Obstetric Multi-Professional Training Course Manual*, 3e. Cambridge: Cambridge University Press.

World Health Organization (WHO) (2023). Epilepsy. https://www.who.int/news-room/fact-sheets/detail/epilepsy (accessed November 2023).

Yger, M., Weisenburger-Lile, D., and Alamowitch, S. (2021). Cerebrovascular events during pregnancy and puerperium. *Revue Neurologique* 177 (3): 203–214. https://doi.org/10.1016/j.neurol.2021.02.001.

Yousif, D., Bellos, I., Penzlin, A.I. et al. (2019). Autonomic dysfunction in preeclampsia: a systematic review. *Frontiers in Neurology* 10: 816. https://doi.org/10.3389/fneur.2019.00816.

Further Resources

National Institute for Health and Care Excellence (NICE). www.nice.org.uk/guidance (accessed November 2023).

Action on Pre-Eclampsia. www.action-on-pre-eclampsia.org.uk (accessed November 2023).

Epilepsy Action. www.epilepsy.org.uk (accessed November 2023).

MS Society (UK). www.mssociety.org.uk (accessed November 2023).

MS Society (USA). www.nationalmssociety.org (accessed November 2023).

Stroke Association. www.stroke.org.uk (accessed November 2023).

Royal College of Obstetrics and Gynaecology (RCOG). www.rcog.org.uk (accessed November 2023).

Glossary

Low molecular weight heparin (LMWH)	A class of anticoagulant medication used in the prevention of blood clots and treatment of venous thromboembolism
Parasympathetic nervous system (PNS)	Responsible for rest and digest actions
Peripheral nervous system (PNS)	All other nervous tissue outside of the brain and spinal cord. This includes the cranial nerves, sensory and motor neurons as well as the enteric plexuses. These nerves carry impulses to and from the spinal cord
Sympathetic nervous system	Responsible for the fight or flight actions

CHAPTER 12

The Vascular System and Associated Disorders

Annabel Jay and Cathy Hamilton

University of Hertfordshire, Hatfield, UK

AIM

This chapter aims to provide insight and understanding to the reader concerning the vascular system and associated disorders in pregnancy.

LEARNING OUTCOMES

On completion of this chapter the reader will be able to:

- Describe the main vascular changes that occur in pregnancy, labour and the puerperium
- Outline the common vascular disorders affecting women in the childbearing period
- Outline the causes and effects of hypertensive disorders
- Identify the signs indicative of pre-eclampsia

Test Your Prior Knowledge

1. Name the four chambers of the heart.
2. List three differences between arteries and veins.
3. List three physiological factors that affect adult blood pressure.
4. Name two vascular disorders commonly affecting pregnant women.

During pregnancy the vascular system undergoes many physiological changes as the woman's body adapts to accommodate the needs of the growing fetus. Most changes are benign and rapidly resolve following the birth. However, occasionally complications arise that may threaten the well-being of both mother and baby. This chapter provides an overview of the vascular system and blood pressure and how they adapt to pregnancy. Disorders of the vascular system will be outlined. This is not intended to provide an in-depth guide to managing vascular conditions, but to give a general overview.

Structure and Function of the Cardiovascular System

The heart pumps blood to the whole body, via the blood vessels. From the moment of the first breath, oxygenated blood is carried from the lungs to the heart, which then pumps blood to the organs and tissues via large arteries and smaller arterioles. Veins and venules bring deoxygenated blood back from the body tissues to the heart and thence to the lungs for carbon dioxide (CO_2) to be released and oxygen to be absorbed.

Structure of the Adult Heart

The heart is situated slightly to the left in the thoracic cavity (Figure 12.1). It contains four chambers: the right atrium (plural atria) and right ventricle and the left atrium and left ventricle. On each side, the atrium and ventricle are separated by valves to prevent backflow of blood. The ventricles are divided by a fibrous septum and surrounded by thick muscle walls (the myocardium). The main vessels include the aorta, the pulmonary arteries and veins and the inferior and superior vena cava. These vessels take blood to and from the lungs and body. The heart's own blood supply, which keeps it functioning, is via the coronary vessels (not depicted). The pumping rhythm of the heart is regulated by electrical impulses arising from the sinoatrial node (or pacemaker) situated in the right atrium.

A non-pregnant woman has approximately 4.5 l of blood, which the heart pumps at approximately 4.5–5 l/min (Gopalan and Kirk 2022). An average heart rate is between 60 and 90 beats/min in a healthy adult when resting. This rises on exertion. A normal heartbeat consists of two sounds: a shorter sound (S1), followed by a longer sound (S2). These are caused by the opening and closing of the valves as the ventricles pump blood into the aorta and pulmonary arteries.

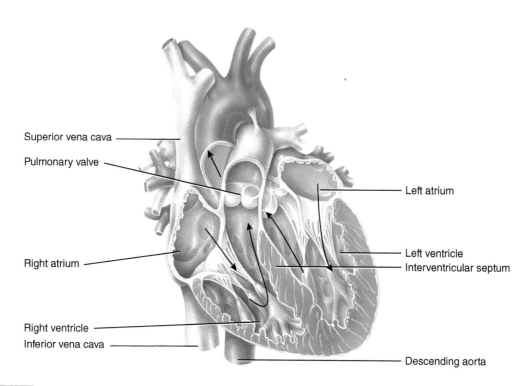

FIGURE 12.1   Structure of the adult heart.

Physiology of the Cardiovascular System

The cardiovascular system comprises the heart and blood vessels. It is designed to meet the homeostatic needs of the body at a cellular level by maintaining an adequate blood supply. This depends on the differing physiological requirements of the body at any given time. For example, blood flow to muscles increases during a period of exercise and to the gastrointestinal system following a meal. The system is controlled overall by nerve centres situated in the brain, but reflexes and local events are also involved in regulation

The main functions of the cardiovascular system are:

- To deliver oxygen and nutrients to the cells and vital organs.
- To remove metabolic waste products including CO_2.
- To ensure the dispersal of heat from active tissues and the redistribution of heat around the body.

Blood Circulation

Blood flows through vessels that run between the heart and the peripheral tissues. The circulatory system can be divided into two distinct pathways: pulmonary circulation and systemic circulation.

Pulmonary circulation transports deoxygenated blood from the right side of the heart to the lungs and then returns blood that has been oxygenated in the lungs to the left side of the heart. Following this, the systemic circulatory pathway transports oxygenated blood from the left side of the heart to all the tissues and vital organs of the body. Deoxygenated blood then returns to the right side of the heart via the systemic circulation. In addition, the exchange of metabolic waste products and nutrients also occurs within the systemic circulatory pathway.

In an average adult woman at rest, the amount of blood circulating within the heart is 4.5 l/min. This is the same as the amount of blood contained within the circulation system.

Overview of Blood Vessels

Usually veins and venules transport deoxygenated blood towards the heart. The exception is the pulmonary veins, which transport oxygenated blood.

Arteries and arterioles are the blood vessels transporting blood away from the heart. These vessels usually carry oxygenated blood, with the exception of the pulmonary arteries that transport deoxygenated blood. Capillaries are tiny blood vessels situated between the venous and arterial systems. They remain very close to the tissues, providing an extensive network of interconnected vessels. Blood vessels have the ability to dilate and contract while providing a closed transport system for the blood, which starts and finishes at the heart.

The main function of blood vessels is to transport blood around the body, but the large blood vessels also receive a blood supply via a network of other vessels called the vasa vasorum. This system provides oxygen and nutrients to the large vessels, removing metabolic waste products. However, smaller blood vessels with very thin walls receive oxygen and nutrients directly from the blood by diffusion as it passes through their lumina.

The heart itself comprises separate pumps providing the force to propel blood around the body through the network of blood vessels (Figure 12.2). The left side of the heart feeds into the systemic circulation while the right side feeds into the pulmonary circulation.

Structure of the Blood Vessels

The anatomical structure of blood vessels alters depending on their specific function within the body. However, the walls of most blood vessels (apart from the capillaries) consist of the same three layers of tissues surrounding a central lumen (Figure 12.3). These are as follows:

- **Tunica interna or intima:** the innermost layer consisting of flattened epithelial cells, supported by a basement membrane along with some elastic and connective tissue. This lining provides a smooth inner surface, meaning that there is reduced friction when blood flows through.

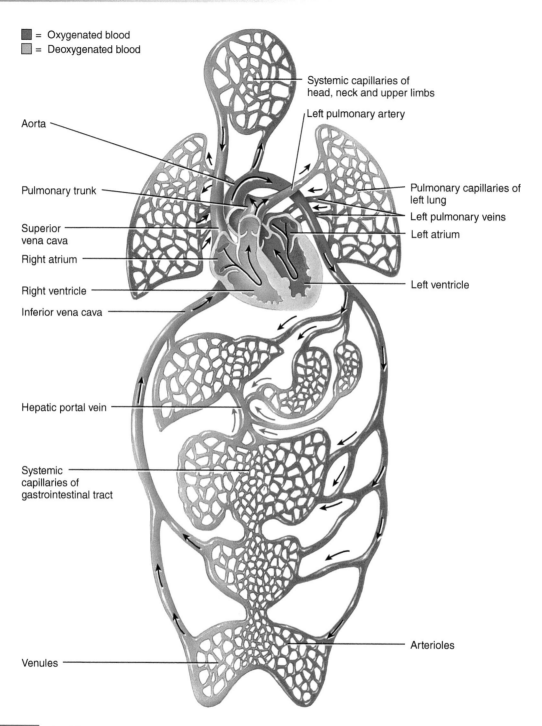

= Oxygenated blood
= Deoxygenated blood

Systemic capillaries of
head, neck and upper limbs

Left pulmonary artery

Aorta

Pulmonary trunk

Pulmonary capillaries of
left lung

Left pulmonary veins

Superior
vena cava

Left atrium

Right atrium

Right ventricle

Left ventricle

Inferior vena cava

Hepatic portal vein

Systemic
capillaries of
gastrointestinal tract

Arterioles

Venules

FIGURE 12.2   Blood flow.

- **Tunica media:** the middle layer composed of elastic tissue and some smooth muscle. The sympathetic nervous system feeds into the smooth muscle layer and affects the diameter of the blood vessel when stimulated. This leads to blood pressure increasing when the blood vessel contracts or decreasing when the blood vessel dilates.
- **Tunica externa** (previously known as the tunica adventitia): the outermost layer, consisting of collagen, fibrous connective tissue and fibroblasts. These fibres support the blood vessels and bind them to the surrounding tissue. This outer layer is supplied with sympathetic nerve fibres and lymphatic vessels. The larger veins also contain elastic fibres.

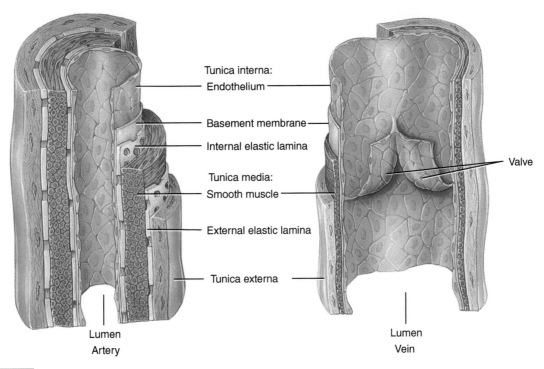

Tunica interna:
Endothelium

Basement membrane

Internal elastic lamina

Tunica media:
Smooth muscle

External elastic lamina

Tunica externa

Valve

Lumen
Artery

Lumen
Vein

FIGURE 12.3 Structure of an artery and a vein.

Arteries

Arteries (Figure 12.4) can be divided into three types:

- **Elastic arteries:** These have thick walls and are usually situated closest to the heart; an example is the aorta. This is the main blood vessel supplying the left ventricle of the heart and the systemic circulation. Elastic arteries contain a

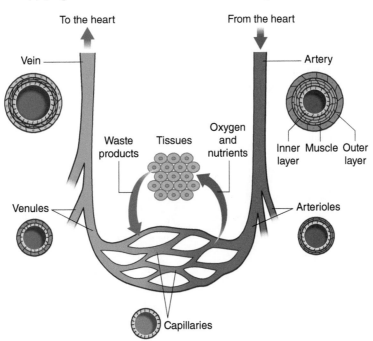

To the heart

From the heart

Vein

Artery

Waste products

Tissues

Oxygen and nutrients

Inner layer

Muscle

Outer layer

Venules

Arterioles

Capillaries

FIGURE 12.4 Interconnections between arteries and Veins in the circulatory system.

high percentage of elastic fibres in the tunica medica. They have large diameters (approximately 2.5 cm), providing lower resistance to blood flow. The elastic walls swell when full of blood and then recoil, pushing blood forwards. This means that blood keeps on flowing even when the left ventricle relaxes. Elastic arteries are also known as conducting arteries, transporting blood from the left ventricle to the smaller arteries.

- **Muscular arteries:** These are smaller, with a diameter of approximately 0.4 cm (Rankin 2017). They consist of more smooth muscle and fewer elastic fibres, enabling them to constrict and dilate to a greater extent and meaning that their resistance to flow is low. As the muscular arteries branch further they decrease in size, leading to a subsequent decrease in elastic fibres and an increase in smooth muscle. They are also referred to as distributing arteries as they transport blood to the vital organs and other areas of the body. This ability to dilate or constrict means that blood can be diverted to the organs where it is most needed at any given time depending on physiological changes. The muscular arteries include the axillary, brachial, splenic, radial, popliteal, femoral and tibial arteries.
- **Arterioles:** Muscular arteries branch further into smaller blood vessels called arterioles, which are the smallest arteries with a diameter of less than 0.3 cm. They have thicker walls composed almost entirely of muscular tissue arranged in concentric layers containing some elastic fibres. They branch down further into tiny vessels called metacapillaries, directing the blood into the capillaries. Metacapillaries are mostly composed of epithelial cells with an incomplete layer of smooth muscle (McCance and Heuther 2018). Arterioles alter the diameter of the capillaries, regulating the volume of blood flowing through them. This means that the overall resistance to blood flow is determined by the diameters of these small vessels and in turn determines the distribution of blood to different parts of the body. When arterioles contract, blood is diverted away from the organs they supply; when they relax, blood flow increases significantly.

Capillaries

Capillaries (Figure 12.5) form a network of narrow, short blood vessels whose walls are usually only one endothelial cell thick. As red blood cells flow in single file through them, they may have to fold in order to pass through the narrow lumen. In the capillary network, water, nutrients, gases and metabolic waste products pass between individual cells and the vascular system. There are approximately 50 million capillaries contained in the body, located throughout apart from in the epidermis and the cornea. When the body is at rest, only 25% of capillaries will be open (Rankin 2017).

Three types of capillaries are described (McCance and Heuther 2018):

- **Sinusoid capillaries** are wider than other capillaries, located mainly in the liver, bone marrow, lymphoid tissue and endocrine organs. Sinusoid capillary walls are lined with phagocytic white blood cells. Blood tends to flow slowly through them to allow further modification of blood content. For example, this is required in the liver when there may be vital nutrients passing through that need to be removed from the blood for distribution around the body.
- **Fenestrated capillaries**, located in the kidneys, are responsible for filtration of the blood in the glomeruli.
- **Continuous capillaries** the commonest type of capillary, distributed throughout most tissues.

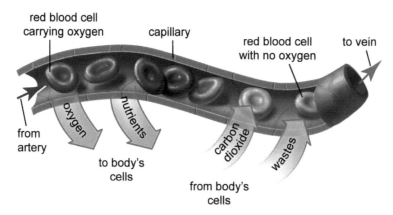

FIGURE 12.5   Flow of blood cells through the capillary.

Venules

Blood flows from the capillaries into venules. These blood vessels consist of endothelium with a small number of fibroblast cells. Venules are very porous, readily permitting the free flow of water, solutes and white blood cells in and out of the cellular fluid surrounding them.

Veins

Venules join together forming veins, which are larger blood vessels consisting of the same three tissue layers as arteries. However, the walls of veins tend to be much thinner than arteries, containing less collagen, elastic fibre and smooth muscle. The diameter of a vein is wider than an artery, and they become much larger and less branched as they move further away from the capillary system towards the heart.

Some veins, for example those situated in the legs, have folds located in the endothelium acting as valves, ensuring blood only flows towards the heart. The highest percentage of blood (at least 60%) is contained within the venous system. Veins may be referred to as capacity vessels, as they have the ability to change their capacity for carrying blood by changing the diameters of the vessels.

Overview of Blood Pressure

Blood pressure (BP) is defined as the force exerted on the walls of blood vessels as blood flows through them (Johnson and Taylor 2021). This force tends to be higher in the large arteries closest to the heart, while decreasing in the smaller blood vessels furthest away from the heart. BP also decreases as blood returns to the heart via the venous system. Although venous blood pressure can be measured, BP measurements usually refer to arterial blood pressure.

BP alters throughout the day, often lowest at night while a person is sleeping and highest first thing in the morning. Neural, chemical and renal processes act within the body to regulate BP, working together to affect cardiac output, peripheral resistance and the volume of blood in circulation.

Neuronal regulation is achieved by a short-term negative feedback system incorporating baroreceptors and chemoreceptors. Baroreceptors are sensitive to alterations in pressure within the arteries situated in the carotid sinus and the aortic arch. Baroreceptors respond to changes in posture and in activity levels. Nerve fibres running from the baroreceptors via the cranial and vagus nerves respond to stretching of the arterial wall. The nerves then exhibit an inhibitory action on the cardiovascular centre located in the medulla oblongata, leading to a slowing of the heartbeat, a decrease in the force of the contraction of the ventricle and arterial vasodilation, leading to the lowering of BP.

Chemoreceptors are sensitive to alterations in oxygen, CO_2 and hydrogen levels and are situated in the aortic and carotid bodies, responding to a decrease in blood oxygen or an increase in the acidity of the blood. This mainly affects the respiratory system, leading to an increased respiratory rate. However, in severe hypoxia this can also result in stimulation of the sympathetic nervous system, leading to an increase in heart rate and BP as the body works to increase oxygen levels within the blood.

Hormonal/chemical regulation of BP involves hormones produced by the adrenal glands, namely adrenaline (epinephrine) and noradrenaline (norepinephrine). These act to stimulate sympathetic activity within the body, known as the 'flight or fight' response. Antidiuretic hormone is also released from the posterior pituitary gland, leading to the retention of fluid within the body when BP is low, for example due to pain or blood loss.

Renal Processes: Renin–Angiotensin System

When blood volume and BP are decreased, renin, a proteolytic enzyme, is released by the kidneys. Renin promotes the conversion of the peptide hormone angiotensin 1 to angiotensin 2. Angiotensin 2 has the effect of causing blood vessels to contract, increasing the BP. Angiotensin 2 also stimulates the release of another hormone, aldosterone, from the adrenal cortex, leading to the retention of sodium and water along with the loss of potassium from the kidneys, which also promotes an increase in BP.

Physiological Factors Influencing the Blood Pressure

A number of factors affect the flow of blood through the vessels that in turn influences the BP:

- The volume of blood circulating around the body. The lower the volume, the lower the BP.
- Cardiac output, defined as a function of the heart rate and stroke volume.
- The viscosity or thickness of a fluid. In blood this is influenced by the ratio of red blood cells and plasma proteins to plasma fluid. Viscosity increases when there is a rise in cell content or a decrease in plasma fluid, which may happen when an individual becomes dehydrated. When plasma fluid is increased, viscosity is decreased. Increased viscosity means that more force is required to propel the blood along a vessel increasing blood pressure.
- Peripheral resistance is associated with the degree of constriction of blood vessels. It is a physiological factor also related to the radius of the blood vessel, its length, the viscosity of the blood and the smoothness of vessel walls. Resistance may also be provided by plasma proteins circulating within the bloodstream. If peripheral resistance is high, a high BP is required to overcome this, ensuring that blood is able to circulate throughout the body. If resistance is low, this leads to lower BP.

Arterial Blood Pressure

This refers to pressure exerted onto the arterial walls as blood flows around the body ensuring that oxygen is delivered to tissues and vital organs. When the ventricle of the heart contracts, the arterial BP increases as the arteries contain the maximum amount of blood. This is known as systole.

Systolic BP is determined by:

- The amount of blood released into the arteries (known as the stroke volume).
- The force of the contraction of the ventricle.
- The capacity of the blood vessel to stretch and expand.

Any increase in the first two factors or a decrease in the third leads to an increase in systolic BP. Conversely, a decrease in the first two factors and an increase in the third leads to a reduction in systolic BP.

When the ventricle relaxes this is known as diastole and there is a corresponding decrease in BP. Diastolic BP is determined by:

- The amount of peripheral resistance from the blood vessel walls.
- The systolic pressure.
- Cardiac output.

Diastolic BP is usually lower when all three of these factors are reduced. This occurs when the heartbeat is slower, as less blood remains in the arteries when the ventricle relaxes.

Arterial BP is measured in millimetres of mercury. When measuring BP the highest and lowest levels should be recorded, as they indicate the different physiological responses of the cardiac cycle. For example, a systolic blood pressure of 120 mmHg and a diastolic measurement of 60 mmHg is recorded as 120 over 60 (120/60 mmHg).

Mean Arterial Pressure

Mean arterial pressure (MAP) is the average pressure required to propel blood through the circulatory system. Rankin (2017) suggests that the MAP is a more accurate indication of tissue perfusion than the systolic/diastolic measurement.

It is stated that a MAP of greater than 60 mmHg indicates that there is sufficient perfusion to supply all the vital organs (DeMers and Wachs 2022). As Johnson and Taylor (2021) highlight, the MAP helps with the interpretation of changes occurring in BP measurements when the diastolic and systolic readings are altering at different rates.

The MAP can be calculated mathematically by doubling the diastolic reading, adding it to the systolic reading and dividing the total by 3.

For example:

BP of 110/65 mmHg has a MAP of 80 mmHg

$$65 \times 2 = 130$$

$$130 + 110 = 240$$

$$240 / 3 = 80 \text{ mmHg}$$

Pulse Pressure

Homan et al. (2022) define pulse pressure as the difference between systolic and diastolic BP. An increase in pulse pressure occurs when the systolic BP is increased or there is a decrease in diastolic BP caused by a combination of increased stroke volume and/or decreased peripheral resistance. This may be associated with bradycardia, infection, pyrexia or physical exercise. A decrease in pulse pressure is due to a decrease in systolic BP and/or an increase in diastolic BP resulting from decreased stroke volume or increased peripheral resistance. This can occur when there is reduced circulating blood volume (hypovolaemia) due to shock or haemorrhage.

Venous Blood Pressure

This is defined as the pressure of blood flowing through veins and measures the venous flow towards the heart. Central venous pressure is defined as pressure in the thoracic vena cava closest to the right atrium; central venous pressure and right atrial pressure are the same reading. Central venous pressure is influenced by:

- The amount of blood returning to the heart via the right atrium.
- The function of the right ventricle.
- Intrathoracic pressure.
- Venous tone.

Changes to the Cardiovascular System in Pregnancy, Labour and the Puerperium

Blood Volume

Blood volume begins to rise from early pregnancy, to meet the needs of the growing uterus, placenta and fetus. Total blood volume increases by up to 45% by the end of pregnancy. However, plasma volume increases by up to 50%, whereas red cell volume increases by a much smaller amount. This results in the blood becoming relatively more dilute, causing haemoglobin (Hb) levels to drop to around 110–130 g/l. This is known as haemodilution, a normal adaptation to pregnancy. The effects of haemodilution can be similar to those of mild anaemia – increasing tiredness and breathlessness on exertion, especially towards the end of pregnancy. These symptoms are also due to the extra weight of the growing fetus and reduced lung volume. Sometimes Hb levels fall below 110 g/l, in which case oral iron supplementation may be prescribed.

Once the baby and placenta have been born, the mother's blood volume begins to return to normal. A rapid volume reduction occurs in the first two weeks postpartum. Some blood is lost in the lochia, but most is excreted via the urinary system. Most women will notice they pass a much larger volume of urine than normal in the first few days postpartum.

Blood Vessels

In order to cope with increased blood volume, the woman's blood vessels undergo changes during pregnancy. Under the influence of the hormones relaxin and progesterone, the resistance of the venous walls is reduced, allowing vasodilation and enabling the vein to carry a greater volume of blood. Side effects may include ankle oedema, haemorrhoids and visibly distended veins, as the venous valves that normally prevent backflow become less efficient. These changes are temporary and normally resolve in the first few weeks after birth.

Heart

During pregnancy the heart increases in size in order to manage the rapidly increasing blood volume and pulmonary blood flow. The muscle wall of the heart grows in size (myocardial hypertrophy) and the four chambers enlarge. The size of the average heart increases over the period of pregnancy. Due to the vasodilatory effects of pregnancy hormones (see earlier) mild valvular regurgitation occurs, but this is usually of no consequence. As the fetus grows, the uterus rises from the pelvic cavity into the abdominal cavity, eventually displacing the diaphragm to a higher position. This in turn causes the heart to move to a slightly higher position and further to the left. By the third trimester, the resulting pressure on the lungs reduces their capacity and may cause the woman to experience breathlessness on exertion and when supine. During labour cardiac output increases by 10–40% above pre-labour levels. Following the birth, the internal organs rapidly return to their pre-pregnant size, shape and position (see Chapter 9 for more information).

Blood Pressure

The effects of vasodilation cause BP to fall slightly from the first trimester of pregnancy, reaching its lowest point at around 24 weeks' gestation. There is a marked decrease in diastolic pressure, but only a slight reduction in systolic pressure. From around 34 weeks of pregnancy, BP gradually begins to rise back to pre-pregnant levels. BP is influenced by many factors, such as stress, eating and drinking, exercise and intra-abdominal pressure from a full bladder.

In pregnancy, postural changes that affect cardiac output can alter BP. In late pregnancy, the enlarged uterus compresses the inferior vena cava and lower aorta (aorto-caval compression) when the woman is supine. This affects blood returning to the heart and reduces cardiac output. It can result in the woman feeling faint and dizzy, as well as affecting blood supply to the placenta. For these reasons, women are advised to avoid the supine position in late pregnancy. Various disorders of the cardiovascular system can affect BP in pregnancy.

Minor Disorders of the Blood Vessels

Varicose Veins

These appear as swollen, convoluted veins and mainly affect the legs, but can also develop in the vulva and anal canal (see later). During pregnancy, the effect of the hormones progesterone and relaxin reduces the efficiency of the valves in the leg veins, resulting in reduced venous return. This is exacerbated by pressure from the growing uterus, slowing venous return from the lower body and causing the veins below the level of the uterus to become swollen (Lydall et al. 2013). Varicose veins may have a familial tendency and affect around 40% of pregnant women. Varicosities cannot be prevented in those with a predisposition to them, but the discomfort can be relieved by elevating the legs when resting, avoiding prolonged standing and wearing support hosiery. Varicose veins usually become less prominent after pregnancy, but may never completely resolve and may gradually worsen with advancing age.

Leg varicosities are usually harmless, but can predispose to deep vein thrombosis (DVT). Women should be advised to report any pain, redness or swelling of the affected leg.

Haemorrhoids

As pregnancy progresses, the veins in the anal canal may become engorged and dilated, resulting in discomfort, itching and sometimes bleeding. Most haemorrhoids remain within the anal canal, but in some cases prolapse to the exterior. Factors predisposing to haemorrhoids include constipation (straining to defecate increases venous pressure), obesity and a weakened pelvic floor. Women who suffer from haemorrhoids prior to pregnancy may find the condition worsens. Treatment includes use of local analgesic creams, ice packs and measures to avoid constipation, such as a high-fibre diet and laxatives. Codeine-based analgesia should be avoided for its constipating effects. Pelvic floor exercises should be encouraged to promote good venous return.

Haemorrhoids usually resolve spontaneously within six weeks of the birth, but there is a risk of infection if the perineum becomes infected. Careful and sensitive inspection of the perineum and perianal region is required to assess haemorrhoids. In severe cases, medical referral is recommended. Lydall et al. (2013) note that although very common, haemorrhoids can be distressing and embarrassing for women and should not be dismissed as trivial.

Major Disorders of the Blood Vessels

Venous Thromboembolism

Venous thromboembolism (VTE) refers to a clot (thrombus) formed in a vein, which partially or totally occludes blood flow. This may be due to trauma to the vessel wall leading to exaggerated coagulation, blood stasis due to inactivity or one of a number of inherited or acquired conditions associated with thrombophilia, such as Hughes syndrome and Factor V Leiden. DVT is the most common type of VTE and usually develops in the legs or pelvis. VTE is potentially lethal, especially if a clot travels to the lungs, where it is known as a pulmonary embolism. Deaths from blood clots currently account for 1.4 per 100 000 maternities, 16% of all maternal deaths in the perinatal period in the United Kingdom (Knight et al. 2022).

Risk factors for VTE in the general population include smoking, obesity, dehydration, major surgery, previous history of VTE and varicose veins. Pregnancy also increases the risk due to greater blood stasis in the lower limbs, reduced venous tone and an increase in coagulation factors (Elliott and Pavord 2013).

DVT in a leg vein is usually characterised by unilateral redness, swelling and pain. Current guidance states that all women should be formally assessed for risk of thrombosis in early pregnancy, in the event of complications, on admittance to hospital and in labour or immediately afterwards (RCOG 2015). Women at risk, or with a history of VTE/DVT, will be offered thromboprophylaxis in the form of low molecular weight heparin during pregnancy and for six weeks postpartum. Emergency caesarean section increases the risk of VTE and women will be considered for thromboprophylaxis for up to 10 days (RCOG 2015). All pregnant women should be advised on measures to reduce the risk of DVT, such as avoiding dehydration, maintaining a healthy weight and avoiding long, uninterrupted periods of sitting.

Valvular Heart Disease

Valvular heart disease is a condition in which the heart valves become inflamed and scarred, leading to stenosis (narrowing and stiffening). Previous rheumatic heart disease (RHD) is frequently the cause. Symptoms of valvular disease include severe breathlessness and excessive tiredness, due to pulmonary hypertension. Women with valvular heart disease will need ongoing treatment from the cardiac team throughout the childbearing period, including restricted activities, cardiac drugs and possibly oxygen therapy.

Marfan's Syndrome

This disorder affects approximately 1 in 5000 people (NHS 2022). It is usually inherited but can occur by spontaneous gene mutation. It affects the connective tissues in the musculoskeletal system, the respiratory system, the eyes, the heart and blood vessels (McLean et al. 2013). Symptoms vary in their severity but tend to worsen with age. Marfan's syndrome can cause weakening of the elastic fibres of the aortic wall, leading to risk of aneurism or rupture. It can also affect the mitral valve, leading to back flow of blood, resulting in shortness of breath, palpitations and fatigue (McLean et al. 2013).

Pregnancy increases the dangers due to increased demands on the cardiac system. Women with Marfan's syndrome are considered to be high risk and require careful monitoring throughout pregnancy. Prophylactic drug therapy to reduce BP may be prescribed.

Chapter 9 addresses other heart disorders.

Hypertensive Disorders and Pre-eclampsia

High BP (hypertension) is defined as sustained BP measures of $\geq 140/90$ mmHg (NICE 2022). Hypertensive disorders affect around 8–10% of all pregnant women (NICE 2019) and account for 3% of maternal deaths in the United Kingdom (Knight et al. 2022). Hypertensive disorders can cause placental insufficiency, leading to restricted fetal growth, placental abruption and prematurity. These disorders may pre-date pregnancy or be directly caused by pregnancy.

Pre-existing (chronic) hypertension is more common in women who are older, of African ethnicity, those who are obese and/or those with a family history of hypertension (Webster et al. 2013). Alternatively, it may be secondary to another medical condition such as renal disease or an endocrine disorder. Chronic hypertension is often asymptomatic and many women will be unaware of it until they become pregnant. It is important to assess BP accurately as early as possible in pregnancy to obtain a baseline against which future readings can be measured. Women with chronic hypertension who book late for antenatal care may appear to have normal BP when what is being measured reflects the physiological fall in BP in mid-pregnancy. In such cases, BP will rise above the hypertensive threshold as pregnancy progresses and fail to return to normal levels by the end of the puerperium.

Some women develop gestational hypertension with no previous history and no other clinical symptoms. In most cases, BP will return to normal in the puerperium. All women with moderate hypertension (BP $\geq 150/100$ but <160/110 mmHg) should be offered referral to a specialist in hypertensive disorders of pregnancy to discuss the risks and benefits of treatment (NICE 2019). Antihypertensive medication may be prescribed, along with lifestyle advice such as weight management and exercise (NICE 2019). BP should be carefully monitored throughout the perinatal period, due to the increased likelihood of developing pre-eclampsia (see next section). Women with severe hypertension (BP $\geq 160/110$) at any stage of pregnancy or the puerperium will normally be referred for hospital assessment (Webster et al. 2013). The NICE guideline on hypertension in pregnancy (NG133) offers clear guidance for the care of women with chronic hypertension and pre-eclampsia (NICE 2019).

Pre-eclampsia

This multisystem disorder affects up to 8% of all childbearing women in the United Kingdom and can present at any time between 20 weeks' gestation and 6 weeks postpartum (RCOG 2022). It is diagnosed when, on at least two occasions, a woman presents with proteinuria of $\geq 1+$ on dipstick urinalysis, systolic BP of >140 mm/Hg and diastolic BP of ≥ 90 mm/Hg (Uzan et al. 2011). Risk factors include nulliparity, pregnancy interval of >10 years, chronic hypertension, obesity, extremes of maternal age and multiple pregnancy (NICE 2019). Pre-eclampsia may have no obvious symptoms, but typically causes increasing hypertension and proteinuria, which if left untreated may result in eclamptic seizures. In rare cases this is fatal for both mother and fetus. Women with pre-eclampsia may present with severe headache, visual disturbances, such as blurring or flashing before the eyes, severe epigastric pain, vomiting and sudden onset of oedema to the face, hands or feet (NICE 2019). Clinical detection of proteinuria and hypertension will confirm the diagnosis.

The exact cause of pre-eclampsia is unknown, but it is thought to be caused initially by abnormal placentation, leading to reduced perfusion of blood and placental hypoxia. Later in pregnancy, the placenta releases factors that damage the endothelial cells lining the maternal blood vessels (Webster et al. 2013). This is thought to cause vasospasm, leading to raised BP and abnormal blood coagulation. The vessel walls become more permeable, resulting in oedema and proteinuria (Uzan et al. 2011). Reduced placental blood flow can cause restricted fetal growth. Complications include prematurity, intrauterine death and placental abruption. In extreme cases, it can lead to renal and liver failure in the mother as well as eclamptic seizures and HELLP syndrome (haemolysis, elevated liver enzymes and low platelets) (Uzan et al. 2011; Webster et al. 2013). This is a medical emergency.

Pre-eclampsia always progresses while pregnancy continues, but can be treated to reduce adverse outcomes. Mild cases (BP $\geq$150/100 but <160/110 mmHg) may be dealt with in the community, provided there are no other risk factors (Webster et al. 2013; NICE 2019), but women with severe symptoms (BP >160/110 mmHg, significant proteinuria and/or other symptoms) will require hospital admission. Pre-eclampsia normally resolves spontaneously once the placenta is delivered and for this reason it is sometimes advisable to induce labour early. The effects can be controlled to some extent by the administration of oral antihypertensives or in severe cases intravenous magnesium sulfate (NICE 2019). However, these are only temporary measures used to stabilise the woman's condition pending delivery of the baby.

Deaths from pre-eclampsia/eclampsia are rare in the United Kingdom due to vigilant maternity care, but account for around 2% of all maternal deaths (Knight et al. 2021). Although the birth of the baby and placenta usually expedites a rapid return to normal BP, nearly half of all eclamptic seizures occur in the postnatal period (Webster et al. 2013; NICE 2019). It is important for midwives to carefully monitor BP in postnatal women, especially those with a known history of pre-eclampsia or chronic hypertension.

Case Study 12.1

Sonia, a 31-year old woman at 36 weeks' gestation, parity 2, gravida 3, arrives at the antenatal clinic for a routine appointment. She is 10 minutes late. Sonia has had two uncomplicated pregnancies in the past and her antenatal history so far has been normal. She has no significant medical history.

Sonia appears flushed and breathless on arrival. Her ankles appear puffy. During routine observations, her BP is measured at 145/95 mm/Hg.

- What might be the possible cause of Sonia's raised BP?
- What other observations should the midwife undertake? Why?
- What questions might the midwife ask Sonia?
- What follow-on care might the midwife recommend?

Consider the following:

- Sonia may have rushed to attend her appointment. She may be stressed due to being late. Increased physical exertion and stress both raise BP.
- The midwife should check Sonia's initial BP measured at her booking visit. Any significant difference between this and her current BP may be a cause for concern. The midwife should carry out a full antenatal assessment, including dipstick testing of Sonia's urine for the presence of protein, which might indicate pre-eclampsia. If proteinuria is detected, a repeat sample will be tested and, if positive, will be sent for laboratory analysis.
- The midwife should ask Sonia when her ankle oedema first presented and whether she has swelling anywhere else. Rapid onset of oedema to the hands, face and legs could be indicative of pre-eclampsia. Sonia's BP should be measured again when she has had a chance to relax and get her breath back – if it is normal, this would suggest that her initially raised BP was simply caused by stress or exertion. The midwife should also assess Sonia's pulse and respiratory rate, to rule out any abnormalities suggestive of an underlying heart condition.
- The midwife should ask whether Sonia often feels breathless or experiences chest pains or palpitations. If so, she should be referred immediately for hospital assessment.
- If all is well, the midwife will arrange to measure Sonia's BP at every antenatal appointment and more frequently if it proves unstable or rises. Assuming no other abnormalities are detected and Sonia's BP remains within normal limits, her midwife may advise her to raise her legs when sitting, or to wear support socks/tights to reduce oedema and increase her comfort. The midwife will advise Sonia on the signs and symptoms of pre-eclampsia and what to do if she has concerns.

Take-Home Points

- The cardiovascular system undergoes extensive changes during pregnancy and the puerperium.
- Some of the changes have symptoms similar to those of pathological conditions, so vigilance is needed at every point of care.
- Women with a history or close family history of cardiac disorders should receive care from a specialist team as well as the midwife.
- Pre-eclampsia affects up to 8% of childbearing women in the United Kingdom. Midwives must be especially alert to the signs and know how to refer women for further investigations.

Conclusion

This chapter has given an overview of the vascular system and highlighted the key changes that occur during the antenatal, intrapartum and postpartum periods. Most of these changes are temporary and will revert to the pre-pregnant state by around six weeks postpartum. A few, such as varicose veins, may remain for life. Most vascular changes cause no more than minor discomfort to the woman, but rarely they can develop into life-threatening conditions. According to the most recent MBBRACE reports, vascular disorders (including eclampsia, heart disease and clots) account for over 40% of maternal deaths, while thrombosis and thromboembolism remain the leading cause of direct maternal death from early pregnancy to six weeks postpartum (Knight et al. 2021, 2022). For this reason, vigilance is required in providing maternity care and a low threshold should be used for medical referral when a vascular disorder is suspected.

References

DeMers, D. and Wachs, D. (2022). Physiology, mean arterial pressure. In: *StatPearls*. Treasure Island, FL: StatPearls Publishing https://www.ncbi.nlm.nih.gov/books/NBK538226.

Elliott, D. and Pavord, S. (2013). Thrombo-embolic disorders. In: *Medical Disorders in Pregnancy: A Manual for Midwives* (ed. S.E. Robson and J. Waugh), 279–297. Oxford: Wiley-Blackwell.

Gopalan, C. and Kirk, E. (2022). *Biology of Cardiovascular and Metabolic Diseases*. London: Elsevier.

Homan, T.D., Bordes, S., and Cichowski, E. (2022). Physiology, pulse pressure. In: *StatPearls*. Treasure Island, FL: StatPearls Publishing https://www.ncbi.nlm.nih.gov/books/NBK482408.

Johnson, R. and Taylor, W. (2021). Assessment of maternal and neonatal vital signs: blood pressure measurement. In: *Skills for Midwifery Practice*, 5e, 37–49. London: Elsevier.

Knight, M., Bunch, K., Tuffnell, D. et al. (ed.) (2021) on behalf of MBRRACE-UK). *Saving Lives, Improving Mothers' Care: Lessons Learned to Inform Maternity Care from the UK and Ireland Confidential Enquiries into Maternal Deaths and Morbidity 2017–19*. Oxford: National Perinatal Epidemiology Unit, University of Oxford https://www.npeu.ox.ac.uk/mbrrace-uk/reports.

Knight, M., Bunch, K., Patel, R. et al. on behalf of MBRRACE-UK(2022). *Saving lives, Improving Mothers' Care Core Report: Lessons Learned to Inform Maternity Care from the UK and Ireland Confidential Enquiries into Maternal Deaths and Morbidity 2018–20*. Oxford: National Perinatal Epidemiology Unit, University of Oxford.

Lydall, R., Khare, M., Farrar, C., and Robson, S.E. (2013). Gastrointestinal disorders. In: *Medical Disorders in Pregnancy: A Manual for Midwives* (ed. S.E. Robson and J. Waugh), 171–198. Oxford: Wiley Blackwell.

McCance, K.L. and Huether, S.E. (2018). *Pathophysiology: The Biologic Basis for Diseases in Adults and Children*, 8e. St Louis: Mosby.

McLean, M., Bu'Lock, F.A., and Robson, S.E. (2013). Heart disease. In: *Medical Disorders in Pregnancy: A Manual for Midwives* (ed. S.E. Robson and J. Waugh), 43–74. Oxford: Wiley Blackwell.

National Health Service (NHS) (2022). Marfan's syndrome. https://www.nhs.uk/conditions/marfan-syndrome (accessed November 2023).

National Institute for Health and Care Excellence (NICE) (2019). Hypertension in pregnancy: diagnosis and management. NG133. https://www.nice.org.uk/guidance/ng133 (accessed November 2023).

National Institute for Health and Care Excellence (NICE) (2022). Hypertension: what is it? https://cks.nice.org.uk/topics/hypertension/background-information/definition (accessed November 2023).

Rankin, J. (2017). *Physiology in Childbearing with Anatomy and Related Biosciences*, 4e. London: Elsevier.

Royal College of Obstetrics and Gynaecology (2015). RCOG Green top guideline no. 37. https://www.rcog.org.uk/guidance/browse-all-guidance/green-top-guidelines/reducing-the-risk-of-thrombosis-and-embolism-during-pregnancy-and-the-puerperium-green-top-guideline-no-37a (accessed November 2023).

Royal College of Obstetrics and Gynaecology (2022). Information for you: Pre-eclampsia. www.rcog.org.uk/media/rnulgc5d/pi_pre-eclampsia-2022.pdf (accessed November 2023).

Uzan, J., Carbonnel, M., Piconne, O. et al. (2011). Pre-eclampsia: pathophysiology, diagnosis, and management. *Vascular Health and Risk Management* 2011 (7): 467–474. https://doi.org/10.2147/VHRM.S20181.

Webster, S., Dodd, C., and Waugh, J. (2013). Hypertensive disorders. In: *Medical Disorders in Pregnancy: A Manual for Midwives* (ed. S.J. Robson and J. Waugh), 27–41. Oxford: Wiley Blackwell.

Further Resources

Cardiomyopathy. www.cardiomyopathy.org (accessed November 2023).
Cardiac Risk in the Young. www.c-r-y.org.uk (accessed November 2023).
British Heart Foundation. www.bhf.org.uk (accessed November 2023).

Glossary

227

Term	Definition
Anaemia	A condition in which haemoglobin levels are abnormally low
Aneurism	A localised bulge in a blood vessel due to a weakened muscle wall
Angiotensin 1	A peptide hormone that acts as a precursor molecule for angiotensin 2
Angiotensin 2	The peptide hormone that directly acts on blood vessels causing them to contract and increase the blood vessel
Antihypertensive	A general term for drugs used to lower blood pressure
Aorto-caval compression	Compression of the aorta and vena cava due to maternal posture
Arrythmia	An abnormal or irregular heart rate
Atrial septal defect (ASD)	An opening between the right and left atria, causing turbulence of blood flow
Atrium	Plural atria, one of the two upper chambers of the heart
Baroreceptor	A sensory nerve ending located in the walls of the large arteries that is sensitive to alterations in blood pressure
Cardiac output	The volume of blood the heart pumps out, usually measured in litres per minute
Carotid sinus	A neurovascular structure located in the area where the common carotid artery branches out and at the beginning of the internal carotid artery
Chemoreceptor	A sensory cell that responds to chemical stimulation
Collagen	Tissue comprising protein molecules made up of amino acids, provides structural support to connective tissues and is rigid and resistance to stretching
Coronary vessels	Blood vessels that supply the heart
Diastole	The resting phase of the cardiac cycle, represented by the lower figure on a blood pressure reading

Electrocardiogram (ECG)	A recording of the heart's rhythm and electrical activity
Factor V Leiden	An inherited disorder due to a genetic mutation of one of the clotting factors in the blood, leading to an increased tendency to clot
Fibroblast	A cell that is involved in the formation of connective tissue, the fibrous substance that supports other tissues within the body; also secretes collagen.
Glomerulus	Plural glomeruli, a cluster of capillaries located around the end of a kidney tubule
Haemodilution	An increase in blood plasma levels, leading to a relatively lower concentration of red blood cells
Haemodynamic	A term referring to the mechanisms of blood circulation
Haemorrhoids	Varicose veins around the anus and anal canal
Homeostatic/ homeostasis	The self-regulatory process whereby biological systems maintain stability despite changing external conditions
Hughes syndrome	Also known as antiphospholipid syndrome, an acquired clotting disorder associated with a previous history of thrombosis
Hypertrophy	The enlargement of an organ or tissue beyond its usual size
Hypoxia	A shortage of oxygen in tissues, organs or the entire body
Lumen	From Latin meaning 'an opening', plural lumina, the inner space of a tubular structure such as a blood vessel
Lymphoid	Relating to tissue in the body responsible for producing lymphocytes (white blood cells) and antibodies; this tissue is located in the lymph nodes, the spleen and other areas of the body
Magnesium sulfate	A drug that can be administered intravenously or intramuscularly to reduce the risk of eclamptic seizure
Medulla oblongata	A long stem-like structure making up the lowest part of the brainstem; it is where the brain and spinal cord connect and is involved in the control of vital processes such as breathing, heartbeat and blood pressure
Myocardial infarction	'Heart attack', a condition in which the blood supply to the heart is suddenly blocked, usually by a blood clot
Perinatal	The period of time shortly before, during and after birth; exact definitions vary
Peptide hormones	A class of proteins that can be bound by receptor proteins to activate or deactivate a biological pathway
Placental abruption	A condition in which the placenta begins to separate from the uterine wall prior to the birth of the baby; an emergency situation
Placentation	The early stages of placental development
Plasma	The fluid content of blood, accounting for around 55% of total blood volume
Postpartum haemorrhage (PPH)	Blood loss of over 500 ml occurring within the first 24 hours after giving birth
Progesterone	A steroid hormone primarily responsible for regulating the female reproductive system
Prophylactic	A drug given to prevent disease or an unwanted occurrence
Proteinuria	Protein detected in the urine
Puerperium	The first six weeks after giving birth
Pulmonary hypertension	High blood pressure in the pulmonary arteries carrying deoxygenated blood from the heart to the lungs
Relaxin	A hormone produced chiefly by the ovaries and placenta that relaxes the pelvic ligaments and softens the cervix prior to labour; also causes vasodilation
Septum	A band of tissue dividing parts of an organ, e.g. the heart ventricles

Sino-atrial node	An area of cardiac muscle in the right atrium that produces an electrical impulse, causing the heart to contract and setting the rhythm of contractions
Solute	A dissolved substance, the minor component in a solution
Stenosis	The narrowing of a blood vessel or other tubular organ
Stroke volume	The volume of blood pumped out of the left ventricle of the heart when the heart contracts during systole
Supine	Lying on the back
Thrombophilia	A disorder of haemostasis, leading to an increased risk of thrombosis
Vagus nerve	The longest of the cranial nerves, responsible for the regulation of internal organ functions, e.g. heart rate and respiratory rate, as well as various reflex actions such as coughing and swallowing
Valvular regurgitation	A condition in which a valve (usually of the heart) fails to close properly, causing backflow of blood
Vasodilation	Dilation (widening) of the veins
Vasospasm	Sudden constriction of the muscular walls of an artery
Ventricle	One of the two lower chambers of the heart

CHAPTER 13

The Blood and Associated Disorders

Thomas McEwan[1] and Suzanne Crozier[2]

[1] *NHS Education for Scotland, Glasgow, UK*

[2] *School of Health and Social Care, Edinburgh Napier University, Edinburgh, UK*

AIM

The aim of this chapter is to provide a comprehensive overview of the main disorders associated with the blood during pregnancy.

LEARNING OUTCOMES

On completion of this chapter the reader will be able to:

- Describe the major formed elements of the blood
- Discuss the factors affecting coagulation and haemostasis in pregnancy
- Explain the ABO and Rh systems of blood groups and the implications of rhesus incompatibility in pregnancy
- Discuss the main blood disorders in pregnancy
- Explain the management of these blood disorders

Test Your Prior Knowledge

1. What is the function of the red blood cell?
2. How many types of white blood cells are there?
3. What are the names of the white blood cells?
4. What do you understand by the term blood groups?

Blood is a type of connective tissue consisting of cells and cell fragments suspended in plasma. The cells and the cell fragments are described as the formed elements of the blood (see Figure 13.1) and the liquid or unformed part is called the plasma. Plasma accounts for 55% of blood volume and red blood cells (RBCs; erythrocytes) make up 45% (Waugh and Grant 2018). The remaining 1% consists of white blood cells and platelets. The volume of blood is constant in a healthy

Fundamentals of Maternal Pathophysiology, First Edition. Edited by Claire Leader and Ian Peate.
© 2024 John Wiley & Sons Ltd. Published 2024 by John Wiley & Sons Ltd.
Companion website: www.wiley.com/go/leader/maternalpatho

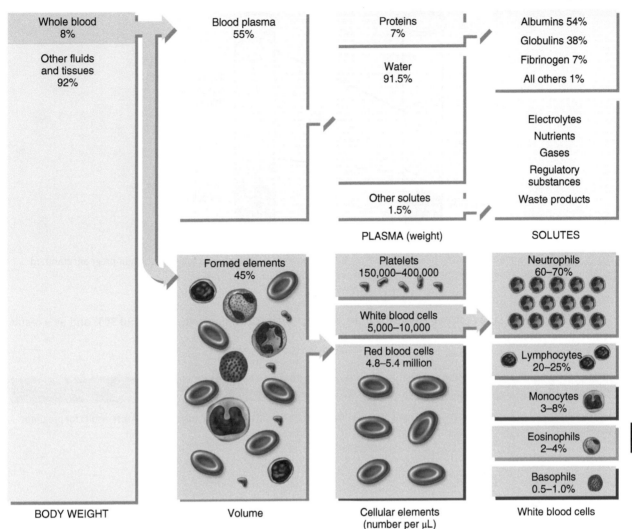

FIGURE 13.1 Cells of the blood before physiological changes in pregnancy.

person unless physiological problems arise because of illness or injury. The process that ensures the constancy of blood volume is known as haemostasis. This chapter provides an overview of the composition and functions of blood, and the physiological changes during pregnancy and disorders of the blood relevant to midwifery practice.

Composition of Blood

Blood is composed of plasma, a yellowish liquid containing nutrients, hormones, minerals and various cells, mainly RBCs, white blood cells and platelets. Both the formed elements and the plasma play an important role in homeostasis. There are significant changes to the blood during pregnancy to facilitate fetal growth and to maintain maternal well-being (Blackburn 2018) (Figure 13.2).

Plasma

Plasma is the liquid part of the blood and is composed of water (91%), proteins (8%) and salts (0.9%); the remaining 0.1% is made up of organic materials, such as fats and glucose. During pregnancy plasma volume increases by

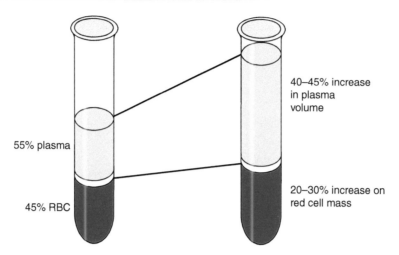

FIGURE 13.2   Components of clotted blood following centrifugal separation – comparison between the non-pregnant standard and following peak plasma volume expansion at around 24 weeks of pregnancy.

40–45%. The increase in the formed elements of the blood (mainly RBCs) is between 20% and 30% and as a result haemodilution occurs.

Orange Flag: Haematological Changes

Haemodilution increases over the course of the pregnancy and must be considered when analysing blood test results for pregnant women.

Plasma Protein

Proteins make up 8% of the plasma and are responsible for creating the osmotic pressure of blood. Due to haemodilution plasma protein levels decrease in the first trimester of pregnancy and then reduce more gradually until term (Murray and Murray 2020). When plasma proteins are lost from the circulation, fluid moves into tissues, causing oedema as the osmotic pressure alters. Peripheral oedema of the legs and feet in late pregnancy is however a physiological response to lowered osmotic pressure and in an otherwise well woman should not cause concern.

Formed Elements of Blood

The formed elements of the blood consist of RBCs (erythrocytes), white blood cells (leucocytes) and platelets (thrombocytes).

Red Blood Cells

RBCs, also known as erythrocytes, are small biconcave discs. During pregnancy the production and number of red blood cells increase by between 15% and 30% depending on the available iron stores (Coad et al. 2020). The increase in production is reliant on a supply of the essential components for red blood cell synthesis, which are:

- Iron
- Folic acid
- Vitamin B_{12}

White Blood Cells

White blood cells, or leucocytes, are a key component of the immune system. Two main types of leucocytes exist: the granulocytes (neutrophils, eosinophils and basophils) and the agranulocytes (monocytes and lymphocytes). There is an initial small increase in white blood cells during pregnancy that is like the response to other physiological stresses (Coad et al. 2020).

Platelets

Platelets have a vital role in reducing blood loss by forming platelet plugs to seal holes in vessel walls. Due to haemodilution the platelet count falls slightly during pregnancy, although coagulability increases.

Haemostasis

Haemostasis involves vasoconstriction, platelet aggregation and coagulation. These elements are crucial in preventing blood loss from damaged or injured tissue. Pregnancy is recognised as being a period of hypercoagulability that increases the risk of thrombosis and coagulopathies. This state is characterised as the Virchow triad as it includes hypercoagulability, potential for venous stasis and endothelial injury, which promote thrombosis (Devis and Knuttinen 2017).

Blood Groups

The distinctive antigens on the RBCs provide the blood group categories of A, B, AB and O (see Table 13.1). With the addition of the Rhesus (Rh) factor these describe the main groups of concern for blood transfusion. In addition, factor D (Rhesus) is present on the blood cell (Rhesus positive) in 85% of the UK population.

233

Learning Event

Explore the most recent Mothers and Babies: Reducing Risk through Audits and Confidential Enquiries across the UK (MBRRACE-UK) report (https://www.npeu.ox.ac.uk/mbrrace-uk). Are disorders of the blood featured? If so, what learning is important to you as a student midwife for your practice?

TABLE 13.1   **Blood groups.**

Blood type	Antigens	Antibodies	Can donate blood to	Can receive blood from
A	Antigen A	Anti-B	A, AB	A, O
B	Antigen B	Anti-A	B, AB	B, O
AB	Antigen A Antigen B	None	AB	A, B, AB, O
O	None	Anti-A	A, B, AB, O	O
		Anti-B		

Red Flag: Rhesus Incompatibility

Rhesus incompatibility describes a situation whereby the maternal and fetal Rhesus types are different. This becomes clinically significant where the mother is Rhesus negative (without the Rh D antigen) and the fetus is Rhesus positive and a sensitising event has occurred, leading to the mother's immune system being triggered into developing anti-D antibodies. These can cross the placenta freely and destroy the Rhesus-positive RBCs of the fetus, leading to haemolytic disease of the newborn (HDN). This condition can result in a range of outcomes for the fetus and newborn, from jaundice and anaemia to severe hydrops fetalis.

Disorders of the Blood

Within this section disorders of the blood and how these manifest in pregnancy and relate to obstetric complications are discussed.

As a general introduction, Figure 13.3 identifies where some of these conditions may present in relation to the stages of the childbearing continuum. A number of those discussed will manifest across several stages, while others will precede and persist beyond these stages.

Anaemia

Anaemia, a Greek word meaning 'without blood', refers to a reduction in RBCs and is a significant global public health problem (Lopez et al. 2016). Anaemia results in a reduced ability of the blood to transport oxygen to the tissues, causing hypoxia. The normal level of haemoglobin in a non-pregnant adult female is approximately $140 \pm 20\,g/l$ of blood (Blackburn 2018).

Anaemia can result from:

- Loss of blood through haemorrhage or in women who are menstruating.
- Destruction of RBCs (haemolysis).
- Deficient RBC production due to red bone marrow failure.
- Infections such as malaria.
- Insufficient dietary intake of iron, folic acid and vitamin B.
- Increased demand for iron and micronutrients during pregnancy.

The most common symptoms of anaemia in pregnancy include pallor, fatigue, light-headedness, tachycardia and headache, with shortness of breath a more significant sign. It can be difficult to differentiate anaemia from these common symptoms that many women will experience during their pregnancy.

There are three major types of anaemia:

- **Microcytic anaemia** (with abnormally small RBCs).
- **Macrocytic anaemia** (with abnormally large RBCs).
- **Normocytic anaemia** (with normal-sized RBCs).

Microcytic Anaemia

Microcytic anaemia is characterised by small RBCs, primarily due to insufficient haemoglobin production. There are several types of microcytic anaemia, of which iron-deficiency anaemia (IDA) is the most common. Iron is a component of haem. A deficiency of iron leads to decreased haemoglobin synthesis, resulting in impairment of oxygen transport. In IDA, the RBCs are small (microcytic) and pale (hypochromic).

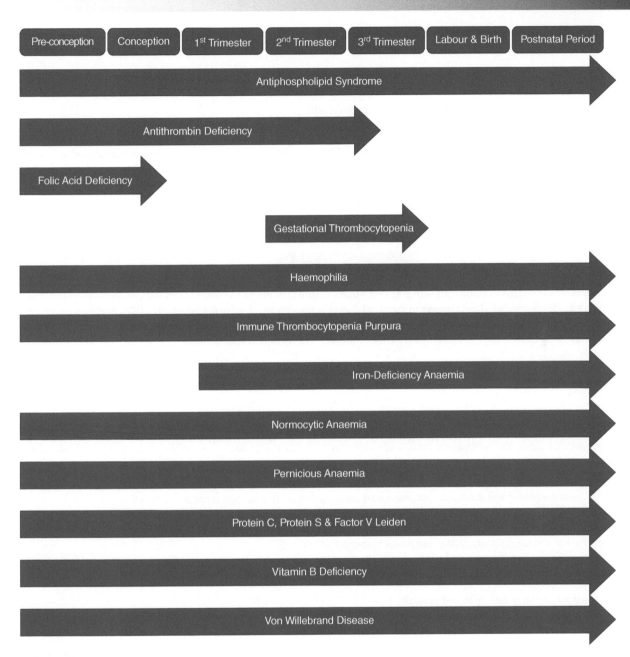

FIGURE 13.3 Blood disorders and stages of pregnancy and childbirth.

Iron-Deficiency Anaemia

In pregnancy IDA is caused by:

- Dietary deficiency of iron.
- Poor absorption of iron from the gastrointestinal tract.
- Increased demands from the developing fetus, increased RBC production and growth of maternal tissue.

All pregnant women are offered a full blood count (FBC) as part of routine antenatal screening. The FBC will identify women who have anaemia and further investigations, advice and/or treatment can be discussed with the general practitioner or obstetrician. The haematological changes during pregnancy mean that the normal values for blood tests including FBC are different to those in the general population and diagnosing IDA can be difficult. Further investigations may include:

- Careful examination of the additional information within the FBC, e.g. haemoglobin concentration, mean cell volume (MCV), haematocrit.
- Serum ferritin, serum iron, serum transferrin, serum folate.
- Vitamin B_{12} levels.

Iron is constantly used in the production of new RBCs. It is obtained from food sources and conserved within the body when RBCs are broken down. Excess iron is stored in the liver and muscle cells and is readily available to produce RBCs. Dietary intake of iron is often poor, and it is estimated that globally 80% of women enter pregnancy without adequate iron stores to support their pregnancy (Blackburn 2018).

Woman-Centred Care

Midwives should discuss all blood tests with pregnant women to gain their informed consent. This also provides a good opportunity to include information about changes to the blood during pregnancy and to raise the possibility of IDA. Reassurance should be offered that the fetus will be unaffected unless the IDA is severe (Blackburn 2018). Good sources of iron in the diet should be discussed while considering individual needs such as cultural preferences, financial situation and access to good-quality food sources.

Medicines Management: Iron Tablets

Iron supplements may be taken as capsules, tablets and liquids. The most common tablet dose is 325 mg of ferrous sulfate. There is no elimination route for iron in the body, and taking more than required can cause serious medical problems. Iron toxicity can cause nausea, vomiting and diarrhoea. Left untreated it can cause irreversible damage to the liver and brain.

Blood counts usually return to normal after two months of iron therapy for most people. During pregnancy women should be advised to take iron with a small amount of food to avoid gastric irritation. Milk calcium and antacids should not be taken at the same time as iron supplements, as they can inhibit absorption of iron.

Constipation and diarrhoea are common side effects of iron supplementation. If constipation becomes a problem a stool softener may be advised. Black stools are normal when taking iron tablets, but women should be advised to seek medical advice if:

- The stools are tarry-looking as well as black.
- The stools have red (blood) streaks.
- Cramps, sharp pains or soreness in the stomach occur.

Macrocytic Anaemia

Macrocytic anaemia is also termed megaloblastic anaemia and is characterised by defective deoxyribonucleic acid (DNA) synthesis, resulting in the production of unusually large RBCs in the circulation. The cells that are produced are fewer in number and contain less haemoglobin, reducing oxygen-carrying capability.

Macrocytic anaemia results from:

- Folate deficiency.
- Vitamin B_{12} deficiency.

Both these micronutrients are coenzymes essential for DNA maturation. Vegans and vegetarians are at risk of developing macrocytic anaemia due to a lack of vitamin B_{12}, which is primarily found in animal products.

Folate Deficiency

Folic acid (folate) is an essential vitamin for the production and maturation of cells, including RBCs. Folate is a water-soluble vitamin and is not stored in the body, so there must be an adequate daily intake to avoid deficiency. Deficiency of folate during the embryonic phase of development can lead to congenital abnormalities such as neural tube defects. Folic acid supplementation is therefore recommended in the pre-conception period for those planning a pregnancy and for the first trimester once the pregnancy is confirmed (NICE 2021).

Red Flag: Epilepsy and Folic Acid

Some antiepileptic drugs interact with folic acid metabolism, increasing the risk of fetal abnormalities in women who have epilepsy. Women with epilepsy must not stop taking or change their medication when pregnant without medical supervision as the increased incidence of seizures poses a higher risk.

Examination Scenario: Serum Ferritin

Ferritin is found in the serum in low concentrations. Its level is directly proportional to the iron stores within the body. It is useful in distinguishing IDA caused by low iron stores from inadequate iron utilisation. It is important to note that serum ferritin values may be elevated due to other conditions including inflammation, liver disease and some malignancies. In general, a serum ferritin level below 30 µg/l should prompt treatment for IDA.

Health Promotion: Folic Acid

Folate and folic acid are forms of a water-soluble B vitamin. Folate occurs naturally in food and folic acid is the synthetic form of this vitamin. Folic acid has been added to cold cereals, flour, breads, paste, bakery items, cookies and crackers as a supplement in the United Kingdom and many other nations.

Foods naturally high in folate and safe to consume during pregnancy include leafy green vegetables (such as spinach, broccoli, kale and cabbage), beans and legumes (such as lentils, peas, kidney beans), yeast and beef extract, oranges and orange juice, wheat bran (and other whole-grain foods), poultry and pork.

Vitamin B_{12} Deficiency

The absorption of vitamin B_{12} in the intestine requires the presence of intrinsic factor (IF), which is produced by the gastric mucosa. IF binds to vitamin B_{12} in food, protecting it from gastrointestinal enzymes and facilitating its absorption. Pernicious anaemia (PA) is an autoimmune condition where insufficient IF is produced, resulting in anaemia and neurological symptoms. While PA is rare in women of childbearing age, dietary vitamin B_{12} deficiency may occur in women who are obese, have undergone bariatric surgery, follow a vegan diet or have a restrictive eating disorder (Shand et al. 2020). Deficiency may also be detected in women who have excessive alcohol intake or who have an inflammatory disease such as Crohn's. PA is managed via intramuscular injections of cobalamin (Mohamed et al. 2020).

Normocytic Anaemia

Normocytic anaemia is characterised by RBCs that are relatively normal in size but insufficient in number. It is less common than microcytic and macrocytic anaemias. Normocytic anaemias include:

- Aplastic anaemia (AA)
- Haemolytic anaemia

AA is a rare form of anaemia that results from either iatrogenic damage to the bone marrow following, for example, chemotherapy, radiation and chemical poisoning, or idiopathic changes often thought to be autoimmune in origin (Young 2018). Stem cells in the bone marrow that should produce RBCs are replaced by fat and the number of RBCs is significantly reduced. Pregnancy-associated aplastic anaemia (pAA) occurs when diagnosis is made for the first time during pregnancy (Jaime-Pérez et al. 2021). The diagnosis of pAA is difficult in pregnancy because of the haematological changes taking place. When AA is present or diagnosed during pregnancy, close monitoring and care by a specialised multidisciplinary team are required. Treatment usually involves blood transfusions and treatment of any infections that occur alongside close monitoring of the pregnancy (Jaime-Pérez et al. 2021).

Haemolytic anaemia occurs when RBCs are haemolysed more rapidly than they can be replaced. Causes include inherited haemoglobinopathies, infection, malignancies, some medicines, mismatched blood transfusions and autoimmune disorders.

Midwives will be familiar with the inherited haemoglobinopathies, sickle cell disease (SCD) and thalassaemia, screened for during pregnancy and in the neonate. In SCD the haemoglobin molecule does not develop correctly, causing the shape of RBCs to change from a disc into a stiff sickle shape when they become deoxygenated. The normal disc shape returns once the RBC reaches the lungs, but the process of sickling repeats. The repetition damages the RBCs and the vessels carrying them, sometimes blocking the blood supply completely. Damaged RBCs are removed from the circulation causing a haemolytic anaemia.

People living with SCD may develop severe anaemia, infections and strokes (Blackburn 2018). There may also be periods of intense pain known as 'crises' when sickling cells block small blood vessels. Crises can be severe and require emergency admission to hospital and are more likely to occur if the person is dehydrated or blood oxygen levels are low. Pregnancy is associated with a higher risk of mortality and morbidity (Oteng-Ntim et al. 2021) and there may be an increase in sickle cell crises due to haematological changes. Pregnancy with SCD increases the risk of:

- Pregnancy loss
- Infection, pre-eclampsia
- Intrauterine growth restriction
- Preterm labour

In the antenatal period genetic counselling will be offered and any crises or infection must be managed promptly and effectively by a specialist centre. Labour and birth should also take place within a specialist centre, with attention paid to hydration and providing effective analgesia.

Thalassaemia is also an inherited disease resulting in the abnormal production of haemoglobin and RBC haemolysis. As with SCD the incidence in the United Kingdom is increasing due to global mobilisation. It is most common in people who originate from the Mediterranean, Middle East or Asia. The severity depends on the number of abnormal genes that are inherited and the way in which they are expressed. Women with beta-thalassaemia minor should be managed in a similar way to those with SCD. Beta-thalassaemia major is a serious condition affecting the spleen and bone marrow and few successful pregnancies have been reported (Shannon et al. 2023).

Expert Midwife: Sickle Cell Disease

SCD and other haemoglobinopathies occur most often in those whose ethnic origin can be traced to parts of the world where malaria is endemic. Being a carrier of SCD offers some protection from malaria, however when both parents are carriers there is a 1 in 4 chance their offspring will inherit the disease. Around 200 women with SCD become pregnant every year in the United Kingdom and SCD is one of the most common inherited disorders. A report presented to the UK Government in 2021 called 'No One's Listening' highlighted failings in care for people with SCD attributed to poor awareness among professionals and negative attitudes. In areas of high prevalence of SCD, specialist midwives are employed to work with multidisciplinary teams to improve outcomes and women's experiences. Women and families are living with SCD across the United Kingdom. It is important that all midwives understand the disease and how to recognise and meet women's additional care needs.

Consider the blood investigations obtained at the booking appointment. How do you explain the purpose of these to the woman to obtain informed consent for these investigations?

Coagulation Disorders in Pregnancy

For a detailed synopsis of blood coagulation, refer to the appropriate section in Peate and Leader (2024), particularly the chapter on the circulatory system (Chapter 9). This section focuses on disorders within the clotting system as well as conditions that predispose a woman to bleeding or coagulation disorders during pregnancy and the perinatal period.

Thrombocytopenia during pregnancy can be linked to two main categories: gestational or autoimmune (Fogerty 2018). A platelet count below 20×10^9/l of blood may lead to haemorrhage from trauma or spontaneous bleeding in the non-pregnant population. A value of less than 150×10^9/l in pregnancy is common, affecting 7–11% of all pregnancies, predominantly in the third trimester (Reese et al. 2018).

Gestational thrombocytopenia (GT) is an asymptomatic, benign diagnosis of exclusion. Presenting in the mid-trimester onwards, the platelet count will self-resolve by about two weeks postpartum (Ciobanu et al. 2016). It is not associated with increased maternal or fetal risks, with only a moderate thrombocytopenia recorded at between 130 and 150×10^9/l. Repeat platelet count should be obtained prior to epidural anaesthesia.

The most common autoimmune cause is immune thrombocytopenia purpura (ITP), which is suspected with the presence of purpura and bruising without known injury, petechiae and nosebleeds. The key difference between this and GT is its presentation in the first and second trimesters and its potential to precede pregnancy (Stavrou and McCrae 2009). Specific antiplatelet antibodies for ITP can be measured, but diagnosis remains one of exclusion, based on the onset and clinical course. Alternatively, the measurement of thrombopoietin (TPO) has been identified as a potential indicator for ITP (Zhang et al. 2016). Different to GT is the potential for fetal and neonatal complications. The antiplatelet antibodies responsible for ITP can readily cross the placenta but rarely cause serious consequences. This must be differentiated from the condition neonatal alloimmune thrombocytopenia (NAIT), which is caused by the generation of maternal antibodies to the specific paternally inherited human platelet antigens (HPAs) on the surface of the fetal platelets (de Vos et al. 2021). The mainstay of treatment for NAIT is corticosteroids and intravenous immunoglobulin (IVIg) (Fogerty 2018).

239

Red Flag: Platelet Count Before Epidural

Although there is no evidence from randomised controlled trials or non-randomised studies on which to base an assessment of the correct platelet threshold prior to insertion of an epidural catheter, the risk of epidural haematoma is increased where severe thrombocytopenia is present in the pregnant woman, with most of these occurring in cases where the platelet count is $<50 \times 10^9$/l.

Von Willebrand disease (VWD) is an inherited condition affecting the blood's ability to clot. Low levels of the blood protein von Willebrand factor affect the ability of platelets to aggregate to form a clot. They may also affect the levels and function of blood clotting factor VIII. Three main types are:

- **Type 1 (mild)**: Low levels of von Willebrand factor and potentially low levels of factor VIII.
- **Type 2 (moderate)**: The von Willebrand factor is not functioning correctly within the blood. There are four subtypes of type 2, each with differing treatment.
- **Type 3 (severe)**: A rare form where von Willebrand factor is absent from the blood and factor VIII levels are very low.

The main symptom is bleeding, becoming more excessive from type 1 to type 3. In the latter bleeding into the muscles, joints and other body systems can be significant and debilitating. Diagnosis examines a range of standard blood investigations as well as von Willebrand factor antigen and activity levels and factor VIII clotting activity. Treatment can include hormonal (desmopressin), replacement (administration of von Willebrand factor) or using some antifibrinolytic medicines.

Haemophilia, a bleeding disorder, is inherited through a gene in the X chromosome for type A and B. It manifests as insufficient clotting factors to prevent excessive bleeding. The three main forms are:

- **Haemophilia type A**: Also known as 'classic' haemophilia, referring to a lack of blood clotting factor VIII.
- **Haemophilia type B:** Also known as 'Christmas disease', referring to a lack of blood clotting factor IX.
- **Haemophilia type C:** A non-inherited condition that refers to a lack of blood clotting factor XI. This type causes few problems other than an increased risk of bleeding after surgery.

If the mother has the haemophilia gene on one of her X chromosomes, there is a 50/50 chance that it will be passed to her baby. In this circumstance her son will have the condition while her daughter would be a carrier. If the father has the condition and the mother is neither a haemophiliac nor a carrier of the condition, then none of their sons will have the disease but all daughters will be carriers. However, one-third of those with haemophilia have no family history. Although carriers will have normal clotting factor levels, they can experience frequent nosebleeds, heavier menstrual bleeding, bruise easily and bleed more after surgery or trauma.

Diagnosis is based on medical and family histories as well as a clinical examination. Specific tests include FBC, coagulation screening (including prothrombin time [PT] and partial thromboplastin time [PTT]) and genetic testing if indicated. Management of this condition will include avoiding situations involving trauma, injury or surgery. Treatment includes replacing low levels of blood clotting factors, blood transfusion following blood loss or hormone treatment (e.g. desmopressin to stimulate factor VIII production).

Antiphospholipid syndrome (also known as Hughes syndrome, sticky blood syndrome or antiphospholipid antibody syndrome) is an autoimmune disorder classified within the rheumatic diseases including lupus and rheumatoid arthritis. Where a woman has a rheumatic disease, careful pre-conception planning and multidisciplinary care during pregnancy and after birth are essential, as some diseases will be exacerbated, particularly the risk of venous thromboembolism (VTE).

Learning Event

What does your local policy advise for VTE risk and prophylaxis?

Antiphospholipid syndrome results in antibodies that attack phospholipids (fats) in the body cells, causing inappropriate clotting in the blood. It may also cause the formation of anticardiolipin antibodies that affect another type of fat within the cells. This disease can cause thrombosis (blood clot formation that can be life threatening), thrombocytopenia and miscarriage (often recurrent). It is typically difficult to diagnose, and tests to identify any lupus anticoagulant, anticardiolipin antibodies or anti-beta-2 glycoprotein will usually be undertaken. Treatment is primarily with a suitable anticoagulant therapy.

Orange Flag: Miscarriage

Pregnancy loss at any stage can have a profound and lasting impact on the psychological well-being of women, their partners and wider families. Even if the current pregnancy is progressing well, memories of past experiences and the fear that miscarriage may recur can have a significant effect on the health and well-being of the woman. Midwives play a key role in providing support and guidance and should be aware of referral pathways to psychological support services and other healthcare professionals in their area, should this be required. In addition, organisations such as the Miscarriage Association (www.miscarriageassociation.org.uk) can offer tailored support to women and their families.

Red Flag: Venous Thromboembolism/Pulmonary Embolism

Pregnancy increases the risk of a VTE, with the highest risk in the immediate postnatal period. All women must undergo a documented assessment of risk factors for VTE in early pregnancy. This should be repeated intrapartum and immediately postnatally, and if the woman is admitted to hospital for any reason. The risk increases further following periods of immobility, for instance after a surgical procedure, or with a diagnosis of pre-eclampsia. The symptoms of a pulmonary embolism (PE) include sudden breathing difficulty or collapse, tightness in the chest or coughing up blood (haemoptysis).

Source: Adapted from RCOG (2015).

Examination Scenario: Ventilation-Perfusion Scan

A ventilation–perfusion (VQ) scan uses radiopharmaceutical material to examine airflow (ventilation) and blood flow (perfusion) in the lungs. It is an effective method of identifying evidence of a blood clot in the lung, known as a PE. This poses a low risk to the fetus if performed antenatally. If conducted postnatally, the woman should avoid close contact (>30 minutes) with her baby for 12 hours after the scan. If breastfeeding, a feed should be offered immediately before the scan. Expressed breast milk should also be collected prior to the scan and used in the 12 hours following the scan.

Antithrombin deficiency (ATD) may be inherited or acquired and is characterised by a tendency to develop venous thrombosis. It is a blood disorder known as a thrombophilia whereby a predisposition to thrombosis exists. This includes protein C, protein S and factor V Leiden, discussed later in this section.

The function of antithrombin is to limit coagulation through the inhibition of factor Xa, factor Ixa and thrombin, required for clot formation. The risk of clot formation is increased in the inherited condition only. The acquired variant is usually the consequence of some other condition and will typically resolve as the predisposing problem improves. It is associated with placental dysfunction and abruption due to placental thrombosis, increased rates of late pregnancy loss, intrauterine growth restriction and pre-eclampsia/eclampsia (White and Hunt 2021). Treatment in pregnancy is usually with subcutaneous low molecular weight heparin, with high levels often required; intravenous infusion of antithrombin concentrates may also be required.

Disseminated intravascular coagulopathy (DIC) is a serious and life-threatening condition that can arise from obstetric and non-obstetric causes. It is a complex condition and readers are directed to the references within this section for more detailed explanations of the pathophysiology. Essentially it is the result of four mechanisms occurring simultaneously:

- The generation of thrombin (a procoagulant), mediated by tissue factor (TF).
- A depressed antithrombin and protein C system (reduced inhibition of thrombin and reduced natural anticoagulant).
- Defective fibrinolysis (reduced ability to inhibit clot formation or remove thrombi) due to increased plasminogen activator inhibitor type 1.
- Inflammatory system stimulated by proinflammatory cytokines (a hypercoagulable state develops).

The main obstetric risks include acute peripartum haemorrhage, placental abruption, pre-eclampsia, infection, sepsis and acute fatty liver disease (Erez et al. 2015). Although relatively rare, DIC that results from peripartum bleeding that cannot be controlled remains a leading cause of maternal mortality worldwide (Rabinovich et al. 2019).

The condition represents the uninhibited, systemic activation of the haemostatic system (Levi and Ten Cate 1999). This results in the formation of widespread microvascular thrombosis that can impede blood flow and perfusion to different organs and may lead to organ failure. Simultaneously there is increased degradation and consumption of coagulation factors and associated anticoagulant proteins, with impaired replenishment of both (Levi and van der Poll 2013). This can lead to uncontrollable bleeding in a setting where clotting is happening, albeit inappropriately.

In pregnancy, two phases that may lead to DIC have been characterised: non-overt and overt overactivation of the haemostatic system (Erez 2022). Non-overt describes a stage where the overactivation of the haemostatic system is

241

compensated, which prevents microthrombi formation or organ dysfunction (Alhousseini et al. 2022). This is most associated with retained stillbirth, retained placenta accreta or chronic placental abruption. Conversely, the overt phase represents the decompensated state where organ failure can develop following small- and medium-vessel thrombosis. This leads to consumption of available coagulation factors and platelets and life-threatening bleeding, and is most associated with placental abruption, HELLP syndrome (haemolysis, elevated liver enzymes and low platelets) and amniotic fluid embolism.

Recognising these phases and their associated presentation have been included within a scoring system for the risk of developing DIC (Taylor et al. 2001; Bakhtiari et al. 2004), modified for the physiological changes of pregnancy (Erez et al. 2014). However, the regular use of this in obstetrics and maternity care is unclear. Laboratory diagnosis of DIC is further complicated by pregnancy due to the physiological increase in clotting and decreased fibrinolytic capacity. The trend and pace of changes are more useful than a single result, with increasing PT and activated PTT times, increasing fibrinogen degradation and D-dimer concentrations with progressively reduced platelet and fibrinogen levels (Rabinovich et al. 2019).

Effective management of DIC relies on early recognition, management of the underlying causative disorder and supportive care to the haemostatic system with close monitoring. Midwives must be familiar with their local protocols for the management of DIC and major obstetric haemorrhage. The use of blood component replacement will be a primary treatment. This may include fresh frozen plasma (FFP), cryoprecipitate (fibrinogen) and platelets. If bleeding is not controlled, surgical intervention including hysterectomy or ligation of the major pelvic vessels may be required.

Expert Midwife: Disseminated Intravascular Coagulopathy

Although DIC is rare, a midwife must always be alert to its possibility. This condition is always secondary to an underlying disorder. In pregnancy the complications that may lead to DIC include HELLP syndrome, pre-eclampsia, acute fatty liver, amniotic fluid embolism, sepsis and postpartum haemorrhage. It has a complex pathophysiology and represents a systematic pathological overactivation of coagulation and fibrinolytic systems. In effect, it leads to microvascular thrombosis that consumes and depletes the available platelets and coagulation proteins. These clots can disrupt blood flow to major organs and increase the risk of severe bleeding. Prompt diagnosis is key and is considered with signs or symptoms of occult bleeding, cardiovascular instability and uncontrollable bleeding. Other signs can include chest pain, skin abnormalities and confusion or disorientation. Successful management of this condition requires a local multidisciplinary team approach that includes haematology and blood transfusion colleagues to access prompt advice, laboratory testing and provision of blood products as required.

Additional disorders of the blood are protein C deficiency, protein S deficiency and factor V Leiden. Protein C deficiency, a vitamin K-dependent coagulation factor, is an inherited disorder characterised by the abnormal formation of blood clots and pulmonary emboli (Dinarvand and Moser 2019). Protein S deficiency is another inherited disorder characterised by the formation of recurrent blood clots and emboli. Protein S is also a vitamin K-dependent coagulation factor. Factor V Leiden is one of the most common genetic variants and leads to an increased risk of venous thrombosis.

Medicines Management: Enoxaparin (Clexane®)

Enoxaparin is an anticoagulant medication used for prophylaxis against and treatment of VTE in pregnancy. This remains a major direct cause of maternal death in the United Kingdom. The use of enoxaparin can prevent the formation of a deep vein thrombosis and PE during pregnancy where there are pre-existing risk factors (previous VTE, thrombophilia, obesity) or obstetric risk factors (pre-eclampsia/eclampsia, multiple pregnancy, caesarean section birth). Its use is not associated with an increased risk of severe postpartum haemorrhage. The appropriate dose is based on booking or early pregnancy weight. This medication is not known to be harmful, as low molecular weight heparins do not cross the placenta and the risks from passage into breast milk and absorption by the baby are negligible.

Source: Adapted from BNF (2022).

Case Study 13.1

Chris is 30 years old and pregnant for the first time. The 12-week scan confirmed a twin pregnancy. At booking the FBC was normal. Chris is now 28 weeks' pregnant and during a routine visit to the midwife she tells you that she is feeling excessively tired, breathless at times and her partner regularly comments on how pale she looks. You repeat her FBC, and these are the results:

Full blood count	
Haemoglobin (Hb)	100 g/l
White blood cells (WBC)	4.5×10^9/l
Platelets (Plt)	240×10^9/l
Red cell count (RBC)	3.6×10^{12}/l
Haematocrit (HCT)	0.34 l/l
Mean cell volume (MCV)	65 fl
Mean cell haemoglobin (MCH)	23 pg

- What will you be telling Chris about these results?
- What will be your plan to meet Chris's additional care needs?
- Why are women with multiple pregnancies more prone to anaemia?
- What types of anaemia might develop in pregnancy?
- What is the role of the midwife in supporting women to maintain a normal Hb level?

Case Study 13.2

Aadya is 36 years old and attending her booking appointment in her fourth pregnancy. Her previous pregnancies and births happened outside of the United Kingdom. A booking scan is awaited, but based on her last normal menstrual period (LNMP) she is currently 12 weeks. Aadya is attending with her sister Prisha, who is interpreting for her as she does not speak English. During your discussion on medical history, Prisha attempts to communicate that her sister has had investigations for a blood disorder that increases her risk of developing clots. At this visit you take some initial vital signs, height and current weight. These are:

Measurements/recordings	
BP	140/95 mmHg.
Pulse	80 beats/minute
Temperature	37.2°C
Urinalysis	Protein ++
Height	160 cm
Weight	90 kg
BMI	35.2 kg/m²

- What disorders of the blood can lead to clots forming? What additional risk factors does Aadya have for thrombosis based on these results?
- Where might you find additional local information on VTE risk in pregnancy?
- What additional investigations or referrals may be required at this time?
- What are the challenges when a family member provides interpretation during a consultation?

> ## Take-Home Points
>
> - There are significant changes to the blood during pregnancy to facilitate fetal growth and to maintain maternal well-being.
> - Pregnancy is recognised as being a period of hypercoagulability, increasing the risk of thrombosis and coagulopathies.
> - The haematological changes during pregnancy mean that the normal values for blood tests are different to those in the general population, so diagnosing disorders can be difficult.
> - Anaemia in pregnancy is common but can take many forms.
> - Midwives must be familiar with the inherited haemoglobinopathies, SCD and thalassaemia.
> - Coagulation disorders in pregnancy can be complex, e.g. DIC, and can manifest as either an inability to form clots or a predisposition to clot formation.
> - VTE remains a major cause of maternal death.

Conclusion

It is essential that the midwife or maternity care professional has a robust understanding of the composition and function of the blood. This must incorporate knowledge and understanding of the physiological adaptations during pregnancy, common and rare disorders of the blood and the implications for clinical care. The case studies presented within this chapter provide realistic examples to help consolidate your understanding of the relevant physiology and how this could be interpreted and applied in practice. Given the essential contribution of the blood to the other body systems, this chapter provides a connective element for your broader understanding of maternal pathophysiology.

References

Alhousseini, A., Romero, R., Benshalom-Tirosh, N. et al. (2022). Nonovert disseminated intravascular coagulation (DIC) in pregnancy: a new scoring system for the identification of patients at risk for obstetrical hemorrhage requiring blood product transfusion. *Journal of Maternal-Fetal & Neonatal Medicine* 35 (2): 242–257.

Bakhtiari, K., Meijers, J.C., de Jonge, E., and Levi, M. (2004). Prospective validation of the International Society of Thrombosis and Haemostasis scoring system for disseminated intravascular coagulation. *Critical Care Medicine* 32 (12): 2416–2421.

Blackburn, S.T. (2018). Haematologic and haemostatic systems. In: *Maternal Fetal and Neonatal Physiology*, 5e, 215–246. S.T. Blackburn. St Louis: Elsevier.

British National Formulary (BNF) (2022). Enoxaparin sodium. https://bnf.nice.org.uk/drugs/enoxaparin-sodium (accessed November 2023).

Ciobanu, A.M., Colibaba, S., Cimpoca, B. et al. (2016). Thrombocytopenia in pregnancy. *Maedica (Bucur)*. 11 (1): 55–60.

Coad, J., Pedley, K., and Dunstall, M. (2020). *Anatomy and Physiology for Midwives*. London: Elsevier.

Devis, P. and Knuttinen, M.G. (2017). Deep venous thrombosis in pregnancy: incidence, pathogenesis and endovascular management. *Cardiovascular Diagnosis and Therapy* 7 (Suppl 3): S309.

Dinarvand, P. and Moser, K.A. (2019). Protein C deficiency. *Archives of Pathology & Laboratory Medicine* 143 (10): 1281–1285.

Erez, O. (2022). Disseminated intravascular coagulation in pregnancy: new insights. *Thrombosis Update* 6: 100083.

Erez, O., Novack, L., Beer-Weisel, R. et al. (2014). DIC score in pregnant women—a population based modification of the International Society on Thrombosis and Hemostasis score. *PloS One* 9 (4): e93240.

Erez, O., Mastrolia, S.A., and Thachil, J. (2015). Disseminated intravascular coagulation in pregnancy: insights in pathophysiology, diagnosis and management. *American Journal of Obstetrics and Gynecology* 213 (4): 452–463.

Fogerty, A.E. (2018). Thrombocytopenia in pregnancy: mechanisms and management. *Transfusion Medicine Reviews* 32 (4): 225–229.

Jaime-Pérez, J.C., González-Treviño, M., and Gómez-Almaguer, D. (2021). Pregnancy-associated aplastic anemia: a case-based review. *Expert Review of Hematology* 14 (2): 175–184.

Levi, M. and Ten Cate, H. (1999). Disseminated intravascular coagulation. *New England Journal of Medicine* 341: 586–592.

Levi, M. and van der Poll, T. (2013). Disseminated intravascular coagulation: a review for the internist. *Internal and Emergency Medicine* 8 (1): 23–32.

Lopez, A., Cacoub, P., Macdougall, I.C., and Peyrin-Biroulet, L. (2016). Iron deficiency anaemia. *Lancet* 387 (10021): 907–916.

Mohamed, M., Thio, J., Thomas, R.S., and Phillips, J. (2020). Pernicious anaemia. *BMJ* 369: m1319. https://doi.org/10.1136/bmj.m1319.

Murray, I. and Murray, J. (2020). Change and adaptation in pregnancy. In: *Myles' Textbook for Midwives* (ed. M.D. Raynor and J.E. Marshall), 197–245. London: Elsevier.

National Institute for Health and Care Excellence (NICE) (2021). Scenario: Pre-conception advice for all women. https://cks.nice.org.uk/topics/pre-conception-advice-management/management/advice-for-all-women (accessed November 2023).

Oteng-Ntim, E., Pavord, S., Howard, R. et al. (2021). Management of sickle cell disease in pregnancy. *British Journal of Haemotology* 194: 908–995. https://doi.org/10.1111/bjh.17671.

Peate, I. and Leader, C. (2024). *Fundamentals of Anatomy and Physiology for Midwives*. Chichester, UK: Wiley.

Rabinovich, A., Abdul-Kadir, R., Thachil, J. et al. (2019). DIC in obstetrics: diagnostic score, highlights in management, and international registry-communication from the DIC and Women's Health SSCs of the International Society of Thrombosis and Haemostasis. *Journal of Thrombosis and Haemostasis* 17 (9): 1562–1566.

Reese, J.A., Peck, J.D., Deschamps, D.R. et al. (2018). Platelet counts during pregnancy. *New England Journal of Medicine* 379: 32–43.

Royal College of Obstetricians and Gynaecologists (RCOG) (2015). Reducing the risk of venous thromboembolism during pregnancy and the puerperium. Green-top guideline no. 37a. https://www.rcog.org.uk/media/qejfhcaj/gtg-37a.pdf (accessed November 2023).

Shand, A., Austin, K., Nassar, N., and Kidson-Gerber, G. (2020). Pharmacological management of anaemia in pregnancy: a review. *Journal of Pharmacy Practice and Research* 50 (3): 205–212.

Shannon, P.E., Lowdermilk, D.L., Cashion, K. et al. (2023). *Maternal Child Nursing Care*, 7e. Gainesville, FL: Elsevier Health Sciences.

Stavrou, E. and McCrae, K.R. (2009). Immune thrombocytopenia in pregnancy. *Hematology/Oncology Clinics* 23 (6): 1299–1316.

Taylor, F.B. Jr., Toh, C.H., Hoots, K.W. et al. (2001). Towards definition, clinical and laboratory criteria, and a scoring system for disseminated intravascular coagulation. *Thrombosis and Haemostasis* 86 (11): 1327–1330.

de Vos, T.W., Porcelijn, L., Hofstede-van Egmond, S. et al. (2021). Clinical characteristics of human platelet antigen (HPA)-1a and HPA-5b alloimmunised pregnancies and the association between platelet HPA-5b antibodies and symptomatic fetal neonatal alloimmune thrombocytopenia. *British Journal of Haematology* 195 (4): 595–603.

Waugh, A. and Grant, A. (ed.) (2018). *Ross & Wilson Anatomy and Physiology in Health and Illness*, 13e. London: Elsevier.

White, K. and Hunt, B.J. (2021). Inherited antithrombin deficiency in pregnancy. *Thrombosis Update* 6: 100094. https://doi.org/10.1016/j.tru.2021.100094.

Young, N.S. (2018). Aplastic anemia. *New England Journal of Medicine* 379 (17): 1643–1656. https://doi.org/10.1056/NEJMra1413485.

Zhang, X., Zhao, Y., Li, X. et al. (2016). Thrombopoietin: a potential diagnostic indicator of immune thrombocytopenia in pregnancy. *Oncotarget* 7 (7): 7489.

Further Resources

British Dietetic Association. Folic acid food fact sheet. www.bda.uk.com/resource/folic-acid.html (accessed November 2023).

National Institute for Health and Care Excellence (NICE). Risk factors for VTE in pregnancy. www.nice.org.uk/guidance/ng201/evidence/n-risk-factors-for-venous-thromboembolism-in-pregnancy-pdf-331305934361 (accessed November 2023).

Haemophilia Society. Women with bleeding disorders. www.haemophilia.org.uk/bleeding-disorders/women-with-bleeding-disorders (accessed November 2023).

Sickle Cell Society. www.sicklecellsociety.org (accessed November 2023).

Thrombosis UK. www.thrombosisuk.org/index.php (accessed November 2023).

Tommy's. Pregnancy information - anaemia and pregnancy. www.tommys.org/pregnancy-information/pregnancy-complications/anaemia-and-pregnancy (accessed November 2023).

Glossary

Agglutination	A process by which red blood cells adhere to one another
Aggregation	In haematological terms, the process by which platelets will adhere together to form a haemostatic plug at sites of vascular injury
Antigen	A foreign substance (e.g. an infecting microorganism) recognised by the immune system, which generates an antibody response
Autoimmune	When the body's immune system cannot tell the difference between the body's own cells and foreign cells, causing the body to mistakenly attack normal cells
Coagulation	The process of transforming a liquid into a solid (especially a clot) or the hardening of tissue by physical means
Gestation	Used to describe the length of a pregnancy, usually in completed weeks
Haemostasis	The stoppage of bleeding
HELLP syndrome	A life-threatening complication associated with pre-eclampsia comprising haemolysis, elevated liver enzymes and low platelets
Homeostasis	Regulation of body systems
Hydrops fetalis	Excessive abnormal retention of fluid in the fetus
Iatrogenic	Caused by medical treatment
Idiopathic	Without known cause
Intrinsic	Originating or due to causes or factors within the body or organ
Purpura	Purple-coloured spots and patches appearing on the skin or mucous membranes

CHAPTER 14

The Renal System and Associated Disorders

Amanda Waterman

Department of Health and Social Work, University of Hertfordshire, Hatfield, UK

AIM

This chapter aims to support midwifery practice, providing the reader with information regarding the pathophysiology associated with the renal system and how this is altered and reacts during pregnancy, birth and the postnatal period.

LEARNING OUTCOMES

On completion of this chapter the reader will be able to:

- Describe the structure and function of the kidneys
- Explore the effects of pregnancy on the kidney function
- Understand the kidney function during pregnancy complications such as pre-eclampsia and acute kidney injury

Test Your Prior Knowledge
1. Describe the location of the kidneys.
2. Describe the structure of the renal system.
3. List the functions of the kidneys.
4. What is the loop of Henle?
5. Discuss the role of the renin–angiotensin system.

The kidneys are bean-shaped organs, comprising a two-layered capsule, the cortex and the medulla, surrounded by perinephric fat, the renal fascia, the Zuckerkandl fascia and paranephric fat (Grigoraş et al. 2021). The kidney has a length of 10–12 cm, width of 5–7 cm and 3–5 cm thickness, weighing approximately 120–135 g in females and 150–200 g in males.

Fundamentals of Maternal Pathophysiology, First Edition. Edited by Claire Leader and Ian Peate.
© 2024 John Wiley & Sons Ltd. Published 2024 by John Wiley & Sons Ltd.
Companion website: www.wiley.com/go/leader/maternalpatho

Kidneys are situated retroperitoneally between the T12 and L3 transverse processes of the vertebrae. The left kidney is located posterior to the descending colon, with the renal hilum (centre of the kidney) aligned to the tail of the pancreas. The right kidney sits posteriorly to the liver, duodenum and hepatic flexure of the ascending colon, forcing it to sit lower than the left kidney. The renal hilum is described as an indentation on the medial border of the kidney, opening into the renal pelvis and sinus. The renal pelvis attaches to the ureters, transporting urine to the urinary bladder. The main function of the kidneys include:

- Removal of waste products.
- Elimination of neurotoxins and drugs.
- Blood pressure control.
- Production of vitamin D and calcium management.
- Erythropoiesis.

Kidney Structure

Kidneys comprise two regions, the cortex and the medulla. The cortex is 1 cm thick forming the outer rim of the kidney, containing the juxtaglomerular apparatus. Other structures, the nephrons and collecting ducts extend into the medulla. There are between 8 and 18 renal pyramids within the medulla, with the wider part of the pyramid in the cortex section and the apex in the medulla section. The pyramids contain the long loops of Henle, collecting ducts and a network of straight arterioles and venules around the loop of Henle, called the vasa recta. The papillae openings at the apex of the pyramid allow urine to pass through the collecting ducts. From the collecting ducts urine pools into the corresponding minor calyces in an area called the **cribosa**. From here urine drains into the renal pelvis, the ureter and to the urinary bladder to be excreted (Soriano et al. 2022). See Figures 14.1 and 14.2.

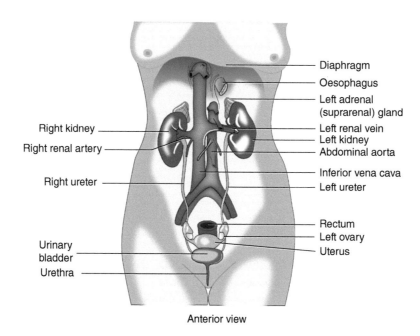

Anterior view

FIGURE 14.1   Organs of the renal system.

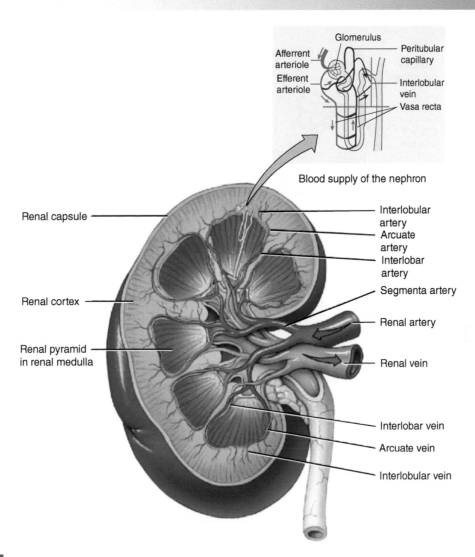

Blood supply of the nephron

Renal capsule

Renal cortex

Renal pyramid
in renal medulla

Interlobular
artery
Arcuate
artery
Interlobar
artery
Segmenta artery
Renal artery
Renal vein
Interlobar vein
Arcuate vein
Interlobular vein

FIGURE 14.2 Internal structure showing blood vessels.

Nephrons

Nephrons can be categorised into **cortical** nephrons and **juxtamedullary** nephrons. Juxtamedullary nephrons make up 15% of the total nephrons with an extra-long loop of Henle extending deeply into the medulla, with the aim of concentrating the urine. See Figure 14.3 on the nephron.

In the kidney renal filtration takes place at the glomerulus, a bundle of capillaries situated within the Bowman's capsule of the nephron (see Figure 14.3). Blood supply transporting filtrates from the renal artery flows into the arcuate arteries within the kidneys, then via the afferent arteriole to the glomerulus apparatus housed within the Bowman's capsule. The Bowman's capsule of the nephron is composed of podocyte cells with villi projections of cytoplasm, fenestrated endothelium and a basement membrane designed to filter substances according to sizes of approximately 60–80 nm and an electrical charge, making it freely permeable to small molecules, but not permitting blood cells or molecules greater than 100 nm – that is, large proteins – to pass. The layers of the Bowman's capsule are made up of

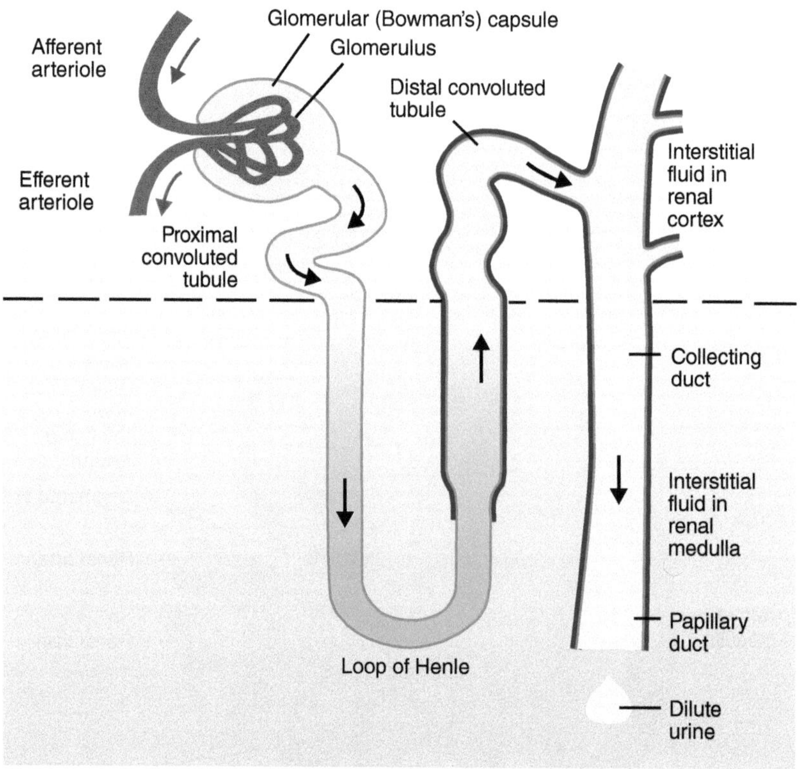

FIGURE 14.3   The nephron.

negatively charged glycoproteins deflecting negatively charged molecules, such as albumin. Filtrates from the glomerular capillaries enter the Bowman's space and are taken up by the Bowman's capsule (Falkson and Bordoni 2022; Veiga-Matos et al. 2020).

The glomerular filtration rate (GFR) is defined as the volume filtered from the glomerulus into the Bowman's capsule per minute (ml/min). It is often used by clinicians as an indicator of renal function. Nerve activity or changes in blood pressure can decrease pressure in the glomerular capillaries by constricting the afferent arteriole or dilating the efferent arteriole. This lower pressure is not effective in pushing out the filtrate into the Bowman's capsule (Falkson and Bordoni 2022).

Proximal Convoluted Tubule

Filtrate from the glomerulus passes through to the proximal convoluted tubule, which consists of epithelial cells made up of microvilli to increase the apical surface area for absorption. Proximal tubule cells use an active transport mechanism such as sodium–potassium (Na^+–K^+) ion pumps and passive transport. Sodium–potassium pumps reabsorb electrolytes, vitamins, bicarbonate and small proteins from the filtrate. Approximately 30% of the water is reabsorbed passively through paracellular transport water channels consisting of proteins called **aquaporin**, such as aquaporin-2 (AQP2) (Klussmann et al. 2000). Reabsorption of solutes, such as electrolytes, helps create a higher osmotic gradient for passive reabsorption of water into the interstitium, also known as the interstitial space, to then be collected by the peritubular capillaries surrounding the nephrons, carrying the reabsorbed elements back into the system.

Loop of Henle

From the proximal convoluted tubules, filtrate is transferred to the descending loop of Henle, which is permeable to water. As the water is reabsorbed into the interstitial space around the descending loop, the filtrate within the loop of Henle becomes more concentrated with the solutes; that is, sodium and potassium. In the ascending loop of Henle (or distal straight tubule), which is not permeable to water, the main function here is to actively reabsorb potassium and chlorine from the filtrate via membrane pumps and deposit them in the surrounding interstitium to create a higher salt concentration within the medulla.

The ascending loop is not permeable to water, so water cannot follow the osmotic pull of sodium and potassium, however as the ascending loop of Henle sits in close proximity to the descending loop of Henle, where water can be reabsorbed, the sodium and potassium actively pumped into the interstitium by the ascending limb help create a high osmolarity environment, pulling water via osmosis from the permeable descending loop (Kamal et al. 2014).

Distal Convoluted Tubule

Of the original glomerular filtrate volume, 10% is transferred to the distal convoluted tubule and has a lower osmolarity and solute concentration (100 mOsm/l) compared to plasma (280 mOsm/l). Much of the reabsorption processes in the distal tubule are influenced by hormonal release, in particular **aldosterone** and **angiotensin II**. In contrast, **urodilatin** (a non-glycosylated peptide and paracrine mediator) and **atrial natriuretic peptide** (ANP) can inhibit reabsorption (Forssmann et al. 2001).

Distal convoluted tubules run very closely to the afferent and efferent arterioles situated at the Bowman's capsule. The macula densa cells lining the distal convoluted tubule act as salt sensors and when salt levels in the filtrate are low, macula densa cells generate paracrine chemical signals, COX-2 (a macula densa-derived prostaglandin), that act on the juxtaglomerular apparatus within the afferent arteriole cell walls, releasing renin to control renal blood flow and glomerular filtration (Peti-Peterdi and Harris 2010).

251

Collecting Duct

Collecting ducts accumulate filtrate from several distal tubules and transcend through the medulla region towards the renal pelvis and ureters. The collecting ducts contain principal cells, which make up the majority of cells, responding to antidiuretic hormone (ADH), helping to reabsorb over 99% of the original filtrate, creating up to 60 ml of concentrated urine per hour collected and excreted from the urinary bladder. The intercalated cells are epithelial cells, which regulate the acid–base balance by secreting acid and reabsorbing bicarbonate. (Peti-Peterdi and Harris 2010).

Counter-current System

The reabsorption of solutes in the ascending loop of Henle creates an interstitial osmolarity, which progressively increases from the cortex (300 mOsm/l) to about 1200 mOsm/l nearer the medulla. This interstitial osmolarity gradient promotes water reabsorption from the parallel descending loop of Henle and the collecting ducts within the medulla as they travel to the renal pelvis. This parallel system with an opposite flow of different concentrations of solutes creates a counter-current. In addition, a counter-current system occurs between the vasa recta blood vessels running parallel to the loops of Henle. The vasa recta has a slower blood flow, which prevents wash-out of solutes from the medulla, it also absorbs interstitial water from the medulla without affecting the solute concentration. This process minimises dilution of the interstitial osmolality, known as the counter-current exchange mechanism (Kriz and Kaissling 2008).

Renal Pelvis

The renal pelvis, located within the pelvicalyceal system of the kidney, occupies most of the renal sinus, which consists of the renal calyces, blood vessels and nerves. The convergence of two or three major calyces, formed from several minor calyces, filters into the renal pelvis, which is a funnel-shaped chamber that then narrows and filters urine into the ureter (Bazira 2022; Ryan et al. 2011).

Ureters

The ureters are positioned at the hilum of the kidney and vertically extending along the psoas fascia and psoas major muscle within the retroperitoneal space, emptying into the bladder. Each ureter is approximately 25–30 cm in length and the two regions are described in relation to their position, so the abdominal segment is positioned near the posterior abdominal wall and the pelvic segment is positioned within the pelvic cavity below the pelvic brim. The ureter is composed of an inner mucosal epithelium layer and an outer layer of interweaved smooth muscle fibres assisting with peristalsis and transportation of urine to the bladder. The narrowest diameter of no more than 1 mm is at the pelvic brim. In the pregnant female the weight of the uterus and the narrow diameter are potential obstructions, which can lead to retention of urine in the ureters, resulting in urinary tract infections (Bazira 2022).

Blood Supply

Kidney blood supply is provided from the main abdominal aortic artery, running through to the renal arteries entering at the renal hilum and branching out throughout the kidneys, via the interlobar arteries and arcuate arteries, to the interlobular arteries in the renal cortex. Blood flows from the arcuate arteries into the narrower afferent arteries and afferent arterioles, forming the glomerulus capillaries bundles within the glomerulus, exiting at the efferent arterioles. The efferent arterioles join to the peritubular capillaries, which network around the nephrons and vasa recta renis (the straight arterioles and the straight venules) of the kidney. Blood is returned to the renal veins and the inferior vena cava (Dalal et al. 2022).

Nerves

Sensory nerves within the kidney are concentrated within the renal pelvis, with the renal sympathetic nerves regulating glomerular filtration, renin release and sodium reabsorption. When increased renal sympathetic nerve activity occurs, this decreases GFR and increases sodium absorption. It is theorised that the overactivity of the renal sympathetic nerves can result in hypertension and other cardiometabolic diseases. Sympathetic nerves can activate the renin–angiotensin–aldosterone system (RAAS) to cause constriction of the peripheral vasculature circulation and sodium retention. Treatments of hypertension using catheter-based renal nerve ablation (CBRNA) to actively destroy the sympathetic and sensory nerves to the kidneys have resulted in an antihypertensive response (Osborn and Banek 2018; Osborn et al. 2021).

Other Kidney Functions

Though the main function of the kidneys is to remove waste products, other key functions include regulation of blood pressure, production of vitamin D and calcium reabsorption, production of red blood cells (erythropoiesis) and elimination of neurotoxins and drugs.

Release of Hormones That Regulate Blood Pressure

The RAAS is initiated when there is a decrease in blood pressure, blood volume or renal sympathetic activation. A decrease in sodium concentration detected by the macula densa cells in the distal tubule activates the juxtaglomerular cells in the close-by afferent arterioles to release renin. Renin converts angiotensin (produced in the liver) to angiotensin I. The angiotensin-converting enzyme (ACE, produced in the lungs), converts angiotensin I to angiotensin II. One role of angiotensin II is to bind to angiotensin II receptors, located in the kidney, vascular smooth muscle cells, adrenal gland and the heart, platelets, adipocytes and placenta. The binding of the angiotensin II to the receptors on the blood vessels causes vasoconstriction, thereby narrowing the vessels, creating an increase in blood pressure (Dalal et al. 2022). See Figures 14.4 and 14.5.

The process can also constrict the efferent arterioles, increasing filtration in the Bowman's space, thereby improving the GFR (Singh and Karnik 2016; Burnier 2001). This is a necessary action to maintain blood pressure, vital for cardiovascular function.

Red Flag

In obstetrics, when blood volume is reduced significantly, for example in the management of hypovolaemic shock from a postpartum haemorrhage or septic shock, it is vital that blood pressure is maintained.

Source: Adapted from Galvagno et al. (2009).

253

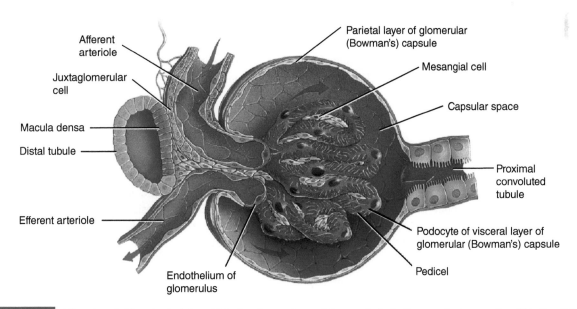

FIGURE 14.4 Afferent and efferent arterioles within the glomerulus and the proximity to the macula densa cells within the distal convoluted tubules.

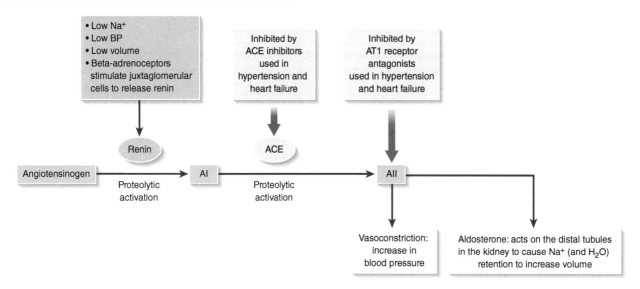

Angiotensin II also initiates aldosterone, a steroid produced in the adrenal cortex to control the balance of water and salts. Aldosterone increases sodium and potassium pump activity, reabsorbing potassium and hydrogen from the tubules. In turn, this creates a higher osmolarity in the interstitium, encouraging water to be drawn from the nephrons to maintain hydration. Angiotensin II can also increase ADH produced in the posterior pituitary gland, which expresses the aquaporin channels in principal cells within the distal convoluted tubule to promote water reabsorption, at the same time stimulating the hypothalamus to increase thirst as a reaction to dehydration (Dalal et al. 2022; Singh and Karnik 2016).

Production of an Active Form of Vitamin D and Calcium Reabsorption

The kidneys play a key role in regulating calcium and phosphorus homeostasis and require the active form of vitamin D, which, along with the parathyroid hormone (PTH), are essential for the control of the transporters transferring the calcium and phosphorus into the kidneys.

Control of the Production of Red Blood Cells

Erythropoietin (EPO), a glycoprotein also known as the erythroid-stimulating hormone, is required to initiate the production of red blood cells (erythropoiesis) and is produced by the liver in the fetus. However, after birth and in adults this function occurs in the peritubular cells within the interstitium of the kidneys. Erythropoiesis is activated by a number of factors, primarily hypoxia, triggering the peritubular cells and proximal tubules cells to produce EPO, which then stimulates marrow progenitors to commence the erythropoiesis process (Bunn 2013).

Renal Elimination of Drugs

The first step of the elimination of drugs is through glomerular filtration, which removes a large number of water-soluble drugs and drug metabolites. As GFR progressively increases during pregnancy, drugs that are solely excreted by the kidneys can be cleared at a faster rate. However, there can be differences in the tubular transport, which can affect the rate of clearance of some drugs. Efflux transporters draw the drugs from the filtrate back into the blood or urine.

Adrenal Glands in Relation to Kidney Function

The adrenal glands, two pyramidal structures located above the kidneys, measure 4–6 cm long and less than 1 cm wide, weigh 4–5 g, and are covered by a fibrous capsule and fat. Similarly to the kidneys they are composed of two regions. The adrenal cortex originates from the mesodermal cells and is responsible for the production and release of cortisol, a hormone regulating the body's stress responses. The zona glomerulosa within the cortex produces aldosterone, which activates sodium and potassium absorption to manage blood volume and blood pressure. This action also maintains homeostasis in blood pH levels. The adrenal medulla is made from neural crest cells and its main function is to produce epinephrine (adrenaline) and norepinephrine (noradrenaline) (Berry 2009; Kanczkowski et al. 2017).

Changes in Physiology of the Renal Function in Pregnancy

Physiological changes in pregnancy affect the renal system and haemodynamics, with the increase of renal plasma flow by up to 80% and GFR by 50%. This state of haemodilution results in a 50% decrease of serum creatinine. Creatinine is a chemical exclusively removed by the kidneys, therefore any severe issues with the kidney function will result in a significant rise in serum creatinine levels. Changes in tubular function occur during pregnancy altering the absorption of water and electrolytes and decreasing the reabsorption of glucose and calcium, resulting in mild glycosuria and calciuria. Mild proteinuria may occur up to 300 mg/d, without microalbuminuria.

The epithelium in the renal tubular network is extremely sensitive to hypoxia and pro-coagulation factors and can lead to tubular necrosis and renal cortex necrosis, resulting in poor renal function and poor urine output. In obstetrics, common causes of hypoxia may be from episodes of hypovolaemia, as a result of hyperemesis or postpartum haemorrhage and sepsis, pre-eclampsia causing glomerular endotheliosis and amniotic fluid embolism causing an occlusion of the renal vasculature (Vijayan et al. 2019).

Orange Flag

Visual disturbances, headaches, epigastric pain, vomiting and oedema are common signs and symptoms of hypertension and pre-eclampsia, which need timely escalation. Women should be aware that they should contact a health professional if these signs present. They can affect the health and well-being of the woman.

255

Pathophysiology of the Renal Function During Pregnancy

With the normal changes in the physiology of the renal system in pregnancy, additional challenges may present in obstetric conditions, such as hyperemesis, pre-eclampsia, haemolysis, elevated liver enzymes and low platelets (HELLP) syndrome, acute fatty liver, diabetes and intrahepatic cholestasis (ICP). They may cause severe dehydration, hypoxia and display pathophysiological factors leading to kidney injury, by having a direct effect on the renal blood flow (RBF) and GFR to the kidneys. The following discussion explores some of these conditions and the effect on kidney function.

Case Study 14.1

Rina is 43 years old and is having her first baby. She is eight weeks pregnant and is meeting you at her booking appointment. She conceived via in vitro fertilisation (IVF). Her body mass index (BMI) at booking is 40 kg/m², with no significant medical history.

- What other information about Rina's clinical history would you like to know?
- You have been asked to do Rina's urinalysis. Explain why you are doing the urinalysis and explain abnormal findings.
- What advice would you offer Rina in the prevention of developing pre-eclampsia?
- Outline a plan of care for Rina.

Urinary Tract Infection: Cystitis and Pyelonephritis

The hormone progesterone produced by the placenta, naturally increases in pregnancy to primarily maintain the pregnancy, but progesterone has a relaxing effect on smooth muscle (the ureters and the urethra are composed of this). The weight and compression on the ureters by the uterus can result in poor return or retention of urine, accompanied by elevated levels of glucose in the urine in pregnancy, creating an ideal environment for bacteria to multiple. In pregnancy the overall incidence of urinary tract infections (UTIs) is approximately 8%, with about 30% of women with asymptomatic bacteriuria (ASB) developing acute cystitis during their pregnancy (Habak and Griggs 2023). Treatment for pregnant women with UTIs or cystitis is oral antibiotics, such as cephalexin, ampicillin and nitrofurantoin. Fluoroquinolones are not recommended in pregnancy as they are teratogenic. If group B *Streptococcus* (GBS) presents in a urine culture at the time of delivery or labour, intravenous (IV) antibiotic therapy should be offered to mitigate the development of early-onset GBS sepsis in the infants of women diagnosed with GBS (Habak and Griggs 2023; NICE 2018a,b; Widmer et al. 2015).

Health Promotion: Urinary Tract Infection

Pregnant women should be alerted to the possible signs of UTI in pregnancy to prevent reoccurrence and treat appropriately. Key signs are frequency and urgency in passing urine, nocturia, pain or burning when passing urine, blood in the urine or abdominal pain. A urine culture should always be requested and antibiotics prescribed. Women should be encouraged to drink adequate fluids but to reduce fizzy drinks or caffeine that may irritate the bladder. Simple analgesia may also be appropriate to relieve any discomfort.

Ascending infection through the ureters, commonly *Escherichia coli* (*E. coli*), occurs in approximately 83% of cases of pyelonephritis, an infection in the kidneys affecting up to 2% of pregnancies, especially women with pre-disposing risk factors such as diabetes, sickle cell anaemia, those who smoke or who those who are immunosuppressed (Wing et al. 2014). In view of *E. coli* colonising regions around the anus and genitalia, promotion of personal hygiene should be discussed in pregnancy, as well as promoting adequate hydration. A diagnosis of pyelonephritis requires close monitoring and IV antibiotics for at least 48 hours within a hospital setting. Prior to discharge, monitoring of pyrexia and a negative urine culture should be achieved. Other complications may include sepsis and pulmonary complications, as seen in 10% of patients having treatment for pyelonephritis, which can lead to endotoxin-mediated alveolar damage resulting in acute respiratory distress or pulmonary oedema (Habak and Griggs 2023).

Hyperemesis Gravidarum

Approximately 0.3–3.6% of pregnant women develop hyperemesis gravidarum (HG). The condition presents with severe vomiting during the first trimester and the main concerns are severe electrolyte imbalance and acute kidney injury (AKI) (Florentin et al. 2020). In early pregnancy, nausea and vomiting in pregnancy (NVP) affects up to 80% of pregnant women in the United Kingdom and is a common reason for hospital admission in the first trimester. Care management includes IV fluid therapy, monitoring hydration and close monitoring of urea and serum electrolytes with a fluid balance rate of 0.5 ml/kg/h.

Medicines Management: Hyperemesis

HG can cause severe dehydration, therefore treatment is offered to prevent this. First-line treatments include oral cyclizine (anti-emetic) or promethazine (antihistamines), prochlorperazine or chlorpromazine (phenothiazines), or the combination drug doxylamine/pyridoxine (Xonvea®). Reassessment should be carried out after 24 hours.

Source: Adapted from NICE (2021b).

The severe dehydration causes changes in kidney function by reducing the GFR and affecting filtrate volumes. The severe hydration leads to lower blood volume and lower blood pressure, causing changes in kidney function by reducing the GFR and affecting filtrate volumes absorbed by the kidneys. Commonly, investigations present with elevated serum creatinine and blood urea nitrogen. Levels of potassium, sodium, calcium, magnesium and bicarbonate may be affected by reduced oral intake of fluids (Jennings and Mahdy 2023). Oral cyclizine or promethazine should be considered as a first-line treatment (NICE 2021b). Ondansetron is safe and effective, but as there is limited research on this medication and its use in pregnancy, it can be considered as second-line treatment (RCOG 2016).

Learning Event: Hyperemesis

- Can you recall a case when a woman presented with hyperemesis in pregnancy?
- What investigations does your Trust use to diagnose the condition?
- What care and support did you offer the woman?

Case Study 14.2

Parveen is a 38-year-old women attending triage. This is her second pregnancy. She has gestation diabetes, which is medicated. She complains of headaches and visual disturbances and you notice her ankles and feet are swollen. In routine admission investigations, Parveen's blood pressure is 146/92 mmHg and her urinalysis shows 2+ proteinuria.

- What other information about Parveen's clinical history would you like to know? What further investigations may you consider?
- Relating to the anatomy and physiology, explain the significance of protein found in the urinalysis.
- What is the relationship between gestation diabetes and developing pre-eclampsia?
- Outline a plan of care for Parveen.

Pre-eclampsia: Effects on Kidneys

The effects of pre-eclampsia (see Chapters 7 and 12) on the kidneys are complex. Pre-eclampsia has close associations with chronic kidney injury and can result in a reduction of the GFR by up to 40%. This significant reduction in GFR may not be sufficient in filtering serum creatinine, resulting in an increase. It is theorised that the podocyte cells in the Bowman's capsule are damaged by pre-eclampsia factors, which affects the initial absorption of filtrates and GFR from the glomerular capillaries (Fakhouri et al. 2012). Women with pre-eclampsia have been found to have lower levels of renin, angiotensin II and aldosterone, factors within the RAAS to manage blood pressure (Kattah 2020).

257

Medicines Management: Pre-eclampsia

With different types of hypertension in pregnancy, it is important to diagnose the type before recommending treatment and medication. For example, chronic hypertension existing prior to the pregnancy and gestational hypertension developing after 20 weeks do not present with proteinuria. They may be managed by lifestyle modification or medication if blood pressure exceeds a certain threshold, normally 140/90 mmHg. Review medication if the woman becomes pregnant, since some hypertensive medications can affect the growing fetus or be less effective as the physiology changes in pregnancy. Common medications include labetalol, nifedipine and in some cases hydralazine.

Source: Adapted from NICE (2019b).

In a meta-analysis of seven cohort studies comparing women with pre-eclampsia and those with uncomplicated pregnancies, 31% of women with pre-eclampsia had microalbuminuria (albumin present in the urine), an eightfold increase compared to 7% of women with uncomplicated pregnancies. Albumin is a large molecule and is not commonly found in the kidneys in normal conditions, but may pass through if blood pressure is higher. NICE (2019b) suggests that an albumin: creatinine levels urine dipstick of 1 g/l on dipstick testing screening is positive makes albuminuria a useful marker for kidney dysfunction (Kumar et al. 2012; Kattah 2020).

Learning Event: Pre-eclampsia

- Explore the guidelines within your Trust for managing gestational hypertension, pre-eclampsia and AKI. Are there any differences compared to the National Guidance (NICE)?
- What is the escalation policy for a woman with raised blood pressure of over 140/90 mmHg?
- Can you recall a case when a woman presented with pre-eclampsia in pregnancy? What investigations does your Trust use to diagnose the condition?
- Can you recall a case when a woman presented with pre-eclampsia in labour? What investigations does your Trust use to diagnose the condition?

Acute Kidney Injury

Pregnancy-related AKI (Pr-AKI) is associated with diminished kidney function leading to chronic kidney disease and end-stage kidney disease, with an increased risk of adverse cardiovascular events, maternal mortality and higher incidences of prematurity and perinatal death (Taber-Hight and Shah 2020; Vijayan et al. 2019; Saad et al. 2016). Pr-AKI can result from multiple factors and can be complicated further by underlying pregnancy conditions such as pre-eclampsia, which can develop potential complications of coagulopathy (deficiency in clotting), resulting in bleeding, hypovolaemia and acute tubular necrosis in the kidney. Though rates of Pr-AKI/AKI in pregnancy globally are falling and are low in the United Kingdom, the number of mortalities from AKI remains unacceptably high. The increased incidence of Pr-AKI in developed countries is mainly attributed to advanced maternal age and co-morbidities during pregnancy. In developing countries, the misdiagnosis or late identification of Pr-AKI may be due to inadequate antenatal care, as well as a higher frequency of septic abortions (Taber-Hight and Shah 2020). Other pregnancy conditions predisposing women to Pr-AKI are discussed later.

Diagnosis of Acute Kidney Injury in Pregnancy

The categorisation of AKI is generalised into prerenal, intrarenal and postrenal aetiologies to help identify the appropriate management. Prerenal is the most common cause in obstetric patients, involving a haemodynamic disturbance, such as massive haemorrhage, acute fatty liver of pregnancy (AFLP), chorioamnionitis, amniotic fluid embolism, septic abortion, pyelonephritis or puerperal sepsis. Intrarenal cases also include pre-eclampsia, HELLP, thrombotic thrombocytopenic purpura (TTP), atypical haemolytic uremic (aTHU) syndrome, pyelonephritis and pulmonary embolism. These conditions have contributing factors often causing primary damage to other organ systems, such as the cardiovascular or hepatic systems. However, as the role of the kidneys is to remove waste and toxins, the process of handling these factors within the renal system is causing damage to the kidneys, such as a reduction in GFR, ischaemic acute tubular injury and irreversible cortical necrosis. The postrenal category is less common and occurs if there is injury to ureters or bladder during C-section or an obstruction in bladder outlet. Pr-AKI is often difficult to diagnose due to the similarity of symptoms of these other underlying conditions in the obstetric patient (Taber-Hight and Shah 2020; Jim and Garovic 2017). See Figure 14.6.

Red Flag

Serum creatinine is exclusively filtered by the kidneys. Injury to the kidneys will affect the filtration and extraction of creatinine, resulting in an increase of serum creatinine levels. Levels of serum creatinine are a good marker for kidney injury.

Investigations

Evaluation for Pr-AKI should include a personalised care management plan led by a multidisciplinary team to include a specialist-trained midwife or midwifery team, consultant obstetrician and consultant nephrologist to review the patient's history and identify any cases of chronic hypertension, diabetes, pre-eclampsia in prior pregnancies, systemic lupus erythematous and pre-existing glomerular diseases.

The GFR should be monitored and the NICE Evidence Review Report (NICE 2019a), suggests that the values used to access chronic kidney disease in adults in NICE Guideline CG182 (now superseded by NG203) are appropriate for use in pregnancy (NICE 2021a). A 24-hour urine protein monitoring of more than 300 mg/d and urine sediment showing casts

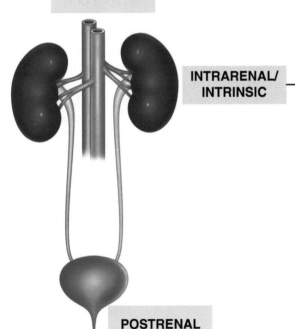

Transient decrease in renal perfusion→↓GFR
• Intravascular volume depletion = hypovolaemia
    • Hyperemesis gravidarum
    • OHSS
    • Diarrhoea
    • Blood loss   — extrarenal loss
      Miscarriage
      Antepartum haemorrhage
      Postpartum haemorrhage
    • Diuretics (renal loss from overuse)
• Decreased arterial pressure/decreased effective circulating volume
      Sepsis postabortal, puerperal, urosepsis
      Heart failure
• Impaired renal autoregulation/intrarenal vasoconstriction
      NSAIDs
      ACE inhibitors, ARB
      Cyclosporin, tacrolimus

PRERENAL

INTRARENAL/ INTRINSIC

Glomerulonephritis
• Acute glomerulonephritis

Interstitial
• Sepsis/Infection postabortal, puerperal, urosepsis,
                pyelonephritis
• Ischemia
    • miscarriage/abortion
    • antepartum haemorrhage-placenta praevia.
         abruptio placentae, uterine rupture
    • postpartum haemorrhage – atonia, perineal
         tears and lacerations

Vascular
    • vasculitis
    • hypertension – Pre-eclampsia/HELLP
    • thrombotic microangiopathy (TMA)
      thrombotic thrombocytopenic purpura (TTP)
      atypical haemolytic uraemic syndrome (aHUS)
      disseminated intravascular coagulation (DIC)

Medication - nephrotoxicity, acute interstitial nephritis
        antibiotic aminoglycosides, iodinated contrast
Acute fatty liver of pregnancy (AFLP)
Lupus nephritis
Antiphospholipid syndrome (APS)
Pulmonary embolism
Amniotic fluid embolism

259

POSTRENAL

Bilateral obstruction and hydronephrosis due to uterine compression of ureters/bladder
Unilateral ureter obstruction due to nephrolithiasis
Bladder outlet obstruction (tumour, lithiasis)
Iatrogenic injury of the bladder/ureter/urethra during caesarean section or vaginal delivery
Spontaneous injury of the urethra/bladder during vaginal delivery

FIGURE 14.6 This is Categorisation of Kidney Injury in Pregnancy.

(blood in urine) should be escalated for a diagnosis of Pr-AKI. Also include investigations into acid–base and electrolyte abnormalities. These non-invasive investigations are recommended as first-line management, but a kidney biopsy diagnosis can potentially suggest more specific treatment (Taber-Hight and Shah 2020; Vijayan et al. 2019; Wiles et al. 2019).

Care and Management

Investigations into haemodynamics, biochemical laboratory investigations and blood pressure measurement should be considered. If required, the management of hypovolaemia involving prompt replacement of IV fluids to restore renal and uterine perfusion should be commenced; however, consider risks of fluid overloading and pulmonary oedema in conditions such as pre-eclampsia. Avoid the administration of nephrotoxins, such as non-steroidal anti-inflammatory drugs (NSAIDs), ACE inhibitors and angiotensin receptor blockers, as prostaglandin antagonists can result in glomerular dysfunction (Jim and Garovic 2017; Taber-Hight and Shah 2020; Lin and Chen 2012; Vijayan et al. 2019; Al-Naimi et al. 2019).

HELLP Syndrome

HELLP (Hemolysis, Elevated Liver enzymes and Low Platelets) is a rare liver and blood clotting pregnancy-related disorder. HELLP syndrome may present with hypertension with or without proteinuria and is primarily associated with liver dysfunction. It has close associations with the pathophysiology of pre-eclampsia, in particular the coagulation cascade, which depletes platelets, hence the low platelet levels in HELLP (Weiner et al. 2016). Pre-eclampsia is known to activate a proinflammatory response that can cause a maternal–fetal immune imbalance, leading to endothelial dysfunction. This initiates a process of platelet activation and aggregation, resulting in the depletion and lowering of platelet levels (Zhou et al. 2002).

Up to 15% of women who develop HELLP syndrome go on to develop Pr-AKI; however, kidney recovery is likely after recovery from HELLP. Thrombotic microangiopathy and glomerular endotheliosis (swelling of glomerulus cells) can result in ineffective filtration by decreasing the size of the pores for filtration and acute tubular necrosis has been found following kidney biopsies from women with HELLP. Some other case studies have found that kidney injury caused nephrosclerosis, a hardening of the kidneys, and glomerulonephritis, an acute inflammatory response, also affecting the function of the kidneys (Gupta et al. 2012; Taber-Hight and Shah 2020).

Expert Midwife: Emergencies and Potential Complications

Pre-eclampsia, HELLP, acute fatty liver of pregnancy predispose a woman potentially to postpartum haemorrhage following birth. If uncontrolled this can lead to hypovolaemic shock, affecting kidney function, leading to acute kidney injury. Emergencies such as postpartum haemorrhages are often anticipated, however anyone who has dealt with an emergency knows how quickly things can escalate. Ensuring the woman is in the right place for birth and has the appropriate team around them and close monitoring are important to prevent more serious conditions such as AKI developing.

Red Flag

Blood pressure is associated with pre-eclampsia and in some cases of HELLP and AFLP. Raised blood pressure poses risks to the mother. Severe high blood pressure in a pre-eclamptic woman may lead to eclampsia. Raised blood pressure reduces the efficiency of placental diffusion, affecting fetal growth.

Acute Fatty Liver of Pregnancy

The cause of AFLP is thought to be related to an abnormality in fetal fatty acid metabolism. AFLP is diagnosed late in the third trimester, commonly from 30 weeks. Signs and symptoms include abdominal pain, nausea and vomiting. Investigations of AFLP are similar to those of HELLP syndrome and pre-eclampsia, such as liver function (LFT) derangements.

When examining a woman's legs for oedema, the following steps are commonly followed:

- Ensue privacy and comfort, wash hands, seek consent.
- **Positioning:** Ask and, if needed, assist the woman to lie down, ensuring she is not completely flat for a long period and is supported by a raised back rest or moved to a left lateral position, legs extended or slightly elevated to facilitate observation.
- **Inspection:** Visually assess the woman's legs for any noticeable swelling. Look for puffiness, tightness or any changes in skin texture or colour. Oedema usually presents as bilateral swelling.
- **Palpation:** Gently press your fingers on various areas of the legs (ankles, shins, calves) to check for the presence of pitting oedema. If there is oedema, you will observe a temporary indentation or pit that remains after pressure is applied and released. Wash hands when finished.
- It is important to monitor and to document as per local policy and procedure the extent and location of the swelling. Note any changes or worsening of the oedema over time.
- Undertake a comprehensive holistic assessment of the woman. If you suspect pre-eclampsia or have concerns, undertake onward referral and help and advice.

Pr-AKI is common in AFLP, affecting between 20% and 100% of women. Pr-AKI in AFLP usually presents similarly to a hepatorenal syndrome, and is more commonly seen in patients with severe liver impairment such as liver failure and ascites (fluid collecting in abdomen) and characterised as reduced renal blood flow and GFR to the kidneys, resulting in inadequate kidney function due to poor perfusion of filtrate. Direct infiltration of fatty cells through the kidneys can contribute to injury (Naoum et al. 2019; Simonetto et al. 2020).

Effects of Medicines on Kidneys

Medications can also affect GFR. NSAIDs can restrict the formation of prostaglandins, which act on dilating the afferent arteriole to increase GFR. ACE inhibitors are commonly used to treat hypertension in diabetes or heart failure, but can also inhibit the formation of angiotensin II. Angiotensin II is required for the vasoconstriction of efferent arterioles to increase blood pressure to achieve an effective GFR.

Patients with chronic kidney disease undergoing anaesthesia will need to be monitored, ensuring that renal perfusion pressures are maintained. Consider seeking early consultation with an anaesthetist if there are concerns over kidney function and the administration of medication (Lucas et al. 2019).

Conditions Associated with the Renal System

The following are a list of conditions that are associated with the renal system. Take some time and write notes about each of the conditions. Think about the medications that may be used in order to treat these conditions. Remember to include aspects of patient care. If you are making notes about people you have offered care and support to, you must ensure that you have adhered to the rules of confidentiality.

The condition	Your notes
Acute renal failure	
Chronic kidney disease	
Cystitis	
Nephrolithiasis	
Glomerular nephritis	

> ## Take-Home Points
>
> - Understanding the pathophysiological changes that occur in pregnancy is essential if the midwife is to offer safe, effective, personalised care to women.
> - The renal system is a complex body system, with a key role to play in maintaining homeostasis, including during pregnancy.
> - Pregnancy and kidney disease can present complications to a person's current and future health.
> - Women with chronic kidney disease are at higher risk for complications such as pre-eclampsia, restricted fetal growth, preterm delivery and a need for caesarean section.
> - Monitoring kidney function is essential to identify and reduce any potential complications.
> - When challenges arise, the midwife has to carefully assess the woman and manage her care, with the woman at the centre of all that is done.
> - A specialist midwife and midwifery care team may be needed to manage any complications that may arise, including a nephrologist, obstetrician and intensivist.

Conclusion

Kidney function generally adapts well in pregnancy, but it is influenced by hormones and changes in blood volume, blood pressure, hypoxia and renal filtration. The role of the midwife is to understand the normal anatomy and physiology of the kidneys and recognise signs and symptoms of Pr-AKI and significant changes in kidney function when caring for women who present with or develop other co-morbidities, such as hyperemesis, pre-eclampsia, HELLP, AFLP and others. Care and management of kidney disease and guidelines for Pr-AKI are being developed. Care plans primarily rely on a multidisciplinary team approach, ensuring that each individual case is managed appropriately. It is the role of the midwife to explore local guidelines and manage cases in a suitable way, seeking further training and knowledge within their roles. There is consensus on investigations into serum creatinine, review for fluid replacement therapy, electrolyte management, kidney biopsies as needed and renal replacement therapy. Guidelines are being developed to accommodate the pregnant woman.

References

Al-Naimi, M.S., Rasheed, H.A., Hussien, N.R. et al. (2019). Nephrotoxicity: role and significance of renal biomarkers in the early detection of acute renal injury. *Journal of Advanced Pharmaceutical Technology & Research* 10 (3): 95–99. https://doi.org/10.4103/japtr.JAPTR_336_18.

Bazira, P.J. (2022). Anatomy of the kidney and ureter. *Surgery (Oxford)* 40 (8): 481–488.

Berry, M.E. (2009). *Adrenal Gland Disorders.* Albuquerque: American Society of Radiologic Technologists.

Britannica (2023). Renin-angiotensin system. https://www.britannica.com/science/renin-angiotensin-system (accessed November 2023).

Bunn, H.F. (2013). Erythropoietin. *Cold Spring Harbor Perspectives in Medicine* 3 (3): a011619. https://doi.org/10.1101/cshperspect.a011619.

Burnier, M. (2001). Angiotensin II type 1 receptor blockers. *Circulation* 103 (6): 904–912.

Dalal, R., Bruss, Z.S., and Sehdev, J.S. (2022). Physiology, renal blood flow and filtration. In: *StatPearls.* Treasure Island, FL: StatPearls Publishing https://www.ncbi.nlm.nih.gov/books/NBK482248.

Fakhouri, F., Vercel, C., and Fremeaux-Bacchi, V. (2012). Obstetric nephrology: AKI and thrombotic microangiopathies in pregnancy. *Clinical Journal of the American Society of Nephrology: CJASN* 7 (12): 2100–2106.

Falkson, S.R. and Bordoni, B. (2022). Anatomy, abdomen and pelvis: Bowman capsule. In: *StatPearls.* Treasure Island, FL: StatPearls Publishing https://www.ncbi.nlm.nih.gov/books/NBK554474.

Florentin, M., Parthymos, I., Agouridis, A.P., and Liamis, G. (2020). Hyperemesis gravidarum: a benign condition of pregnancy or a challenging metabolic disorder? *European Journal of Case Reports in Internal Medicine* 7 (12): 001979. https://doi.org/10.12890/2020_001979.

Forssmann, W.G., Meyer, M., and Forssmann, K. (2001). The renal urodilatin system: clinical implications. *Cardiovascular Research* 51 (3): 450–462. https://doi.org/10.1016/S0008-6363(01)00331-5.

Galvagno, S.M., Camann, D.O. Jr., and William, M.D. (2009). Sepsis and acute renal failure in pregnancy. *Anesthesia & Analgesia* 108 (2): 572–575. https://doi.org/10.1213/ane.0b013e3181937b7e.

Grigoraş, A., Balan, R.A., Căruntu, I.D. et al. (2021). Perirenal adipose tissue—current knowledge and future opportunities. *Journal of Clinical Medicine* 10 (6): 1291. https://doi.org/10.3390/jcm10061291.

Gupta, A., Ferguson, J., and Rahman, M. (2012). Acute oliguric renal failure in HELLP syndrome: case report and review of literature. *Renal Failure* 34 (5): 653–656. https://doi.org/10.3109/0886022X.2012.660856.

Habak, P.J. and Griggs, R.P. Jr. (2023). Urinary tract infection in pregnancy. In: *StatPearls*. Treasure Island, FL: StatPearls Publishing https://www.ncbi.nlm.nih.gov/books/NBK537047.

Jennings, L.K. and Mahdy, H. (2023). Hyperemesis gravidarum. In: *StatPearls*. Treasure Island, FL: StatPearls Publishing https://www.ncbi.nlm.nih.gov/books/NBK532917.

Jim, B. and Garovic, V.D. (2017). Acute kidney injury in pregnancy. *Seminars in Nephrology* 37 (4): 378–385. https://doi.org/10.1016/j.semnephrol.2017.05.010.

Kamal, E.M., Behery, M.M., Sayed, G.A., and Abdulatif, H.K. (2014). RIFLE classification and mortality in obstetric patients admitted to the intensive care unit with acute kidney injury: a 3-year prospective study. *Reproductive Sciences* 21 (10): 1281–1287.

Kanczkowski, W., Sue, M., and Bornstein, S.R. (2017). The adrenal gland microenvironment in health, disease and during regeneration. *Hormones (Athens, Greece)* 16 (3): 251–265. https://doi.org/10.14310/horm.2002.1744.

Kattah, A. (2020). Pre-eclampsia and kidney disease: deciphering cause and effect. *Current Hypertension Reports* 22: 91. https://doi.org/10.1007/s11906-020-01099-1.

Klussmann, E., Maric, K., and Rosenthal, W. (2000). The mechanisms of aquaporin control in the renal collecting duct. *Reviews of Physiology, Biochemistry and Pharmacology* 141: 33–95. https://doi.org/10.1007/BFb0119577.

Kriz, W. and Kaissling, B. (2008). Structural organization of the mammalian kidney. In: *Seldin and Giebisch's The Kidney*, 4e (ed. R.J. Alpern and S.C. Hebert), 479–563. Cambridge, MA: Academic Press.

Kumar, R., Tebben, P.J., and Thompson, J.R. (2012). Vitamin D and the kidney. *Archives of Biochemistry and Biophysics* 523 (1): 77–86. https://doi.org/10.1016/j.abb.2012.03.003.

Lin, C.Y. and Chen, Y.C. (2012). Acute kidney injury classification: AKIN and RIFLE criteria in critical patients. *World Journal of Critical Care Medicine* 1 (2): 40–45. https://doi.org/10.5492/wjccm.v1.i2.40.

Lucas, G.N.C., Leitão, A.C.C., Alencar, R.L. et al. (2019). Pathophysiological aspects of nephropathy caused by non-steroidal anti-inflammatory drugs. *Jornal Brasileiro de Nefrologia* 41 (1): 124–130. https://doi.org.10.1590/2175-8239-JBN-2018-0107.

Naoum, E.E., Leffert, L.R., Chitilian, H.V. et al. (2019). Acute fatty liver of pregnancy: pathophysiology, anesthetic implications, and obstetrical management. *Anesthesiology* 130 (3): 446–461. https://doi.org/10.1097/ALN.0000000000002597.

National Institute for Health and Care Excellence (NICE) (2018a). Urinary tract infection (lower): antimicrobial prescribing. NG109. https://www.nice.org.uk/guidance/ng109 (accessed November 2023).

National Institute for Health and Care Excellence (NICE) (2018b). Urinary tract infection (recurrent): antimicrobial prescribing. NG112. https://www.nice.org.uk/guidance/ng112 (accessed November 2023).

National Institute for Health and Care Excellence (NICE) (2019a). Intrapartum care for women with existing medical conditions or obstetric complications and their babies. NG121. https://www.nice.org.uk/guidance/ng121 (accessed November 2023).

National Institute for Health and Care Excellence (NICE) (2019b). Hypertension in pregnancy: diagnosis and management. NG133. https://www.nice.org.uk/guidance/ng133 (accessed November 2023).

National Institute for Health and Care Excellence (NICE) (2021a). Chronic kidney disease: assessment and management. NG203. https://www.nice.org.uk/guidance/ng203 (accessed November 2023).

National Institute for Health and Care Excellence (NICE) (2021b). Nausea/vomiting in pregnancy: Scenario: Management. https://cks.nice.org.uk/topics/nausea-vomiting-in-pregnancy/management/management/#drug-treatments (accessed November 2023).

Osborn, J.W. and Banek, C. (2018). Catheter-based renal nerve ablation as a novel hypertension therapy, lost, and then found, in translation. *Hypertension* 71 (3): 383–388.

Osborn, J.W., Tyshynsky, R., and Vulchanova, L. (2021). Function of renal nerves in kidney physiology and pathophysiology. *Annual Review of Physiology* 10 (83): 429–450. https://doi.org/10.1146/annurev-physiol-031620-091656.

Peti-Peterdi, J. and Harris, R.C. (2010). Macula densa sensing and signaling mechanisms of renin release. *Journal of the American Society of Nephrology: JASN* 21 (7): 1093–1096. https://doi.org/10.1681/ASN.2009070759.

Royal College of Obstetricians and Gynaecologists (RCOG) (2016). The management of nausea and vomiting of pregnancy and hyperemesis gravidarum. https://www.rcog.org.uk/media/y3fen1x1/gtg69-hyperemesis.pdf (accessed November 2023).

Ryan, S., McNicholas, M., and Eustace, S.J. (2011). *Anatomy for Diagnostic Imaging e-Book*. St Louis: Elsevier Health Sciences.

Saad, A.F., Roman, J., Wyble, A., and Pacheco, L.D. (2016). Pregnancy-associated atypical hemolytic-uremic syndrome. *AJP Reports* 6 (1): e125–e128. https://doi.org/10.1055/s-0036-1579539.

Simonetto, D.A., Gines, P., and Kamath, P. (2020). Hepatorenal syndrome: pathophysiology, diagnosis, and management. *BMJ* 370: m2687. https://doi.org/10.1136/bmj.m2687.

Singh, K.D. and Karnik, S.S. (2016). Angiotensin receptors: structure, function, signaling and clinical applications. *Journal of Cell Signaling* 1 (2): 111. https://doi.org/10.4172/jcs.1000111.

Soriano, R.M., Penfold, D., and Leslie, S.W. (2022). Anatomy, abdomen and pelvis: kidneys. In: *StatPearls*. Treasure Island, FL: StatPearls Publishing https://www.ncbi.nlm.nih.gov/books/NBK482385.

Taber-Hight, E. and Shah, S. (2020). Acute kidney injury in pregnancy. *Advances in Chronic Kidney Disease* 27 (6): 455–460. https://doi.org/10.1053/j.ackd.2020.06.002.

Veiga-Matos, J., Remião, F., and Motales, A. (2020). Pharmacokinetics and toxicokinetics roles of membrane transporters at kidney level. *Journal of Pharmacy & Pharmaceutical Sciences* 2020 (23): 333–356. https://doi.org/10.18433/jpps30865.

Vijayan, M., Avendano, M., Chinchilla, K.A., and Jim, B. (2019). Acute kidney injury in pregnancy. *Current Opinion in Critical Care* 25 (6): 580–590. https://doi.org/10.1097/MCC.0000000000000656.

Vinturache, A., Popoola, J., and Watt-Coote, I. (2019). The changing landscape of acute kidney injury in pregnancy from an obstetric perspective. *Journal of Clinical Medicine* 8: 1396.

Weiner, E., Schreider, L., Grinstein, E. et al. (2016). The placental component and obstetric outcome in severe pre-eclampsia with and without HELLP syndrome. *Placenta* 47: 99–104.

Widmer, M., Lopez, I., Gülmezoglu, A. et al. (2015). Duration of treatment for asymptomatic bacteriuria during pregnancy. *Cochrane Database of Systematic Reviews* 2015 (11): CD000491. https://doi.org/10.1002/14651858.CD000491.pub3.

Wiles, K., Chappell, L., Clark, K. et al. (2019). Clinical practice guideline on pregnancy and renal disease. *BMC Nephrology* 20: 401. https://doi.org/10.1186/s12882-019-1560-2.

Wing, D.A., Fassett, M.J., and Getahun, D. (2014). Acute pyelonephritis in pregnancy: an 18-year retrospective analysis. *American Journal of Obstetrics and Gynecology* 210 (3): 219.e1–219.e6.

Zhou, Y., McMaster, M., Woo, K. et al. (2002). Vascular endothelial growth factor ligands and receptors that regulate human cytotrophoblast survival are dysregulated in severe pre-eclampsia and hemolysis, elevated liver enzymes, and low platelets syndrome. *American Journal of Pathology* 160 (4): 1405–1423. https://doi.org/S0002-9440(10)62567-9.

Further Resources

National Institute for Health and Care Excellence Kidney Conditions. https://www.nice.org.uk/guidance/conditions-and-diseases/kidney-conditions.

Peate, I. and Hamilton, C. (2022). *Fundamentals of Pharmacology for Midwives*. Chichester, UK: Wiley.

Glossary

Aquaporin	Membrane proteins, which serve as channels in the transfer of water
Bowman's capsule	Made up of three layers, endothelial cells, basement membrane and podocytes
Bowman's space	Space that allows filtrate to be extracted from the arterioles
Cortex	Forms the outer rim of the kidney, containing the glomerular apparatus
Electrolytes	Chemicals that conduct electricity when dissolved in water
Erythropoietin	A hormone produced by the kidneys, which stimulates the production of red blood cells
Fenestrated	The presence of gaps in the cell walls, which allow filtrates of a certain size to pass through
Haemodilution	An increase in blood fluids, resulting in lowering of the concentration of red blood cells
Medulla	Inner part of the kidney, contains collecting ducts and renal pyramids
Osmolarity	Concentration of a solution expressed as the total number of solute particles per litre
Papillae	The openings at the apex of the renal pyramids
Placental growth factor (PIGF)	In blood plasma or serum, a protein involved in placental angiogenesis (the development of new blood vessels)
Pyramids	Consist of collecting tubules, collecting ducts, long loops of Henle and vasa recta
Renin	A proteolytic enzyme released into the circulation primarily by the kidneys
Starling equation	Describes the net flow of fluid across a semipermeable membrane
Vasa recta	The straight arterioles and the straight venules of the kidney

CHAPTER 15

The Respiratory System and Associated Disorders

Alison Anderson

South Tees NHS Foundation Trust, Middlesbrough, UK

AIM

This chapter will explore the respiratory system, the adaptations to its function during pregnancy and the pathophysiology of a range of respiratory disorders.

LEARNING OUTCOMES

On completion of this chapter the reader will be able to:

- Describe the anatomy of the upper and lower respiratory systems
- Identify the functions of the structures found in the respiratory system
- Describe the respiratory changes occurring in pregnancy
- Explain the processes of internal and external respiration
- Describe the pathophysiology of a range of respiratory disorders

Test Your Prior Knowledge

1. Describe the pathway of inhaled air from nose to alveoli.
2. Name five parts of the respiratory system and their associated adaptations during pregnancy.
3. Describe the processes of internal and external respiration.
4. Describe the chemical and nervous control of respiration and identify the associated organs.

The respiratory system ensures that the oxygen needed for cellular respiration is taken from the air we breathe in to all the cells of the body where cellular respiration takes place. Many disorders can affect the respiratory system, ranging from the common cold to more severe conditions such as asthma, tuberculosis, pneumonia, Covid-19 and pulmonary embolism. It is important for the midwife to be aware of any changes in the respiratory function of a woman they are caring for and to take the appropriate action.

Fundamentals of Maternal Pathophysiology, First Edition. Edited by Claire Leader and Ian Peate.
© 2024 John Wiley & Sons Ltd. Published 2024 by John Wiley & Sons Ltd.
Companion website: www.wiley.com/go/leader/maternalpatho

Overview of the Respiratory System

The respiratory system provides the exchange of gases needed for cellular respiration. Air is inhaled from the atmosphere into the lungs, and oxygen is then transported via the cardiovascular system to the tissues. Carbon dioxide, metabolic waste from respiration, is returned to the lungs and excreted in the air expired. The demand for oxygen and removal of carbon dioxide are greater during pregnancy, labour and the postnatal period due to increased workload, but a healthy respiratory system can cope with these demands (Wylie 2005). The respiratory system can be divided structurally into the upper and lower respiratory systems or functionally into the conducting and respiratory parts.

Figure 15.1 shows the respiratory system.

Upper Respiratory Tract

The upper respiratory tract is made up of the nose, pharynx, larynx and associated structures. Air enters the airway through the nose or mouth. The nose is made up of bone and cartilage and is divided into two by the nasal septum. Ciliated columnar epithelial cells, containing mucous-secreting goblet cells, line the nasal cavity and filter, warm and moisten the air. The nasal cavity opens posteriorly into the pharynx. The ciliated cells in the nasal cavity provide a gentle current moving any trapped mucus towards the pharynx, where it is swallowed, passed to the stomach and digested.

The pharynx is a funnel-shaped tube made up of three regions: the nasopharynx, oropharynx and laryngopharynx. As well as transporting air, food and water, the pharynx warms and moistens air further, protects the tympanic membrane or eardrum from changes in atmospheric pressure, acts as a resonance chamber for sound, and produces antibodies for infection prevention. The pharyngeal tonsil or adenoids are found in the upper region of the nasopharynx and the palatine and lingual tonsils are situated in the oropharynx. The laryngopharynx lies inferiorly to the oropharynx and divides into two: anteriorly, the larynx and trachea transport air into the lungs; posteriorly, the oesophagus transports food and liquid

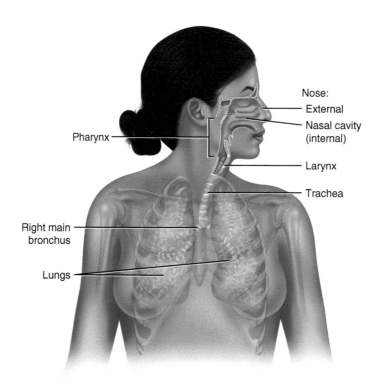

Nose:
External
Nasal cavity
(internal)

Pharynx

Larynx

Trachea

Right main
bronchus

Lungs

FIGURE 15.1   The respiratory system.

into the stomach. The epiglottis is made of fibroelastic cartilage, closing off the larynx during swallowing to prevent food or fluids entering the trachea. The vocal cords, a pair of folds in the mucous membrane, are also found in the larynx. The vocal cords can vibrate when air passes over them, causing sound waves, allowing speech.

Lower Respiratory Tract

The lower respiratory tract includes the trachea, bronchi and lungs. After the larynx, air enters the trachea, where it then passes through one of two bronchi. The bronchi divide repeatedly into smaller bronchioles before ending in air sacs, called alveoli (Figure 15.2).

Trachea → bronchi → bronchioles → terminal bronchioles → respiratory bronchioles → alveoli ducts → alveoli

The trachea lies in front of the oesophagus and is held open by 16–20 horseshoe-shaped or C-shaped rings of hyaline cartilage. The trachea wall has three layers: an outer fibrous and elastic tissue layer, a middle layer of cartilage, bands of smooth muscle and some areolar tissue containing blood vessels, lymph vessels and autonomic nerves, and an inner lining consisting of a mucous membrane containing ciliated epithelium that moves mucus, dust and microorganisms upwards and out of the lungs. The C-shaped cartilage rings have two main functions: keeping the trachea patent during pressure changes associated with breathing and allowing for the slight expansion of the oesophagus during swallowing of food or fluid.

The lungs are large, cone-shaped organs with a broad concave base, found in the thoracic cavity (Figure 15.3). The heart, in the mediastinum, separates the two lungs. At the mediastinal surface of the lungs a triangular area can be found, called the hilum, where the bronchus, blood vessels, nerves and lymphatic vessels enter the lungs. The superior-most part of the lung, the apex, extends just above the clavicles. The base of the lungs is concave and lies just above the

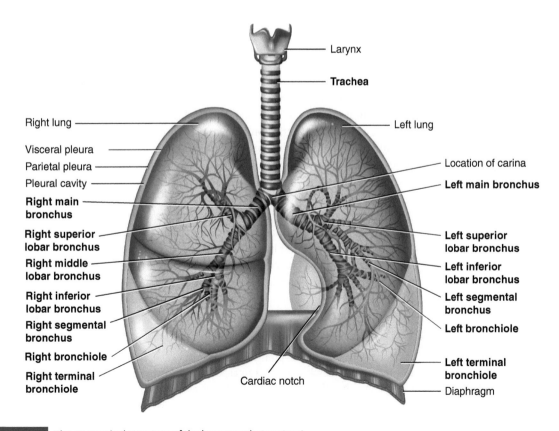

FIGURE 15.2 The anatomical structure of the lower respiratory tract.

267

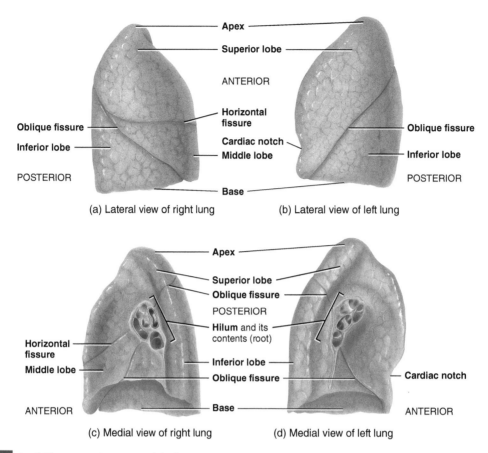

Apex

Superior lobe

ANTERIOR

Horizontal fissure

Oblique fissure

Cardiac notch

Inferior lobe

Middle lobe

POSTERIOR

Oblique fissure

Inferior lobe

POSTERIOR

Base

(a) Lateral view of right lung   (b) Lateral view of left lung

Apex

Superior lobe

Oblique fissure

POSTERIOR

Hilum and its contents (root)

Horizontal fissure

Middle lobe

Inferior lobe

Oblique fissure

Cardiac notch

ANTERIOR   Base   ANTERIOR

(c) Medial view of right lung   (d) Medial view of left lung

FIGURE 15.3   (a–d) The external anatomy of the lungs.

268

diaphragm. The costal surface of the lungs presses against the costal cartilages, intercostal muscles and rib cage. The lungs are surrounded by a two-layered pleural membrane secreting pleural fluid from the epithelial cells, aiding the movement of the lungs against the thoracic wall without friction and preventing the pleural layers from separating due to the surface tension that exists. The membrane covering the surface of the lungs is the visceral or pulmonary pleura and the part of the membrane covering the thoracic wall and diaphragm is the parietal pleura (Figure 15.2).

The trachea subdivides into two main branches, the right and left bronchus, dividing repeatedly into smaller and smaller tubes called bronchi and then, finally, bronchioles. The trachea, bronchi and bronchioles contain smooth muscle that enables them to constrict. The bronchioles lead ultimately to numerous alveoli, where most of the gaseous exchange takes place. The right bronchus is wider, shorter (approximately 25 mm long) and straighter than the left bronchus (approximately 50 mm long), due to the position of the heart in the left side of the chest. The bronchi enter the lungs at the hilum. The same three layers existing in the trachea can be found in the bronchi. The smaller bronchi have smaller cartilage plates rather than rings present in their walls, alongside smooth muscle.

Health Promotion: Vaccination in Pregnancy

Midwives are ideally placed to offer health education advice and promotion to pregnant women in their care. Pregnancy is one of the rare times when a woman will encounter health professionals on a regular basis for an intense period of time (DOH 2010). There are two vaccinations that a pregnant woman may be offered in her pregnancy: the pertussis or whooping cough vaccine and the seasonal flu vaccine. The midwife needs to fully understand the reasons these vaccinations are offered in pregnancy, the timing of the vaccinations, the side effects and the contra-indications to the vaccinations, as well as the mode of administration.

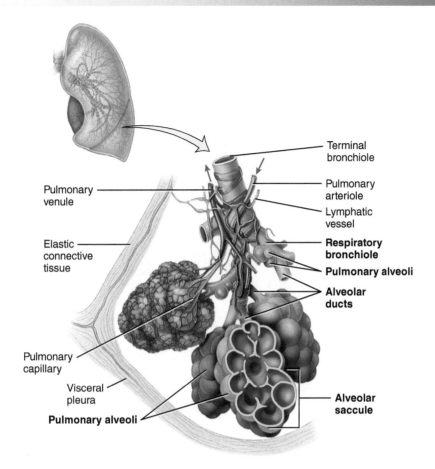

Pulmonary venule

Elastic connective tissue

Pulmonary capillary

Visceral pleura

Pulmonary alveoli

Terminal bronchiole

Pulmonary arteriole

Lymphatic vessel

Respiratory bronchiole

Pulmonary alveoli

Alveolar ducts

Alveolar saccule

FIGURE 15.4 The structure of a lobule of the lung.

As the bronchi divide into the smaller bronchioles, the rings of cartilage supporting the airways are replaced by smooth muscle. The rings of cartilage reduce in size as the bronchi divide. The lower bronchioles have no cartilage present as it would interfere with the exchange of gases and the expansion of lung tissue. For airflow to be regulated within each lung, the amount of smooth muscle in the bronchioles increases as the cartilage decreases. This smooth muscle increases and decreases the diameter of the airways, in response to stimuli, through contraction and relaxation under the control of the autonomic nervous system. The sympathetic nervous system causes bronchodilation and the parasympathetic nervous system causes bronchoconstriction. As the bronchi divide, eventually the smaller passageways are termed terminal bronchioles, then respiratory bronchioles, and finally alveoli ducts that lead to the alveoli or air sacs (Figure 15.4). Alveoli are not part of the conducting region of the respiratory system.

The lungs form a very efficient gas exchange surface, for which they are specially adapted. They provide a large surface area by the presence of an estimated 200–400 million alveoli or air sacs; they have a network of capillaries surrounding each alveolus and they have a thin exchange surface. There are only two layers of cells, known as the respiratory membrane, between the air in the alveolus and the blood in the capillaries through which oxygen and carbon dioxide diffuse in a process called gaseous exchange (Figure 15.5). These are the alveolar epithelium (squamous epithelial cells) and the cells forming the capillary wall. Alveoli are minute, bubble-like air sacs lined with moisture and are liable to collapse, causing their sides to stick together because of surface tension. Septal cells in the alveolar epithelium secrete surfactant that greatly reduces the surface tension of the alveoli and keeps them open during expiration, thereby preventing their collapse.

Oxygen and carbon dioxide are exchanged at the respiratory membrane by a process called diffusion, relying on pressure gradients between the lungs and atmospheric pressure.

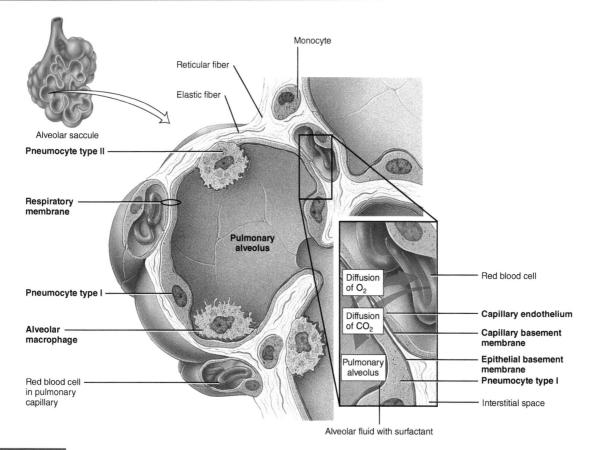

Monocyte

Reticular fiber

Elastic fiber

Alveolar saccule

Pneumocyte type II

Respiratory membrane

Pulmonary alveolus

Pneumocyte type I

Alveolar macrophage

Red blood cell in pulmonary capillary

Diffusion of O_2

Diffusion of CO_2

Pulmonary alveolus

Red blood cell

Capillary endothelium

Capillary basement membrane

Epithelial basement membrane

Pneumocyte type I

Interstitial space

Alveolar fluid with surfactant

FIGURE 15.5   The structure of the alveolus.

Respiratory Muscles

Diaphragm

Forming the floor of the thoracic cavity, separating it from the abdominal cavity, is the strong dome-shaped muscle of the diaphragm. The diaphragm muscle fibres radiate from a central tendon, attaching to the vertebral column, sternum and lower ribs. Contraction of this muscle causes the diaphragm to move downwards and flatten, lifting the rib cage and enlarging the thoracic cavity, causing a decrease in pressure in the thoracic cavity (Figure 15.6). During contraction, the central tendon moves downwards to be level with the ninth thoracic vertebrae; when the diaphragm muscle is in its relaxed state, the central tendon is level with the eight thoracic vertebrae.

Intercostal Muscles

There are 11 pairs of intercostal muscles lying between the 12 pairs of ribs and these are the accessory muscles of respiration. There are two layers: the external and internal intercostal muscles. The external intercostal muscles are involved in inspiration, extending downwards and forwards from the lowest edge of the rib above to the uppermost edge of the rib below. The internal intercostal muscles are involved in expiration during phases of activity, extending downwards and backwards from the lowest edge of the ridge above to the uppermost edge of the rib below. They lie at right angles to the external intercostal muscles.

The role of the intercostal muscles is primarily to stabilise the rib cage during expansion of the thoracic cavity. However, during physical exertion or upper airway obstruction, when there is an increased need for oxygen, the intercostal muscles help to enlarge the rib cage, allowing for further lung expansion. As the first rib is fixed, when the external intercostal muscles contract they move the ribcage upwards and outwards towards the first rib.

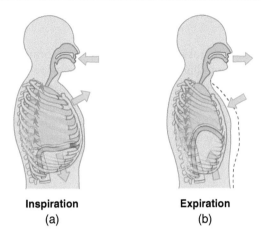

Inspiration
(a)

Expiration
(b)

FIGURE 15.6 Changes in chest size, intercostal muscles, diaphragm and rib cage positions during (a) inspiration and (b) expiration.

Pulmonary Ventilation (Breathing)

The process of breathing, or pulmonary ventilation, moves air in and out of the lungs. The average adult has a respiratory rate of 12–15 breaths/min. Breathing is made up of two phases: inspiration and expiration. Inspiration is the movement of air into the lungs and expiration is the movement of air out of the lungs. Gases flow from regions of high pressure to regions of low pressure until the pressure gradient is equal, according to Boyle's law. For inspiration to occur, the gas pressure in the alveoli must be less than that in the atmosphere. For expiration, the gas pressure in the alveoli must be greater than that in the atmosphere (Kent 2000).

Inspiration

Inspiration is an active process, requiring energy, which occurs by enlarging the thoracic cavity (the intercostal muscles contract, drawing the rib cage upwards and outwards, and the diaphragm contracts and moves downwards), increasing the volume of the lungs. As the ribcage and diaphragm move, the parietal and visceral pleura, and consequently the lungs, are pulled with them, causing lung expansion. This reduces the gas pressure in the alveoli to below atmospheric pressure, creating a pressure gradient, drawing air into the lungs until alveolar pressure equals atmospheric pressure.

Expiration

During the relatively passive process of expiration, the respiratory muscles relax, reducing the volume of the thoracic cavity, resulting in an elastic recoil of the lungs and an associated temporary rise in alveolar pressure to above atmospheric pressure. This rise in alveolar pressure causes air to be pushed out of the lungs. Three factors can affect ventilation: compliance and elasticity of the lung tissue, and airway resistance.

Health Promotion: Covid-19 in Pregnancy

Women with Covid-19 are more likely to get seriously ill, which can lead to pregnancy problems, for example preterm birth or having a baby with a low birth weight.

Look at the research on Covid-19 in pregnancy and associated outcomes for women and their babies and describe how you would support and advise a woman in your antenatal clinic to make an informed decision about whether she should have the Covid-19 vaccine while pregnant.

- Pregnancy and coronavirus (Covid-19) (NHS 2022).
- Covid-19 during pregnancy (Centers for Disease Control and Prevention 2022).
- SARS-CoV-2 and pregnancy rapid report March–May 2020 (Knight et al. 2020).
- SARS-CoV-2 and pregnancy rapid report June 2020–March 2021 (Knight et al. 2021).

Gaseous Exchange

Diffusion is the movement of a substance across a semi-permeable membrane from an area of high concentration to an area of low concentration to reach equilibrium. Diffusion determines the movement of gases in external and internal respiration. The pressure exerted by an individual gas in a mixture is known as its partial pressure, PO_2 or PCO_2.

Alveolar air is saturated with water vapour and contains decreased oxygen and increased carbon dioxide levels. Gaseous exchange (external respiration) between the alveoli and surrounding blood capillaries is constant.

External Respiration

External respiration is the exchange of gases at the alveolar surface between the alveoli and blood capillaries that surround them (Figure 15.7). Blood arriving at the alveoli in the pulmonary artery from tissue cells of the body has high levels of carbon dioxide (5.8 kPa) and low levels of oxygen (5.3 kPa) compared to alveolar air (PO_2 13.3 kPa, PCO_2 5.3 kPa). Carbon dioxide diffuses down a concentration gradient into the alveoli, and oxygen diffuses from the alveoli to the blood in the capillaries. Blood leaving the alveoli has equal carbon dioxide and oxygen concentrations to that of the air in the alveolar space.

Internal Respiration

Internal respiration is the exchange of gases at the level of the cells in the tissues between the systemic capillaries and tissue cells (Figure 15.8). Blood arriving at the cells in the body from the lungs has high levels of oxygen (13.3 kPa) and low levels of carbon dioxide (5.3 kPa). This creates a concentration gradient between the capillaries and tissue cells of the

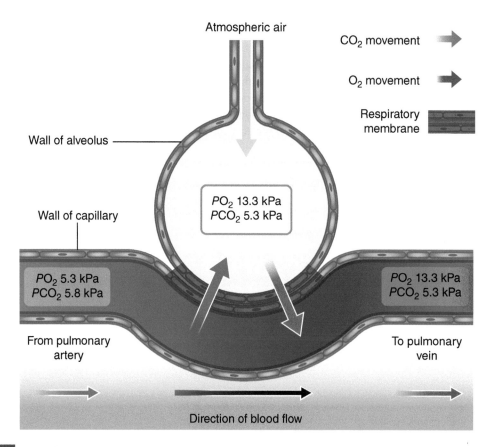

FIGURE 15.7   External respiration.

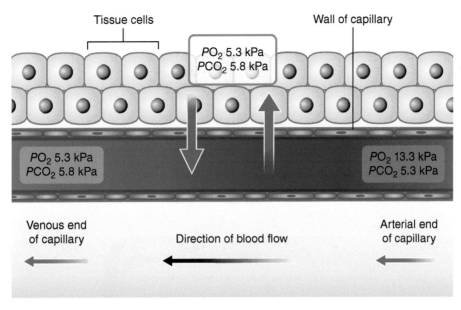

Tissue cells

Wall of capillary

PO_2 5.3 kPa
PCO_2 5.8 kPa

PO_2 5.3 kPa
PCO_2 5.8 kPa

PO_2 13.3 kPa
PCO_2 5.3 kPa

Venous end
of capillary

Direction of blood flow

Arterial end
of capillary

FIGURE 15.8 Internal respiration.

body. Oxygen diffuses down a concentration gradient from the capillaries into the cell, and carbon dioxide diffuses from the cells into the blood in the capillaries.

Figure 15.9 summarises internal and external respiration processes.

Transport of Gases

The two gases involved in respiration, oxygen and carbon dioxide, are carried in the blood in different ways. **Oxygen** is mostly (99%) transported attached to haemoglobin molecules in the erythrocytes in the form of oxyhaemoglobin, a reversible reaction. A small amount of oxygen is also carried dissolved in the plasma.

$$\text{Oxygen} + \text{haemoglobin} \rightleftharpoons \text{oxyhaemoglobin}$$

Carbon dioxide is a waste product of metabolism and is mostly (70%) transported in the plasma of blood as bicarbonate ions (HCO_3^-). About 23% of the carbon dioxide is transported in the erythrocytes as carbaminohaemoglobin. Approximately 7% of the carbon dioxide is carried in simple solution in plasma.

Control of Respiration

Respiration is normally under involuntary control as the body responds to varying changes in conditions. Voluntary control can be exerted as the need arises, for example due to speaking. However, involuntary control resumes if carbon dioxide levels in the blood rise (hypercapnia), disrupting homeostasis.

Nervous control of respiration is via the respiratory centre, a group of nerves found in the medulla oblongata in the brainstem that control the rate and depth of breathing via inspiratory neurons (Figure 15.10). The pneumotaxic centre (inhibitory, preventing overinflation of the lungs) and the apneustic centre (stimulatory, prolonging inhalation) situated in the pons, higher in the brainstem, adjust the activity of the respiratory centre (Stables and Rankin 2010; Waugh and Grant 2018).

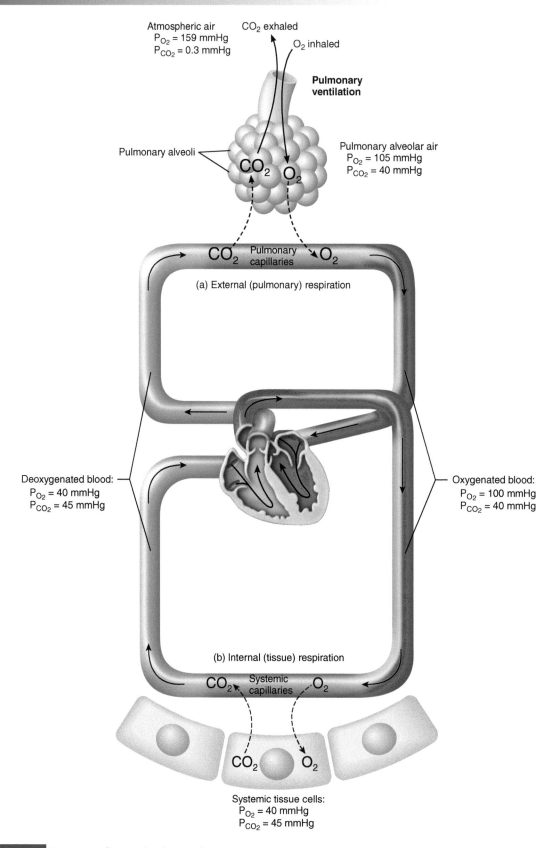

Atmospheric air
P_{O_2} = 159 mmHg
P_{CO_2} = 0.3 mmHg

CO_2 exhaled

O_2 inhaled

Pulmonary ventilation

Pulmonary alveoli

CO_2 O_2

Pulmonary alveolar air
P_{O_2} = 105 mmHg
P_{CO_2} = 40 mmHg

CO_2 Pulmonary capillaries O_2

(a) External (pulmonary) respiration

Deoxygenated blood:
P_{O_2} = 40 mmHg
P_{CO_2} = 45 mmHg

Oxygenated blood:
P_{O_2} = 100 mmHg
P_{CO_2} = 40 mmHg

(b) Internal (tissue) respiration

CO_2 Systemic capillaries O_2

CO_2 O_2

Systemic tissue cells:
P_{O_2} = 40 mmHg
P_{CO_2} = 45 mmHg

FIGURE 15.9   Summary of internal and external respiration.

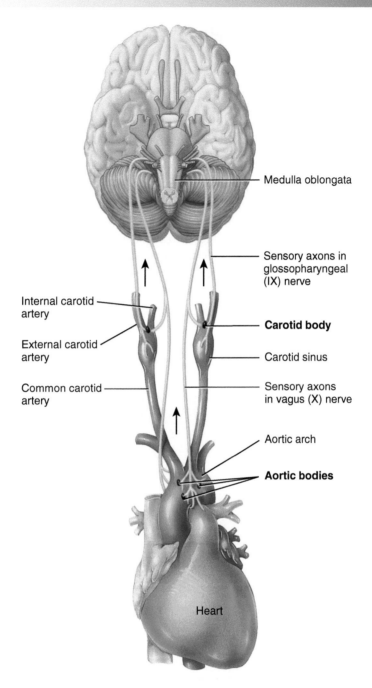

Medulla oblongata

Sensory axons in glossopharyngeal (IX) nerve

Internal carotid artery

Carotid body

External carotid artery

Carotid sinus

Common carotid artery

Sensory axons in vagus (X) nerve

Aortic arch

Aortic bodies

Heart

FIGURE 15.10 Structures involved in the control of respiration. Source: Reproduced by permission from Waugh and Grant (2018) / Elsevier.

Chemical control is via centrally and peripherally located receptors that detect changes in arterial partial pressures of oxygen and carbon dioxide. Peripheral chemoreceptors can be found in the carotid bodies and in the arch of the aorta. They send impulses to the respiratory centre to alter ventilation when they detect changes to PO_2, PCO_2 and H^+. Central chemoreceptors are found on the surface of the medulla oblongata, primarily responding to hypercapnia (excessive carbon dioxide levels). An increase in hydrogen ions detected by central chemoreceptors causes impulses to be sent to the respiratory centre to increase the ventilation rate, thereby decreasing the PCO_2.

275

Physiological Changes in Pregnancy

During pregnancy, there are increased metabolic demands of the maternal and fetal tissues. To compensate for this, there is an increase in metabolic rate and maternal respiratory effort whereby minute ventilation increases by 15% and approximately 16–20% more oxygen is consumed (Table 15.1). The expanding uterus also affects the respiratory system as it grows. The elevation of the maternal diaphragm in late pregnancy results in functional residual capacity falling by 20% in the third trimester. However, movement of the diaphragm and therefore vital capacity remain unchanged.

The upper respiratory tract and airway mucosa are affected also by hormonal changes in pregnancy. Although airway patency and gaseous exchange across the alveoli remain stable in pregnancy, increasing oestrogen levels cause airway mucosal hyperaemia, oedema, hypersecretion and friability (Koehler et al. 2005).

Oestrogen also plays a part in increasing the number and sensitivity of progesterone receptors in the hypothalamus and medulla. Increasing progesterone levels in pregnancy increases the sensitivity of the respiratory centre to carbon dioxide levels. Both hormones also increase the hypoxic sensitivity of peripheral chemoreceptors. A relaxation of the bronchioles can also result from increased levels of progesterone, sometimes leading to some dyspnoea.

During labour, an increase in tidal volume and respiratory rate may be caused by pain levels. After delivery, the changes in the respiratory system rapidly return to normal due to delivery of the placenta leading to a fall in progesterone levels.

TABLE 15.1   Physiological changes in respiratory function in pregnancy.

Physiological variable	Change
Oxygen consumption	Increases by approximately 20%
Metabolic rate	Increases by approximately 15%
Minute ventilation	Increases by approximately 15%
Tidal volume	Increases
Functional residual capacity	Decreases by approximately 20% in third trimester
Vital capacity	Unchanged
Partial pressure of oxygen (PaO_2)	Increases
Partial pressure of carbon dioxide ($PaCO_2$)	Decreases
Arterial pH	Increases

Respiratory Conditions in Pregnancy

Breathlessness or Dyspnoea in Pregnancy

The sensation of feeling out of breath or the inability to catch your breath is known as breathlessness or dyspnoea. Breathlessness is common and occurs in approximately three-quarters of women at some time during pregnancy, but is most common during the third trimester. Approximately 50% of women experience breathlessness by 20 weeks and around 70% by 30 weeks of pregnancy (Mehta et al. 2015; Stone and Nelson-Piercy 2012). It can potentially cause diagnostic confusion (Nelson-Piercy 2020). Breathlessness can be due to many diagnoses, for example generalised dyspnoea, asthma, cardiac disease, arrhythmia, pulmonary embolism.

Considerations for Pregnancy: Breathlessness

Antenatal Period

Breathlessness in pregnancy is usually due to a physiological response. If symptoms are severe or worsening, a pathological cause must be considered. Investigations must be discussed and evaluated regarding benefit and risk for the woman and her unborn baby. Antenatal education and support from the midwife are essential.

Intrapartum Period

Breathlessness in labour not associated with contractions needs an early referral to an obstetrician by the midwife. Maternal observations (MEWS) will guide frequency and escalation processes in addition to the need for the baby to be continuously monitored.

Postnatal Period

Postnatal breathlessness is unusual and should be escalated appropriately. Causes may include pulmonary embolism, haemorrhage or anaemia.

Asthma

Asthma is a common chronic inflammatory condition of the lung airways and affects approximately 7% of childbearing-age women, occasionally being first diagnosed in pregnancy (Stone and Nelson-Piercy 2012). Asthma is caused by allergen exposure or triggers initiating an inflammatory response, for example smoking, pollen allergy, exercise, drugs or pollution.

Exposure to allergens or triggers causes an overactivity in the inflammatory response of the bronchioles in the lungs. T lymphocytes overproduce cytokines that stimulate the production and release of the antibody immunoglobulin E (IgE). These antibodies bind to mast cells in the lungs leading to the release of histamine, prostaglandin and thromboxane A_2. These chemicals cause the mucous membrane and muscle layers of the bronchioles to thicken, reducing airflow in the lungs and the muscles go into spasm (bronchospasm) (Figure 15.11). The mucous glands also enlarge and there is an excessive secretion of thick sticky mucus that exacerbates the airway narrowing. The cytokine increases also cause leucocytes, such as eosinophils and platelets, to accumulate in the airways, which lead to epithelial damage (Hazeldine 2013).

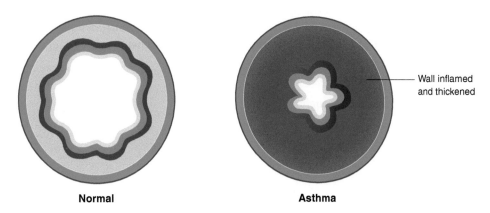

Normal   **Asthma**

Wall inflamed and thickened

FIGURE 15.11 Changes to the diameter of the bronchioles in asthma.

If asthma is well controlled in pregnancy, there is a low risk of adverse maternal and fetal complications. Therapy should be optimised in pregnancy to reduce the risk of acute asthma attacks. There is more of a risk to the pregnant woman and her fetus from poorly controlled severe asthma than from the medications used to prevent or treat it.

Common symptoms of asthma, which are usually worse at night and in the early morning, include:

- Shortness of breath
- Chest tightness
- Episodes of wheeziness
- Cough

Medicines Management: Asthma – A Stepwise Approach

Step	Severity	Preferred treatment	Notes
One	Mild, intermittent	No daily medication needed	Short-acting bronchodilators as needed during episodes of symptoms
Two	Mild, persistent	Low-dose inhaled corticosteroids	
Three	Moderate, persistent, daily symptoms	*Either* low-dose inhaled corticosteroids and long-acting beta2-agonist *or* medium-dose inhaled corticosteroids	Alternatively, can use a medium-dose inhaled corticosteroid and long-acting inhaled beta2-agonist if a woman has recurring severe exacerbations
Four	Severe persistent, continual symptoms, frequent nocturnal symptoms	High-dose inhaled corticosteroids and long-acting inhaled beta2-agonist *and*, if needed, corticosteroid tablets long term	

Source: Adapted from National Institutes of Health and National Heart, Lung, and Blood Institute (2005).

Pneumonia

Although there is no increased frequency of pneumonia occurring in the pregnant population compared to the general population, pneumonia in pregnancy can be more virulent with increased mortality. Women with a pre-existing history of asthma, cystic fibrosis, anaemia, smoking and an immunosuppressive state have an increased risk of contracting pneumonia. Of antenatal admissions to intensive care units, 40% are for pneumonia (Nelson-Piercy 2020). Preterm delivery and low-birth-weight infants are associated with severe pneumonia in pregnancy (Stone and Nelson-Piercy 2012).

Common symptoms of pneumonia include:

- Dry cough developing into a productive cough
- Purulent sputum
- Malaise
- Pyrexia
- Tachycardia
- Rigors in severe cases
- Tachypnoea
- Pleuritic pain on inspiration

Red Flag: Pneumonia and Antibiotic Therapy

If a pregnant or postnatal woman is diagnosed with pneumonia, consideration of which antibiotic to commence is important according to gestation in pregnancy and whether the woman is breastfeeding if postnatal.

Aminoglycosides, tetracycline and quinolones are contra-indicated in pregnancy and breastfeeding.

If amoxicillin is prescribed, a higher dose is needed in pregnancy (500 mg three times daily).

Tuberculosis

Tuberculosis is a major health concern worldwide, in particular in low-income countries where prevention or treatment may not be readily available. Approximately 1.5 million deaths to tuberculosis are estimated to occur worldwide and tuberculosis is the 13th leading cause of death (WHO 2021). *Mycobacterium tuberculosis* is the main bacteria causing caseating granulomas within the lungs. Little evidence exists as to the effects between pregnancy and tuberculosis and treatment should not be delayed. BCG vaccination should be recommended to all neonates at risk of tuberculosis due to contact in pregnancy or parental origin from a high-risk country.

Learning Event: Tuberculosis and BCG Immunisation of the Neonate

Conduct research on:

- The countries of parental origin that would be at high risk for tuberculosis and therefore would require a BCG vaccination to be offered to the neonate.
- The immunisation schedule for the BCG vaccination in the neonate.

You may find the following resources useful:

- TB, BCG vaccine and your baby (UKHSA 2021a).
- BCG vaccination programme (UKHSA 2021b).

Common symptoms of tuberculosis include:

- Cough
- Haemoptysis
- Weight loss
- Night sweats

Medicines Management: Tuberculosis

Treatment of tuberculosis in pregnancy is recommended due to the increased risk of maternal and fetal morbidity and mortality (Mehta et al. 2015). The disease is associated with an increased risk of:

- Prematurity
- Low birth weight
- Stillbirth

Usual first-line treatment is triple or quadruple therapy for the first two months followed by a course of more than one drug that the organism is sensitive to:

- Isoniazid
- Rifampicin
- Pyrazinamide
- Ethambutol

Pulmonary Embolism

A pulmonary embolism (PE) is a thromboembolic event caused by a blockage, usually a blood clot, in the pulmonary artery, therefore potentially preventing blood flow to the lungs (Figure 15.12). Usually, the cause is from a deep vein thrombosis (DVT) in the leg or pelvis that travels through the circulation to the lungs to cause a PE. Damage to blood vessels can cause the formation of a blood clot.

Common symptoms of a pulmonary embolism are:

- Dyspnoea
- Tachypnoea
- Pleuritic pain
- Cough
- Haemoptysis

Learning Event: Diagnosis of a Pulmonary Embolism

Symptoms of a PE are like those of other respiratory conditions and the severity of the PE can vary. This can make diagnosis difficult. Different tests can be carried out to help confirm a diagnosis of a PE.

- What care plan would you put in place if a woman with symptoms of a PE arrived at maternity triage?
- List the different diagnostic tests that could be performed.
- What are the considerations for the mother and the fetus around having these different diagnostic tests?

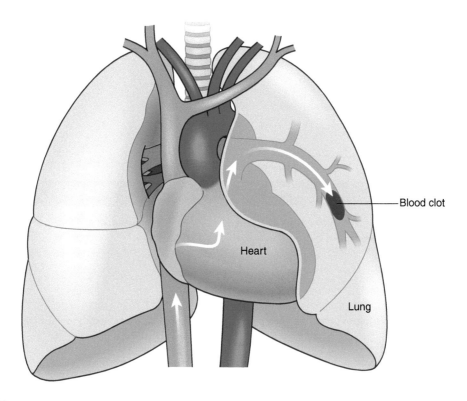

FIGURE 15.12 Pulmonary embolism.

Medicines Management: Prophylactic Low Molecular Weight Heparin

Thrombosis and thromboembolism remain the leading direct cause of maternal deaths as reported by MBRRACE-UK (Knight et al. 2022). Royal College of Obstetricians and Gynaecologists (RCOG 2015b) guidelines recommend prophylaxis treatment from either the first trimester, 28 weeks' gestation or postnatally depending on several risk factors.

Review the venous thromboembolism (VTE) risk assessment charts in your area of work.

- What would be your recommended prophylaxis treatment for a woman with a body mass index (BMI) of 32 kg/m², who smoked 10 cigarettes a day and had three children already?
- Why do you think MBRRACE-UK recommends reweighing pregnant women at 28 weeks' gestation?

Expert Midwife: D-dimer Testing in Pregnancy

D-dimer testing is often used to investigate acute VTE in the non-pregnant state. Due to the progressive rise in D-dimer levels during pregnancy to 'abnormal' levels at term in a healthy woman, a positive D-dimer test in pregnancy is not necessarily consistent with a VTE. D-dimer levels are also raised further in:

- Multiple pregnancies
- Following caesarean section
- Major postpartum haemorrhage

Consequently, D-dimer testing in pregnancy is not recommended (RCOG 2015a).

Cystic Fibrosis

Cystic fibrosis (CF) is a genetic, autosomal recessive disorder affecting the exocrine glands, leading to an increase in mucus secretions and ion transport, particularly sodium and chloride, at the epithelial cells of these glands. It results when the CF transmembrane conductance regulator protein (CFTR) is either not made at all or is not made correctly. The respiratory, gastrointestinal, endocrine and reproductive systems are all affected by this disorder (Figure 15.13). It affects 1 in 25 Caucasian people.

Common symptoms of CF are:

- Repetitive and persistent lung infections
- Wheezing, coughing and shortness of breath
- Malnutrition affecting weight gain and growth
- Jaundice
- Diarrhoea or constipation
- Salty sweat

A multidisciplinary approach is key when planning the care of a woman with CF. Risks to the fetus include preterm birth, intrauterine growth restriction and CF diagnosis.

Orange Flag: Cystic Fibrosis and Pregnancy

Pre-pregnancy counselling is essential if a woman has CF. Since the woman is homozygous for the disorder, all offspring will be carriers of the CF gene. Partner genetic testing is advised to determine if they are also a carrier.

Although the median survival age of CF sufferers has increased over the years due to medical advancements allowing better management of symptoms, women with CF are still unlikely to live long enough to see their children into adulthood.

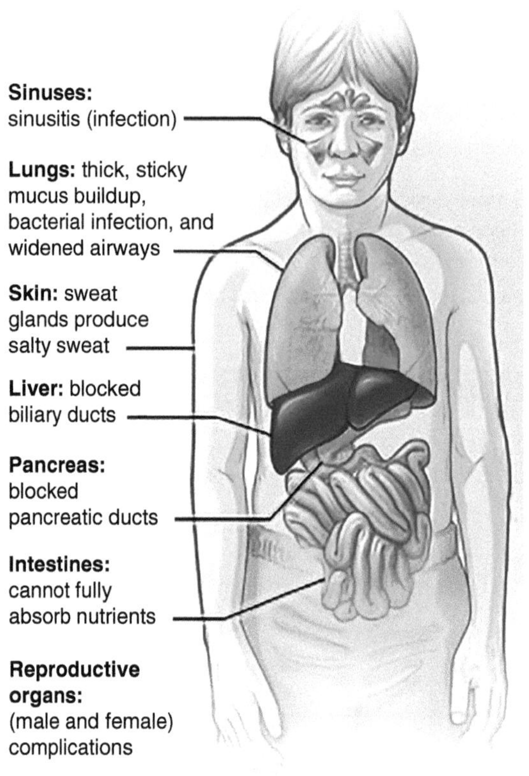

Sinuses:
sinusitis (infection)

Lungs: thick, sticky
mucus buildup,
bacterial infection, and
widened airways

Skin: sweat
glands produce
salty sweat

Liver: blocked
biliary ducts

Pancreas:
blocked
pancreatic ducts

Intestines:
cannot fully
absorb nutrients

Reproductive
organs:
(male and female)
complications

FIGURE 15.13   Organs affected by cystic fibrosis.

Considerations for Pregnancy: Cystic Fibrosis

Antenatal Period

- Ensure an appointment has been made with a consultant after antenatal booking with a midwife.
- Regular growth scans are advised to monitor for signs of intrauterine growth restriction.
- Promote a healthy lifestyle and nutritious diet, including dietary supplements where prescribed.
- Monitor for signs of breathlessness and escalate accordingly.

Intrapartum Period

- Anaesthetic review is advised as if a caesarean section is required, general anaesthesia may be contra-indicated.
- Ensure oxygen supplementation is available in the delivery room should it be required.
- Continuous fetal monitoring is advised.
- Prolonged active second stage of labour should be avoided.
- If preterm birth is likely, a paediatrician should be alerted to be ready for delivery.

Postnatal Period

- The woman should continue her normal CF management routine, including dietary supplements.
- CF testing is included in the newborn blood spot screen that is part of the UK National Screening Programme.

Cigarette Smoking in Pregnancy

It has long been established that smoking is linked to maternal and infant mortality and morbidity (Patrick and Bauman 1997; Bai et al. 2000). Maternal smoking has been shown to decrease the amount of oxygen being transported to the fetus in utero. Carbon monoxide from the cigarette smoke binds with haemoglobin instead of oxygen to make carboxyhaemoglobin, reducing the number of binding sites on haemoglobin molecules for oxygen (Chappell and Lilley 1994). Studies have linked maternal smoking in pregnancy and the postnatal period to the following neonatal outcomes:

- Reduced level of pulmonary function (Cook and Strachan 1999; Stocks and Dezateux 2003).
- Increased risk of asthma (Gililand et al. 2001; Milner et al. 2007).
- Increased risk of respiratory infection (Taylor and Wadsworth 1987).
- Low birth weight (Secker-Walker and Vacek 2003).
- Premature birth (Secker-Walker and Vacek 2003).

Case Study 15.1   Smoking in Pregnancy

Martha attended an antenatal booking appointment for her pregnancy. She has a BMI of $26\,kg/m^2$, suffers from asthma, has a 2-year-old child at home who had a low birth weight comparable to their gestation, on the second centile, and Martha had a normal blood pressure. The midwife asked if she could take Martha's carbon monoxide reading and Martha accepted. Her carbon monoxide level was 12 ppm. The midwife explained she would refer Martha to the local smoking-cessation service and discussed how smoking could affect her pregnancy.

1. Why do you think the NHS has now adopted an 'opt-out' system for smoking cessation?
2. All health professionals should offer very brief and brief interventions as part of their role in health promotion. Explain what very brief and brief interventions are and how they can be beneficial in supporting a woman to stop smoking.
3. Read 'Saving babies' lives: a care bundle for reducing stillbirth' to ensure you can give evidence-based advice to a woman on the importance of smoking cessation in pregnancy.

Source: Adapted from NHS England (2016).

The Respiratory System and the Neonate

In utero, the fetus's lungs are fluid filled and gaseous exchange is carried out by the placenta. Respiratory movements can be seen on ultrasound scan in pregnancy, drawing small amounts of amniotic fluid into the fetal air passages, causing development of lung tissue. The lung fluid begins to be absorbed by the alveolar epithelial cells at the onset of labour, triggered by hormonal changes. Passage through the vagina during the second stage of labour allows for the remainder of the amniotic fluid present in the fetal lungs to be removed. Babies born by elective caesarean section are two to three times more likely to suffer respiratory morbidity as these hormonal and physical changes are not triggered (Hansen et al. 2008; Kamath et al. 2009). Various stimuli at delivery (change in temperature, touch, noise, lights) cause the baby to take their first breath and cry, resulting in any remaining fluid being absorbed by the epithelial cells.

Surfactant

Surfactant is a phospholipid fluid secreted by septal cells in the lungs. Surfactant reduces surface tension in the alveoli, preventing their collapse during expiration. From 35 weeks' gestation a fetus starts secreting surfactant into the distal air passages and alveoli.

Respiratory Distress Syndrome in the Neonate

Without surfactant the lungs cannot function effectively and severe breathing problems can develop. A baby born before 34 weeks of pregnancy may not have accumulated enough surfactant to cope with breathing, may have immature lungs and can suffer from respiratory distress syndrome (RDS). RDS occurs when the alveoli collapse during expiration due to the lack of surfactant. Once collapsed, an increased effort is needed to reinflate the alveoli. Damage to the alveoli epithelium and capillary walls causes plasma to leak into the alveoli air spaces, making breathing extremely difficult. Surfactant can be introduced artificially into the lungs of premature babies to help minimise the effects of respiratory distress syndrome (Jena et al. 2019). A baby with RDS may need to be treated with a ventilator in addition to administration of surfactant.

Woman-Centred Care: Premature Birth and Respiratory Distress Syndrome

Having a baby at an early gestation who may need neonatal resuscitation and admittance to the neonatal unit can be extremely scary and worrying for both parents. If premature birth is likely, the best course of action would be to fully inform the parents of what might need to happen to support their baby's transition to air breathing. If birth is imminent, then a full explanation needs to be given as soon as possible after the baby has been stabilised. Ideally resuscitation should take place where the parents are so that they can see their baby. Some hospitals have mobile resuscitation trolleys so that this can be carried out at the bedside of the mother. Once the baby has been stabilised and is maintaining their temperature, the parents preferably need time to see, touch and hold their child before the baby is taken to the neonatal unit.

Conditions Associated with the Respiratory System

The following is a list of conditions that are associated with the respiratory system. Take some time and write notes about each of the conditions. Think about the medications that may be used to treat these conditions and be specific about the pharmacokinetics and pharmacodynamics. Remember to include aspects of patient care. If you are making notes about women you have offered care and support, to you must ensure that you have adhered to the rules of confidentiality.

The condition	Your notes
Asthma	
Tuberculosis	
Pulmonary embolism	
Influenza	
Breathlessness	
Amniotic fluid embolism	
Cystic fibrosis	

Take-Home Points

- Respiration is the process whereby gaseous exchange occurs at the lungs (oxygen is taken from the atmosphere) and the cells of the body (carbon dioxide is returned to the lungs to be expired) to provide the essential reactants for cell metabolism.
- The respiratory system can be divided structurally into the upper and lower respiratory systems and functionally into the conducting and respiratory parts.
- Pregnancy, labour and the postnatal period increase demand on the respiratory system due to increased metabolic demands of the mother and fetus.
- In utero, the functions of the fetal respiratory system are carried out by the placenta; after birth the respiratory system begins to function in a healthy term neonate.
- There are many diseases affecting the respiratory system and pregnancy is an added risk factor if a woman has any pre-existing respiratory condition or develops a respiratory disease in her pregnancy or the postnatal period.
- Treatment and medication for respiratory conditions should always follow policy and protocol for any contra-indications in pregnancy.

Conclusion

The respiratory system provides the oxygen needed for cellular respiration. Many disorders can affect the respiratory system, for example asthma, Covid-19 and pulmonary embolism, and can cause increased concern in a pregnant woman. The midwife needs to ensure she is aware of any changes affecting a woman or her baby's respiratory system and escalate accordingly to the obstetric or neonatal team.

References

Bai, J., Wong, F.W.S., Gyaneshwar, R., and Stewart, H.C. (2000). Profile of maternal smokers and their pregnancy outcomes in southwestern Sydney. *Journal of Obstetrics and Gynaecology Research* 26: 127–132.

Centers for Disease Control and Prevention (2022). Pregnant and recently pregnant people at risk increased risk for severe illness from COVID-19. https://www.cdc.gov/coronavirus/2019-ncov/need-extra-precautions/pregnant-people.html (accessed November 2023).

Chappell, C. and Lilley, G. (1994). Effects of smoking on the fetus and young children. *British Journal of Midwifery* 2 (12): 587–591.

Cook, D.G. and Strachan, D.P. (1999). Health effects of passive smoking. 10. Summary of effects of parental smoking on the respiratory health of children and implications for research. *Thorax* 54: 357–366.

Department of Health (DOH) (2010). *Midwifery 2020: Delivering Expectations*. London: Department of Health.

Gililand, F.D., Li, Y.F., and Peters, J.M. (2001). Effects of maternal smoking during pregnancy and environmental tobacco smoke on asthma and wheezing in children. *American Journal of Respiratory and Critical Care Medicine* 163: 429–436.

Hansen, A.K., Wisborg, K., Uldbjerg, N. et al. (2008). Risk of respiratory morbidity in term infants delivered by elective caesarean section: cohort study. *British Medical Journal* 336: 85–87.

Hazeldine, V. (2013). Pharmacological management of acute asthma exacerbations in adults. *Nursing Standard* 27 (33): 43–49.

Jena, S.R., Bains, H.S., Pandita, A. et al. (2019). Surfactant therapy in premature babies: SurE or InSurE. *Pediatric Pulmonology* 54 (11): 1747–1752.

Kamath, B.D., Todd, J.K., Glazner, J.E. et al. (2009). Neonatal outcomes after elective caesarean delivery. *Obstetrics and Gynecology* 113: 1231–1238.

Kent, M. (2000). *Advanced Biology*. Oxford: Oxford University Press.

Knight, M., Bunch, K., Cairns, A. et al. on behalf of MBRRACE-UK. (2020). Saving lives, improving mothers' care rapid report: learning from SARS-CoV-2-related and associated maternal deaths in the UK March–May 2020. Oxford: National Perinatal Epidemiology Unit, University of Oxford.

Knight, M., Bunch, K., Cairns, A. et al. on behalf of MBRRACE-UK. (2021). Saving lives, improving mothers' care rapid report 2021: learning from SARS-CoV-2-related and associated maternal deaths in the UK June 2020–March 2021. Oxford: National Perinatal Epidemiology Unit, University of Oxford.

Knight, M., Bunch, K., Patel, R. et al. on behalf of MBRRACE-UK(2022). *Saving lives, improving mothers' care: lessons learned to inform maternity care from the UK and Ireland Confidential Enquiries into Maternal Deaths and Morbidity 2018–20*. Oxford: National Perinatal Epidemiology Unit, University of Oxford.

Koehler, K.F., Helguero, L.A., Haldosén, L.A. et al. (2005). Reflections on the discovery and significance of oestrogen receptor beta. *Endocrine Reviews* 26: 465–478.

Mehta, N., Chen, K., Hardy, E., and Powrie, R. (2015). Respiratory disease in pregnancy. *Best Practice and Research Clinical Obstetrics and Gynaecology* 29: 598–611.

Milner, A.D., Rao, H., and Greenough, A. (2007). The effects of antenatal smoking on lung function and respiratory symptoms in infants and children. *Early Human Development* 83: 707–711.

National Health Service (NHS) (2016). Saving babies' lives: a care bundle for reducing stillbirth. https://www.england.nhs.uk/wp-content/uploads/2016/03/saving-babies-lives-car-bundl.pdf (accessed November 2023).

National Health Service (NHS) (2022). Pregnancy and coronavirus (COVID-19). https://www.nhs.uk/conditions/coronavirus-covid-19/people-at-higher-risk/pregnancy-and-coronavirus (accessed November 2023).

National Institutes of Health and National Heart, Lung, and Blood Institute (2005). Managing asthma during pregnancy. Recommendations for pharmacologic treatment. http://www.nhlbi.nih.gov/files/docs/astpreg_qr.pdf (accessed November 2023).

Nelson-Piercy, C. (2020). Respiratory disease. In: *Handbook of Obstetric Medicine*, 6e (ed. C. Nelson-Piercy), 64–87. London: CRC Press.

Patrick, P.L. and Bauman, A. (1997). How well does epidemiological evidence hold for the relationship between smoking and adverse obstetric outcomes in New South Wales? *Australian and New Zealand Journal of Obstetrics and Gynaecology* 37: 168–173.

Royal College of Obstetricians and Gynaecologists (RCOG) (2015a). Chickenpox in pregnancy. Green-top guideline no. 13. https://www.rcog.org.uk/guidance/browse-all-guidance/green-top-guidelines/chickenpox-in-pregnancy-green-top-guideline-no-13 (accessed November 2023).

Royal College of Obstetricians and Gynaecologists (RCOG) (2015b). Thromboembolic disease in pregnancy and the puerperium: acute management. Green-top guideline no. 37b. https://www.rcog.org.uk/media/wj2lpco5/gtg-37b-1.pdf (accessed November 2023).

Secker-Walker, R.H. and Vacek, P.M. (2003). Relationships between cigarette smoking during pregnancy, gestational age, maternal weight gain, and infant birthweight. *Addictive Behaviour* 28: 55–66.

Stables, D. and Rankin, J. (2010). *Physiology in Childbearing*, 3e. London: Elsevier.

Stocks, J. and Dezateux, C. (2003). The effect of parental smoking on lung function and development during infancy. *Respirology* 8: 266–285.

Stone, S. and Nelson-Piercy, C. (2012). Respiratory disease in pregnancy. *Obstetrics, Gynaecology and Reproductive Medicine* 22 (10): 290–298.

Taylor, B. and Wadsworth, J. (1987). Maternal smoking during pregnancy and lower respiratory tract illness in early life. *Archives of Disease in Childhood* 62: 786–791.

UK Health Security Agency (UKHSA) (2021a). TB, BCG vaccine and your baby. https://assets.publishing.service.gov.uk/government/uploads/system/uploads/attachment_data/file/1017772/UKHSA_12079_TB_BCG_and_your_baby_leaflet.pdf (accessed November 2023).

UK Health Security Agency (UKHSA) (2021b). BCG vaccination programme. https://www.gov.uk/government/collections/bcg-vaccination-programme (accessed November 2023).

Waugh, A. and Grant, A. (2018). *Anatomy and Physiology in Health and Illness*, 13e. London: Elsevier.

World Health Organization (2021). Tuberculosis. https://www.who.int/news-room/fact-sheets/detail/tuberculosis (accessed November 2023).

Wylie, L. (2005). *Essential Anatomy and Physiology in Maternity Care*, 2e. London: Elsevier.

Further Resources

Bhatia, P. and Bhatia, K. (2000). Pregnancy and the lungs. *Postgraduate Medical Journal* 76: 683–689.

Jensen, D., Webb, K.A., and O'Donnell, D.E. (2007). Chemical and mechanical adaptations of the respiratory system at rest and during exercise in human pregnancy. *Applied Physiology, Nutrition, and Metabolism* 32 (6): 1239–1250.

LoMauro, A., Aliverti, A., Frykholm, P. et al. (2019). Adaptation of lung, chest wall, and respiratory muscles during pregnancy: preparing for birth. *Journal of Applied Physiology* 127 (6): 1640–1650.

Tan, E.K. and Tan, E.L. (2013). Alterations in physiology and anatomy during pregnancy. *Best Practice and Research Clinical Obstetrics and Gynaecology* 27: 791–802.

Glossary

Alveoli	Tiny air sacs at the end of the alveoli ducts where gaseous exchange occurs
Blood plasma	A straw-coloured liquid component of blood in which blood cells are absent
Chemoreceptors	Sensors that detect changes in the carbon dioxide, oxygen and pH levels in the body, can be central or peripheral
Cilia	Tiny, threadlike projection from the surface of a cell body
Diffusion	The movement of a substance from an area of high concentration to an area of low concentration
Dyspnoea	Difficult or laboured breathing, e.g. breathlessness
Erythrocyte	A red blood cell, which is biconcave in shape, usually without a nucleus. Contains haemoglobin
Eustachian tubes	Connect the middle ears to the back of your throat. They help equalise air pressure inside your ears and drain fluid
Haemoptysis	Coughing up blood
Hyperaemia	An excess of blood in the vessels supplying an organ or other part of the body
Hypercapnia	An increase in the partial pressure of carbon dioxide (PCO_2) in the blood
Intercostal muscles	Accessory muscles to respiration, found in between the 12 ribs
Mediastinum	The central portion of the thoracic cavity that contains a group of structures related to the respiratory system including the trachea, nerves and blood vessels
Medulla oblongata	The lowest part of the brainstem connected to the midbrain by the pons. It plays a critical role in transmitting signals between the spinal cord and the brain in controlling activities such as respiration
Metabolism	A series of chemical reactions in the body that provide energy for the body's vital processes
Oestrogen	A sex hormone responsible for the development and regulation of the female reproductive system
Oxygenated blood	Blood rich in oxygen
Pleural membrane	A serous membrane that folds back on itself to form a two-layered membranous pleural sac around the lungs
Pleuritic pain	A sharp chest pain when breathing
Pons	Part of the brainstem lying inferior to the midbrain and superior to the medulla oblongata. Controls unconscious processes such as breathing
Progesterone	A sex hormone released from the ovary responsible for control of the menstrual cycle and in maintaining the early stages of pregnancy
Purulent sputum	Sputum that is off-white, yellow or green and opaque in appearance
Surfactant	A compound of phospholipids and proteins that decreases surface tension in the lungs
Tachypnoea	Increased respiratory rate
Ventilation	The flow of air into and out of the alveoli of the lungs during inspiration and expiration

CHAPTER 16

The Gastrointestinal System and Associated Disorders and Nutrition

Clare Gordon[1] and Claire Leader[2]

[1] *College of Nursing, Midwifery and Healthcare, University of West London, London, UK*

[2] *Department of Nursing, Midwifery and Health, Northumbria University, Newcastle upon Tyne, UK*

AIM

The aim of this chapter is to provide an overview of the pathophysiology and disorders associated with the gastrointestinal system in pregnancy and the postnatal period, and to offer the reader some insight into the considerations for nutrition for the mother and the developing fetus.

LEARNING OUTCOMES

On completion of this chapter the reader will be able to:

- Identify the anatomy of the gastrointestinal system
- Describe the function of the organs contained within the gastrointestinal system and the associated pathophysiology leading to disorders
- Discuss the processes involved in digestion and associated pathophysiology
- Describe the way in which associated disorders manifest in pregnancy and consider appropriate care pathways and public health interventions

Test Your Prior Knowledge

1. What are the key organs of the gastrointestinal system?
2. What is obstetric cholestasis?
3. When should women begin supplementing with folic acid?
4. What are some of the risks associated with a raised body mass index (BMI)?

Fundamentals of Maternal Pathophysiology, First Edition. Edited by Claire Leader and Ian Peate.
© 2024 John Wiley & Sons Ltd. Published 2024 by John Wiley & Sons Ltd.
Companion website: www.wiley.com/go/leader/maternalpatho

The gastrointestinal (GI) system is also referred to as the digestive system, GI tract or alimentary canal; these terms are interchangeable. See Figure 16.1 for an overview of the digestive system.

In order to function effectively, human cells require nutrients. The GI tract is responsible for processing food into the right nutrients through a complex interplay of mechanical and physiological processes that aim to break down raw material (food and drink).

The digestive system plays an essential role in the digestion of food and the absorption of nutrients. It is also responsible for removing waste products from the body.

The GI tract is a long muscular tube where food passes through from the point at which it is ingested in the mouth. It then passes through several different organs with different functions that break down the food ready for absorption into nutrient molecules and where any remaining matter, usually fibre and waste, are finally eliminated or egested through the anus as faeces. The constituents of digestion are amino acids, mineral salts, fats and vitamins. Enzymes within the digestive system are responsible for this process and also created in the GI tract by specialist glands. The GI tract is around 5 m in length from the mouth, where it starts, to the anus, where it finishes. There are various organs that play a vital role in the digestion process along the length of the tract. Disorders of the GI system are relatively common due, in part, to its considerable length and the range of organs involved. During pregnancy, these disorders may arise or be exacerbated as a result of the growing uterus displacing the organs of the GI tract, as well as physiological adaptations made by the body that cause changes in the endocrine system, disrupting normal physiological processes.

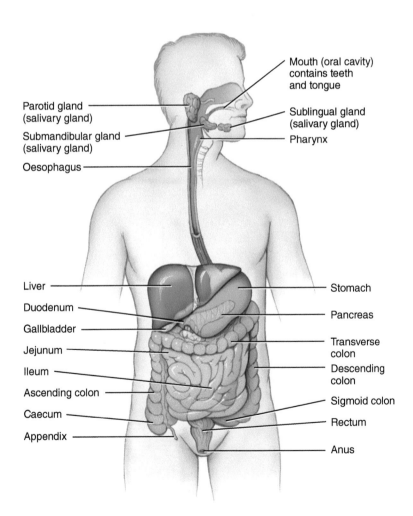

FIGURE 16.1 The digestive system.

The GI tract consists of:

- The mouth
- The pharynx   } Upper GI tract
- The oesophagus
- The stomach

- The small intestine
- The large intestine   } Lower GI tract
- The rectum and anal canal

There are three additional accessory organs that play a major part in the digestive process and these are the pancreas, the liver and the gall bladder. Ingestion, propulsion, digestion, absorption and elimination are the key activities that take place in the digestive system.

There are two mechanisms of digestion: mechanical, which uses movement or a mechanism; and chemical, which is a result of the action of enzymes and secretions in the digestive tract.

Structure of the Gastrointestinal Tract

See Figure 16.2.

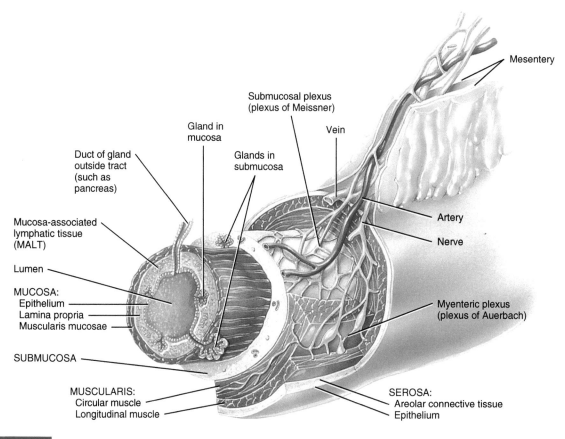

FIGURE 16.2   Structure of the gastrointestinal tract.

Mouth

The mouth or the oral cavity is made up of muscular cheeks (at the sides), the hard and soft palates (the roof) and the tongue and soft tissues (floor of the mouth). The entrance to the mouth is surrounded by the lips. See Figure 16.3 on the oral cavity. Behind the lips are the ridges of the maxilla and mandible, which are covered with a mucous membrane called the gingiva or gum. Approximately 60–75% of pregnant women can experience gingivitis in pregnancy and this is when the gums become swollen and spongy. Women may experience bleeding gums when brushing their teeth and this is due to the elevation of progesterone and oestrogen levels that result in increased vascular permeability.

Learning Event

Investigate the information you can give a woman about dental care during pregnancy.

Teeth

Teeth form part of the oral cavity and are embedded into the ridges of the mandible and maxilla (Figure 16.4). Babies are born with two sets of teeth, which develop in the maxilla and mandible. These are known as deciduous (temporary or baby teeth) and permanent teeth and there are usually 20 deciduous teeth, 10 in each jaw. The deciduous teeth erupt through the gum into the oral cavity from around the sixth month of life. The permanent teeth begin to replace the deciduous teeth from around the age of 6 years and this process is usually complete by the age of 13 years. In an

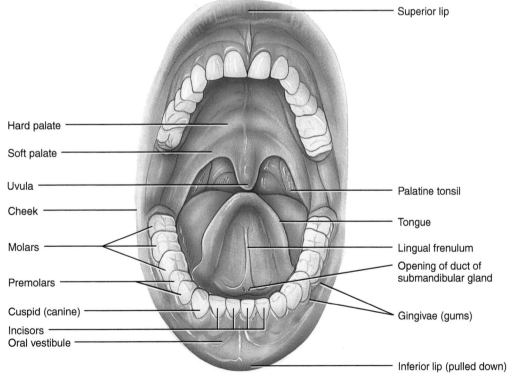

Anterior view

FIGURE 16.3 The oral cavity.

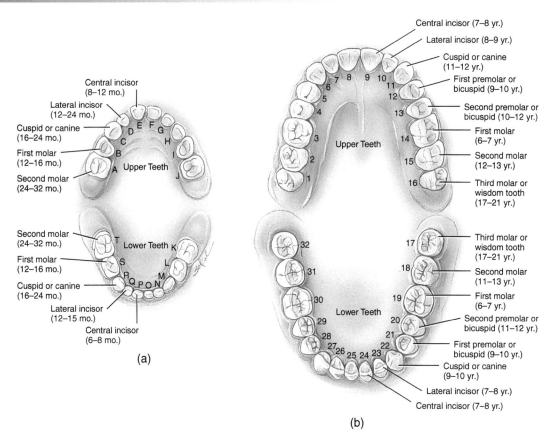

Central incisor (7–8 yr.)
Lateral incisor (8–9 yr.)
Cuspid or canine
(11–12 yr.)
First premolar or
bicuspid (9–10 yr.)
Second premolar or
bicuspid (10–12 yr.)
First molar
(6–7 yr.)
Second molar
(12–13 yr.)
Third molar or
wisdom tooth
(17–21 yr.)

Upper Teeth

Third molar or
wisdom tooth
(17–21 yr.)
Second molar
(11–13 yr.)
First molar
(6–7 yr.)
Second premolar or
bicuspid (11–12 yr.)
First premolar or
bicuspid (9–10 yr.)
Cuspid or canine
(9–10 yr.)
Lateral incisor (7–8 yr.)
Central incisor (7–8 yr.)

Lower Teeth

Central incisor
(8–12 mo.)
Lateral incisor
(12–24 mo.)
Cuspid or canine
(16–24 mo.)
First molar
(12–16 mo.)
Second molar
(24–32 mo.)

Upper Teeth

Second molar
(24–32 mo.)
First molar
(12–16 mo.)
Cuspid or canine
(16–24 mo.)
Lateral incisor
(12–15 mo.)
Central incisor
(6–8 mo.)

Lower Teeth

(a)

(b)

FIGURE 16.4   Tooth structure. (a) Deciduous (primary) dentition. (b) Permanent (secondary) dentition.

adult, the dentition consists of 32 teeth, with the wisdom teeth (third molars) being the last to erupt. There are two types of teeth: incisors and canines, used for cutting and biting; and premolars and molars, used for grinding and chewing.

Palate

The palate forms the roof of the mouth and is divided into two parts: the hard anterior palate and the soft posterior palate. The hard palate is formed by the maxilla and palatine bones. The soft palate is composed of muscle and is at the back of the roof of the mouth. A small muscular protrusion hangs down at the rear of the soft palate known as the uvula. Either side of the uvula are four folds of mucous membrane. The two anterior ones are the palatoglossal arches and the two posterior ones are the palatopharyngeal arches. There is a collection of lymphoid tissue on each side known as the palatine tonsils.

Tongue

The tongue is a large muscular structure attached to the floor of the mouth. It is attached to the hyoid bone at the posterior and by a mucous membrane called the frenulum to the floor of the mouth. The surface of the tongue is covered in stratified epithelium with lots of tiny projections known as papillae, some of which contain taste-sensitive nerve endings that stimulate the sense of taste in taste buds. Glands are also found on the surface of the tongue and these secrete digestive enzymes. The muscular action of the tongue plays an important role in chewing (mastication), swallowing, speech and taste.

Salivary Glands

Saliva is produced by three pairs of salivary glands that release their digestive enzymes into the ducts that lead into the mouth: the parotid glands, the submandibular glands and the sublingual glands. These contain clusters of cells known as acini.

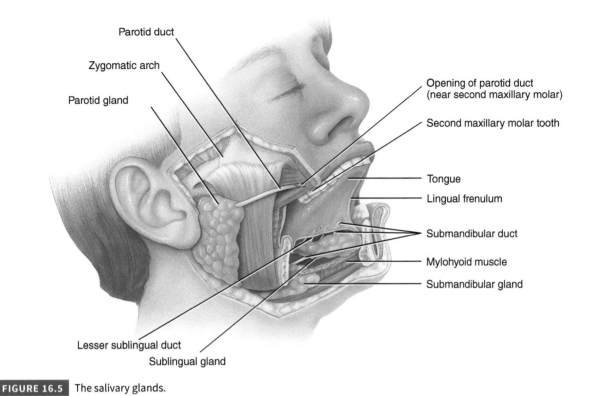

FIGURE 16.5 The salivary glands.

Saliva is made up of a combination of secretions from the six saliva glands and the many small mucus secretin glands that are found in the mouth in the oral mucosa. See Figure 16.5 for an outline of the salivary glands.

Approximately 1–1.5 l of saliva is produced daily. It is made up mainly of water (99.5%), mineral salts, salivary amylase, mucus and antimicrobial substances such as immunoglobulins and the enzyme lysozyme. Saliva has several functions including keeping the mouth clean and moist, mixing with foods to stimulate the sense of taste and lubricating food for easier swallowing. The presence of lysozyme and immunoglobulins helps combat infection in the mucous membranes and helps prevent tooth decay and the start of the chemical breakdown of food. The salivary enzyme amylase starts the breakdown of complex sugars including starches. The pH range for salivary amylase is between 5.8 and 7.4; the optimum level for salivary action is around a pH of 6.8.

Pharynx

The pharynx is described in three parts: the nasopharynx, which is involved in respiration (see Chapter 15), and the oropharynx and laryngopharynx, which are associated with the GI tract. Food passes from the mouth to the pharynx and through the oesophagus in a continuous process.

Swallowing happens in three phases once chewing is complete and a bolus is formed: oral, pharyngeal and oesophageal phases (see Figure 16.6 for illustration on swallowing).

- **Oral phase:** The voluntary action of the tongue and cheek muscles pushes the food bolus to the rear of the mouth towards the pharynx. Food is taken into the mouth and then chewed (masticated) by the teeth and then mixed with saliva and formed into a bolus (small mass) in preparation for swallowing (deglutition). The saliva coats the bolus to provide a slippery surface to make the passage of the bolus smoother. The tongue and cheeks help to move the food into position.

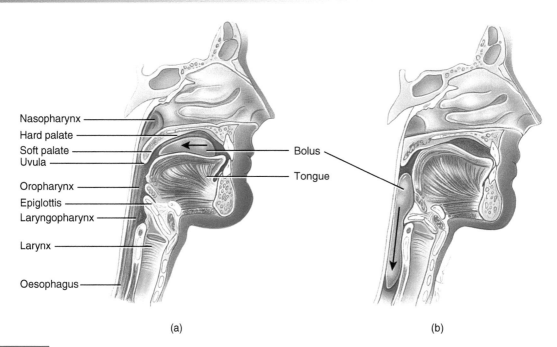

Nasopharynx

Hard palate

Soft palate

Uvula

Bolus

Tongue

Oropharynx

Epiglottis

Laryngopharynx

Larynx

Oesophagus

(a)

(b)

FIGURE 16.6   Swallowing. (a) Position of structures before swallowing. (b) During the pharyngeal stage of swallowing.

- **Pharyngeal phase:** The nasopharynx is occluded as the soft palate rises upwards. The tongue and pharyngeal folds block the bolus coming back into the mouth and the larynx is moved upwards and forwards, occluding the epiglottis thus preventing the food bolus entering the trachea. This action is a reflex action that is stimulated by the deglutition centre in the medulla. The swallowing reflex is initiated as the bolus reaches the posterior pharyngeal wall. These coordinated actions ensure that the bolus of food moves into the correct tube.
- **Oesophageal phase:** The action of peristalsis moves the food bolus through the oesophagus and into the stomach.

Oesophagus

The oesophagus runs continuously from the pharynx to the stomach and is approximately 25 cm long. It passes through the muscle fibres of the diaphragm and then curves sharply upwards before joining the stomach. This anatomical feature is thought to be one of the factors that prevents the regurgitation of gastric contents into the oesophagus. There are also two sphincters at either end of the oesophagus. The cricopharyngeal sphincter or upper oesophageal sphincter prevents air passing into the oesophagus during inspiration; and the cardiac sphincter or lower oesophageal sphincter prevents the regurgitation or reflux of gastric contents into the oesophagus. The food bolus passes through the oesophagus by the process of peristalsis (see Figure 16.7).

Stomach

The stomach is a J-shaped portion of the GI tract and it is continuous with the oesophagus at the lower oesophageal sphincter and with the duodenum at the pyloric sphincter (see Figure 16.8). The stomach is made up of the four basic layers of tissue that are seen in the GI tract. However, the muscle layer consists of three layers of smooth muscle fibres, whereas elsewhere in the GI tract there are only two layers. There is an outer layer of longitudinal fibres, a middle layer of circular fibres and an inner layer of oblique fibres. This additional layer of muscle allows for the churning action that is required for digestion.

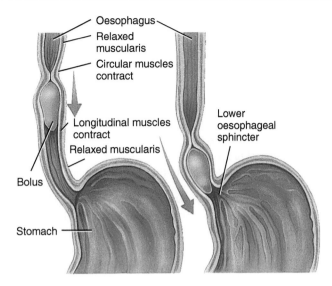

FIGURE 16.7 Peristalsis in the oesophagus. Anterior view of frontal sections.

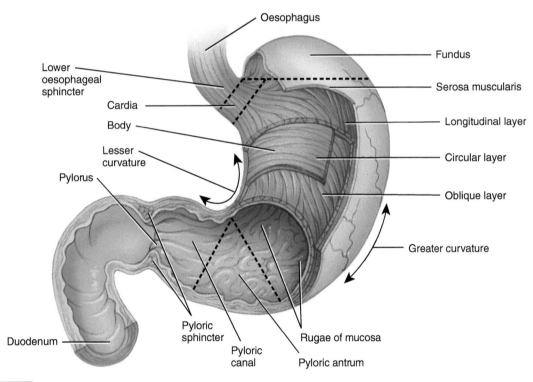

FIGURE 16.8 The stomach. Anterior view.

Functions

The functions of the stomach are:

- Acting as a reservoir for food.
- Mechanical digestion – churning up food to mix with gastric juices, facilitated by the strong muscular contractions of the smooth muscle. The mixed contents are liquefied to chyme.

- Defence against microbes and other harmful microorganisms – provided by hydrochloric acid in the gastric juice.
- Chemical digestion – pepsins breaking proteins into polypeptides.
- Production and secretion of intrinsic factor required for the absorption of vitamin B_{12}.
- Secretion of gastrin.
- Regulation of the passage of gastric contents into the duodenum.

The stomach has three main regions:

- The fundus, which is above the cardiac sphincter.
- The body, which makes up the main part of the stomach.
- The pylorus, at the lower end of the stomach, leading to the duodenum.

When food enters the stomach it is broken down by a wave-like muscle action, churned and mixed with gastric secretions. As it reduces to a more fluid-like substance, it becomes known as chyme. The action of peristalsis moves the contents towards the pylorus. This rhythmical contraction of smooth muscle is responsible for motility and is under the influence of the sympathetic and parasympathetic nerves. The pyloric sphincter between the stomach and the duodenum is relaxed and open when the stomach is inactive. When the stomach contains food the sphincter is closed.

Secretions

The gastric juices are made up of water, mucus and hydrochloric acid, which makes the stomach contents highly acidic and helps to protect against any ingested harmful microorganisms. It also enables enzymes to begin the process of protein digestion. Pepsinogen, which is the precursor of pepsin responsible for the breakdown of proteins and intrinsic factor, is required for the absorption of vitamin B_{12} (Figure 16.9).

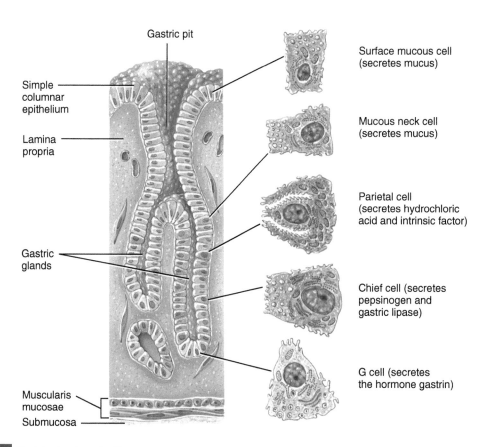

FIGURE 16.9 Gastric glands and cells.

Small Intestine

The small intestine is continuous with the stomach from the pyloric sphincter and is approximately 6 m in length. The lumen of the small intestine is approximately 2.5 cm in diameter. It is situated in the abdominal cavity and opens into the large intestine (see Figure 16.10).

There are four layers to the small intestine, but the mucosa and submucosa layers are modified to facilitate digestion and absorption. The surface area of the mucosal layer is increased by circular folds called plicae circulars, with further folding of the epithelial cells that produce villi and hair-like projections known as microvilli. Microvilli form what is known as a brush border (see Figure 16.11).

The functions of the small intestine are:

- Completion of chemical digestion of carbohydrates, proteins and fats.
- Absorption of nutrients.
- Mechanical digestion by the process of segmentation and peristalsis.
- Continued onward movement of the contents of the small intestine by the action of peristalsis.
- Secretion of intestinal juices and pancreatic juices from the pancreas, increasing the pH of chyme that facilitates the action of the enzymes.
- Secretion of secretin and cholecystokinin (CCK).

The digestion of food is completed in the small intestine and absorption of most nutrients takes place here. The small intestine is divided into three parts:

- **Duodenum:** This is the entrance to the small intestine and is the shortest section, measuring around 25 cm. The common bile duct and the pancreas open into the duodenum. The duodenum empties into the jejunum.
- **Jejunum:** This is the mid-section of the small intestine and measures approximately 2.5 m. It empties into the ileum.
- **Ileum:** This is the last section of the small intestine and measures about 3.5 m. It is joined to the large intestine at the ileocecal sphincter. This valve prevents products of digestion from the large intestine backflowing into the small intestine.

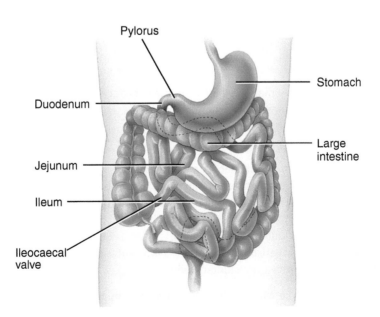

Pylorus

Duodenum

Stomach

Large intestine

Jejunum

Ileum

Ileocaecal valve

FIGURE 16.10 The small intestine.

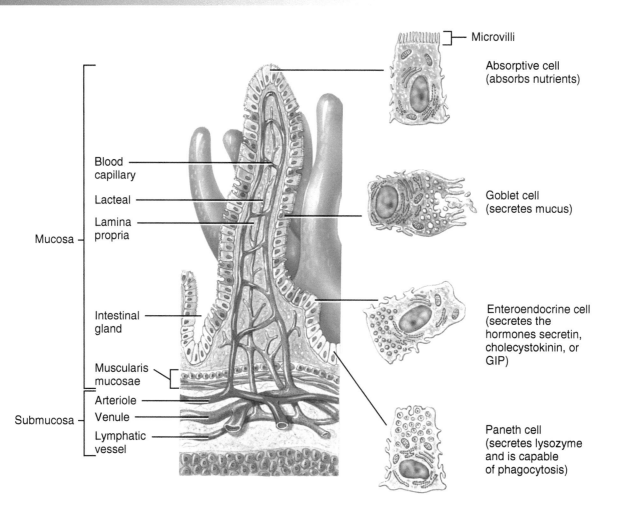

Microvilli

Absorptive cell
(absorbs nutrients)

Blood
capillary

Lacteal

Lamina
propria

Mucosa

Goblet cell
(secretes mucus)

Intestinal
gland

Enteroendocrine cell
(secretes the
hormones secretin,
cholecystokinin, or
GIP)

Muscularis
mucosae

Arteriole

Venule

Submucosa

Lymphatic
vessel

Paneth cell
(secretes lysozyme
and is capable
of phagocytosis)

FIGURE 16.11   The cells within the villi of the small intestine. Enlarged villus showing lacteal, capillaries, intestinal glands and cell types. GIP, gastric inhibitory polypeptide.

Large Intestine

The large intestine is continuous from the small intestine from the ileocaecal valve to the rectum and anal canal. it is approximately 1.5 m in length. The lumen of the large intestine is approximately 6.5–7 cm in diameter (see Figure 16.12).

The functions of the large intestine are:

- Absorption of water by osmosis until semi-solid faeces are formed.
- Heavy colonisation of bacteria, which synthesises vitamin K and folic acid.
- Bacterial fermentation of unabsorbed nutrients, particularly carbohydrates, which produces hydrogen, carbon dioxide and methane. These gases are eliminated from the bowel in the form of flatus (wind).
- Further breakdown of bile pigment bilirubin to urobilinogen.
- Mass movement through the action of peristalsis as a result of food entering the stomach.
- The process of defecation that occurs by an involuntary reflex.

The large intestine is divided into the caecum, the colon, the rectum and the anal canal, contained within the abdominal cavity. The caecum is the first part of the large intestine and is separated from the ileum by the ileocaecal sphincter.

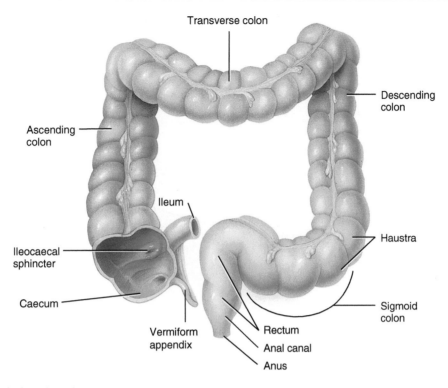

FIGURE 16.12 The large intestine.

Accessory Structures

There are three accessory structures associated with the GI tract (see Figure 16.13).

Pancreas

The pancreas is a soft pinkish-coloured gland approximately 12–15 cm in length. It consists of a head, body and tail. It is situated across the posterior abdominal wall behind the stomach, with the head tucked into the curve of the duodenum and the body and the tail lying behind the stomach (see Figure 16.13). The abdominal aorta and inferior vena cava lie behind the pancreas. The pancreas is supplied by the splenic and mesenteric arteries. The splenic and mesenteric veins provide venous drainage and join other veins to form the portal vein. The pancreas is an exocrine and an endocrine organ (see Chapter 17 for a detailed outline of pancreatic function).

Liver

The liver is a large gland in the body. It is reddish brown in colour and weighs between 1 and 2 kg. It lies in the upper part of the abdominal cavity under the diaphragm, protected by the ribs. The upper and anterior surfaces of the liver are smooth and curved. The posterior surface is irregular. The liver has four unequal-sized lobes. The right and left lobes are

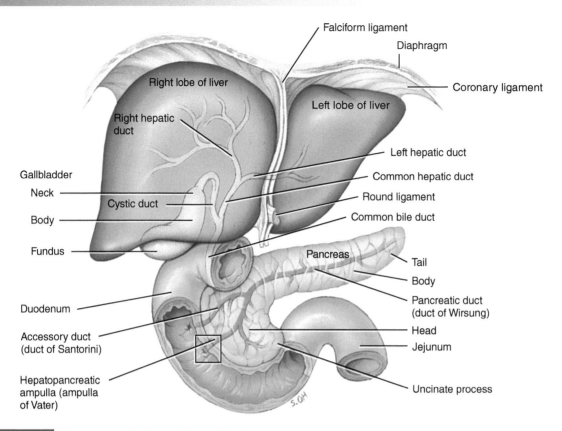

FIGURE 16.13   The pancreas, the liver and the gallbladder. Anterior view.

separated by a deep fissure and by the falciform ligament. The ligamentum teres, the fibrous remanent of the left umbilical vein, runs alongside the free edge of the falciform ligament (see Figure 16.13).

The functions of the liver are:

- **Metabolism:** Blood sugar is regulated by converting glucose to glycogen as a response to insulin. Glycogen is converted back to glucose when glucagon is present and as required. The liver uses fatty acids and glycerol that are the products of the breakdown of fats to provide energy and heat. Excess amino acids are broken down and converted to urea and uric acid.
- **Storage:** The liver acts as a store for vitamins A, B_{12}, D, E and K. The liver also stores glucose in the form of glycogen, and elements of iron and copper.
- **Secretion:** Bile that is produced by the liver is secreted by the gallbladder into the GI tract and aids in the breakdown of fats.

Gallbladder

The gallbladder is a small, pear-shaped organ that lies to the posterior of the liver. It is a reservoir for bile (see Figure 16.13). It contains the same layers of tissue as the rest of the GI tract, but there is an additional layer of oblique muscle fibres and the mucous membrane has small folds or rugae when the gallbladder is empty. When the gallbladder is filled and distended, these rugae disappear. The gallbladder is approximately 3–4 cm long. A branch of the hepatic artery known as the cystic artery provides blood supply to the gallbladder. The cystic vein, which joins the portal vein, drains blood away from the gallbladder. Bile is excreted into the bile ducts when the muscle wall of the gallbladder contracts. This is stimulated by the hormone CCK. When the gallbladder contracts the sphincter at the entrance of the bile duct relaxes. This sphincter is known as the hepatopancreatic sphincter (sphincter of Oddi).

Disorders of the Gastrointestinal Tract in Pregnancy

Heartburn

Heartburn, which may also be termed gastro-oesphageal reflux disease (GORD) or acid reflux, is experienced by up to 80% of women in pregnancy and, while it can develop at any stage, is more common in the second and third trimesters. It is characterised by a burning sensation in the epigastric region, behind the sternum or throat, and can cause a bitter taste in the mouth caused by the regurgitation of gastric acid (Bharj and Daniels 2017).

The hormone progesterone that is produced in pregnancy is responsible for the relaxation of smooth muscle tissue throughout the body. This enables the uterus to stretch and grow as pregnancy progresses and the fetus develops. Under normal circumstances the sphincter muscle that is connected to the oesophagus will act like a valve, allowing passage of food into the stomach, while preventing stomach acid from leaking up into the oesophagus. The relaxing effect of progesterone makes this muscle less effective in pregnancy, causing acid reflux. Additionally, later in pregnancy, as the uterus and fetus grow, there is increasing pressure on the stomach, which also causes acid to leak into the oesophagus.

There are a number of non-pharmacological approaches to the prevention and treatment of acid reflux in pregnancy and women should be advised to try these before medication (NICE 2022):

- Eat smaller meals more frequently.
- Avoid food that exacerbates the heartburn (common irritants include caffeine, fruit juice, spicy food, carbonated drinks, chocolate and fatty foods).
- Avoid excessive weight gain.
- Sleep on the left side.
- Stop smoking.

Medicines Management: Acid Reflux in Pregnancy

Lifestyle changes should always be advised to pregnant women as a first-line treatment for acid reflux. However, if symptoms persist, antacids containing combinations of aluminium and magnesium (such as co-magaldrox) or alginate products (such as Gaviscon Advance) may be used on an 'as required' basis. While calcium-containing products may be used occasionally or in the short term, products containing sodium bicarbonate or magnesium trisilicate are not recommended for use in pregnancy.

Where women are taking iron or folate supplements, antacids should be avoided within two hours of taking these as they can affect absorption.

Acid-suppressing drugs should only be used as a last resort and may be more appropriate in secondary care. There is a paucity of evidence of their safety in pregnancy.

Appendicitis

The vermiform appendix (more often known as the appendix) is a fine, narrow tube-like structure that is closed at the distal end and leads from the inferior aspect of the caecum. It is approximately 8–9 cm in length and has the same structure as the rest of the GI tract, but it contains more lymphoid tissue. The appendix plays no part in digestion, but it can become problematic if it becomes inflamed.

Red Flag: Appendicitis

Appendicitis can be very difficult to diagnose. The appendix can become inflamed, a likely cause of which is from a blockage of faecoliths (hardened faeces), or it can become twisted or kinked. Its common presentation is pain in the centre of the abdomen that after several hours moves to the right side and is localised around the site of the appendix. However, in pregnancy it may present as gastric reflux, constipation, diarrhoea, urinary symptoms and a general feeling of being unwell. In some cases the pain will

301

settle, but in more severe cases where microbial infection is present, an abscess can form and in the worst case can perforate. In pregnant women it is more difficult to diagnose due to the growing uterus and the abdominal wall being stretched away from the site of the appendix. Differential diagnosis may include ectopic pregnancy, threatened miscarriage, gastroenteritis, pyelonephritis, pre-eclampsia, placental abruption or chorioamnionitis.

Obstetric Cholestasis

Obstetric cholestasis (OC) is also referred to as intrahepatic cholestasis of pregnancy (ICP). It most commonly occurs after the 28th week of pregnancy when the levels of oestrogen are at their highest and will stop in the first or second week postpartum. It affects approximately 1 in 140 pregnancies in the United Kingdom. Women of Native Indian descent in areas of Chile and Bolivia appear to have a genetic trait that predisposes them to OC. In Europe, particularly Finland, Sweden and Portugal, rates of OC appear to increase in the winter months, which may be indicative of seasonal dietary requirements; this is also seen in Chile. There is a higher incidence seen in twin pregnancies where oestrogen levels are higher and following in vitro fertilisation. It is also more common if the woman's mother or sister developed OC.

The symptoms of OC include intense pruritus (itching) starting on the hands and soles of the feet, which can spread to other parts of the body. There is no visible rash present with OC. The itching is described as unbearable in the worst cases and can prevent women from sleeping well and have an effect on their mental health. Raised serum bile acids and abnormal liver function tests are the other key features of OC. Serum bilirubin can be raised in a small number of cases. Rarely women present with jaundice, dark urine and pale stools. Due to the impairment of the function of the liver, there can be an effect on the fetus and this includes premature delivery, fetal distress and intrauterine death/stillbirth, and meconium-stained liquor. The woman may be at a higher risk of pre-eclampsia and gestational diabetes, a postpartum haemorrhage, gallstones and malabsorption of vitamin K. Close monitoring of both the mother and the baby is essential throughout the remainder of the pregnancy and in the immediate postnatal period.

The role of any treatment is to try to reduce the maternal itching. Topical emollients such as aqueous cream with or without menthol can be used. Although there is very little high-quality evidence to support their use, they have no known harmful effects and it may relieve some of the discomfort from the itching. Antihistamines such as chlorphenamine that also has a sedative effect may be useful for women who are struggling to sleep, but they have not been evaluated for effectiveness in women with OC. Ursodeoxycholic acid is not routinely offered as there is no clear evidence of significant benefit. The Royal College of Obstetricians and Gynaecologists (RCOG 2022) recommends considering a planned birth at 38–39 weeks in women with moderate OC with peak bile acids of 40–99 μmol/l and no other risk factors. Where peak bile acids are 100 μmol/l or more and the risk of stillbirth is higher, planned birth between 35 and 36 weeks is recommended. OC should not affect a woman's choice of mode of birth and she should be supported in making an informed decision.

Diet and Nutrition in Pregnancy

Good diet and nutritional intake before, during and following pregnancy form the cornerstone of good health and offer a better start for babies. Ensuring a healthy, balanced diet with recommended supplements optimises health and supports improved pregnancy outcomes for women and babies. Additionally, maintaining a healthy weight is also important as this can reduce the risk of complications. However, nutritional advice can be contrary and confusing for pregnant women as well as health professionals. To support women to make good choices, midwives must have a fundamental under-standing of the requirements of a good diet and the most up-to-date evidence on vitamin supplementation in pregnancy.

The Eatwell guide offers advice on how to eat a balanced diet that incorporates the key food groups and nutrients (see Figure 16.14). Currently there is limited evidence specifically around diet in pregnancy and research on effective ways of improving the nutritional status of women pre-conception, during pregnancy and while breastfeeding is much needed, particularly in lower income and Black and minority ethnic (BME) groups (National Institute for Health Research 2017).

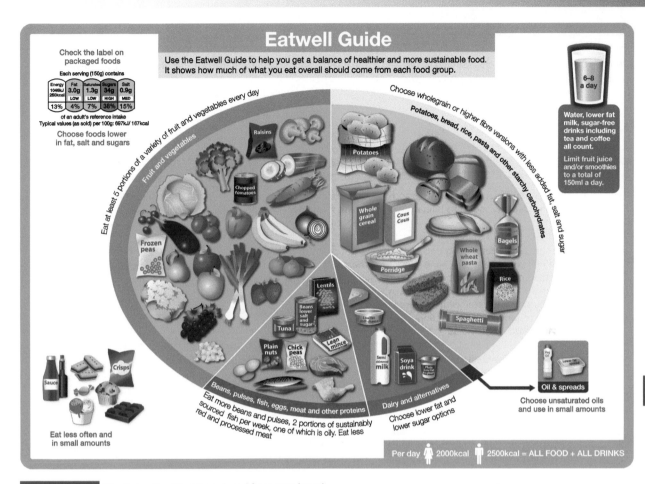

FIGURE 16.14 The Eatwell guide. Reproduced from PHE (2016).

Pre-conception

Public health initiatives have stressed the importance of building health before pregnancy in improving outcomes. Pre-conception care is often a missed opportunity to begin to discuss aspects of diet and supplementation in preparation for pregnancy. With 45% of pregnancies and one-third of births (PHE 2018) being unplanned, it is clear that this is a challenge. Current evidence shows a strong association between folic acid supplementation and the reduction of neural tube defects such as spina bifida. Women are advised to take 400 µg folic acid pre-conception up to 12 weeks' gestation (NICE 2008). This dose will be higher where there are risk factors such as if either parent or a previous child has a neural tube defect (or there is a family history), if the woman has diabetes or is taking medications for epilepsy or antiretroviral for HIV. Supplements should be taken in addition to a diet rich in folate such as peas, beans, green leafy vegetables, lentils and orange juice.

During Pregnancy

Throughout pregnancy women should be offered the best available dietary advice to optimise the health and well-being of themselves and their baby. While the dietary advice offered to the general population will support this (see PHE 2016), women also need to be aware of supplementation as well as foods to avoid. Table 16.1 highlights the recommended vitamins and minerals for pregnancy and their functions. Table 16.2 highlights food to avoid in pregnancy and while breastfeeding.

Orange Flag

Women from lower income groups should be directed to the Healthy Start scheme as if they are eligible, they will be offered financial support towards food and supplements.

TABLE 16.1   Vitamins and minerals important for pregnancy.

Name	Function	Source	Daily intake guidance
Folic acid	Prevention of neural tube defects such as anencephaly and spina bifida	Green leafy vegetables, peas, beans, fortified breakfast cereals, orange juice	400 µg daily pre-conception and up to 12 weeks (higher doses indicated where there are risk factors)
Vitamin D	To support calcium absorption and maintain normal growth, bone and teeth formation Deficiency can lead to rickets in children and osteomalacia in adults Also associated with increased risk of respiratory tract infections such as influenza and Covid-19	Synthesis by ultraviolet rays of the sun Some found in oily fish, eggs and red meat Also in fortified foods such as spreads and cereals	Offered to all pregnant and breastfeeding women 10 µg/d (400 IU)
Vitamin A	Vision, immune function, skin	Cheese, eggs, oily fish, milk, yoghurt, red and leafy green vegetables, yellow fruits	600 µg Pregnant women should *not* supplement as can be harmful to developing fetus
Calcium	For healthy teeth and bone formation, blood clotting, nerve conduction and muscle function	Broccoli, tempeh, leafy greens, tofu, almonds, beans, lentils, oranges, seeds, dairy, sardines, calcium-fortified foods	Not currently recommended as can be obtained through diet in sufficient amounts

Source: Adapted from NICE (2008, 2014) and NIHR (2017).

TABLE 16.2   Foods to avoid in pregnancy and while breastfeeding.

Food to avoid	Why
Dairy Unpasteurised milk or foods such as soft cheese Mould-ripened cheeses such as brie, camembert Soft blue cheeses such as Danish blue	May contain listeria bacteria that may lead to listeriosis, which can cause miscarriage, stillbirth or infant morbidity
Meat Cold cured meats such as salami, pepperoni, chorizo, prosciutto (unless thoroughly cooked) Raw or uncooked meats Liver and liver products Pâté (including vegetarian pâté) Game meats such as goose, partridge or pheasant	Raw or undercooked meats (including cured meats) may contain parasites that cause toxoplasmosis, which can lead to miscarriage Liver and liver products contain high levels of vitamin A that can be harmful to the fetus
Eggs Raw or partially cooked hen's eggs that are not British Lion marked Raw or partially cooked duck, goose or quail eggs	Increased risk of salmonella that can cause food poisoning

(Continued)

304

TABLE 16.2 *(Continued)*

Food to avoid	Why
Fish To limit: Smoked fish such as salmon and trout No more than two portions of oily fish such as salmon, trout, mackerel or herring No more than two tuna steaks or four cans of tuna per week To avoid: Swordfish, marlin, shark, raw shellfish	Tuna has higher levels of mercury than other fish, which can be harmful to the fetus Oily fish may contain pollutants such as polychlorinated biphenyls that can harm the fetus Raw shellfish may contain harmful bacteria, viruses or toxins that may cause food poisoning
Alcohol Current guidelines recommend that women who are trying to conceive or are pregnant should avoid alcohol completely	Increases the risk of miscarriage, preterm birth, low birth weight and fetal alcohol spectrum disorder (FASD)

Source: Adapted from NHS (2023).

Obesity

Of women whose body mass index (BMI) was recorded at booking, 49% were classified as overweight or obese. There is a significant variation between ethnic groups, with two-thirds of Black women recorded as overweight or obese, compared to 51% of Asian women and 48% of white women (Public Health England 2019). There are several factors associated with obesity such as gender (more women than men are obese), social deprivation, ethnicity, genetics, mental health and lifestyle.

There are many complications associated with obesity in pregnancy for both the mother and the fetus. Obesity can have a direct influence on the outcome of a pregnancy. Women can experience intrinsic problems such as gestational diabetes, hypertension and pre-eclampsia, venous thromboembolism, anaesthetic problems and interventional issues such as difficulty in performing certain screening tests during pregnancy like amniocentesis, chorionic villus sampling or ultrasound scans where it is more difficult to detect fetal anomalies and growth, difficulty in auscultation of the fetal heart during pregnancy and labour and difficulty in abdominal palpation. Women are also more likely to experience a more medicalised birth – instrumental birth or caesarean section, prolonged labour, shoulder dystocia during birth, postpartum haemorrhage and difficulty with breastfeeding. They are at a higher risk of developing wound infections and longer postoperative recovery times. The fetus is at a higher risk of anomalies such as neural tube defects, fetal macrosomia, fetal trauma, stillbirth, neonatal death and there is a higher rate of neonatal unit admissions (Denison et al. 2018).

Women with obesity should be counselled during pregnancy on these risks and be given opportunities to discuss them with a midwife and obstetrician to make informed choices about their individualised care plan.

Expert Midwife: Obesity in the Antenatal Period

At the booking appointment, I recorded Jasmin's height and current weight and calculated her BMI and recorded it in her maternity records. I calculated her BMI to be 40.1. Due to this, I had a conversation with Jasmin about the care pathway I would recommend. I would like to refer her to the consultant obstetrician and talk to her about some of the additional care I would be putting in place as her community midwife. I talked to Jasmin about the risk of gestation diabetes and what that is and that we would like to do a screening test (glucose tolerance test – GTT) at 28 weeks.

We talked through some of the risk factors in our Trust's leaflet on obesity in pregnancy. Jasmin found some of the information quite scary, so I talked through some of the risks and how we can try and help manage them. She is really worried about having a large baby or having to have a caesarean section. I also talked to Jasmin about making simple changes to her diet and physical activity to help her have the healthiest pregnancy and birth she can. Jasmin asked me about what a healthy weight gain in pregnancy is, but at present there is no consensus about this so I suggested she focus on trying to eat as healthy a diet as she can. She is due to see the obstetrician after her first ultrasound scan. I also talked to Jasmin about the scan, as it can sometimes be more difficult to obtain the nuchal translucency measurements via a transabdominal scan so she may be offered a transvaginal scan.

Jasmin is aware that she will have an appointment during her pregnancy with an anaesthetist who specialises in obstetrics. This appointment is there to pre-empt any potential concerns that may arise during labour and birth should Jasmin need any interventions. These would be documented in her notes. We talked about the large amount of information that Jasmin had received and we agreed that if she had any questions before the next appointment she could contact me via the community midwives office.

Woman-Centred Care

Think about how you can address obesity with a woman in your care.

- What would be the appropriate language to use?
- How would you address this in a sensitive but professional manner?

Expert Midwife: Obesity in the Postnatal Period

Jasmin had her baby a week ago and all being well I will be discharging her to the care of the health visitor and her GP. She had a normal vaginal birth following a healthy pregnancy and has a baby boy weighing 3760 g. She has been breastfeeding successfully and her son is back to his birth weight. I carried out all the usual postnatal checks and everything was normal and as expected and as part of the ongoing care, I talked to Jasmin about weight loss. Jasmin had made some healthy changes to her diet during her pregnancy by reducing her fat and sugar intake and she had started to exercise gently by walking and to swim. She was very keen to continue to do this. We talked about different support groups like walk and talk for new mums or a weight management service in the community. The GP and health visitor would be able to signpost Jasmin to these if she would like to pursue them.

Jasmin has been doing some reading and is aware that even a small amount of weight retained after a pregnancy can potentially lead to higher risk factors in subsequent pregnancies, and we talked about the risk of hypertensive disorders and diabetes. At the end of the visit, all was well and I was able to discharge Jasmin.

Conditions Associated with the Gastrointestinal Tract

The following is a list of conditions associated with the GI tract. Take some time and write notes about each of the conditions. Think about the anatomy and physiology associated with these conditions. Remember to include aspects of patient care. If you are making notes about people you have offered care and support to, you must ensure that you have adhered to the rules of confidentiality.

The condition	Your notes
Haemorrhoids	
Hyperemesis gravidarum	
Oral candidiasis	
Hepatitis A	

> ## Take-Home Points
>
> - The digestive system carries out six process from ingestion, propulsion, mastication, digestion and absorption through to elimination. During pregnancy the action of progesterone on smooth muscle causes several adaptations to the gastrointestinal tract that can cause women to experience some common disorders of pregnancy, such as delayed gastric emptying time, constipation, acid reflux and changes in appetite.
> - Gastrointestinal health and optimum nutrition play an important role during pregnancy and can have an impact on the health and well-being of the mother and the fetus.

Conclusion

This chapter has offered an overview of the GI system and the key functions that support health and well-being, specifically in the pre-conception, pregnancy and postnatal periods. GI disorders can range from mild symptoms such as heartburn or constipation to more serious problems for the woman and fetus, such as obstetric cholestasis or appendicitis. It is essential that midwives have an understanding of the importance of GI health, supported by optimum nutrition and the maintenance of a healthy weight in order to optimise outcomes for women and their babies.

References

Bharj, K. and Daniels, L. (2017). Confirming pregnancy and care of the pregnant woman. In: *Mayes Midwifery*, 15e (ed. S. McDonald and G. Johnson), 503–536. Edinburgh: Elsevier.

Denison, F.C., Aedla, N.R., Keag, O. et al., on behalf of the Royal College of Obstetricians and Gynaecologists(2018). Care of women with obesity in pregnancy. Green-top guideline no. 72. *British Journal of Obstetrics and Gynaecology* 126 (3): e63–e106.

National Health Service (NHS) (2023). Foods to avoid in pregnancy. https://www.nhs.uk/pregnancy/keeping-well/foods-to-avoid (accessed November 2023).

National Institute for Health and Care Excellence (NICE) (2008). Maternal and child nutrition. https://www.nice.org.uk/Guidance/PH11 (accessed November 2023).

National Institute for Health and Care Excellence (NICE) (2014). Vitamin D: supplement use in specific population groups. https://www.nice.org.uk/guidance/ph56/chapter/What-is-this-guideline-about (accessed November 2023).

National Institute for Health and Care Excellence (NICE) (2022). Dyspepsia – pregnancy-associated: scenario: management. https://cks.nice.org.uk/topics/dyspepsia-pregnancy-associated/management/management (accessed November 2023).

National Institute for Health Research (NIHR) (2017). Better beginnings – improving health for pregnancy. https://evidence.nihr.ac.uk/themedreview/better-beginnings-improving-health-for-pregnancy (accessed November 2023).

Public Health England (PHE) (2016). The Eatwell Guide. https://www.gov.uk/government/publications/the-eatwell-guide (accessed November 2023).

Public Health England (PHE) (2018). Health matters: reproductive health and pregnancy planning. https://www.gov.uk/government/publications/health-matters-reproductive-health-and-pregnancy-planning/health-matters-reproductive-health-and-pregnancy-planning (accessed November 2023).

Public Health England (PHE) (2019). Health of women before and during pregnancy: health behaviours, risk factors and inequalities. https://assets.publishing.service.gov.uk/media/5dc00b22e5274a4a9a465013/Health_of_women_before_and_during_pregnancy_2019.pdf (accessed November 2023).

Royal College of Obstetricians and Gynaecologists (RCOG) (2022). Intrahepatic cholestasis of pregnancy. Green-top guideline no. 43. https://obgyn.onlinelibrary.wiley.com/doi/pdf/10.1111/1471-0528.17206 (accessed November 2023).

Further Resources

Knight, J., Bayram-Weston, Z., and Nigam, Y. (2019). Gastrointestinal tract 6: the effects of the gut microbiota on human health. *Nursing Times* 115 (11): 46–50.

Peate, I. and Hamilton, C. (2022). *Fundamentals of Pharmacology for Midwives*. Chichester, UK: Wiley.

Glossary

Absorption	The uptake of digested food by the intestine into the blood stream
Amylase	An enzyme that digests carbohydrate
Bile	Produced by the liver and required for the digestion of fat
Bile duct	A small tube that carries bile from the liver
Bilirubin	A product of the breakdown of haemoglobin excreted in bile
Canine	A type of tooth
Carbohydrate	One of the major food groups
Cardiac sphincter	A circle of muscle at the lower end of the oesophagus – also known as the lower oesophageal sphincter
Cholecystokinin	A digestive hormone
Cholesterol	A fat-like material present in the blood and most tissues
Chyme	A semi-fluid mass of partially digested food mixed with gastric secretions
Defecation	The expulsion of faeces through the anus
Deglutition	Swallowing
Digestion	The chemical and mechanical breakdown of food
Duodenum	The first part of the small intestine
Faeces	The waste material eliminated through the anus
Fat	A substance in which energy is stored by the body
Fatty acids	A fundamental constituent of important lipids including triglycerides
Flatus	Intestinal gas composed of swallowed air and bacterial fermentation from the intestinal contents
Frenulum	The fold between the lip and the gum
Fundus	The base of the hollow organ: the furthest part from the opening
Gastric juices	Liquid secreted by the gastric glands containing hydrochloric acid, pepsinogen, mucin and rennin
Gastrin	The hormone produced in the mucous membrane of the pyloric region of the stomach
Gingivitis	Inflammation of the gums
Glucagon	Produced by the pancreas, causes an increase in blood sugar level
Glycogen	The principal form in which carbohydrate is stored in the liver and muscles
Heartburn	Discomfort or burning that is felt behind the breast bone, often caused by regurgitation of the stomach contents into the oesophagus
Hepatocytes	Liver cell
Hydrochloric acid	An acid produced by parietal cells in the stomach
Hypochondriac region	The upper lateral divisions of the abdominopelvic cavity
Ileocecal valve	The point at which the small and large intestines meet
Ileum	The end of the small intestine
Incisors	A type of tooth
Insulin	Produced in the pancreas and required to regulate blood sugar

Intrinsic factor	Substance required for the absorption of vitamin B_{12}
Jejunum	The mid-part of the small intestine between the duodenum and the ileum
Kupffer cell	Hepatic macrophage
Laryngopharynx	The point at which the larynx and pharynx meet
Lower oesophageal sphincter	Also known as the cardiac sphincter
Lysozyme	An antimicrobial enzyme
Mastication	Chewing
Meissner's plexus	Nerves of the small intestine
Mesenteric plexus	Digestive track innervation
Microvilli	Cytoplasmic extensions of the villi
Molar	A type of tooth
Monosaccharides	A simple sugar
Mucosa	A layer of the digestive tract
Nasopharynx	The part of the pharynx that lies above the soft palate
Oesophagus	The muscular tube from the laryngopharynx to the stomach
Oral cavity	The first part of the digestive system
Oropharynx	Part of the pharynx closest to the oral cavity
Osmosis	The passage of water across a semi-permeable membrane from a weak to a strong solution
Parasympathetic nerves	Autonomic nervous system nerve fibres
Pepsin	Enzyme required for the breakdown of protein
Pepsinogen	The enzyme precursor to pepsin
Peristalsis	Wavelike contractions that move food through the digestive tract
Peritoneum	The serous membrane that lines the abdominal cavity
Peyer's patches	Lymphatic tissue of the small intestine
Plicae circulars	Folds in the small intestine
Portal triad	Corner of a liver lobule
Premolar	A type of tooth
Protein	A large polypeptide
Pyloric sphincter	The valve that controls the passage of food from the stomach to the small intestine
Rectum	The final portion of the large intestine
Rugae	Folds or ridges found in the digestive tract
Saliva amylase	Carbohydrate-digesting enzyme found in saliva
Secretin	The hormone that regulates the secretion of pancreatic juice
Segmentation	The movement of chyme in the small intestine
Serosa	The outer layer of the digestive tract
Stercobilin	Product of the breakdown of bilirubin
Stomach	The reservoir where the digestion of protein begins in the digestive tract
Sublingual glands	Saliva glands situated in the floor of the mouth
Submandibular glands	Saliva glands situated below the jaw on both sides
Submucosa	The connective tissue layer of the digestive tract
Superior mesenteric artery	The blood vessel that supplies the small intestine with arterial blood
Taeniae coli	Muscle bands in the large intestine
Urea	The main breakdown product of protein metabolism
Uvula	A small piece of tissue that protrudes from the soft palate
Vermiform appendix	The blind-ended tube that is connected to the caecum
Villi	Tiny finger-like projections found on the surface of the mucosa in the small intestine

CHAPTER 17

The Endocrine System and Associated Disorders

Rosalind Haddrill

School of Health and Social Care, Edinburgh Napier University, Edinburgh, UK

AIM

This chapter provides an overview of pathophysiology in relation to the endocrine system and its impact on conception, pregnancy and birth, as well as maternal and infant well-being in the postnatal period. Diagnosis and management are considered.

LEARNING OUTCOMES

By the end of the chapter the reader will be able to:

- Identify the most common endocrine disorders related to pregnancy, both pre-existing and occurring during the perinatal period
- Explain the pathophysiology of these endocrine disorders and relate this to the normal anatomy and physiology of the endocrine system
- Describe the risks for the woman, fetus and neonate associated with these disorders
- Discuss the principles of management of endocrine disorders during pregnancy, birth and postnatally

Test Your Prior Knowledge

1. List three major types of diabetes mellitus relevant to women of reproductive age. How do they differ in their cause, onset and effect? How is diabetes managed to reduce the risks to the pregnant woman, her fetus and newborn?
2. Explain the difference between hypothyroidism and hyperthyroidism and the hormones involved. What is the impact of these conditions on pregnancy, for the mother, fetus and newborn? What are the risks? How are they managed?
3. List the different hormones that may contribute to hyperemesis gravidarum. What are their actions and how do they contribute to nausea and vomiting in pregnancy?
4. List as many of the hormones produced by the anterior pituitary gland as you can and their functions. How might the loss of these hormones affect a woman who suffers from Sheehan's syndrome after a major postpartum haemorrhage? What would be the symptoms?

Fundamentals of Maternal Pathophysiology, First Edition. Edited by Claire Leader and Ian Peate.
© 2024 John Wiley & Sons Ltd. Published 2024 by John Wiley & Sons Ltd.
Companion website: www.wiley.com/go/leader/maternalpatho

An understanding of the anatomy and physiology of the endocrine system is required to fully appreciate the pathophysiological changes that may occur during conception, pregnancy and birth.

The endocrine system works with the nervous and immune systems, coordinating and regulating the body's physiology in response to changes inside and outside the body. This chapter considers the diverse pathophysiology of the endocrine system in relation to reproduction, exploring some of the major disorders, including pre-existing endocrine conditions, but also those that may develop during pregnancy, birth and postnatally and the role of hormones in each. This includes diabetes mellitus, hyperemesis gravidarum and disorders of the adrenal, thyroid and pituitary glands and the hypothalamic–pituitary–adrenal (HPA) axis. Many of these have a genetic component and are linked together.

Women with pre-existing endocrine disorders may experience reduced fertility and their pregnancies are likely to be complex, with increased risk of morbidity and mortality. Alongside women who develop endocrine complications during pregnancy, their care is managed by a multidisciplinary team including obstetricians and medical specialists. The primary aim of such care is to reduce the maternal, fetal and neonatal risks associated with each condition. Midwives play a pivotal role coordinating care and providing continuity of carer for woman and family.

Diabetes Mellitus

In the islets of Langerhans in the pancreas, alpha cells secrete glucagon when blood glucose levels are low, which converts glycogen, stored in the liver and muscles, into glucose. Beta cells secrete insulin when blood glucose levels are high. Insulin converts glucose into glycogen for storage and increases the uptake of glucose by cells, especially muscle cells, and the storage of fats in adipose tissue.

Diabetes mellitus can be defined as a group of metabolic diseases characterised by hyperglycaemia (high blood glucose) resulting from defects in insulin secretion, insulin action or both (American Diabetes Association 2013). Diabetes is one of the most common endocrine disorders affecting women of reproductive age. The three major types of diabetes are shown in Table 17.1.

311

Type 1 Diabetes

Type 1 diabetes (T1DM) accounts for about 8% of all diabetes in the United Kingdom (Diabetes UK 2022). Its cause is unclear, although a childhood virus (coxsackie B4) has been implicated in the onset of T1DM, with a peak incidence around 12 years. The virus destroys cells in the pancreas and triggers an autoimmune response in those genetically

TABLE 17.1 The three major types of diabetes mellitus in women of reproductive age.

Type of diabetes	Onset/ diagnosis	Cause/risk factors	Key characteristics	Treatment/ management
Type 1 diabetes mellitus (T1DM)	Childhood	Viral illness in childhood	Autoimmune – destruction of cells in pancreas: insulin production reduced/ ceases	Insulin dependent
Type 2 diabetes mellitus (T2DM)	Adulthood	Obesity, age, ethnicity, family history	Cardiometabolic – insulin resistance, insufficient insulin produced	Diet, exercise, oral treatment, insulin if required
Gestational diabetes mellitus (GDM)	During pregnancy	More common in those at risk of T2DM: obesity, ethnicity, family history	Insufficient additional insulin produced to compensate for increased resistance in pregnancy Disappears after birth but significantly increased risk of recurrence and T2DM in future	Diet, exercise, oral treatment, insulin if required

susceptible. Progressive destruction of beta cells occurs, often over an extended period, resulting in an almost complete lack of insulin production and impaired alpha cell function, leading to an excess of glucagon. This results in hyperglycaemia, causing damage at cellular and organ levels. Insulin treatment is essential to prevent cardiovascular and microvascular damage resulting from hyperglycaemia.

Type 2 Diabetes

Type 2 diabetes (T2DM) accounts for about 90% of diabetes in the United Kingdom (Diabetes UK 2022). Onset is usually later in life, associated with obesity, age and ethnicity. Rates of T2DM in pregnancy are increasing (NICE 2015). In T2DM there is increased insulin resistance and insulin has a reduced capability to influence cellular uptake of glucose, due to a reduction in insulin receptors on cells. Cell destruction in the islets of Langerhans also leads to reduced insulin production. These result in sustained hyperglycaemia. T2DM is associated with an increased risk of long-term health complications.

Gestational Diabetes Mellitus

Gestational diabetes (GDM) is defined as any degree of glucose intolerance with onset or first recognition during pregnancy (American Diabetes Association 2013). It has been estimated that globally in 2021, 13.9% of live births were affected by GDM (International Diabetes Federation 2021). The prevalence of women with GDM is increasing, due to higher rates of obesity and women becoming pregnant when they are older. After birth GDM usually disappears, but the recurrence rate in a subsequent pregnancy is around 50% (Schwartz et al. 2015). In addition, women with GDM have a substantially increased risk of T2DM (up to 17-fold compared to women without GDM), with the risk highest during the 3–6 years after GDM and aged less than 40 years, but remaining markedly elevated thereafter (Song et al. 2018). Risk factors for GDM are shown in Table 17.2.

In England, the proportion of births complicated by diabetes mellitus, in any form, increased from 5% to 8% between 2013–2014 and 2018–2019 (NHS England 2020). While this increase may be linked to increases in maternal obesity, it may also partly be an indication of improved identification and recording of the condition during pregnancy. Of women in the United Kingdom who have diabetes during pregnancy, it is estimated that approximately 87.5% have GDM, 7.5% have T1DM and the remaining 5% have T2DM (NICE 2015).

TABLE 17.2   **Risk factors for gestational diabetes (GDM).**

Previous GDM
Body mass index (BMI) above 30 kg/m^2
Previous baby weighing ≥4.5 kg
First-degree relative with diabetes
Ethnicity with high prevalence of diabetes
Polycystic ovary syndrome (PCOS)
Previous unexplained stillbirth
Glycosuria during pregnancy *may* indicate GDM and warrants further testing
Smoking and significant inter-pregnancy weight gain also increase the risk

Pregnancy Physiology and Diabetes

Pregnancy has a diabetogenic effect on the body, altering glucose metabolism. This has an impact on maternal metabolism, especially in the third trimester, with progressive insulin resistance due to the placental hormones oestrogen and human placental lactogen (hPL), which decrease insulin efficiency. The resulting hyperglycaemia increases plasma glucose availability to the fetus, thus favouring fetal growth. This increase in insulin resistance is normally countered by an increased production of insulin, stimulated by progesterone (Figure 17.1). Gestational diabetes (GDM) results from a reduced capacity to compensate for this insulin resistance, perhaps due to a genetic predisposition for diabetes. Glucose metabolism becomes unstable and pre-existing diabetes becomes more difficult to control too.

Risks to the Woman and Fetus/Neonate

The longer-term effects of diabetes include diabetic neuropathy, microvascular disease such as retinopathy and nephropathy, atherosclerosis leading to hypertension and risk of stroke, peripheral vascular disease and an increased risk of infection, due to raised blood glucose and impaired white cell function. GDM is associated with increased risk of morbidity and mortality in the immediate pregnancy and subsequent pregnancies, as well as long-term risks concerning the metabolic health of the woman and offspring. Women with previous GDM are more likely to develop serious health conditions that can reduce life expectancy such as cardiovascular disease or non-alcoholic fatty liver disease, regardless of whether they develop T2DM (Daly et al. 2018; Lavrentaki et al. 2019); their infants are predisposed to future obesity, T2DM and neurological impairment (Sheiner 2020).

If pre-existing diabetes is well controlled before, during and after pregnancy, the impact on maternal and fetal morbidity and mortality is significantly reduced. However, where control is poor, adverse outcomes are more common for both the woman and the fetus/infant (see Table 17.3). For all women with diabetes, management of diet and exercise and/or drug therapy will be required to minimise risks to the fetus, for example from excessive fetal growth (macrosomia) as a result of hyperglycaemia, resulting in injury at birth. Studies suggest that GDM is associated with adverse psychosocial outcomes for women too, resulting from the shock of diagnosis and loss of normality and control in their pregnancies (Morrison et al. 2014)

313

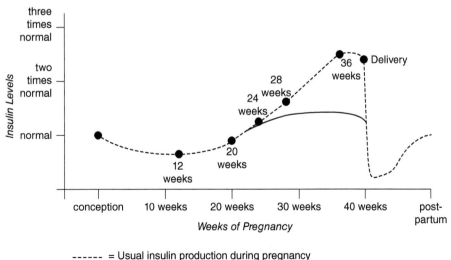

----- = Usual insulin production during pregnancy

——— = Shortage of insulin production during pregnancy with gestational diabetes

FIGURE 17.1 Changing insulin requirements during pregnancy. Source: Reproduced by permission from Marcinkevage and Narayan (2011) / Elsevier.

TABLE 17.3   Risks associated with diabetes during childbearing, for woman and fetus/neonate.

Increased risks for the woman	Increased risks for the fetus/neonate
Perinatal health	
Pregnancy-induced hypertension Pre-eclampsia	Fetal growth restriction – with pre-eclampsia or nephropathy
Worsening of retinopathy and nephropathy (T1DM and T2DM)	Fetal and congenital malformations
Polyhydramnios – excess amniotic fluid	Fetal macrosomia – excessive growth
Premature labour and birth	Neonatal asphyxia/respiratory distress
Induction of labour	Birth injury as a result of shoulder dystocia, e.g. Erb's palsy
Instrumental/operative birth	Neonatal hypoglycaemia
Birth injury (e.g. third-degree perineal tear)	Admission to neonatal unit
Infection	Polycythaemia leading to neonatal jaundice
Not breastfeeding successfully	Miscarriage, stillbirth and neonatal death
General health	
T2DM after GDM	T2DM as an adult
Hypertension, cardiovascular disease	Metabolic and cardiovascular disease in adulthood
Non-alcoholic fatty liver disease	Obesity
Neuropathy	Neuropsychiatric disease, neurodevelopmental impairment
Retinopathy	
Nephropathy	

GDM, gestational diabetes; T1DM, type 1 diabetes; T2DM, type 2 diabetes.

Maternal Risks Associated with Diabetes in Pregnancy

Hypoglycaemia results from an imbalance between insulin and glucose; those with insulin-dependent diabetes are most at risk. As blood glucose levels fall, brain cells are depleted and a loss of consciousness can occur. Hypoglycaemia results in the secretion of glucagon, adrenaline and growth hormone, leading to tachycardia, tremors/shaking, pallor and anxiety. It also results in headaches, dizziness and confusion. Treatment is with oral or intravenous glucose to prevent coma. Women with insulin-treated diabetes are advised to maintain their blood glucose level above 4 mmol/l and to carry a fast-acting form of glucose, and may be offered continuous subcutaneous insulin infusion during pregnancy (NICE 2015).

Ketoacidosis is another acute life-threatening complication of T1DM, linked to severe illness/infection and poor diabetic control. It results from the breakdown of fatty acids (ketones) as a result of a deficit of insulin, leading to extreme hyperglycaemia (>9 mmol/l). It usually occurs in the second or third trimester because of increasing insulin resistance and is more common in pregnancy, when it can occur at a lower blood glucose level. If untreated it can lead to dehydration, electrolyte imbalance and acidosis, resulting in shock, coma and eventually death. Emergency treatment aims to stabilise the woman and lower her blood glucose levels using insulin.

Red Flag

Any hospital admission of an unwell pregnant woman with hyperglycaemia requires urgent testing for ketoacidosis, due to the increased risk of maternal and fetal mortality.
What actions should be taken to manage ketoacidosis in a pregnant woman with diabetes?

Management and Care

Pre-conception
Women with pre-existing diabetes are offered advice, renal and retinal assessment and optimisation of blood glucose control to minimise the risks of fetal loss, congenital anomalies and fetal macrosomia. High-dose folic acid (5 mg) daily is prescribed prior to conception to reduce the risk of neural tube defects.

Antenatal
An oral glucose tolerance test (OGTT) is offered to all women with risk factors for GDM at around 24–28 weeks' gestation (see Table 17.2). If women have had GDM previously they are offered self-monitoring or an OGTT early in pregnancy, and a further OGTT at 24–28 weeks if the results of the first test are normal (NICE 2015). Measurement of HbA1C (glycosylated – having glucose attached to it – haemoglobin) provides an indicator of blood glucose control over the previous 8–12 weeks: the life span of the red blood cell. Measured in early pregnancy and throughout, HbA1C can be used to monitor pre-existing diabetes and identify those at risk of GDM and T2DM.

Care is provided to all women with diabetes by a multidisciplinary team (see Case Study 17.1). Monitoring and interventions during pregnancy and labour aim to reduce the risks to the woman and fetus/neonate. In women with pre-existing diabetes, close blood glucose self-monitoring and control are advised to prevent ketosis and hypoglycaemia, which may be challenging during early pregnancy due to nausea and vomiting. Modification of insulin requirements as pregnancy progresses will be necessary, as insulin resistance increases. Women with GDM are offered initial monitoring, dietary and exercise advice. While some find that GDM can be controlled with changes in diet and exercise, most will need oral blood glucose-lowering agents such as metformin, or insulin, at some point in pregnancy (NICE 2015). Close monitoring of fetal growth occurs.

Medicines Management

Metformin acts to reduce blood glucose levels by:

- Increasing insulin sensitivity.
- Reducing glucose production by the liver.
- Increasing glucose dispersal into the muscle cells (i.e. out of the blood).
- Reducing intestinal absorption of glucose.

How is metformin administered? What dose is given to pregnant women with GDM?
When should women stop taking metformin?

Intrapartum
Birth should take place in a consultant-led unit with neonatal facilities. If there are no complications antenatally, women will be offered induction of labour between 37 and 40 weeks' gestation, depending on the type of diabetes. In more complex cases women will be offered an elective caesarean section.

Neonatal

The newborn infant of a diabetic mother is at increased risk of hypoglycaemia in the 24 hours after birth, due to increased glucose levels during pregnancy. Women are encouraged to undertake antenatal colostrum expression and storage after 37 weeks' gestation to prevent this. Close monitoring, skin to skin, effective early feeding and measurement of pre-feed blood glucose levels are an important part of early care.

Red Flag

The newborn infant of a diabetic mother is at increased risk of hypoglycaemia.

- What are the signs and symptoms of neonatal hypoglycaemia and why is it dangerous?
- How should the infant be cared for in the first 24 hours of life to reduce this risk?

Postnatal

Insulin requirements fall immediately after birth and there is no requirement to continue blood glucose monitoring in women with GDM. However, close monitoring of blood glucose and diet is needed with T1DM if breastfeeding, as energy requirements are higher. Women with pre-existing diabetes are given opportunities to discuss further pregnancies and pre-conception care. After having GDM, women are offered postnatal lifestyle advice, including weight control, diet and exercise, and blood glucose assessment at 6–13 weeks postnatal and annually, to assess for signs of T2DM.

Learning Event

Reflect on your experience of meeting a woman in early pregnancy who has risk factors for GDM.

- How would you explain to her what GDM is and why it occurs during pregnancy?
- What are the risks associated with it for the woman and her baby?

Case Study 17.1

Miriam is aged 27 years and has T1DM. She is pregnant with her first baby. Prior to pregnancy Miriam received pre-conceptual advice from her diabetic consultant. Her HbA1C was measured to confirm good diabetic control and retinopathy and nephropathy screening was undertaken. She was prescribed 5 mg folic acid to take until 12 weeks' gestation.

After attending her booking appointment with her community midwife, Miriam is referred to a joint diabetes clinic, which includes specialist diabetic nurses and midwives, dieticians, diabetic and obstetric consultants. She attends the diabetes clinic and is offered:

- Contact with the clinic every one to two weeks throughout pregnancy.
- A dating ultrasound scan at the first appointment to confirm the pregnancy.
- Measurement of HbA1C.
- Real-time continuous glucose monitoring.
- Blood ketone testing strips and a meter.
- Retinal and renal assessment, to be repeated at 28 weeks' gestation.
- An ultrasound scan at 20 weeks to detect fetal structural abnormalities.
- Ultrasound monitoring of fetal growth and amniotic fluid volume every 4 weeks from 28 to 36 weeks.
- Induction of labour between 37 weeks and 38 weeks and 6 days or (if indicated) caesarean section.

Miriam is advised about:

- The importance of good diabetic control to minimise the risks to herself and her baby.

- Testing her fasting, pre-meal, one-hour post-meal and bedtime blood glucose levels daily, to maintain a fasting blood glucose of 5.3 mmol/l and a one-hour level of 7.8 mmol/l.
- The signs and risks of hypoglycaemia and ketoacidosis during pregnancy.
- The timing, mode and management of birth, including analgesia, anaesthesia and insulin.

Postnatal care, initial care of the neonate and breastfeeding.

Source: Adapted from NICE (2015).

Thyroid Disorders

The main thyroid hormones are thyroxine (T_4) and triiodothyronine (T_3). These are produced by the thyroid gland in response to thyroid-stimulating hormone (TSH) being released from the anterior pituitary gland, which is turn is produced in response to thyrotropin-releasing hormone (TRH) being released from the hypothalamus. A negative feedback system controls levels: high levels of TSH result in low secretion of T_4 and T_3 and vice versa (see Figure 17.2). T_4 circulates in the blood in two forms: T_4 that is protein bound, and free T_4 (fT_4) that is unbound and can enter and affect target cells and tissues. Free T_4 is a more accurate indicator of thyroid function and is used for laboratory testing.

Although the thyroid gland increases in size and activity in pregnancy, overall thyroid function remains normal during most pregnancies. Thyroid hormones are important for the neurological development of the fetus. The fetal thyroid starts functioning around 12 weeks' gestation, therefore during early pregnancy the fetus relies on maternal thyroid hormones for its development. Thyroid function is balanced by changes in the metabolism of iodine, the requirement for which doubles in pregnancy. Iodine deficiency may result in increased hypothyroidism and pregnancy-induced goitre (thyroid gland hypertrophy) (Baragwanath and Vaidya 2017).

Hypothyroidism

Hypothyroidism consists of a lack of T_3 and T_4 and occurs because of a defect either in the thyroid gland or in the control pathway for TRH or TSH. Hypothyroidism reduces fertility if untreated. It is associated with increased TRH and TSH, which

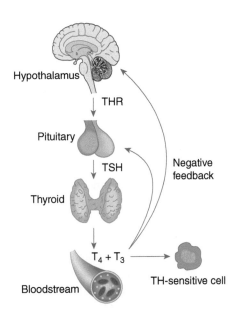

FIGURE 17.2 Negative feedback control of thyroid hormone (TH) production. TRH, thyrotropin-releasing hormone; TSH, thyroid-stimulating hormone.

raise levels of prolactin in the blood (hyperprolactinaemia), preventing ovulation. It is also a relatively common pregnancy-related thyroid disorder, affecting approximately 3% of all pregnant women.

Causes

A common cause of hypothyroidism in the United Kingdom is chronic autoimmune thyroiditis, with or without goitre (Hashimoto's thyroiditis). Hypothyroidism can also result from subacute thyroiditis, a temporary inflammation of the thyroid gland triggered by viral infections such as mumps or influenza, or a result of thyroidectomy or radioactive iodine treatment. Hypothyroidism during pregnancy can also occur as a result of treatment for Grave's disease (see later). Autoimmune thyroiditis is familial and is associated with other autoimmune disorders such as T1DM.

Symptoms and Confirmation

Symptoms of hypothyroidism include weight gain, constipation, alopecia, dry skin, lethargy and cognitive impairment, although many women are asymptomatic when diagnosed. Hypothyroidism is confirmed through the thyroid function test (TFT), with high TSH and normal or low fT_4 and fT_3 levels.

Hypothyroidism and Pregnancy

Pregnancy complications include pregnancy-induced hypertension and GDM, and impaired brain development and physical growth in the fetus, resulting in low birth weight. There is an increased risk of premature and stillbirth (Teng et al. 2013). There may also be an association between thyroid dysfunction and depression during pregnancy and in the postpartum period (Schmidt et al. 2022).

Management and Care

Midwives should ensure accurate booking information and early referral to specialist endocrine and obstetric teams. Treatment is with oral thyroxine (levothyroxine), with the dose adjusted to maintain TSH within the normal range. Requirements are likely to increase in early pregnancy, so early medical input is recommended as soon as possible after pregnancy confirmation, ideally pre-conception (Teng et al. 2013). Treatment with levothyroxine during pregnancy is associated with decreased risks of pregnancy loss and neonatal death; requirements may increase by up to 40% (Bein et al. 2021; NICE 2021). Regular measurement of thyroid function during pregnancy, using TFTs, should occur to enable adjustment. Body mass index (BMI) estimation, diet and exercise are also important, as weight gain and lethargy are associated with hypothyroidism. Midwives should be alert for signs of impaired fetal growth and hypertension, and ensure that regular TFTs are taken.

Demand for thyroxine will reduce postnatally and should be checked 6–12 weeks after birth. The condition can result in congenital hypothyroidism in the newborn, which requires treatment in the neonatal period to prevent permanent neurological damage. Congenital hypothyroidism is screened for on day 5 as part of the UK Newborn Screening Programme.

Hyperthyroidism (Thyrotoxicosis)

Hyperthyroidism results from excessive production of thyroid hormones. Severe hyperthyroidism is associated with infertility, but pregnancy may occur if the condition is mild or successfully treated.

Causes

Hyperthyroidism in pregnancy is mainly caused by transient gestational hyperthyroidism or Graves' disease (autoimmune hyperthyroidism); other causes are rare (Nguyen et al. 2018). Transient gestational hyperthyroidism is usually mild and affects 1–3% of pregnancies, occurring in the first half of pregnancy. It is caused by stimulation of thyroid follicular cells by placental human chorionic gonadotropin (hCG), structurally similar to TSH, which peaks around 10 weeks' gestation. As women with hyperemesis gravidarum tend to have high levels of hCG, they are at increased risk (see section on hyperemesis). It resolves by 20 weeks' gestation and treatment is not usually required.

Graves' disease affects about 1 in 500 pregnant women (Baragwanath and Vaidya 2017). Thyroid-stimulating antibodies activate TSH receptors, leading to increased production of thyroid hormones. In some cases Graves' disease is associated with other autoimmune conditions such as T1DM and pernicious anaemia due to vitamin B_{12} deficiency. Trophoblastic tumours such as hydatidiform mole may rarely cause hyperthyroidism (see Case Study 17.1), as can overtreatment of hypothyroidism.

Symptoms and Confirmation

Symptoms include heat intolerance, sweating, palpitations, weight loss, hypertension, insomnia and anxiety. The condition is confirmed through the TFT, with raised fT_4 and low TSH levels.

Hyperthyroidism and Pregnancy

In women with pre-existing disease, the condition may get worse in the first trimester but generally improves throughout the rest of the pregnancy. Graves' disease tends to improve in pregnancy; 30–40% of women may be able to stop antithyroid medication after 30 weeks' gestation (Nguyen et al. 2018).

Hyperthyroidism is associated with severe adverse effects for mother and fetus, such as pre-eclampsia and heart failure in the woman, and growth restriction, miscarriage, premature birth and stillbirth/neonatal death. There are also risks of the transfer of thyroid antibodies resulting in neonatal thyroid dysfunction. This may get worse initially and may require temporary treatment, but resolves within three months of birth. Treatment of hyperthyroidism may also result in fetal hypothyroidism.

Care and Management

Ideally, women should receive pre-conception counselling prior to pregnancy and ensure their hyperthyroidism is well controlled, to reduce the risk of complications. Management of hyperthyroidism in pregnancy is complex, requiring early referral to specialist multidisciplinary care.

Outside of pregnancy, treatment includes antithyroid drugs that block the manufacture of thyroid hormones, with close monitoring of dosages and levels of fT_4 to keep within the normal range and prevent iatrogenic hypothyroidism. These drugs are associated with congenital anomalies, especially if taken in the first trimester, though the risk is very small (Morales et al. 2021). The lowest possible dose should be used, with regular measurement of fT_4 and TSH levels. Some women may be able to reduce or stop taking antithyroid drugs in pregnancy, especially in the third trimester, but there is a high risk of recurrence postnatally.

Fetal growth should be assessed regularly using ultrasound. Close monitoring during labour and close observation of mother and infant in the immediate postnatal period are also essential. Antithyroid drugs can be taken while breastfeeding but should be taken after feeding. The infant's thyroid function may need to be monitored; signs of neonatal hyperthyroidism include weight loss, tachycardia, irritability and poor feeding, which may require admission to a neonatal unit.

Postnatal thyroiditis (inflammation of the thyroid) is a temporary autoimmune condition that can occur in the first 12 months after birth. It is usually mild but can lead to hyperthyroidism or hypothyroidism; testing is recommended for women experiencing postnatal depression, lactation problems or other symptoms of hyper- or hypothyroidism (Epp et al. 2021).

Medicines Management

Hypo- and hyperthyroidism are treated with levothyroxine and antithyroid drugs such as carbimazole and propylthiouracil, respectively.

- How are these drugs administered?
- How is the correct dose determined?
- What are the risks for the fetus of such medication?

Hyperemesis Gravidarum

Many women will experience nausea and vomiting in the early part of pregnancy, resolving around the end of the first trimester. However, hyperemesis gravidarum results in excessive nausea and vomiting that is often prolonged. Hyperemesis is defined as nausea and vomiting that is associated with weight loss of more than 5% during early pregnancy (Lee and Saha 2011). The incidence is around 0.5% of pregnancies and for approximately 10% of these women it resolves only after birth (Verberg et al. 2005). Hyperemesis can result in severe dehydration and metabolic imbalance, requiring hospital treatment to correct and prevent poor pregnancy outcomes, such as poor fetal growth and premature birth. Maternal complications include liver and kidney damage, resulting in jaundice, and also vitamin deficiency and thromboembolism. It is a leading cause of hospitalisation during pregnancy.

Numerous hypotheses exist about the aetiology of hyperemesis. These include gut infections, vitamin deficiency, overactivity of the HPA axis and the psychological impact of the pregnancy. However, the endocrine influence is the most likely, with several hormones implicated directly and indirectly.

Progesterone

During pregnancy the sex hormones, particularly progesterone, cause abnormal activity in gastric and colonic smooth muscle. This leads to slower gastric emptying and relaxation of the lower oesophageal sphincter, which may result in nausea and vomiting.

Human Chorionic Gonadotrophin

hCG peaks at the same time as the highest incidence of hyperemesis in early pregnancy (Figure 17.3). It is more common in pregnancies associated with elevated levels of hCG, such as twin pregnancies and also hydatidiform mole (molar pregnancy; see Case Study 17.1). However, other conditions associated with high hCG levels, such as choriocarcinoma, do not result in nausea and vomiting, and many pregnant women with high hCG levels do not experience hyperemesis. In addition, a significant number of women with hyperemesis experience symptoms that continue beyond the first trimester, when hCG levels are falling. One hypothesis is that hyperemesis is not simply caused by elevated hCG levels but by specific isoforms (variants) of hCG, suggesting that there might be genetic/ethnic variations among women experiencing hyperemesis (Lee and Saha 2011).

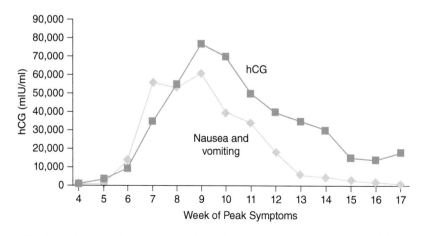

FIGURE 17.3   The relationship between hCG and nausea and vomiting in pregnancy. Source: Adapted from Niebyl (2010).

Oestrogen

High oestrogen levels also contribute to slower intestinal transit time and gastric emptying. Hyperemesis is associated with a number of pregnancy factors linked to high oestrogen levels, such as a higher BMI and first pregnancies. However, these do not explain why the symptoms in women with hyperemesis are so much more severe or why it is most prevalent during the first trimester, given that oestrogen levels rise progressively during pregnancy (Lee and Saha 2011).

Thyroid Hormones

hCG is a TSH agonist. During peak hCG levels in the first trimester of normal pregnancy serum TSH levels fall, mirroring the hCG peak, and free T_3 and T_4 levels are significantly elevated. TSH returns to normal throughout the duration of pregnancy. Because of the structural similarity to TSH, increased hCG levels can cause excessive stimulation of the thyroid gland, resulting in transient hyperthyroidism (thyrotoxicosis). This is common among women with hyperemesis, occurring in approximately one-third of cases, particularly in cases of molar (see Case Study 17.2) and multiple pregnancies, conditions associated with higher hCG levels (Verberg et al. 2005). However, while hyperthyroidism is more prevalent, it is not exclusive to women with hyperemesis, as many women with hyperemesis do not experience hyperthyroidism. The combination of hyperthyroidism and hyperemesis is particularly serious, as it is associated with elevated levels of miscarriage, premature birth and complications during pregnancy such as pre-eclampsia.

Case Study 17.2

Esmé is 37 years old and 12 weeks pregnant with her first baby. She is attending her hospital appointment for a dating ultrasound scan. She has experienced severe nausea and vomiting since finding out she is pregnant and has lost a lot of weight.

During the scan the sonographer explains that the embryo has not developed properly and that Esmé has a molar pregnancy. They arrange for a doctor to come and speak to Esmé and her partner. The doctor explains that a hydatidiform mole or molar pregnancy is a rare complication, occurring in about 1 in 600 pregnancies, and is characterised by the abnormal growth of trophoblast cells, cells which normally develop into the placenta. A complete molar pregnancy is where abnormal cells grow in the uterus after conception, without an embryo; a partial molar pregnancy is where there may be early signs of an embryo, but it does not develop. It is more common in women under 20 or over 35 years. Complete molar pregnancies have up to a 15% chance of developing into a choriocarcinoma, a malignant cancer of the trophoblast cells; 50% of all cases of choriocarcinoma result from complete molar pregnancies. The removal of the conceptus – products of conception – must take place.

Molar pregnancies result in elevated hCG levels that may subsequently result in transient hyperthyroidism, which may be contributing to Esme's symptoms. The doctor explains that hCG levels will be monitored frequently, through blood and urine tests, after the removal of the conceptus, to ensure that levels return to normal. Esmé will be followed up in a specialist centre for months afterwards. Some women will require chemotherapy to treat a persistent gestational tumour. Esmé is advised that molar pregnancy does not affect fertility and that many women go on to have healthy babies afterwards.

The aetiology of hyperemesis remains unclear. Although some of the proposed mechanisms could provide a reasonable explanation, conclusive evidence for any single cause remains unconvincing and further research is required.

Care and Management

Midwives need to be able to distinguish between women with minor nausea and vomiting due to pregnancy and those with hyperemesis. Women with hyperemesis show signs of significant dehydration, such as oliguria (reduced urine output), ketones and low levels of sodium and chloride in the urine; also low blood pressure, raised pulse, paleness (perhaps due to anaemia) and lethargy. Women require admission to stabilise their condition, in order to receive rehydration, close monitoring and investigations to rule out urinary tract infections, which have similar symptoms, and molar pregnancy. Management includes intravenous fluids, antiemetics, vitamins and minerals. Most women respond quickly and oral fluids and solid food may be recommended eventually.

Learning Event

Reflect on your experience of supporting a woman who has nausea and vomiting in early pregnancy.

- Can you explain why she might be feeling this way?
- What advice can you give to her to manage her symptoms?
- How would you know if she had hyperemesis gravidarum?

Adrenal Disorders

Polycystic Ovary Syndrome

Polycystic ovary syndrome (PCOS) is one of the most common endocrine disorders in women of reproductive age (Yu et al. 2016). Its prevalence can vary from 2% to 26%, with a higher incidence among women of South Asian origin (RCOG 2014). PCOS is associated with infertility due to the absence of ovulation (anovulation), infrequent periods (oligomenorrhoea) and an excess of male hormones (androgens) such as testosterone, a condition known as hyperandrogenism (see Figure 17.4). Women with PCOS are more likely to need to use assisted reproductive technology to conceive (Roos et al. 2011). Many women with PCOS are obese and have a higher incidence of conditions associated with poor cardiovascular health, such as hypertension, insulin resistance and raised levels of insulin in the blood (hyperinsulinaemia). The cause of PCOS is not fully understood, but evidence of a genetic component has been recognised.

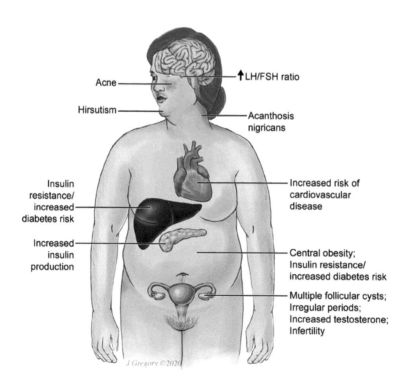

Acne

Hirsutism

↑LH/FSH ratio

Acanthosis nigricans

Insulin resistance/ increased diabetes risk

Increased insulin production

Increased risk of cardiovascular disease

Central obesity; Insulin resistance/ increased diabetes risk

Multiple follicular cysts; Irregular periods; Increased testosterone; Infertility

J Gregory ©2020

FIGURE 17.4   Symptoms of polycystic ovary syndrome. FSH, follicle-stimulating hormone; LH, luteinising hormone.

PCOS is also associated with congenital adrenal hyperplasia, where the synthesis of cortisol is blocked, leading to infertility that requires treatment with glucocorticoids, enabling ovulation and pregnancy to occur.

Women with PCOS are significantly more likely to experience pregnancy complications, irrespective of how they conceive. These include pre-eclampsia, gestational diabetes and premature birth, linked to some of the common features of PCOS Palomba et al. (2015). Some studies suggest an increased risk of impaired fetal growth, miscarriage, caesarean birth and perinatal death (Kjerulff et al. 2011; Yu et al. 2016). There is also some suggestion that the offspring of women with PCOS have an increased risk of metabolic and reproductive dysfunction too. The underlying pathophysiology of these pregnancy complications and those of the child are unclear, but are likely to be linked to obesity and increased levels of androgens (Roos et al. 2011).

Management and Care

Women with PCOS may need increased monitoring during pregnancy and childbirth. In terms of managing diabetes risk, all women with PCOS who are planning a pregnancy should be offered a 75 g OGTT pre-conception or in early pregnancy. Pregnant women with PCOS should also be offered screening for GDM at 24–28 weeks' gestation, with referral to a specialist obstetric diabetic service if needed. During pregnancy changes to drug treatment(s) should be made, for example any hormonal treatment should be stopped (NICE 2022).

Addison's Disease (Adrenal Insufficiency)

Addison's disease is caused by inadequate secretion of corticosteroids (glucocorticoids and mineralocorticoids). This rare condition occurs as a result of autoimmune destruction of the adrenal cortex, often in combination with other autoimmune endocrine disorders such as Grave's disease or T1DM, or as a result of tuberculosis or Sheehan's syndrome (see the section on pituitary disorders). Symptoms include persistent nausea and vomiting, weight loss, hypotension and reduced fertility. It is diagnosed with low morning plasma cortisol levels among other biochemical changes.

Management and Care

Oral or intravenous hydrocortisone can prevent acute adrenal crisis, for example as a result of surgery or infection (situations where corticosteroids would naturally increase). Increased doses are therefore required for labour and birth. Vomiting in early pregnancy may have an impact on oral absorption. During labour continuous fetal monitoring and close monitoring of the woman are needed, including blood pressure and strict fluid balance with intravenous fluids, to prevent hypovolaemia and hypotension. Continued close monitoring is required postnatally and a tapered dose of hydrocortisone should be given over several days (Anand and Beuschlein 2018).

Cushing's Syndrome

Cushing's syndrome occurs because of excessive levels of corticosteroids as a result of pituitary or adrenal carcinoma. Like PCOS, it is associated with amenorrhoea and anovulation, so is rare in pregnancy. Where pregnancy does occur there is a high chance of morbidity and mortality. Elevated cortisol levels during pregnancy may result in a higher risk of maternal hypertension, impaired glucose tolerance and pre-eclampsia, also increased rates of premature birth, miscarriage and stillbirth, and neonatal complications too (Tang et al. 2020).

Pituitary Disorders

Sheehan's Syndrome

Sheehan's syndrome is postpartum partial or complete hypopituitarism caused by necrosis (cell injury that results in the premature death of cells) of the anterior pituitary gland. This occurs as a result of severe hypovolaemic shock and hypotension, for example due to postpartum haemorrhage. During pregnancy, an increased amount of the hormone oestrogen in the body causes an increase in the size of the pituitary gland and the volume of blood flowing through it. This makes the anterior pituitary susceptible to damage from ischaemia (loss of blood and oxygen to tissues). The posterior pituitary has a separate blood supply so is not affected.

Sheehan's syndrome is now rare in developed countries, where improved maternity care usually prevents extreme blood loss during birth. An Icelandic study estimated prevalence to be 5 in 100 000, but noted that this was likely to be an underestimation, due to delayed diagnosis or misdiagnosis (Kristjansdottir et al. 2011). The condition is still common in developing countries, however: in India a prevalence of 3% was estimated in one study (Shivaprasad 2011). Prevention of excessive blood loss during labour and appropriate management of postpartum haemorrhage are an essential part of preventing Sheehan's syndrome.

The diverse symptoms of Sheehan's syndrome are due to the loss of anterior pituitary hormones, such as prolactin, follicle-stimulating hormone (FSH) and luteinising hormone (LH), TSH and adrenocorticotrophin (ACTH), which stimulates the functioning of the adrenal cortex (see Figure 17.5). There are both chronic and acute forms of the condition, depending on the degree of damage to the pituitary gland. In the acute form symptoms may become apparent shortly after birth; in the chronic form symptoms may not appear, or be diagnosed, for months or years after giving birth. The acute form is most dangerous and associated with persistent low blood pressure, tachycardia and hypoglycaemia, as a result of hypocortisolism (lack of cortisol). It is sometimes evident immediately after birth and can result in adrenal crisis, which can be fatal. With both acute and chronic forms the most common symptom is difficulty with or absence of lactation, which is important for early diagnosis and intervention. Other symptoms include headache and visual disturbances, nausea, amenorrhoea, lethargy and atrophy of the genitalia and breasts (Diri et al. 2016).

Blood tests confirm hormone levels, followed by referral to an endocrinologist if needed, and imaging (computed tomography [CT] or magnetic resonance imaging [MRI]) of the pituitary gland to rule out tumours. Hormone replacement is required, including lifelong treatment with ovarian (e.g. oestrogen), thyroid and adrenocortical hormones, for example hydrocortisone. Another condition with similar symptoms is lymphocytic hypophysitis, where lymphocytes enter the pituitary gland, resulting in pituitary enlargement and impaired function. It most often occurs in late pregnancy or postnatally.

324

HYPOTHALAMUS HORMONE	ANTERIOR PITUITARY GLAND HORMONE RELEASED/INHIBITED	TARGET ORGAN OR TISSUES	ACTION
Growth-hormone-releasing factor	Growth hormone (GH)	Many (especially bones)	Stimulates growth of body cells
Growth-hormone-release-inhibiting factor	Growth hormone (inhibits release)	Many	Inhibits hormone production in many parts of the body
Thyroid-releasing hormone (TRH)	Thyroid-stimulating hormone (TSH)	Thyroid gland	Stimulates thyroid hormone release
Corticotropin-releasing hormone (CRH)	Adrenocorticotropic hormone (ACTH)	Adrenal cortex	Stimulates corticosteroid release
Prolactin-releasing hormone	Prolactin	Breasts	Stimulates milk production
Prolactin-inhibiting hormone (Dopamine)	Prolactin (inhibits release)	Breasts	Inhibits milk production
Gonadotropin-releasing hormone	Follicle-stimulating hormone (FSH) Luteinising hormone (LH)	Gonads	Various reproductive functions

Adapted from Peate (2017). Reproduced with permission of John Wiley & Sons.

FIGURE 17.5   The diverse functions of the anterior pituitary gland.

Prolactinoma

A prolactinoma is a pituitary adenoma (non-cancerous tumour) formed as a result of the proliferation of lactotroph cells in the anterior pituitary gland. Prolactinomas synthesise and secrete prolactin, resulting in hyperprolactinaemia, with impacts on oestrogen release. This affects ovulation and results in infertility and sometimes galactorrhoea, the production of a milk-like discharge from the breasts not linked to lactation. Larger tumours can compress the pituitary cells, affecting the release of several hormones and resulting in hypothyroidism. Other symptoms occur because of pressure in the brain, such as headaches and visual disturbances. Prolactinomas may grow during pregnancy or as a result of contraceptive use, in response to increased oestrogen levels. Treatment with a dopamine agonist restores normal prolactin levels and may shrink the tumour.

Chronic Stress

Evidence exists that chronic hyper- as well as hyposecretion of glucocorticoid hormones such as cortisol, as a result of stress exposure, is involved in the development of a range of metabolic, immune, endocrine and neuropsychiatric disorders. Stress has an impact on human fertility, due to suppression of gonadotropin release from the anterior pituitary gland and subsequent impact on the ovaries and testes, as a result of elevated glucocorticoid levels (Whirledge and Cidlowski 2010). Recurrent pregnancy loss may be linked to stress inhibiting progesterone synthesis too, again as a result of elevated glucocorticoid levels, as they share the same synthesis pathway (Solano and Arck 2019).

The maternal HPA axis is integral to increased cortisol exposure in the fetus (Figure 17.6). The HPA axis undergoes dramatic changes during pregnancy and postnatally. Cortisol levels rise threefold in pregnancy by the third trimester, due

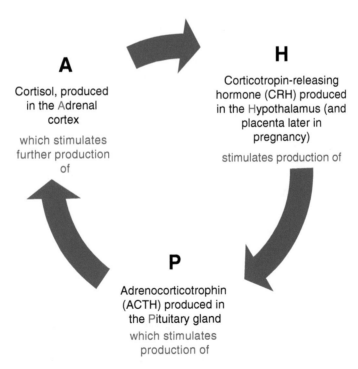

A

Cortisol, produced in the Adrenal cortex

which stimulates further production of

H

Corticotropin-releasing hormone (CRH) produced in the Hypothalamus (and placenta later in pregnancy)

stimulates production of

P

Adrenocorticotrophin (ACTH) produced in the Pituitary gland

which stimulates production of

FIGURE 17.6 The hypothalamic–pituitary–adrenal (HPA) axis.

to increased oestrogen and placental production of corticotropin-releasing hormone (CRH). The HPA axis returns to pre-pregnant levels with a drop in CRH following the birth of the placenta. However, the fetus is partially protected from elevated cortisol in pregnancy by a specific enzyme (HSD11B2) that converts active cortisol into inactive cortisone, preventing overexposure (Duthie and Reynolds 2013).

The maternal HPA axis is modified by chronic and acute stress and disease, including anxiety and depression. High maternal cortisol levels exhaust the protective mechanism of HSD11B2, resulting in a greater transfer of glucocorticoids to the fetus, evident in amniotic fluid. Increased cortisol levels are associated with growth restriction and shorter gestation at birth. There is also evidence of epigenetic changes in the placenta due to chronic stress, which may act as a biomarker for future disease (Jahnke et al. 2021). Animal and human studies show that prenatal exposure to chronic maternal stress increases the risk to the fetus of behavioural and mental health problems later in life, and of cardiometabolic disease (such as diabetes) as an adult, through fetal programming (Van den Bergh et al. 2020). In the United Kingdom maternity services, family healthcare, perinatal mental health services and social care work together to try to minimise stress during the childbearing period for women and families.

Take-Home Points

- Disorders of the endocrine system result from the impaired production, release and functioning of a wide range of hormones in the body, affecting many body systems. Many are autoimmune disorders, with a genetic influence, and are inter-related.
- Such disorders have an impact on fertility and on the well-being of the woman and the fetus during pregnancy and birth, as well as the neonate, with increased risk of pregnancy loss and morbidity due to impaired fetal growth and premature birth.
- Pregnancy may exacerbate pre-existing conditions and some disorders may have longer-term or lifelong consequences for both woman and child.
- Effective maternity care involves multidisciplinary collaboration from a range of specialisms, reducing risks and optimising the childbearing experience, even in the most complex circumstances.

Conclusion

The endocrine system works with the nervous and immune systems, coordinating and regulating the body's physiology. Disorders of the endocrine system related to childbearing result from the impaired production, release and/or functioning of a wide range of hormones in the body. Pregnancy may exacerbate pre-existing conditions, many of which are autoimmune disorders, with a genetic influence, which are inter-related.

Such disorders have an impact on a woman's ability to conceive, but also on the well-being of the woman and the fetus during pregnancy and birth, as well as the neonate. There is an increased risk of pregnancy loss and morbidity, and the potential for long-term consequences for both woman and child. Effective maternity care involves careful monitoring and management, through multidisciplinary collaboration from a range of medical specialisms, alongside midwifery care. The aim is to reduce risks and optimise the childbearing experience for women and their families, even in the most complex circumstances.

References

American Diabetes Association (2013). Diagnosis and classification of diabetes mellitus. *Diabetes Care* 36 (Suppl 1): S67–S74. https://doi.org/10.2337/dc13-S067.

Anand, G. and Beuschlein, F. (2018). Management of endocrine disease: fertility, pregnancy and lactation in women with adrenal insufficiency. *European Journal of Endocrinology* 178 (2): R45–R53. https://doi.org/10.1530/eje-17-0975.

Baragwanath, G. and Vaidya, B. (2017). Thyroid disorders in pregnancy. *British Journal of Family Medicine* https://pavilionhealthtoday.com/fm/thyroid-disorders-in-pregnancy.

Bein, M., Yu, O.H.Y., Grandi, S.M. et al. (2021). Levothyroxine and the risk of adverse pregnancy outcomes in women with subclinical hypothyroidism: a systematic review and meta-analysis. *BMC Endocrine Disorders* 21 (1): 1–17.

Daly, B., Toulis, K.A., Thomas, N. et al. (2018). Increased risk of ischemic heart disease, hypertension, and type 2 diabetes in women with previous gestational diabetes mellitus, a target group in general practice for preventive interventions: a population-based cohort study. *PLoS Medicine* 15 (1): e1002488. https://doi.org/10.1371/journal.pmed.1002488.

Diabetes UK (2022). Position statements report: statistics. https://www.diabetes.org.uk/professionals/position-statements-reports/statistics (accessed November 2023).

Diri, H., Karaca, Z., Tanriverdi, F. et al. (2016). Sheehan's syndrome: new insights into an old disease. *Endocrine* 51 (1): 22–31. https://doi.org/10.1007/s12020-015-0726-3.

Duthie, L. and Reynolds, R.M. (2013). Changes in the maternal hypothalamic-pituitary-adrenal axis in pregnancy and postpartum: influences on maternal and fetal outcomes. *Neuroendocrinology* 98 (2): 106–115. https://doi.org/10.1159/000354702.

Epp, R., Malcolm, J., Jolin-Dahel, K. et al. (2021). Postpartum thyroiditis. *BMJ* 372: n495. https://doi.org/10.1136/bmj.n495.

International Diabetes Federation (2021). *IDF Diabetes Atlas 2021*, 10e. https://diabetesatlas.org/atlas/tenth-edition.

Jahnke, J.R., Terán, E., Murgueitio, F. et al. (2021). Maternal stress, placental 11β-hydroxysteroid dehydrogenase type 2, and infant HPA axis development in humans: psychosocial and physiological pathways. *Placenta (Eastbourne)* 104: 179–187. https://doi.org/10.1016/j.placenta.2020.12.008.

Kjerulff, L.E., Sanchez-Ramos, L., and Duffy, D. (2011). Pregnancy outcomes in women with polycystic ovary syndrome: a metaanalysis. *American Journal of Obstetrics and Gynecology* 204 (6): 558.e1–558.e6.

Kristjansdottir, H.L., Bodvarsdottir, S.P., and Sigurjonsdottir, H.A. (2011). Sheehan's syndrome in modern times: a nationwide retrospective study in Iceland. *European Journal of Endocrinology* 164 (3): 349–354. https://doi.org/10.1530/eje-10-1004.

Lavrentaki, A., Thomas, T., Subramanian, A. et al. (2019). Increased risk of non-alcoholic fatty liver disease in women with gestational diabetes mellitus: a population-based cohort study, systematic review and meta-analysis. *Journal of Diabetes and Its Complications* 33 (10): 107401. https://doi.org/10.1016/j.jdiacomp.2019.06.006.

Lee, N.M. and Saha, S. (2011). Nausea and vomiting of pregnancy. *Gastroenterology Clinics of North America* 40 (2): 309–334. vii. https://doi.org/10.1016/j.gtc.2011.03.009.

Marcinkevage, J.A. and Narayan, K.M.V. (2011). Gestational diabetes mellitus: taking it to heart. *Primary Care Diabetes* 5 (2): 81–88. https://doi.org/10.1016/j.pcd.2010.10.002.

Morales, D.R., Fonkwen, L., and Nordeng, H.M.E. (2021). Antithyroid drug use during pregnancy and the risk of birth defects in offspring: systematic review and meta-analysis of observational studies with methodological considerations. *British Journal of Clinical Pharmacology* 87 (10): 3890–3900. https://doi.org/10.1111/bcp.14805.

Morrison, M.K., Lowe, J.M., and Collins, C.E. (2014). Australian women's experiences of living with gestational diabetes. *Women and Birth* 27 (1): 52–57. https://doi.org/10.1016/j.wombi.2013.10.001.

National Institute of Health and Care Excellence (NICE) (2015). Diabetes in pregnancy: management from pre-conception to the postnatal period. NG3. https://www.nice.org.uk/guidance/ng3 (accessed November 2023).

National Institute of Health and Care Excellence (NICE) (2021). Clinical knowledge summaries: hypothyroidism. https://cks.nice.org.uk/topics/hypothyroidism (accessed November 2023).

National Institute of Health and Care Excellence (NICE) (2022). Clinical knowledge summaries: polycystic ovary syndrome. https://cks.nice.org.uk/topics/polycystic-ovary-syndrome (accessed November 2023).

Nguyen, C.T., Sasso, E.B., Barton, L., and Mestman, J.H. (2018). Graves' hyperthyroidism in pregnancy: a clinical review. *Clincal Diabetes and Endocrinology* 4: 4. https://doi.org/10.1186/s40842-018-0054-7.

NHS England (2020). Better births four years on: a review of progress. https://www.england.nhs.uk/wp-content/uploads/2020/03/better-births-four-years-on-progress-report.pdf (accessed November 2023).

Niebyl, J. (2010). Nausea and vomiting in pregnancy. *New England Journal of Medicine* 363: 1544–1550. https://doi.org/10.1056/NEJMcp1003896.

Palomba, S., de Wilde, M.A., Falbo, A. et al. (2015). Pregnancy complications in women with polycystic ovary syndrome. *Human Reproduction Update* 21 (5): 575–592. https://doi.org/10.1093/humupd/dmv029.

Roos, N., Kieler, H., Sahlin, L. et al. (2011). Risk of adverse pregnancy outcomes in women with polycystic ovary syndrome: population based cohort study. *BMJ* 343 (1) 194: –d6309. https://doi.org/10.1136/bmj.d6309.

Royal College of Obstetricians and Gynaecologists (RCOG) (2014). Long-term consequences of polycystic ovary syndrome. Green-top guideline no. 33. https://www.rcog.org.uk/media/qmtlp2b0/gtg_33.pdf (accessed November 2023).

Schmidt, P.M.D.S., Longoni, A., Pinheiro, R.T., and Assis, A.M.D. (2022). Postpartum depression in maternal thyroidal changes. *Thyroid Research* 15 (1): 6. https://doi.org/10.1186/s13044-022-00124-6.

Schwartz, N., Nachum, Z., and Green, M.S. (2015). The prevalence of gestational diabetes mellitus recurrence—effect of ethnicity and parity: a metaanalysis. *American Journal of Obstetrics & Gynecology* 213 (3): 310–317. https://doi.org/10.1016/j.ajog.2015.03.011.

Sheiner, E. (2020). Gestational diabetes mellitus: long-term consequences for the mother and child grand challenge: how to move on towards secondary prevention? *Frontiers in Clinical Diabetes and Healthcare* 1: https://doi.org/10.3389/fcdhc.2020.546256.

Shivaprasad, C. (2011). Sheehan's syndrome: newer advances. *Indian Journal of Endocrinology and Metabolism* 15 (Suppl 3): S203–S207. https://doi.org/10.4103/2230-8210.84869.

Solano, M.E. and Arck, P.C. (2019). Steroids, pregnancy and fetal development. *Frontiers in Immunology* 10: 3017. https://doi.org/10.3389/fimmu.2019.03017.

Song, C., Lyu, Y., Li, C. et al. (2018). Long-term risk of diabetes in women at varying durations after gestational diabetes: a systematic review and meta-analysis with more than 2 million women. *Obesity Reviews* 19 (3): 421–429. https://doi.org/10.1111/obr.12645.

Tang, K., Lu, L., Feng, M. et al. (2020). The incidence of pregnancy-associated Cushing's disease and its relation to pregnancy: a retrospective study. *Frontiers in Endocrinology* 11: 305. https://doi.org/10.3389/fendo.2020.00305.

Teng, W., Shan, Z., Patil-Sisodia, K., and Cooper, D.S. (2013). Hypothyroidism in pregnancy. *Lancet Diabetes & Endocrinology* 1 (3): 228–237.

Van den Bergh, B.R., van den Heuvel, M.I., Lahti, M. et al. (2020). Prenatal developmental origins of behavior and mental health: the influence of maternal stress in pregnancy. *Neuroscience & Biobehavioral Reviews* 117: 26–64.

Verberg, M.F.G., Gillott, D.J., Al-Fardan, N., and Grudzinskas, J.G. (2005). Hyperemesis gravidarum, a literature review. *Human Reproduction Update* 11 (5): 527–539. https://doi.org/10.1093/humupd/dmi021.

Whirledge, S. and Cidlowski, J.A. (2010). Glucocorticoids, stress, and fertility. *Minerva Endocrinologica* 35 (2): 109.

Yu, H.-F., Chen, H.-S., Rao, D.-P., and Gong, J. (2016). Association between polycystic ovary syndrome and the risk of pregnancy complications A PRISMA-compliant systematic review and meta-analysis. *Medicine (Baltimore)* 95 (51): e4863. https://doi.org/10.1097/MD.0000000000004863.

Further Resources

Autoimmune Association. www.autoimmune.org (accessed November 2023).

British Thyroid Foundation. Pregnancy and fertility in thyroid disorders. www.btf-thyroid.org/pregnancy-and-fertility-in-thyroid-disorders (accessed November 2023).

Diabetes UK. Guide to pregnancy. www.diabetes.org.uk/guide-to-diabetes/life-with-diabetes/pregnancy (accessed November 2023).

Pituitary Foundation. www.pituitary.org.uk (accessed November 2023).

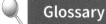

Glossary

Aetiology	The cause or origin of disease
Agonist	A chemical that binds to and activates cell receptors to produce a biological response
Androgen	Male hormones, such as testosterone
Antagonist	A chemical that interferes with or inhibits the physiological action of another
Autoimmune	An abnormal immune response: autoantibodies attack and destroy healthy cells and tissues
Conceptus	Any products of conception, including the embryo, fetus and surrounding tissue
Congenital	Present or evident from birth
Gestational	Occurring during pregnancy
Glucocorticoids	Steroid (cholesterol-based, fat-soluble) hormones such as cortisol, which are produced by the adrenal glands (situated above each kidney)
Goitre	A swelling in the neck resulting from an enlarged thyroid gland
HbA1C	Glycosylated (having glucose attached to it) haemoglobin – measurement indicates blood glucose control over the previous 8–12 weeks
Iatrogenic	A medical disorder, illness or injury resulting from medical treatment
Mineralocorticoids	Include aldosterone, produced by the adrenal gland, which helps to maintain water and electrolyte balance in the body

CHAPTER 18

Pain

Claire Ford and Matthew Robertson

Department of Nursing, Midwifery and Health, Northumbria University, Newcastle upon Tyne, UK

AIM

This chapter aims to support midwifery practice, providing the reader with information about the pathophysiology of pain and how it manifests during pregnancy, birth and the postnatal period.

LEARNING OUTCOMES

On completion of this chapter the reader will be able to:

- Be aware of the pathophysiology associated with pain and the impact this can have on women during the perinatal journey
- Appreciate the importance of understanding the underpinning evidence associated with pharmacological and non-pharmacological analgesic approaches
- Have a greater awareness of the importance of respecting individual choice and the need to provide individualised woman-centred care.

Test Your Prior Knowledge

1. What do you already know about the pathophysiology of pain?
2. How can pain be manifested in women during the perinatal journey?
3. What impacts can pain have on women's well-being?
4. Name as many definitions of pain as you can and indicate how these differ from one another.
5. Discuss some of the assessment strategies that can be used by midwives to assess women's pain.

Pain is one of the most common women's problems and one of the most frequent reasons individuals seek medical advice. It is also synonymously linked with childbirth, labour and postnatal recovery; however, while midwives are frequently faced with this clinical issue, it can often be difficult to assess and manage as it is subjective, unique to each woman and activated by a variety of stimuli, including biological, physical and psychological (Boore et al. 2021). When women state they are in pain, it is, therefore, every midwife's duty to listen to what they say (Nursing and Midwifery Council [NMC] 2018), believe that pain is what they say it is, observe for supporting information using appropriate and varied assessment approaches and act as soon as possible by utilising suitable management strategies.

Fundamentals of Maternal Pathophysiology, First Edition. Edited by Claire Leader and Ian Peate.
© 2024 John Wiley & Sons Ltd. Published 2024 by John Wiley & Sons Ltd.
Companion website: www.wiley.com/go/leader/maternalpatho

Woman-Centred Care

For many women, the anxiety and fear associated with pain during labour and delivery can be significant. It is therefore extremely important to enable women to voice their fears or concerns about pain in advance of the labour and delivery and discuss their past pain histories, as they may already receive treatment for chronic pain and may need further guidance about what possible analgesic approaches would be beneficial. It is also essential to be open-minded and receptive to alternative beliefs and customs around pain and how this should be managed, as the way in which a woman may deal with the pain may differ from what you have previously experienced.

Pain Theories

Knowledge of pain processes has changed considerably over the last 500 years from beliefs that pain is a sensation linked to body fluid imbalance, evil spirits or a punishment from God (Ford 2020). In 1965 Melzack and Wall conceptualised and pioneered a new model of pain, referred to as the 'gate control theory'. They hypothesised that neurons within the superficial dorsal horn of the spinal cord could modulate the flow of signals from the stimulation of peripheral nociceptors (sensory neurons) through the central nervous system (CNS) to the brain, thus effectively increasing or decreasing the amount of pain experienced (Todd 2016). They further postulated that the gate control was influenced by psychological and physiological factors and accordingly have been accredited with taking the first step in recognising the symbiotic relationship and the interactive and interdependent nature of these factors. This psychophysiological theory and its underlying principles have widespread applicability and have consequently laid the foundation for some of the additional altered models that have been developed over the last 50 years (VanMeter and Hubert 2022).

One such model is Engel's 'biopsychosocial model', which has taken the gate theory one step further, reinforcing the uniqueness of individuals' pain experiences and reaffirming that pain often results from the culmination of a myriad of factors that are biological, social and psychological in origin (Engel 1980). These can include stimulus intensity, genetic predisposition, economic and environmental factors, cultural beliefs, and individual pain perception and coping mechanisms (Ford 2020). Ronald Melzack has also advanced and extended the gate control theory of pain, in order to address the original theory's inability to explain phantom limb pain (Keefe et al. 1996). This has resulted in the creation of the 'neuromatrix' theory of pain, and a greater understanding of the role of supraspinal influences and brain function on pain perceptions (Keefe et al. 1996). This supplementary theory proposes that the multidimensional experience of an individual's pain is a result of a unique neurosignature (nerve impulse pattern in the brain) that can be produced by genetic and sensory influences, triggered by sensory stimuli and also when stimuli are absent (Melzack 2001, 2005; Melzack and Katz 2013).

Orange Flag: Fear, Anxiety and Pain

Fear and anxiety have a potential exacerbating influence on the levels of pain experienced. Consequently, without tailored, holistic woman-centred care and perinatal education and reassurance, multitudes of factors can increase women's anxiety levels to such degrees that fear manifests itself in physiological responses, leading to hyperalgesia, over-sensitisation of nociceptors and a heightened receptivity to noxious and psychogenic stimuli. Additionally, anxiety can have detrimental effects on the maintenance and induction of anaesthesia, increasing the need for anaesthetic drugs, and can exacerbate complications in stress responses.

Source: Adapted from Ford (2020).

Pathophysiology of Pain

How pain is transmitted and modulated by the body and received and interpreted by the brain is extremely complex. This process is also associated with a variety of chemicals, neurons and electrical impulses, influenced by psychological and social elements (Ashelford et al. 2019). In order to understand how pain is manifested in women during the perinatal journey, it is important to examine these pain pathways and the underlying anatomy and physiology in greater detail.

Neurons

There are estimated to be over 100 billion neurons within the body, and these are different to other body cells as they can both initiate and conduct nerve impulses; thus, generating an action potential for the sending and receiving of information (Boore et al. 2021). There are three types of neurons: sensory neurons carry signals from the body to the spinal cord and brain and are therefore afferent neurons; motor neurons are efferent pathways, relaying impulses from the brain and spinal cord to either muscle or epithelial tissue; and interneurons are connecting neurons that carry impulses from sensory to motor neurons.

Neurons also have three parts: the cell body, which is considered the core and main part of the neuron; axons, which transfer signals away from the cell body; and dendrites, which forward impulses towards the cell body (Waugh and Grant 2022). The axon is the stalk and is wrapped in myelin, a white fatty protective coat playing an essential role in the conductivity of the impulses, covering sections of the axon length, separated by the nodes of Ranvier. Dendrites are branched projections surrounding the cell body and are shaped in a way that increases the surface area, enhancing the effectiveness and speed of the signal (see Figure 18.1). Neurons communicate with each other by sending nerve impulses, known as action potentials, along the axon and then to another cell across a gap (synaptic cleft) separating two neurons, by a chemical or electrical synaptic relay facilitated by neurotransmitters.

Neuroglia

There are around one trillion neuroglial cells within the CNS that play a huge supporting role, protecting the neurons, holding neurons together and regulating neuron functions (McErlean and Migliozzi 2017). As with the nervous system's overall structure, central and peripheral divisions vary in size and shape (see Figure 18.2). Microglia, as the name suggests, are smaller, playing a large role in the inflammatory process, and oligodendrocytes are longer, producing the myelin sheath that coats the neuron axon and due to its consistency also holds some nerve fibres together.

Spinal Cord

The spinal cord, which is continuous with the medulla oblongata, is cylindrical, suspended in the vertebral canal, extending from the first cervical vertebra to the end of the first lumber vertebra. There are three groups of neurons in the spinal cord: ascending neurons carry signals upwards to the brain; descending neurons carry instructions away from the brain down the spinal cord; and interneurons act as connectors between the ascending and descending neurons. The spinal cord is approximately 42–45 cm long and is surrounded by the meninges and the cerebrospinal fluid (CSF). Grey matter is central, set out in an H shape (see Figure 18.3) and divided into horns (McErlean and Migliozzi 2017). The anterior (ventral) horn contains cell bodies found along the length of the spinal cord, stimulating the skeletal muscle. The posterior (dorsal) horn contains sensory neurons associated with pain signals and the lateral horns contain cells that stimulate smooth muscles (Boore et al. 2021).

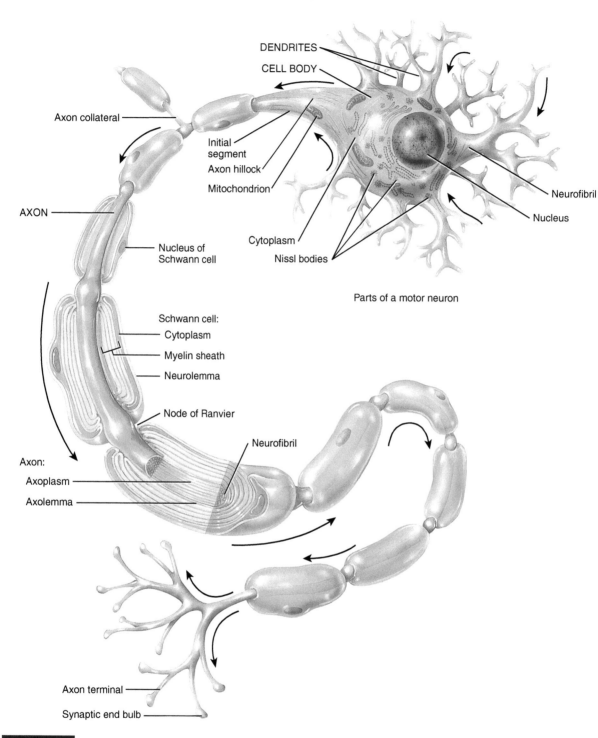

DENDRITES

CELL BODY

Axon collateral

Initial segment

Axon hillock

Mitochondrion

Neurofibril

Nucleus

AXON

Nucleus of Schwann cell

Cytoplasm

Nissl bodies

Parts of a motor neuron

Schwann cell:

Cytoplasm

Myelin sheath

Neurolemma

Node of Ranvier

Neurofibril

Axon:

Axoplasm

Axolemma

Axon terminal

Synaptic end bulb

FIGURE 18.1   A neuron.

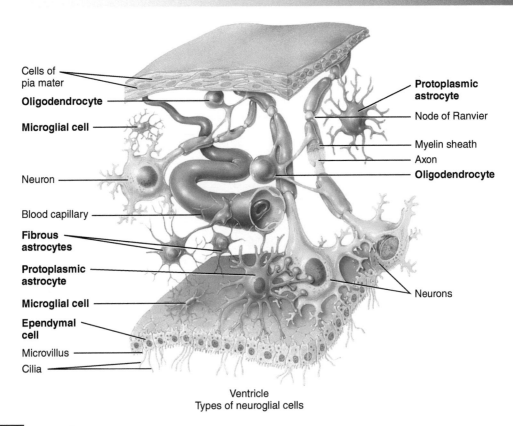

Cells of pia mater

Oligodendrocyte

Microglial cell

Neuron

Blood capillary

Fibrous astrocytes

Protoplasmic astrocyte

Microglial cell

Ependymal cell

Microvillus

Cilia

Protoplasmic astrocyte

Node of Ranvier

Myelin sheath

Axon

Oligodendrocyte

Neurons

Ventricle
Types of neuroglial cells

FIGURE 18.2 A neuroglia.

White matter surrounds the grey matter and also has three columns, the posterior, anterior and lateral columns, which are then divided into tracts. The ascending tract, as the name suggests, transmits signals to the brain, and the descending transmits them away from the brain. Three main pathways on either side of the spinal cord, for sensory information, are the dorsal column tract (fine touch and vibration to the cerebral cortex), the spinothalamic tract (temperature and pain signals to the cerebral cortex) and the spinocerebellar tract (posture and position from all parts of the body).

Spinal Nerves

There are 31 pairs of spinal nerves attached to the subdivisions of the spinal column, often categorised in numerical order and identified by the first letter of the associated section of the spine. Thus, in the cervical sections of the spine you will find eight pairs (C1–C8), within the thoracic segments two pairs (T1–T12) and five pairs in the lumbar region (L1–L5), with another five in the sacral area (S1–S5). The last pair is attached to the coccygeal division (see Figure 18.4). Once these spinal nerves leave the spinal cord, they break off to form the network of nerves in the body and limbs, and some combine and entwine to form braided branches or plexuses. These nerves serve as the highway by which impulses are sent to and from all other areas of the body via the sophisticated pathway referred to as the peripheral nervous system, which contains both sensory and motor fibres (McErlean and Migliozzi 2017). These nerves therefore make possible movement and sensation; thus, if these are injured or impaired it can result in a loss of movement or feeling in specific parts of the body. A detailed map of this network and testing of the body dermatome (Figure 18.5) via sensory block checks are therefore imperative when caring for women with neuraxial anaesthesia in order to confirm injury and reduced sensation.

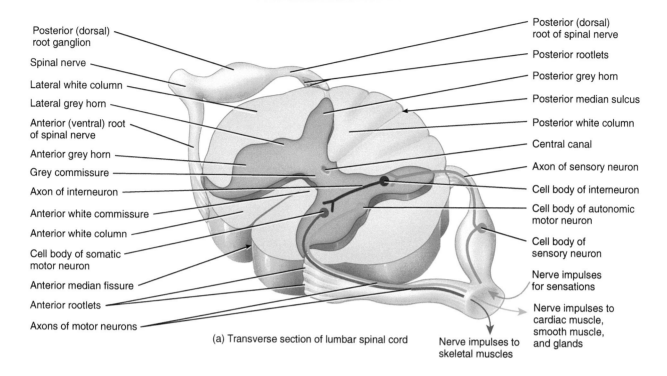

Posterior (dorsal) root ganglion

Spinal nerve

Lateral white column

Lateral grey horn

Anterior (ventral) root of spinal nerve

Anterior grey horn

Grey commissure

Axon of interneuron

Anterior white commissure

Anterior white column

Cell body of somatic motor neuron

Anterior median fissure

Anterior rootlets

Axons of motor neurons

Posterior (dorsal) root of spinal nerve

Posterior rootlets

Posterior grey horn

Posterior median sulcus

Posterior white column

Central canal

Axon of sensory neuron

Cell body of interneuron

Cell body of autonomic motor neuron

Cell body of sensory neuron

Nerve impulses for sensations

Nerve impulses to cardiac muscle, smooth muscle, and glands

Nerve impulses to skeletal muscles

(a) Transverse section of lumbar spinal cord

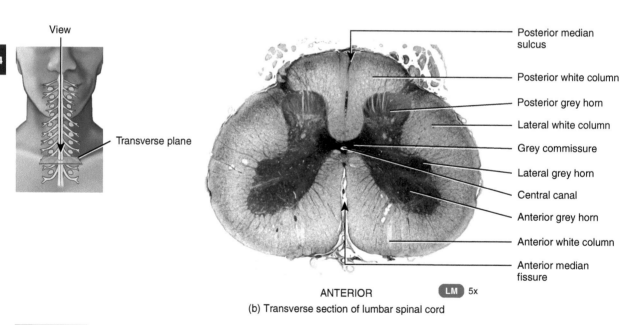

View

Transverse plane

Posterior median sulcus

Posterior white column

Posterior grey horn

Lateral white column

Grey commissure

Lateral grey horn

Central canal

Anterior grey horn

Anterior white column

Anterior median fissure

ANTERIOR

LM 5x

(b) Transverse section of lumbar spinal cord

FIGURE 18.3   The spinal cord.

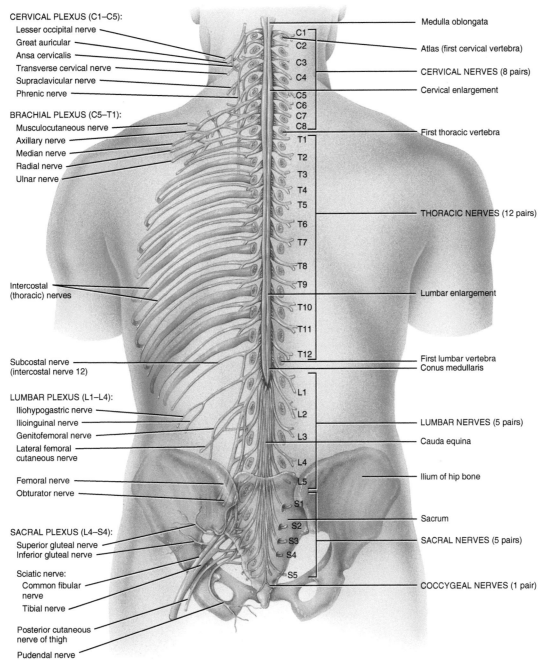

CERVICAL PLEXUS (C1–C5):
Lesser occipital nerve
Great auricular
Ansa cervicalis
Transverse cervical nerve
Supraclavicular nerve
Phrenic nerve

BRACHIAL PLEXUS (C5–T1):
Musculocutaneous nerve
Axillary nerve
Median nerve
Radial nerve
Ulnar nerve

Intercostal
(thoracic) nerves

Subcostal nerve
(intercostal nerve 12)

LUMBAR PLEXUS (L1–L4):
Iliohypogastric nerve
Ilioinguinal nerve
Genitofemoral nerve
Lateral femoral
cutaneous nerve

Femoral nerve
Obturator nerve

SACRAL PLEXUS (L4–S4):
Superior gluteal nerve
Inferior gluteal nerve

Sciatic nerve:
  Common fibular
  nerve
  Tibial nerve

Posterior cutaneous
nerve of thigh

Pudendal nerve

Medulla oblongata
Atlas (first cervical vertebra)
CERVICAL NERVES (8 pairs)
Cervical enlargement

First thoracic vertebra

THORACIC NERVES (12 pairs)

Lumbar enlargement

First lumbar vertebra
Conus medullaris

LUMBAR NERVES (5 pairs)
Cauda equina

Ilium of hip bone

Sacrum

SACRAL NERVES (5 pairs)

COCCYGEAL NERVES (1 pair)

C1, C2, C3, C4, C5, C6, C7, C8
T1, T2, T3, T4, T5, T6, T7, T8, T9, T10, T11, T12
L1, L2, L3, L4, L5
S1, S2, S3, S4, S5

Posterior view of entire spinal cord and portions of spinal nerves

FIGURE 18.4 The spinal nerves.

335

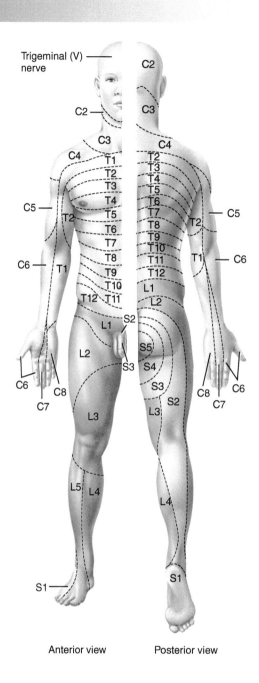

FIGURE 18.5 Dermatomes.

Pain Pathways

Pain pathways are associated with ascending, descending and modulating processes (see Figure 18.6) and while some treatments and management approaches are effective in interfering with the signals that are being sent to the brain, others could play a role in how the body responds to these signals after they are received and interpreted by the brain.

The first part of the pathway is usually associated with the stimulation of sensory nerve endings, known as nociceptors, by chemicals such as histamine and prostaglandins released when tissue injury or irritation occurs (Boyd 2022). Nociceptors are specialised peripheral nervous tissue sensitive to changes in the environment and more

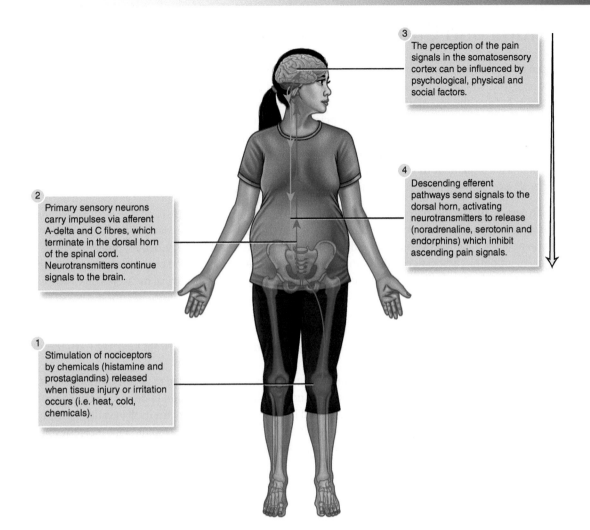

3 The perception of the pain signals in the somatosensory cortex can be influenced by psychological, physical and social factors.

4 Descending efferent pathways send signals to the dorsal horn, activating neurotransmitters to release (noradrenaline, serotonin and endorphins) which inhibit ascending pain signals.

2 Primary sensory neurons carry impulses via afferent A-delta and C fibres, which terminate in the dorsal horn of the spinal cord. Neurotransmitters continue signals to the brain.

1 Stimulation of nociceptors by chemicals (histamine and prostaglandins) released when tissue injury or irritation occurs (i.e. heat, cold, chemicals).

FIGURE 18.6 The pain pathway.

importantly from thermal, mechanical and chemical noxious stimuli. Once activated these primary sensory neurons carry impulses via afferent A-delta fibres (wide, myelinated, fast and associated with localised sharp pain) and C fibres (narrow, non-myelinated and slower) towards the CNS (Todd 2016). These terminate in the dorsal horn of the spinal cord forming synapses, where the action of neurotransmitters (i.e. glutamate and substance P) continue to transfer the signals along relay neurons to the somatosensory cortex (Ashelford et al. 2019).

The perception of the pain signals in the brain can be influenced by a wide array of factors including psychological, physical, social and pharmacological, and the response to the perceived pain signals could be in the form of emotional reactions and physiological responses, activating the descending inhibitory efferent pathways. Signals are transmitted from the brain back to the dorsal horn, where nerve endings are activated to release neurotransmitters (noradrenaline, serotonin and endorphins) that bind to the afferent pain fibres, inhibiting the synaptic transmission to the relay neurons.

It is in the descending pain pathway that opioids have been recognised as being the most effective medication, by inhibiting the synaptic transmission between the pain fibres. However, the way in which this occurs is different from the body's natural inhibitory mechanism. Opioid peptides, once bound to the appropriate receptors (mu – μ, kappa – κ and delta – δ) modulate pain input in two ways: by releasing a large number of calcium ions blocking the presynaptic terminal and by opening potassium channels that flood the synapse and hyperpolarise the neurons, preventing signals from passing across the synapse (Bannister 2019).

Definitions and Categories of Pain

Before pain can be treated, it is necessary to understand and determine which type of pain the woman is experiencing, as the choice of analgesic should be tailored to the type of pain and personal preferences. The first worldwide accepted definition of pain is from the International Association for the Study of Pain (IASP), which declares that pain is 'an unpleasant sensory and emotional experience associated with actual or potential tissue damage' (Merskey and Bogduk 1994, p. 209). However, pain is not always directly linked to the amount of trauma, it can also be associated with psychological and emotional issues (VanMeter and Hubert 2022). It is therefore multilayered and the most commonly used classifications are separated by duration (acute or chronic), type (nociceptive, neuropathic and psychogenic) and site (somatic and visceral) (see Figure 18.7). Some overlap and women may present with one or more.

- **Acute** pain serves a protective purpose, is of short duration (less than three months) and is reversible. Predominantly nociceptive in nature, it involves sensory processes, and can be treated very effectively with analgesics.
- **Chronic** pain serves no protective purpose and persists past the initial healing stage, usually more than three months. It is largely neuropathic, associated with an array of changes to the peripheral and central sensory pathways, is typically connected with chronic disease, and is usually treated alongside psychological measures due to its extremely subjective nature.
- **Nociceptive** pain is the most frequently experienced type of pain. It is a primitive sensation, protective in nature, that involves the passing of information through primary afferent fibres to the cerebral cortex via pain receptors, referred to as nociceptors, which are stimulated and activated by tissue damage resulting from heat, cold, stretch, vibration or chemicals.
- **Neuropathic** pain is more degenerative and usually occurs as a result of pain related to sensory abnormalities that can be caused by damage to the nerves (a nerve infection) or neurological dysfunction (a disease in the somatosensory nervous system). This type of pain may not be diagnosed immediately, it can manifest itself in various ways and it can often be confused with acute persistent pain. Neuropathic pain is often managed via multimodal analgesic approaches.
- **Inflammatory** pain is stimulation of nociceptive processes by chemicals released as part of the inflammatory process.
- **Somatic** pain is a large part of the body's natural defence mechanism and is associated with nociceptive processes activated in skin, bones, joints, connective tissues and muscles.
- **Visceral** pain is a sensation and nociceptive process activated in the organs (i.e. stomach, kidneys, gallbladder) transmitted via the sympathetic fibres and linked to conditions such as irritable bowel syndrome and dysmenorrhoea.
- **Referred** pain is felt in the skin that lies over an affected organ, or in an area some distance from the site of disease or injury.

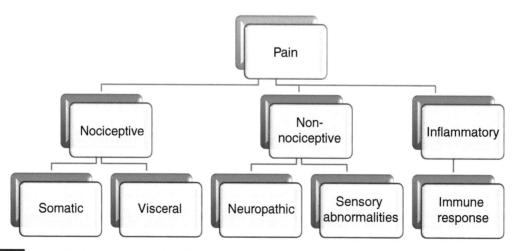

FIGURE 18.7   Types of pain. Source: Reproduced from Cunningham (2017) and VanMeter and Hubert (2022).

Case Study 18.1   Rheumatoid Arthritis and Pregnancy

Felicity is a 29-year-old woman who is speaking to her midwife for the first time after finding out she is pregnant (approximately seven weeks' gestation). She was diagnosed with rheumatoid arthritis in her early 20s and is worried about the effect of her prescribed medications on the fetus. She is otherwise healthy and while this pregnancy was not planned, she and her partner are very happy. She has over the last few months experienced a flare-up of symptoms so is currently prescribed oral methotrexate and ibuprofen.

Rheumatoid arthritis is an autoimmune disease, more common in females, usually affecting the joints, which can become swollen, stiff and painful. For some women the pain and swelling improve throughout pregnancy, but some women's symptoms worsen. Additionally, some of the medications used to control the symptoms can potentially affect fetal development (NRAS 2022).

- How can you differentiate normal pregnancy symptoms (pain and swelling) from worsening symptoms of the underlying disease?
- Who else would you need involved in Felicity's care?
- What would be your recommendations regarding her current medication and analgesic requirements going forward?

Medicines Management: Ibuprofen

One of the most frequently used medications for the treatment of pain from rheumatoid arthritis is a non-steroidal anti-inflammatory drug (NSAID) such as ibuprofen. Ibuprofen is a propionic acid derivative that can be given orally or topically 600 mg four to six times a day, up to a daily maximum of 1.8 g.

Consequences for pregnancy: Ibuprofen should be avoided unless benefits outweigh risks and the risk to the fetus increases after week 32, as it can potentially cause closure of the fetal ductus arteriosus in utero, resulting in persistent pulmonary hypertension of the newborn and lung and kidney damage. It can also delay the onset and progression of labour.

Consequences postnatally: Many women find NSAIDs beneficial to treat pain after childbirth.

Source: Adapted from BNF (2022a).

339

Importance of Individualised Pain Assessments

Women react to pain in varying ways. Some see pain as something that should be endured, for others it can be a debilitating problem that is impeding their ability to function and has negative impacts on their perinatal experiences. Therefore, to ensure that an effective and individually tailored holistic management plan is developed, it is important to understand how pain uniquely affects women from a biopsychosocial perspective. To do this midwives use a range of tools, such as the skills of observation (the art of noticing), questioning techniques, active listening and interpretation. Another strategy often employed by midwifery professionals is the assessment and measurement of vital signs, such as tachypnoea, tachycardia and systolic hypertension, all of which may help in identifying women's pain, especially when they are unable to verbalise it (Erden et al. 2018). It is important to remember that no one skill is superior. Rather, it is the culmination of information gathered via the various methods that enables midwives to determine if a woman is in pain and understand how this pain is affecting them physically, psychologically, socially and culturally (Kettyle 2019) (see Table 18.1).

TABLE 18.1   Example of assessment domains.

Physical appearance	Physical impact
Facial expressions	Bowel habits
Posturing	Insomnia
Guarding	Fatigue
Reduced movement	Vital signs
Abnormal gait	
Body language	

Pain characteristics	Emotional/behavioural
Location	Depression
Duration	Anger
Intensity	Irritability
Precipitating or aggravating factors	Vocalisations

Quality of life	Past experiences
Social activities	Coping strategies
Relationships	Medications
Work	Expectations
Cultural impact	
Religion	

Source: Adapted from Cunningham (2017) and Kettyle (2019).

Red Flag: Abdominal Pain During Pregnancy

During pregnancy is in not uncommon for women to experience some degree of abdominal or pelvic pain and in most cases this is benign. However, midwives need to bear in mind that other abdominal organs can be diseased and that non-pregnancy-related acute emergency conditions such as appendicitis and pancreatitis can occur.

It is important to undertake a thorough assessment of the pain and the onset, location, aggravating and alleviating factors, and other associated signs and symptoms (gastrointestinal, vital signs). You must carry out physical examination and if necessary, make a referral to a pregnancy assessment unit or contact emergency services, depending on the severity of the pain and the level of acuity and associated symptoms.

N.B. Always alleviate the pain, attempt to identify the cause and in the early stages of pregnancy consider ectopic pregnancy.

Source: Adapted from Child and Impey (2016).

Expert Midwife: Pelvic Pain

While we are primarily caring for women who are healthy, we also need to take a holistic approach, which includes consideration of conditions that may arise due to or outside of normal pregnancy. One example that has always stuck with me was a woman who at 31 weeks' gestation attended a routine antenatal appointment. Towards the end of the visit, she mentioned that she had some pain in her right groin and wondered if she needed a referral to a physiotherapist for symphysis pubis dysfunction. Despite having already carried out an abdominal examination and assessment of her blood pressure, I decided to ask further questions about the pain, other associated symptoms and wanted to examine the area in greater detail. Consequently, she needed to remove her trousers and her right leg appeared slightly swollen, and slight erythema was present. This prompted me to suspect a deep vein thrombosis and to make an immediate referral to the pregnancy assessment unit. Venous thromboembolism in her right groin was confirmed and treatment commenced.

Maria, Midwife

Multimodal Management Strategies

The word analgesia, 'to be without the feeling of pain', is derived from the Greek language and in terms of pain management relates to medication and alternative interventions. Hence, pain management plans should incorporate a multimodal approach, using a range of pharmacological and non-pharmacological strategies to successfully and holistically treat women's pain (Baston and Hall 2017). A combination approach is also recommended for pharmacological management, as several drugs have morphine-sparing properties that increase the effect of opioids; therefore, the use of adjuvants is recommended (Boyd 2022). This is an effective way to manage pain, but the decisions about which management strategies to use should also take into consideration the context of the clinical situation, the risks to the mother and child, the environment and the physical space and the availability of resources. Clinical decisions associated with analgesic administration must also be made in line with Royal Pharmaceutical Society (RPS 2019) recommendations, which state that any healthcare professional administering medicines must possess a comprehensive understanding of the drug itself and an awareness of the potential risks and side effects.

Case Study 18.2   Labour Pain

Charlotte, 23 years old, is in spontaneous labour with her first child. She has arrived at the delivery suite and is experiencing back pain and regular contractions every 2–4 minutes, lasting 30–60 seconds. She has taken paracetamol at home and is happy to use whatever methods of pain relief the midwifery team suggest and has no specific requirements in her birth plan.

- What questions will the midwife need to ask and what other assessments will she need to undertake to establish the level of pain and the most appropriate analgesic approach?
- Before reading the remaining sections of the chapter, make a list of the approaches you think could be used now, and also a list of other approaches and in what circumstances these may be used for Charlotte as she progresses through her labour.
- After finishing the chapter, review your list to see if your approaches have changed.

Health Promotion

Vulval varicosities during pregnancy are linked with venous stasis and venous thromboembolic events. It is essential that women are educated about the strategies that can be undertaken to reduce the risk of developing venous thromboembolism.

- To reduce venous stasis, encourage women to regularly change their position, from sitting to standing, and to sit with their legs elevated.
- To increase venous return, advise women they can wear compression hosiery, take regular exercise and encourage calf muscle contraction even when their legs are elevated.
- To reduce the risk of hypercoagulability, stress the importance of drinking water and hydration, stopping smoking and maintaining a healthy diet.

Non-pharmacological Strategies

Pharmacological treatments are not the only strategy at midwives' disposal. True holistic management cannot be achieved without the incorporation of non-pharmacological therapies. Some of these interventions are long-standing, are engrained in some traditional midwifery practices and, when used correctly, can enhance women's feelings of empowerment and involvement (Baston and Hall 2017).

Woman-Centred Care

It is important to be aware of your own beliefs and values, as these may be at odds with those of the women you care for. You may also have specialist skills, such as training in hypnotherapy, reflexology and cognitive behavioural theory. However, despite these being at your disposal, the final decision must be the woman's even if her approaches are not what you are used to.

Expert Midwife: Pain Management Strategies

I have had the pleasure of caring for hundreds of women during the labour and birthing process, and am still to this day sometimes surprised by the innovative ways in which some women manage and react to pain. I remain in awe of a woman's abilities to work with the pain and use non-pharmacological approaches to ensure they remain empowered. Women, their birthing partners and sometimes myself have danced and rocked through contractions. I remember one occasion when I needed to learn a TV theme tune as she and her partner wanted to sing this when she experienced pain.

It is therefore essential that you as midwifery students remain open-minded and take every opportunity to learn and expose yourself to new approaches so you can adapt your future practice depending on the women's unique needs.

Emma, Midwife

Non-pharmacological strategies can be placed into three main groups (see Table 18.2) and the choice of which to use depends on the woman's preferences and existing coping mechanisms. These strategies have been highlighted as they align with the fundamental core values of care and compassion and require very little in terms of resources or time.

- **Distraction:** This basic skill often requires no equipment, can be done anywhere and is a useful way of taking women's minds off their pain. Birth partners and midwives can play a major role in incorporating activities to distract the women from the focus of each contraction, and the use of this approach has been known to reduce the need for pharmacological intervention (Johnson and Taylor 2022).
- **Breathing techniques:** Physical reactions to pain can include altered patterns of breathing, which can become faster and shallower, and some women may even hold their breath. To ensure adequate maternal and fetal oxygenation and assist in the modulation, ascending and descending pathways, it may be necessary to help the woman regulate her breathing with the use of breathing techniques (Baston and Hall 2017).
- **Therapeutic touch and massage:** For centuries, the therapeutic placing on of hands has proven to be a useful skill and has beneficial physiological (stimulation of A-beta fibres that restrict pain pathways) and psychological properties. However, midwives must be cognisant of the woman's personal preferences and past experiences, as she

TABLE 18.2   Example of non-pharmacological management strategies.

Psychological/emotional	Physical	Alternative
Spiritual	Heat and cold pads (used with caution during pregnancy)	Acupuncture
Relaxation	Water immersion	Acupressure
Information	Exercise	Electrostimulation
Breathing	Massage	Herbs
Music	Body position/comfort	Reflexology
Distraction	Art therapy	Biofield therapies (e.g. reiki)
Imagery	Rest	
Cognitive behavioural therapy		
Yoga		
Tai chi		

Source: Adapted from Cunningham (2017) and Johnson and Taylor (2022).

may be averse to physical touching, especially if she has been subject to physical and sexual abuse (Chapman and Charles 2018).

- **Environment**: Sound, lighting and the temperature of the woman's immediate environment has been shown to heighten or reduce perceptions of pain. Building safe nesting environments that are warm, dark and quiet can also reduce fear and anxiety, which in turn has a beneficial impact on pain experiences. Towards the late stages of labour women may also withdraw into themselves, and this is when distraction and touch may not be beneficial (Baston and Hall 2017).
- **Transcutaneous electrical nerve stimulation (TENS):** This involves a pulsed electrical current being delivered to the surface of the skin, usually at specific acupuncture points, to stimulate endorphins and block ascending signals (Johnson and Taylor 2022). However, NICE (2017) stipulates that this should not be used during established labour.
- **Water:** Deep water immersion has many unique benefits: it helps to relieve muscle tension and anxiety, eases backache, has analgesic properties and induces feelings of relaxation (Chapman and Charles 2018). However, the temperature should be regularly monitored to ensure it does not go above 37.5°C (NICE 2017).

Pharmacological Management

One very effective strategy that midwives have within their management arsenal is the use of pharmacological treatments. The choice depends on what stage of the perinatal journey the pain is being experienced in and whether the pain is nociceptive, neuropathic, inflammatory or of mixed origin. There are three main categories: opioids, non-opioids/NSAIDs and adjuvants/co-analgesics. The most efficient pharmacological regimen for moderate to severe pain often incorporates a combined approach by administrating a specific drug in conjunction with adjuvants or co-analgesics.

Woman-Centred Care

It is very important that the most appropriate drug is used to treat women's pain and the decision of which analgesic to choose should (whenever possible) be made in partnership with the woman and the pharmacist or prescriber (NMC 2018; RPS 2019). For example, ibuprofen is not recommended during the antenatal period, but following birth it is suitable for the management of inflammatory pain that may be experienced following perineal trauma. The woman may prefer an alternative medication if she is currently breastfeeding.

343

Non-opioids

The most widely used and safest analgesic (when taken correctly) is acetaminophen (paracetamol), which can also be used as an antipyretic (Boyd 2022). The recommended oral dose is 500 mg–1 g, every 4–6 hours, with a maximum of 4 g in 24 hours (see Table 18.3). There are very few side effects associated with paracetamol; however, if taken in excess it can lead to series hepatotoxicity. When an overdose is suspected the antidote N-acetylcysteine should be administered. Caution is advised for anyone with renal or hepatic impairment and heavy alcohol consumption can increase the risk of hepatotoxicity.

Non-steroidal Anti-inflammatories

NSAIDs are used not only for their anti-inflammatory actions but also for their analgesic and antipyretic properties. They are not effective for women experiencing visceral pain associated with the abdomen and chest, but can be given as an adjuvant for severe pain (especially following a caesarean section) due to their opioid-sparing effects. There are a wide variety of NSAIDs, each with its own chemical composition; however, they are very similar in terms of the analgesic effect (see Table 18.3).

Prostaglandin has beneficial effects in maintaining renal blood flow and keeping the lungs open, therefore care must be taken with women with asthma or poor renal function. Prostaglandin suppression can also result in gastrointestinal damage, nausea, gastritis, dyspepsia and in severe cases gastric bleeding and ulcerations (Boyd 2022). Oral NSAIDs

TABLE 18.3 Examples of non-opioids and non-steroidal anti-inflammatory drugs.

Medication type	Acetaminophen	Salicylic acid derivatives	Propionic acid derivatives	Others
Medication name	Paracetamol	Aspirin	Ibuprofen	Diclofenac
Route of administration	Oral, rectal or intravenous infusion	Oral or rectal	Oral or topical	Oral, intramuscular injection, rectal, topical and intravenous infusion
Dose (oral)	500 mg–1 g up to 4 g daily	300–900 mg	600 mg up to 1.8 g daily	75–150 mg daily
Frequency and timings (oral)	4–6 h	4–6 h	4–6 times a day	1–3 times a day
Onset/duration	15–60 min/6 h	30–60 min or 1–8 h for coated tablets/12 h	1–2 h/5–10 h	1 h/12 h
Common side effects	No common side effects	Indigestion	Heartburn and indigestion	Gastrointestinal disorders
Pregnancy, labour and breastfeeding	Not known to be harmful	Avoid during the third trimester, delivery and also if breastfeeding	Avoid during pregnancy and to be used with caution during breastfeeding	Avoid unless essential, i.e. surgery and severe acute pain

Source: Adapted from BNF (2022b).

should therefore be taken with or after food and the drugs may be enteric coated. For NSAIDs that are COX-2 selective, gastrointestinal side effects can be reduced; however, inhibiting COX-2 can also increase cardiovascular risk and therefore they are not used routinely.

Health Promotion: Buying Over-the-Counter Medications

Some medications such as paracetamol are often found in combination medications (i.e. co-codamol) that can be purchased over the counter. Care must be taken, as they may contain drugs that the woman may be unaware of, which could lead to inadvertent overdose or teratogenic implications for the fetus. It is essential that midwives during antenatal classes and appointments explain to women which common over-the-counter medications they can use for mild pain and stress that they should always speak to the pharmacist before purchasing new medications.

Opioid Agonists

Opioids can be created synthetically and semi-synthetically. Stronger opioids (e.g. morphine) are indicated for the treatment of severe pain and weaker opioids (e.g. codeine) are often prescribed to manage mild to moderate pain (see Table 18.4). For pain relief during labour, the recommended opioids are pethidine and diamorphine (NICE 2017).

Opioids bind to opioid receptors located within the CNS, the brain, the spinal cord and peripherally in the gastrointestinal tract. Once the opioids attach to the receptors, they block pain signals and release large amounts of dopamine throughout the body (Schumacher et al. 2015). There are three classic types of opioid receptors that have designated Greek letters (μ, κ, δ) and different analgesics bind to these receptors in a variety of ways, which explains why there is a wide range of benefits and side effects associated with opioid use.

TABLE 18.4 Examples of opioids.

Medication name	Codeine	Tramadol	Diamorphine	Pethidine
Route of administration	Oral, intramuscular injection	Oral, intramuscular injection, intravenous injection or infusion	Intramuscular, subcutaneous or intravenous injection	Intramuscular or subcutaneous injection
Dose	Oral: 30–60 mg Maximum 240 mg/daily	Oral: 50–100 mg Maximum 400 mg	Intramuscular 5 mg	Injection 50–100 mg maximum 400 mg/day
Frequency and timings	4–6 h orally	4 h orally	Every 4 h	Every 1–3 h
Onset/duration	30–60 min/6 h	Up to 60 min/6 h	6–10 min/4 h	10 min/2–4 h
Common side effects	Nausea and vomiting, constipation, cardiac arrhythmias (prolonged use)	Seizures, serotonin syndrome	Nausea and vomiting, constipation, delirium, dependence, respiratory depression	Nausea and vomiting, constipation, delirium, dependence, respiratory depression
Pregnancy, labour and breastfeeding	Respiratory depression and withdrawal symptoms can occur in neonates. Advised to avoid if breastfeeding	Respiratory depression and withdrawal symptoms can occur in neonates. Advised to avoid if breastfeeding	Respiratory depression and withdrawal symptoms can occur in neonates. A therapeutic dose is unlikely to affect infants if breastfeeding	Respiratory depression and withdrawal symptoms can occur in neonates. A therapeutic dose is unlikely to affect infants if breastfeeding

Source: Adapted from BNF (2022b).

Caution should be taken when administering opioid analgesics, as there are several cautions and contra-indications that need to be considered, especially during labour. First, it is of note that repeated opioid administration could result in opiate dependence. NICE (2019) produced a document specifically focusing on opioid dependence, which states that signs of physical and psychological dependence can appear in as little as 2–10 days. It is also worth recognising that individuals may experience increased tolerance to the potency of an opiate with repeated usage, which may then develop into a dependence where pain cannot be managed with the medication prescribed (BNF 2023a). However, NICE also states that dependence is no deterrent for the control of severe pain, and this must be taken into consideration when caring for women with substance misuse during labour and delivery.

Examination Scenario: Pupil Response and Signs of Substance Misuse

Pinpoint pupils are caused by opioid drugs as they stimulate the oculomotor nerves that shrink the diameter of the pupil. This phenomenon is still utilised as a vital diagnostic tool when testing for opioid overdose and substance misuse.

Red Flag: Respiratory Depression

One of the most serious side effects of opioids is an increase in respiratory depression, which if not treated could result in a significant brain injury, cardiac arrest or death (Lee et al. 2015). To treat respiratory depression, the opioid antagonist naloxone, also known as an opiate reversal agent, should be administered. When injected intravenously, the effects of this agent occur within two minutes of administration. The mode of action for naloxone is not fully understood, but it is thought to be a competitive opioid receptor antagonist, so it has a higher affinity to the receptor sites in the CNS, especially the mu receptor (Wang et al. 2016).

It is imperative that women who are given opioids during delivery are closely monitored and opioids should be avoided if delivery is imminent, as the baby may also develop respiratory depression and drowsiness that could last several days (NICE 2017).

Learning Event

Naloxone is very short-acting, with a half-life of approximately 30–80 minutes, which is shorter than the average half-life of some opiates. As a consequence, repeated administration may be necessary.

Inhalation Analgesics

Nitrous oxide (N_2O), commonly referred to as Entonox, is a well-established anaesthetic and analgesic gas mixture. The combination of 50% N_2O and 50% oxygen is found in obstetric and maternity departments and can be beneficial in all stages of labour, and it is frequently used for the maintenance of anaesthesia (Johnson and Taylor 2022; BNF 2023b). When inhaled it provides pain relief as well as anaesthetic properties such as sedation. Added benefits of its use are that there are few effects on the baby, the woman can control the amount as it is self-administered and she can use it as soon as the contractions start (Johnson and Taylor 2022). The precise mechanism of action for the anaesthetic properties of N_2O remains unknown; however, the most prevalent explanation is that the N_2O inhibits the pain receptors on the ascending pain pathway, blocking the neurons carrying the pain response via the afferent A-delta and C fibres. The analgesic mechanism of N_2O is better understood. It forces the release of opioid peptides binding to the opioid receptors in the brain and CNS. This results in the release of opioids in the brainstem, blocking the pain signals on the descending pain pathway (Huang and Johnson 2016). N_2O is absorbed via diffusion in the lungs and is eliminated and excreted by respiration within approximately five minutes (BNF 2023b).

Local and Regional Anaesthesia

Local and regional anaesthesia is often used in maternity and obstetric units and includes interventions such as epidural and spinal analgesia, as well as local anaesthetic into the subcutaneous tissue during episiotomy procedures and perineal repair. It can be used to manage both acute and chronic pain, which makes it of vital importance when considering individuals with complex pain management needs. Every local anaesthetic has different physicochemical properties, but they all share the same mode of action. They block the voltage-gated sodium channels in the axon of nerve cells, halting the transfer of electrons between the nerve cells and interrupting pain signals.

An epidural is a procedure that involves injecting local anaesthetic, often combined with an opioid, into the space around the spinal nerves known as the epidural space (see Figure 18.8), to provide pain relief (analgesia) or a total block

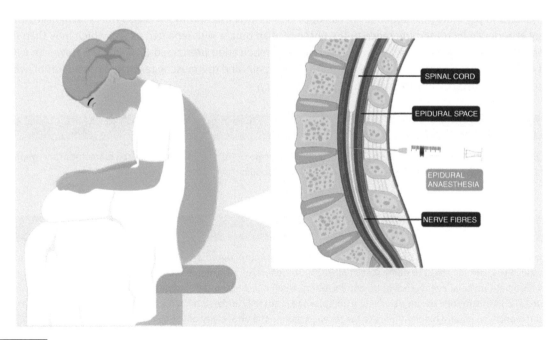

FIGURE 18.8 Placement of epidural and spinal analgesia/anaesthesia.

TABLE 18.5 Side effects and potential complications associated with epidural and spinal analgesia/anaesthesia.

Hypotension
Higher incidence of instrumental delivery
Poor mobility
Urinary retention
Maternal fever
Respiratory depression
Partial block
Dural puncture
Catheter migration
Abscess formation
Haematoma
Meningitis

Source: Adapted from NICE (2017) and Johnson and Taylor (2022).

(anaesthesia). This is administered via an epidural catheter that is inserted between vertebra L3 and L4, enabling the drugs to be continuously infused. An additional benefit of using an epidural catheter is that the analgesia can be 'topped up' as required, allowing for prolonged analgesic effect. A spinal procedure involves the administration of medication through the epidural space, directly into the intrathecal space (subarachnoid space). The benefits of this procedure are that lower doses of drugs can be used and it is considered more effective due to rapid onset. For this reason, it is preferred for emergency caesarean sections (Johnson and Taylor 2022). Combined epidural and spinal analgesia can also be used that combines the advantages of both techniques.

There are side effects associated with epidural and spinal analgesia (see Table 18.5) and it is essential that women should be closely monitored and any side effects reported to the anaesthetic staff immediately. The levels of the block should also be checked (using dermatomes) at least once an hour to ensure the treatment is working and that the block level has not risen past T4 (NICE 2017).

347

Red Flag: Epidural Anaesthesia/Analgesia

While epidurals are considered a safe procedure and used routinely during labour, there are some complications and risks that midwives and midwifery students need to be cognisant of, as delays in recognition and treatment could result in neurological damage. Due to these risks, and the additional levels of skill needed to insert them, epidurals are normally only offered in obstetric units and blood pressure and fetal heart rate need to be closely monitored.

Complications include:

- Hypotension
- Incontinence
- Nausea and vomiting
- Headache
- Bradypnoea
- Temporary or permanent nerve damage
- Infection

Source: Adapted from NICE (2017); Roderick et al. (2017); Yentis et al. (2020).

Examination Scenario: Assessment of Neuraxial Anaesthesia

Roderick et al. (2017) conducted a national survey to examine the monitoring of recovery after neuraxial anaesthesia. They found that within the United Kingdom practice varied widely and only 56% of obstetric units had a policy in place to monitor this treatment.

Reflect on what you have witnessed in practice:

- Have you undertaken checks especially related to the assessment of neuraxial anaesthesia?
- Are there specific documents and tools that are used in practice to assist midwives in assessing the level and effectiveness of the types of anaesthesia and analgesia?
- Would you feel confident using these in practice?
- If you suspected neurological changes in a woman in your care, what would you do?

Toxicity

When undertaking perineal repair and injecting a local anaesthetic into the subcutaneous tissue, it is vital to aspirate and check the position, as injecting the local anaesthetic into a blood vessel can result in complications from the toxic potential of this drug. Early symptoms of mild local anaesthetic toxicity include restlessness, tinnitus, slurred speech and a metallic taste in the mouth (Christie et al. 2015). In the most serious of cases, the toxicity can enter the systemic circulation and cause a cardiac arrest. Initial signs include tachycardia and hypertension, followed by myocardial depression, vasodilation, hypotension and a multitude of cardiac arrhythmias such as sinus bradycardia, conduction blocks, ventricular tachyarrhythmia and eventually asystole.

Learning Event: Treating Local Anaesthetic Toxicity

To treat local anaesthetic toxicity midwives must assess the airway, breathing and circulation in turn and if required commence cardiopulmonary resuscitation procedures. If there is no response a 20% lipid emulsion should be given intravenously, as this reduces the amount of toxin that can bind to the myocardium (Ciechanowicz and Patil 2012). If the woman has a strong cardiac output, 100% oxygen should be administered and the airway secured.

Conditions Associated with Pain

The following is a list of some of the perinatal conditions that can result in pain. Take some time and write notes about each of the conditions. Think about the altered pathophysiology involved. Remember to include aspects of women's care. If you are making notes about people to whom you have offered care and support, you must ensure that you have adhered to the rules of confidentiality.

The condition	Your notes
Placental abruption	
Symphysis pubis dysfunction	
Migraine	
Back pain	
Sickle cell	

Take-Home Points

- When caring for any woman it is important to have a sound understanding of the pathophysiology of pain. This enables midwives to recognise how and when pain can have negative impacts on perinatal journey experiences.
- When assessing pain midwives must use a biopsychosocial approach and be aware of context when choosing a pain assessment tool.
- It is also essential to include women and their partners in their care, as decisions made about how their pain should be managed must be tailored to their individual needs.
- When assessing pain, in addition to normal adaptations during pregnancy, midwives need to consider that the pain experienced by a woman could be unrelated to the pregnancy and liaise with other healthcare professionals to ensure that the underlying cause is investigated and the pain is managed safely and effectively.

Conclusion

Pain management strategies are most successful when they incorporate multimodal approaches that are chosen in partnership with the women. This is not only to take advantage of the pharmacological benefits of a range of drugs, but also to reduce potential side effects and adopt a holistic and woman-centred approach to pain management. To achieve this safely and effectively, midwives and midwifery students must ensure that their knowledge and understanding of pain pathways and analgesic approaches are up to date and if additional advice is required that they consult with specialised pain teams or pharmacists.

References

Ashelford, S., Raynsford, J., and Taylor, V. (2019). *Pathophysiology and Pharmacology for Nursing Students*, 2e. London: Sage.

Bannister, K. (2019). Descending pain modulation: influence and impact. *Current Opinion in Physiology* 11 (1): 62–66.

Baston, H. and Hall, J. (2017). *Midwifery Essentials: Labour*, 2e. London: Elsevier.

Boore, J., Cook, N., and Shepherd, A. (2021). *Essentials of Anatomy and Physiology for Nursing Practice*, 2e. London: Sage.

Boyd, C. (2022). *Clinical Skills for Nurses*. Chichester: Wiley.

British National Formulary (BNF) (2022a). Ibuprofen. https://bnf.nice.org.uk/drugs/ibuprofen (accessed November 2023).

British National Formulary (BNF) (2022b). *BNF – 80*. London: BMJ Group and Pharmaceutical Press.

British National Formulary (BNF) (2023a). Morphine. https://bnf.nice.org.uk/drugs/morphine (accessed November 2023).

British National Formulary (BNF) (2023b). Nitrous oxide. https://bnf.nice.org.uk/drugs/nitrous-oxide (accessed November 2023).

Chapman, V. and Charles, C. (2018). *The Midwife's Labour and Birth Handbook*. Chichester: Wiley.

Child, T. and Impey, L. (2016). *Obstetrics and Gynaecology*, 5e. Chichester: Wiley.

Christie, L., Picard, J., and Weinberg, G. (2015). Local anaesthetic systemic toxicity. *British Journal of Anaesthesia* 15 (3): 136–142.

Ciechanowicz, S. and Patil, V. (2012). Intravenous lipid emulsion – rescued at LAST. *British Dental Journal* 212 (5): 237–241.

Cunningham, S. (2017). Pain assessment and management. In: *Clinical Skills for Nursing Practice* (ed. T. Moore and S. Cunningham), 104–131. Oxford: Routledge.

Engel, G.L. (1980). The clinical application of the biopsychosocial model. *American Journal of Psychiatry* 137 (5): 535–544.

Erden, S., Demir, N., Ugras, G.A. et al. (2018). Vital signs: valid indicators to assess pain in intensive care unit patients? An observational, descriptive study. *Nursing and Health Sciences Journal* 20 (4): 502–508.

Ford, C. (2020). 'Myth or reality?' Preoperative pain planning and management: A critical ethnographic examination and exploration of day surgery preoperative practices. PhD thesis, Northumbria University.

Huang, C. and Johnson, N. (2016). Nitrous oxide, from the operating room to the emergency department. *Current Emergency and Hospital Medicine Reports* 4 (1): 11–18.

Johnson, R. and Taylor, W. (2022). *Skills for Midwifery Practice*, 5e. London: Elsevier.

Keefe, F.J., Lefebvre, J.C., and Starr, K.R. (1996). From the gate control theory to the neuromatrix: revolution or evolution? *Pain Forum* 5 (2): 143–146.

Kettyle, A. (2019). Pain assessment and management. In: *Essential of Nursing Adults* (ed. K. Elcock, W. Wright, P. Newcombe, and F. Everett), 174–192. London: Sage.

Lee, L., Caplan, R.A., Stephens, L.S. et al. (2015). Postoperative opioid-induced respiratory depression – a closed claims analysis. *Journal of Pain Medicine* 122 (1): 649–665.

McErlean, L. and Migliozzi, J.G. (2017). The nervous system. In: *Fundamentals of Anatomy and Physiology for Nursing and Midwives Students*, 2e (ed. I. Peate and M. Nair), 403–438. Chichester, UK: Wiley.

Melzack, R. (2001). Pain and the neuromatrix in the brain. *Journal of Dental Education* 65 (12): 1378–1382.

Melzack, R. (2005). Evolution of the neuromatrix theory of pain. The Prithvi Raj lecture: presented at the Third World Congress of World Institute of Pain, Barcelona 2004. *Pain Practice* 5 (2): 85–94.

Melzack, R. and Katz, J. (2013). Pain. *Wiley Interdisciplinary Reviews: Cognitive Science* 4 (1): 1–15.

Merskey, H. and Bogduk, N., IASP Task Force on Taxonomy(1994). *Classification of Chronic Pain*, 2e. Seattle, WA: IASP Press.

National Institute for Health and Care Excellence (NICE) (2017). *Intrapartum Care for Healthy Women and Babies*. London: NICE.

National Institute for Health and Care Excellence (NICE) (2019). Opioid dependence. https://cks.nice.org.uk/opioid-dependence (accessed November 2023).

National Rheumatoid Arthritis Society (NRAS) (2022). Rheumatoid arthritis and pregnancy. https://nras.org.uk/resource/rheumatoid-arthritis-pregnancy (accessed November 2023).

Nursing and Midwifery Council (NMC) (2018). The Code: professional standards of practice and behaviour for nurses, midwives and nursing associates. www.nmc.org.uk/standards/code (accessed November 2023).

Roderick, E., Hoyle, J., and Yentis, S.M. (2017). A national survey of neurological monitoring practice after obstetric regional anaesthesia in the UK. *Anaesthesia* 72: 755–759.

Royal Pharmaceutical Society and Royal College of Nursing (2019). *Professional Guidance on the Administration of Medicines in Midwives Settings*. London: Royal Pharmaceutical Society.

Schumacher, M., Basbaum, A., and Naidu, R. (2015). Opioid agonists and antagonists. In: *Basic and Clinical Pharmacology* (ed. B. Katzung), 553–574. New York: McGraw-Hill Education.

Todd, A.J. (2016). Anatomy of pain pathways. In: *An Introduction to Pain and Its Relation to Nervous System Disorders* (ed. A.A. Battaglia), 13–34. Chichester: Wiley.

VanMeter, K.C. and Hubert, R.J. (2022). *Gould's Pathophysiology for the Health Professions*, 7e. St Louis: Elsevier.

Wang, X., Zhang, Y., Peng, Y. et al. (2016). Pharmacological characterization of the opioid inactive isomers (+)-naltrexone and (+)-naloxone as antagonists of toll-like receptor 4. *British Journal of Pharmacology* 173 (5): 856–869.

Waugh, A. and Grant, A. (2022). *Ross and Wilson Anatomy and Physiology in Health and Illness*, 14e. London: Elsevier.

Yentis, S.M., Lucas, D.N., Brigante, L. et al. (2020). Safety guidelines: neurological monitoring associated with the obstetric neuraxial block. *Anaesthesia* 75: 913–919.

Further Resources

National Rheumatoid Arthritis Society. www.nras.org.uk/resource/rheumatoid-arthritis-pregnancy (accessed November 2023).

NHS Guide to Pelvic Pain in Pregnancy. www.nhs.uk/pregnancy/related-conditions/common-symptoms/pelvic-pain (accessed November 2023).

Glossary

Action potential	A rapid sequence of changes in the voltage across a membrane
Afferent	Inwards or towards
Anterior	Near the front
Autonomic	Involuntary or unconscious

Efferent	Outwards or away
Epidural	On or around the dura mater
Erythema	Superficial reddening of the skin
Ganglia	A collection of neuronal bodies found in the peripheral nervous system
Gestation	The period related to the development of the fetus inside the womb between conception and birth
Hyperalgesia	An increased sensitivity to feelings of pain
Lateral	Of or relating to the side
Neurotransmitter	A signalling molecule secreted by a neuron to affect another cell across a synapse
Nociceptor	A sensory receptor for painful stimuli
Perinatal	Time immediately before, during and after birth
Posterior	Situated behind
Receptor	An organ or cell able to respond to light, heat or other external stimuli and transmit a signal to a sensory nerve
Synapse	A gap between two nerve cells, where neurotransmitters diffuse from one cell to another

CHAPTER 19

The Musculoskeletal System and Associated Disorders

Suzanne Britt

University of Nottingham, UK

AIM

This chapter aims to provide insight and understanding to the reader concerning a range of disorders associated with the musculoskeletal system in pregnancy.

LEARNING OUTCOMES

On completion of this chapter the reader will be able to:

- Review the musculoskeletal system
- Have an understanding of pathophysiology and the musculoskeletal system
- Be familiar with a number of musculoskeletal system conditions
- Apply their understanding to the care of women

Test Your Prior Knowledge

1. How does pregnancy affect the musculoskeletal system in women?
2. What are some potential musculoskeletal issues that pregnant women may encounter?
3. How might these conditions be managed or prevented?
4. What hormonal changes during pregnancy affect the strength or flexibility of muscles and joints?

The musculoskeletal (MSK) system provides stability, support and movement for the body. It controls cardiac function, respiration, digestion and temperature regulation. This chapter will briefly recap on the structural elements of the MSK system, before examining selected pathological conditions affecting it and the burden they pose to public health. It also explores how particular MSK conditions may affect the childbearing population, outlining considerations for midwifery practice.

The Skeleton

The skeleton is made up of approximately 206 bones and is divided into the axial skeleton and the appendicular skeleton, as shown in Figure 19.1.

The skeletal system supports the framework of the body, its muscles and soft tissue. It protects internal organs, interacts with muscles and joints to produce movement and provides storage for minerals needed for homeostasis. The bones of the skeleton are classified into four types, illustrated in Figure 19.2.

Figure 19.3 shows a typical long bone, like the femur or humerus, consisting of a shaft or diaphysis, two epiphyses (sing. epiphysis) at its extremities, articular cartilage that covers the epiphysis at the point where one bone meets another,

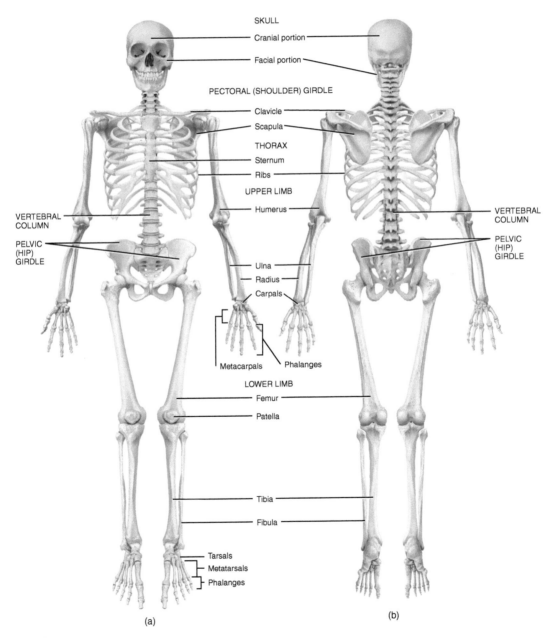

SKULL
Cranial portion
Facial portion

PECTORAL (SHOULDER) GIRDLE
Clavicle
Scapula

THORAX
Sternum
Ribs

UPPER LIMB
Humerus

VERTEBRAL COLUMN

PELVIC (HIP) GIRDLE

Ulna
Radius
Carpals

Metacarpals   Phalanges

LOWER LIMB
Femur
Patella

Tibia
Fibula

Tarsals
Metatarsals
Phalanges

VERTEBRAL COLUMN

PELVIC (HIP) GIRDLE

(a)   (b)

FIGURE 19.1 The skeleton. (a) Anterior view. (b) Posterior view.

Compact bone (long bone):
found in the toes, legs, fingers
and arms

Short bone

Flat bone

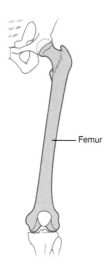

Femur

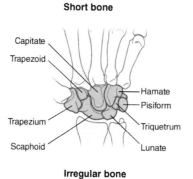

Capitate
Trapezoid
Hamate
Pisiform
Trapezium
Triquetrum
Scaphoid
Lunate

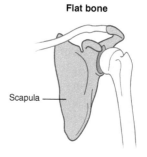

Scapula

Irregular bone

Sesamoid bone

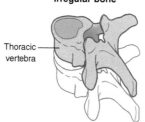

Thoracic
vertebra

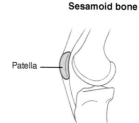

Patella

FIGURE 19.2   Types of bones.

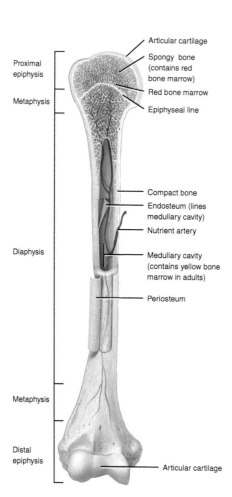

Articular cartilage

Spongy bone
(contains red
bone marrow)

Proximal
epiphysis

Red bone marrow

Metaphysis

Epiphyseal line

Compact bone

Endosteum (lines
medullary cavity)

Nutrient artery

Diaphysis

Medullary cavity
(contains yellow bone
marrow in adults)

Periosteum

Metaphysis

Distal
epiphysis

Articular cartilage

FIGURE 19.3   A long bone – a partially sectioned humerus (arm bone).

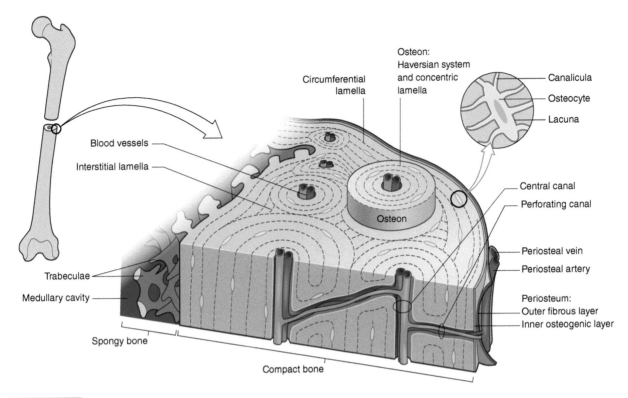

FIGURE 19.4 The osteon and Haversian canal.

and a medullary cavity, the site of yellow marrow production. The long bone is covered by the tough membranous layer, the periosteum, important for blood, nutrient and nerve supply.

Bone tissue is structurally complex, yielding to substantial forces and allowing for delivery of nutrients for cell repair. Spongy or trabecular bone makes up most of the tissue of short flat and irregular bones and most of the epiphyses of long bones. It resembles a spongy meshwork and contains red bone marrow in some locations. Its spongy nature enables it to withstand significant force. Compact or cortical bone forms the superficial layer of bones. Approximately 25% stronger than spongy bone, it comprises cells called osteons with central (Haversian) canals, lamellae and osteocytes in lacunae, maintaining bone health. The osteon is shown in Figure 19.4.

Where Bones Meet: Joints and Articulations

The point where two bones meet is called a joint or articulation. The most abundant and flexible joints are synovial joints, protected by a joint capsule. Inside the capsule, the synovial membrane produces synovial fluid, a lubricant that minimises wear from movement. These joints have smooth, compressible articular cartilage covering the bone ends. Figure 19.5 illustrates the structure of a synovial joint. Figure 19.6 shows the diverse types of synovial joints in the body and their actions.

Muscles

The muscular system facilitates both external and internal movement. External muscles create motion across bones and joints, while internal muscles handle tasks like transporting food in the gastrointestinal system, regulating cardiac and respiratory functions, and making micro-adjustments such as pupil dilation. There are three main types of muscular

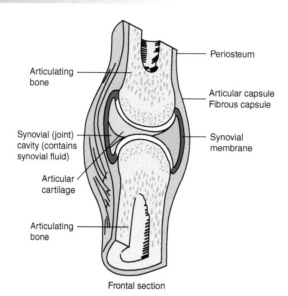

FIGURE 19.5   A synovial joint.

tissue: skeletal striated muscle for skeletal movement; smooth non-striated muscle in the walls of organs, blood vessels and skin; and cardiac striated muscle in the heart. Muscular tissue possesses four key properties: excitability, responding to electrical or chemical signals; contractility, generating forceful contraction for action; extensibility, stretching when needed; and elasticity, returning to its original shape after contraction or extension.

Expert Midwife: Maintaining Good Posture

I think it is really important when working with women to explain to them the importance of maintaining good posture, especially as the pregnancy progresses and the centre of gravity shifts. I would encourage women to stand tall, imagine lifting their bump towards them and evenly distribute their weight on both feet. Additionally, I would suggest to them that they use supportive cushions or even a rolled-up towel to support their back sitting for extended periods.

Carrianne, Midwife

Muscle Groups, Tendons and Ligaments

Movement requires interaction between muscles and skeletal structures across joints. The body's approximately 700 muscles are arranged in groups according to function, shown in Figure 19.7. Most muscles produce movement, but some stabilise the body and even prevent harmful motion.

Muscles attach to bones via strong inelastic connective tendons, which help to generate pulling forces. They are distinguished from ligaments, flexible and elastic fibrous bands connecting bone to bone.

Expert Midwife

If I assess that there are no contra-indications, I might suggest to women that water-based exercise, such as water aerobics or swimming, offers a range of benefits during pregnancy. Water-based exercise is a low-impact workout, the buoyancy of the water supports the growing abdomen, the exercises promote improved blood circulation throughout the body, can help reduce swelling in the legs and are good for strengthening muscles.

I always advise women that they should be mindful of their comfort level and avoid overly strenuous activities or exercises that involve jumping or abrupt movements in water.

Yanabita, Midwife

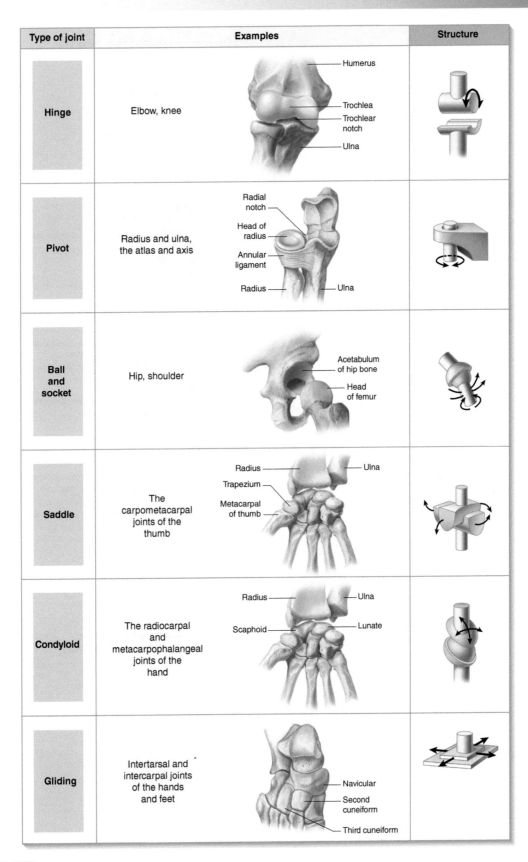

Type of joint	Examples	Structure
Hinge	Elbow, knee	
Pivot	Radius and ulna, the atlas and axis	
Ball and socket	Hip, shoulder	
Saddle	The carpometacarpal joints of the thumb	
Condyloid	The radiocarpal and metacarpophalangeal joints of the hand	
Gliding	Intertarsal and intercarpal joints of the hands and feet	

FIGURE 19.6 Types of synovial joints.

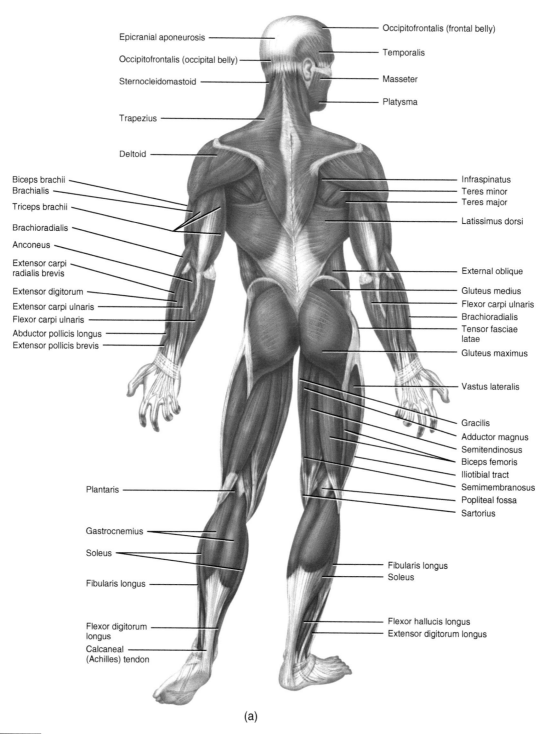

(a)

FIGURE 19.7   The major muscles of the body. (a) Posterior view. (b) Anterior view.

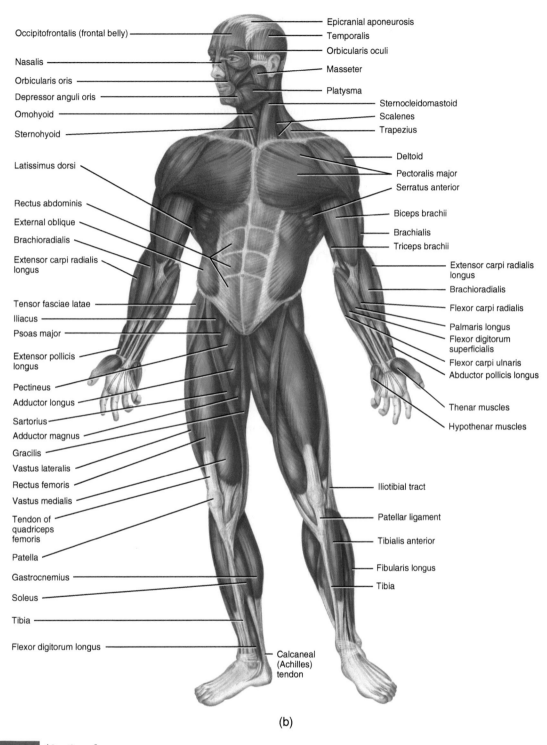

Occipitofrontalis (frontal belly)
Nasalis
Orbicularis oris
Depressor anguli oris
Omohyoid
Sternohyoid
Latissimus dorsi
Rectus abdominis
External oblique
Brachioradialis
Extensor carpi radialis longus
Tensor fasciae latae
Iliacus
Psoas major
Extensor pollicis longus
Pectineus
Adductor longus
Sartorius
Adductor magnus
Gracilis
Vastus lateralis
Rectus femoris
Vastus medialis
Tendon of quadriceps femoris
Patella
Gastrocnemius
Soleus
Tibia
Flexor digitorum longus

Epicranial aponeurosis
Temporalis
Orbicularis oculi
Masseter
Platysma
Sternocleidomastoid
Scalenes
Trapezius
Deltoid
Pectoralis major
Serratus anterior
Biceps brachii
Brachialis
Triceps brachii
Extensor carpi radialis longus
Brachioradialis
Flexor carpi radialis
Palmaris longus
Flexor digitorum superficialis
Flexor carpi ulnaris
Abductor pollicis longus
Thenar muscles
Hypothenar muscles

Iliotibial tract
Patellar ligament
Tibialis anterior
Fibularis longus
Tibia

Calcaneal (Achilles) tendon

(b)

FIGURE 19.7   (*Continued*)

The Burden of Musculoskeletal Impairment

MSK impairment is a term describing approximately 150 different diseases or conditions affecting joints, muscles, bones or other connective tissues (WHO 2022), typically characterised by pain and changes to mobility. They can occur at any stage of life, and many younger people find their working lives blighted and even cut short by poor MSK health. MSK conditions represent a global public health concern, with around 619 million people affected in 2020, predicted to increase to 843 million by 2050 (Cieza et al. 2021). Easy to overlook, because these conditions are rarely fatal, they contribute considerably to an ever-increasing burden of disability and are a significant source of years lived with disability (YLD). In the United Kingdom alone, approximately 20% of the population seek GP advice about an MSK condition every year (Office for Health Improvement and Disparities 2022). In 2020, MSK problems were the second most common cause of sickness absence, which accounted for 20.8 million days lost in work (Office for Health Improvement and Disparities 2022).

Musculoskeletal Conditions

MSK conditions are broadly categorised as follows:

- Conditions affecting joints such as osteoarthritis, rheumatoid arthritis, gout, spondyloarthritis.
- Conditions affecting bones such as osteoporosis, osteopenia, traumatic fractures and fragility fractures.
- Conditions affecting muscles such as sarcopenia or atrophy.
- Conditions affecting multiple elements of the MSK system such as carpal tunnel syndrome (CTS), regional neck and back pain, as well as widespread pain conditions such as fibromyalgia and some autoimmune connective tissue diseases that manifest in MSK pain, e.g. lupus.

The causes of these conditions vary and include overuse injury, trauma, disease processes and inflammation. MSK pain is the most common form of non-cancer pain (WHO 2022), with temporary and lifelong consequences.

Learning Event

Consider for a moment how MSK pain might be a women's health issue.

- What factors do you think might be relevant when looking at these conditions though a gendered lens?
- How do you think gender affects treatment and caregiver response?
- Do you think that we expect men and women to deal with pain differently?
- How do you think this might affect your practice as a midwife?

Musculoskeletal Conditions and Overall Health

Evidence indicates that people with MSK conditions are more likely to have other chronic diseases. A review by Williams et al. (2018), focusing on burdensome MSK conditions such as osteoarthritis and back pain, suggested that early treatment of these conditions might help prevent the development of other chronic ailments, like cardiovascular disease. MSK conditions are mainly characterised by pain, which can be acute, chronic or intermittent. Living with these conditions can have impacts on an individual's life chances, leading to work loss, dependence on others and affecting mental health. Figure 19.8 shows the cycle of pain and poor mental health and underlines the need for holistic assessment when caring for individuals with MSK conditions.

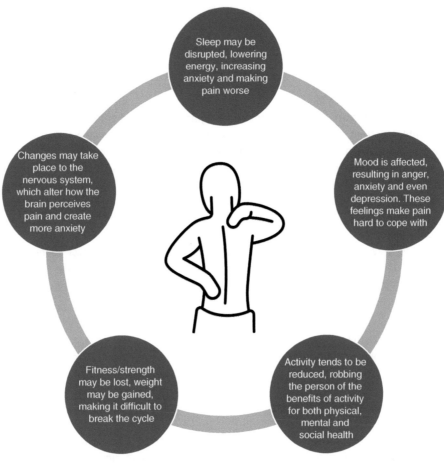

FIGURE 19.8 A potential cycle of pain and poor mental health.

Clinical Investigation: Musculoskeletal Conditions

Following is a list of some common MSK disorders that you might encounter in practice. Make notes and seek out resources to expand your knowledge around how they affect childbearing families.

Condition	How prevalent is it, globally and in the United Kingdom?	Implications for pregnancy and childbearing	How is it treated? What might midwives need to know?
Fibromyalgia			
Arthritis			
Osteogenesis imperfecta			

Use the following resources:

- https://www.brittlebone.org/information-resources/about-oi
- www.arthritisaction.org.uk
- www.fmaware.org
- Bair, M.J. and Krebs, E.E. (2020). Fibromyalgia. *Annals of Internal Medicine* 172 (5): ITC33–ITC48.

Injuries to the Musculoskeletal System

MSK injuries are common and represent a burden to healthcare systems due to restrictions on activities and normal functioning.

Sprains, Strains and Dislocations

A **sprain** occurs where there is an injury to the ligament and the joint capsule, whereas a **strain** affects the tendons or muscles. A sprain resembles a strain, but the pain and the swelling subside more slowly. Sprains are usually caused by abnormal or excessive joint movement and the ligaments may tear completely or incompletely. Signs include pain, swelling, heat, disability and discoloration, with the knee, ankle and elbow being common sites. Treatment for sprains and strains is dependent on the severity of the injury. National Institute for Health and Care Excellence (NICE) guidance (2020) presents comprehensive principles for management to guide practitioners, including referral to emergency medicine for suspected fractures and dislocations, alongside potential self-management including 'PRICE' (protection, rest, ice, compression and elevation).

Dislocations occur when two bones separate at a joint due to a sudden impact, falls or deliberate injury. They can harm surrounding ligaments and tendons and may cause long-term neuromuscular damage if not promptly treated. **Reduction** is the typical treatment, aiming to realign the bones as soon as possible to prevent complications. Common sites for dislocations are the shoulder, fingers, patella, elbow and hip.

Fractures and Bone Healing

Normal bone can withstand significant forces. Bone mass increases when the mechanical demands on bone are increased; conversely, a reduction in load – such as during a period of immobility – results in bone mass reduction, potentially increasing the risk of injury.

Bone formation, repair and remodelling involve osteoblasts, osteoclasts, osteocytes and osteogenic (stem) cells, outlined in Table 19.1.

Bone-lining cells occupy the bone's surface, flat-shaped and quiescent cells, whose function is not fully understood (Florencio-Silva et al. 2015) but that play an important role in bone remodelling, simplified in Table 19.2. **Remodelling**

TABLE 19.1   Bone cells and their function.

Osteogenic cells	Osteoblasts	Osteoclasts	Osteocytes
Precursors to osteoblasts, sometimes called progenitor cells	Anabolic in nature Cuboidal in shape Synthesise the components and constituents of the bone matrix, promoting mineralisation	Catabolic in nature Phagocytic cells Degrade, dissolve and resorb bone material Integral part of remodelling process	Osteoblasts 'trapped' in the lacunae of the bone structure Make up the majority of bone cell matrix (90–95%) Most mature bone cells, maintaining the bone matrix

TABLE 19.2   Bone remodelling process.

Bone needs replacing or remodelling The bone-lining cells seen on the surface are currently preventing the breakdown process	Secretory activity of the bone-lining cells allows the osteoclasts to access bone matrix They now destroy old bone	Site of bone breakdown, awaiting production of new cells and bone matrix	Osteoblasts synthesise new matrix, composed of osteocytes
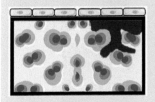	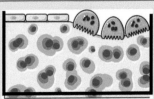	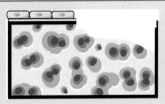	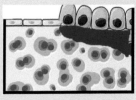

Source: Adapted from https://orthopaedia.com/page/Describe-bone-remodeling.

serves to adjust bone architecture to meet changing mechanical needs and helps to repair microdamage in bone matrix, preventing the accumulation of old bone.

A **fracture** is a break in the bone caused by excessive stress beyond its capacity to withstand. Fractures fall into three main categories: those from sudden traumatic injuries; stress fractures due to repeated wear or overuse; and pathological fractures that happen spontaneously due to underlying conditions, like osteoporosis or cancer, weakening the bones. Figure 19.9 illustrates various types of fractures.

When a fracture occurs, there may be signs and symptoms such as pain, tenderness, swelling, loss of function and possible deformity of the affected part. Nerve function may also be lost temporarily. Bone healing is a complex process that is still open to debate, but is generally understood to involve the phases shown in Figure 19.10.

Factors affecting the healing process include the amount of bone loss, bone type injured (cortical bone is slower to heal), older age, diseases such as diabetes, and modifiable factors like smoking and poor nutritional status (Einhorn and Gerstenfeld 2015).

Childbearing Considerations: Musculoskeletal Injury

Pregnancy may be a time where the potential for sprains and strains increases, due to increases in gestational weight and alterations in the centre of gravity as the pregnancy proceeds. While fractures are not a common complication of pregnancy and the childbearing period, they do result from road traffic crashes, falls and other traumatic impact such as domestic violence. There can be serious consequences for mother and fetus and initial care is from highly specialised trauma teams (Battaloglu et al. 2016). The management of fractures depends on the type, location and cause of the fracture, as well as the gestational age and health status of mother and fetus. General management principles will consider issues of pain management, venous thromboembolism prophylaxis, nutrition and supplementation for healing, physical therapy for rehabilitation, and birth planning around mode of delivery. For cases of fracture reduction, aligning broken bone ends and immobilising them with a splint, brace or cast, management by an obstetric anaesthetic team is crucial (Heesen and Klimek 2016). Midwives also play a role in education around the primary prevention of injuries, especially those resulting from road traffic crashes and seat-belt injuries.

FRACTURE	DESCRIPTION	ILLUSTRATION	RADIOGRAPH
Open (*Compound*)	The broken ends of the bone protrude through the skin. Conversely, a *closed (simple) fracture* does not break the skin.		
Comminuted (KOM-i-noo-ted; *com-* = together; *-minuted* = crumbled)	The bone is splintered, crushed, or broken into pieces at the site of impact, and smaller bone fragments lie between the two main fragments.		
Greenstick	A partial fracture in which one side of the bone is broken and the other side bends; similar to the way a green twig breaks on one side while the other side stays whole, but bends; occurs only in children, whose bones are not fully ossified and contain more organic material than inorganic material.		
Impacted	One end of the fractured bone is forcefully driven into the interior of the other.		
Pott	Fracture of the distal end of the lateral leg bone (fibula), with serious injury of the distal tibial articulation.		

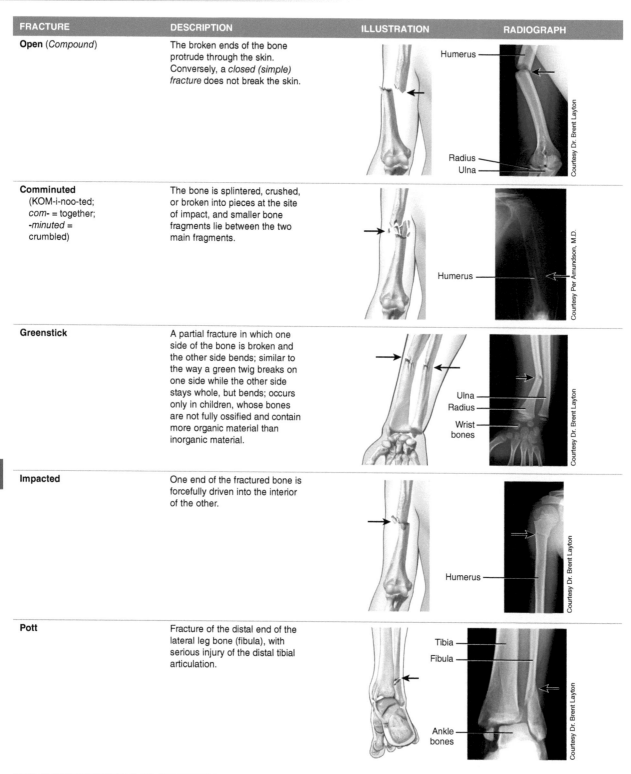

FIGURE 19.9   Some common fracture classifications and x-ray images.

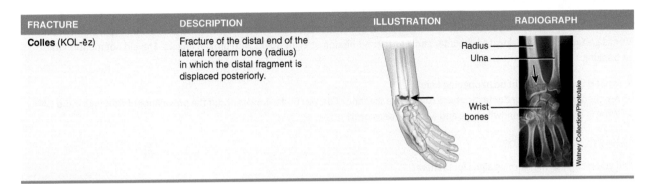

FRACTURE	DESCRIPTION	ILLUSTRATION	RADIOGRAPH
Colles (KOL-ēz)	Fracture of the distal end of the lateral forearm bone (radius) in which the distal fragment is displaced posteriorly.		

FIGURE 19.9 (*Continued*)

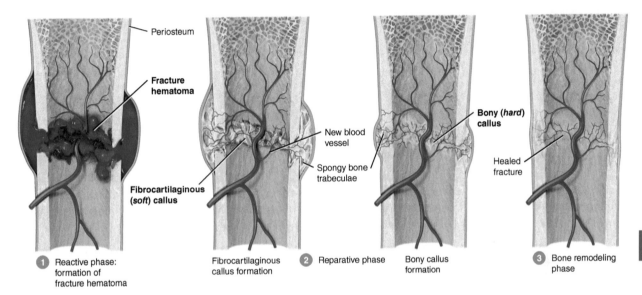

① Reactive phase: formation of fracture hematoma

Fibrocartilaginous callus formation

② Reparative phase

Bony callus formation

③ Bone remodeling phase

FIGURE 19.10 Steps in repair of a bone fracture.

Medicines Management

In some cases pain or discomfort may be severe enough to require medication. When considering medication for pregnant women with MSK conditions, midwives must exercise caution due to potential adverse effects on the woman and also the fetus.

The use of medication for MSK conditions during pregnancy should be approached with caution and a thorough understanding of the potential risks and benefits. Midwives should strive to provide comprehensive care that incorporates non-pharmacological approaches whenever possible, while also using medications judiciously when needed to optimise the health and well-being of pregnant women and their unborn babies.

Case Study 19.1

Ali is a primigravida, 22 years old, attending a routine midwifery appointment at 34 weeks. She has had a straightforward pregnancy. Today she has come to clinic unaccompanied for the first time; she normally brings her partner's 12-year-old daughter with her.

During routine blood pressure checks, you notice a faint bruise on her inside upper arm. Ali notices your reaction and tells you that she has been decorating and banged her arm on the stepladder. You do not probe further.

After the appointment you check the GP record and notice that she had an admission to the emergency department at four weeks gestation with a dislocated shoulder and a further admission at eight weeks with broken fingers. She did not mention these at booking.

- What do you think might be happening here?
- Are there risk factors for domestic abuse (DA) in this scenario? Can you find evidence about the prevalence of MSK injury and DA?
- What is the role of the midwife here and what happens next?

Review Your Learning

Did you recognise the warning signs for DA here?

- Pregnancy
- Accompanied at all visits to date
- Disguised injury
- Previous unexplained injury

Did you recognise the role of the midwife here?

- Enquiry
- Support
- Advocacy
- Multiprofessional working
- Excellent (safe) record keeping

Domestic Abuse

DA is defined as an incident or pattern of incidents of controlling, coercive, threatening, degrading and violent behaviour, including sexual violence, in the majority of cases by a partner or ex-partner, but also by a family member or carer (Women's Aid 2022). It can include, but is not limited to, the following types of acts:

- Intimidation, name calling, isolation from support networks, coercive control by means of threats and degradation, repeated yelling or shouting, mocking.
- Psychological abuse, emotional abuse.
- Financial/economic abuse, withholding money, stealing benefits and/or controlling bank accounts.
- Harming someone while performing caring duties, for example overfeeding, over- or undermedication, restricting access to medical equipment.
- Physical abuse, beating, kicking, non-fatal strangulation.
- Sexual abuse, forced sexual acts, rape.
- Abuse related to faith, including religious marriage and divorce.
- Harassment and stalking.
- Online social cruelty and cyberbullying, stealing passwords, doxxing, using spyware and sniffer software.

Red Flag

Incidences of domestic abuse are known to increase during pregnancy and the postnatal period and midwives play a key role in supporting the identification of those who are at risk of, or already experiencing, abuse (Baird et al. 2013).

The 2021 Domestic Abuse Act includes provisions for addressing 'honour'-based abuse, which may not always involve a personal connection between the perpetrator and the victim but is often carried out by family members. The Act also covers forced marriage and female genital mutilation (FGM).

DA has severe effects on physical, mental and psychological health for both adults and children. While both men and women can be victims, it primarily stems from imbalances of power within relationships, disproportionately

Listen	Listen closely, with empathy, not judging.
Inquire about needs and concerns	Assess and respond to her needs and concerns – emotional, physical, social and practical.
Validate	Show that you believe and understand her.
Enhance safety	Discuss how to protect her from further harm.
Support	Help her connect to services, social support.

FIGURE 19.11 The LIVES framework for healthcare response to violence against women. Source: Adapted from WHO (2021).

affecting oppressed groups. Women, in particular, are at greater risk due to societal inequalities between genders. Various intersecting factors, such as disability, chronic illness, pregnancy or recent childbirth, isolation from support networks, lack of financial resources and poor mental health, can increase an individual's vulnerability to abuse. Few factors reliably predict the risk of violence, but verbal/emotional abuse and forced sex are closely associated with it.

A systematic review (O'Doherty et al. 2015) found that while routinely asking about DA was acceptable to women and was useful in identifying cases, the evidence that it had a positive impact on referral and other key outcomes was weaker. Healthcare professionals – including midwives – find it difficult to ask about violence and abuse (Beynon et al. 2012; Taylor et al. 2013), fearing that doing so is time-consuming and harms relationships with women. Keynejad et al. (2021) propose that practitioners follow the LIVES response, set out in Figure 19.11.

Midwives should respond sensitively and patiently to suspected cases of DA. A meta-synthesis of survivors' needs (Tarzia et al. 2020) found that clinicians must behave proportionately and understand that DA is frequently a chronic situation. Pressure to disclose can worsen the situation, so continuity and follow-up care are crucial when there are no immediate safety concerns. Risks escalate considerably when a victim is planning to leave the relationship or is suspected of doing so. The following factors are important in healthcare responses:

- Consider protocols, training, local links and referral pathways. Staff should know how to contact local DA agencies for referral/advice.
- Display information posters in waiting rooms and toilets, in local languages.
- Consider covert disclosure systems, such as using stickers on urine samples to signal a desire to speak privately.
- Have protocols for DA enquiry, safe documentation on protected platforms inaccessible to perpetrators, and information sharing with relevant professionals to support women in accessing specialist support.

Musculoskeletal Injury and Domestic Abuse

Unexplained MSK injuries should always be explored in the context of DA, especially when other factors, like pregnancy and previous injuries (as in Case 19.1), are considered. Studies show that physical violence often presents as recurrent finger and hand fractures, foot and ankle injuries, and head and neck injuries (Bhandari et al. 2006; Thomas et al. 2021). Healthcare professionals should include attendance at an emergency department for such injuries in any abuse-related risk assessment. Emotional, psychological and sexual abuse often coexist with physical abuse. However, despite the importance of inquiring about DA in MSK injury cases, only 2% of orthopaedic staff in a UK study routinely did so (Downie et al. 2019). There is a need for increased focus on MSK trauma and its connection to the complex issue of domestic violence and abuse.

Key Musculoskeletal Considerations for Public Health, Pregnancy and the Postnatal Period

Low Back Pain

Low back pain (LBP) occurs in the posterior aspect of the body from the lower margin of the 12th ribs to the lower gluteal folds, with or without pain referred into one or both lower limbs and lasting for at least one day (Hoy et al. 2014). Within MSK conditions, LBP represents the leading cause of disability worldwide (Kahere et al. 2022) and is associated with significant loss of productive activity. A systematic review of studies (Hoy et al. 2014) found that LBP was most common in women and people aged 40–80. The burden of LBP is most likely to fall on socioeconomically disadvantaged groups, especially where access to rehabilitation and effective treatments is poor.

The causes of LBP are diverse, often with a non-specific origin. Acute LBP may result from spinal injury or muscle strain. Chronic back pain, lasting over 12 weeks, can stem from ineffective management of acute episodes (Stevens et al. 2021), as well as psychological and social influences, some still being studied (Hartvigsen et al. 2018; Corrêa et al. 2022). Modifiable factors like smoking, obesity and occupational ergonomic conditions play a significant role in LBP (GBD 2021 LBP Collaborators 2023). Figure 19.12 illustrates the condition's complexity.

Medicines Management

Non-steroidal anti-inflammatory drugs (NSAIDs) including ibuprofen, naproxen, indomethacin and diclofenac are often used to treat mild to moderate pain and fever. They are inhibitors of cyclo-oxygenase. In the fetus and newborn, cyclo-oxygenase is a potent dilator of the ductus arteriosus and pulmonary resistance vessels. Its inhibition could potentially cause premature closure of these vessels. For this reason, NSAIDs have always been contra-indicated after 28 weeks of pregnancy.

A review of data from a 2022 study suggests that prolonged use of NSAIDs from the 20th week of pregnancy onwards may be linked to an increased risk of oligohydramnios and fetal renal dysfunction. Some cases of constriction of the ductus arteriosus have also been observed at this stage. If the use of a systemic NSAID after the 20th week of pregnancy is deemed necessary after consulting with a healthcare professional, it should be prescribed at the lowest possible dose for the shortest duration. If used for more than several days, additional neonatal monitoring should be considered. Pregnant individuals should also be advised to discontinue NSAID use in the last trimester of pregnancy.

Midwives should follow the contra-indications and warnings in the product information in relation to pregnancy. Women who are using gel or creams containing NSAIDs during pregnancy should be advised to read the patient information leaflet.

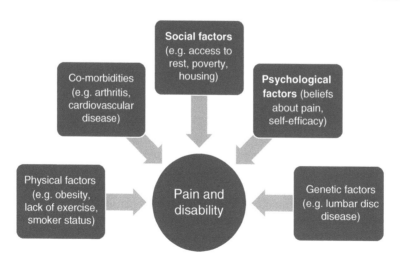

FIGURE 19.12   Contributors to lower back pain and disability. Source: Adapted from: Hartvigsen et al. (2018).

The Perinatal Period and Low Back Pain

Learning Event

Before reading this section, think about the following questions. Note down your answers and then return to them later.

- How often have you encountered LBP in your clinical practice?
- What do you think are the reasons for this being such a common condition in the perinatal period (think about the physiological changes in pregnancy as well as lifestyle factors)?
- How does low and general back pain affect the experience of
  - Labour and birth?
  - Breastfeeding?
  - Caring for a newborn baby?

LBP in the perinatal period often accompanies literature about pelvic girdle pain (PGP) and it can be difficult to determine prevalence, with ranges between 20% and 75% reported (Chen et al. 2021). Katonis et al. (2011) distinguish between PGP and lumbar pain and suggest that early differentiation be part of an overall assessment.

Chen et al. (2021) identify two patterns of pain in pregnancy: pregnancy-related lower back pain and pregnancy-related pelvic girdle pain. They propose the term pregnancy-related lumbo-pelvic pain as an umbrella term to encompass these conditions. Wu et al. (2004) conducted a review on MSK pain in pregnancy and found different pain descriptors for girdle pain ('stabbing' sensation), lower back pain ('dull ache') and thoracic spine pain ('burning'). However, they could not classify the pain further from these descriptors. Pierce et al. (2012) suggest using the term lumbo-pelvic pain (LPP) to support women experiencing generalised MSK pain. Their cross-sectional study shows that women with combined LBP and PGP, or PGP alone, experience higher levels of pain and disability compared to women with LBP alone. They include a useful pain diagram indicating the lumbopelvic regions, reproduced in Figure 19.13.

Daneau et al. (2021) propose a number of development mechanisms for LPP in pregnancy. Predictive risk factors include history of LBP, previous pelvic trauma or pregnancy-related PGP, raised body mass index (BMI), physically demanding occupation and also emotional distress. Proposed underlying mechanisms include significant hormonal and biomechanical changes, muscular adaptations and altered pain sensitivity.

369

The Postnatal Period

Postnatal back and neck pain is a common health concern after childbirth, with potential sources depicted in Figure 19.14. Studies highlight the under-recognition and persistence of maternal morbidity and pain during the postnatal period, particularly backache (Glazener et al. 1995). Research by Schytt et al. (2005) indicates that MSK symptoms, including

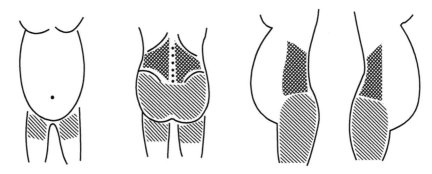

FIGURE 19.13 Possible sites of lumbopelvic pain in pregnancy. Source: Reproduced from Pierce et al. (2012) / Hindawi Publishing Corporation/ CC by 4.0.

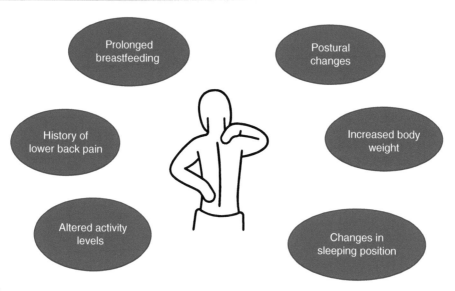

FIGURE 19.14   Potential sources of postnatal back pain.

neck, shoulder and back pain, are prevalent one year after birth. Concerns about epidural analgesia leading to postpartum backache appear unsupported by observational and interventional studies, although research in this area presents challenges (Komatsu et al. 2020).

Orange Flag: Psychological Effects of Pain After Birth

Postnatal pain can challenge the transition to parenthood and impact psychological well-being. Cooklin et al. (2018) found that while a high burden of physical problems had a weak association with poor maternal mood at eight weeks postpartum, when combined with sustained breastfeeding problems there was a significant impact on mental health. While this study does not focus on back pain specifically, it does suggest that a plausible approach for healthcare professionals might be to underpin mental health via strategies to alleviate physical pain alongside breastfeeding support. Zhang et al. (2023) see the perinatal period as a 'teachable moment' where women and families are open to interventions around future well-being. Educating about prevention and mitigation of back pain using non-pharmaceutical methods (exercise therapy, physical therapy, mindfulness-based cognitive behavioural therapy and relaxation) could be explored within antenatal education classes or postnatal parenting groups.

Case Study 19.2

Di, 32 years old, is now 28 weeks pregnant with her second baby. She has been struggling with pain in her lower back since early in her pregnancy but is now describing shooting pains in her pelvis. Walking without pain is becoming impossible. It is difficult getting out of bed and carrying her other child around is very challenging. She is requesting a meeting with her obstetric consultant to discuss an elective lower-segment caesarean section (LSCS).

- What do you think is happening here? What factors may have contributed to her current condition?
- Using your anatomy knowledge, how would you explain the anatomical changes to Di?
- How would you respond to Di's request around elective LSCS?
- What other professionals should be involved here? What is the role of the midwife?

See the Further Resources section for useful resources for your answer.

Formulate a plan to help Di, including issues around birth and breastfeeding, applying the principles of women-centred, holistic care.

Pelvic Girdle Pain

Pelvic girdle pain (PGP), also termed symphysis pubis dysfunction, affects approximately 1 in 5 pregnancies. PGP is defined as pain between the posterior iliac crest and the gluteal fold, particularly around the sacroiliac joint, which may radiate to the thighs and hips (Vleeming et al. 2008). PGP can occur in conjunction with or separately from pain in the pubic symphysis. Figure 19.15 shows the landmarks of the pelvis and Figure 19.16 shows possible sites of pain with PGP. Additional symptoms may include clicking, locking or grinding of the pelvic joints and reduced ability to perform daily activities.

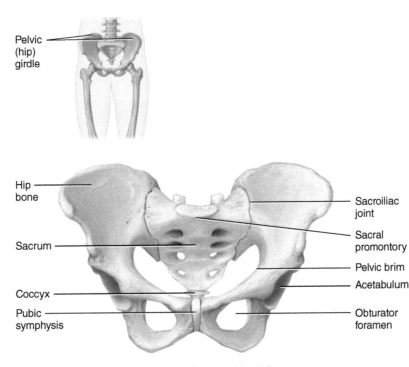

Anterosuperior view of pelvic girdle

FIGURE 19.15 Anterosuperior view of pelvic girdle.

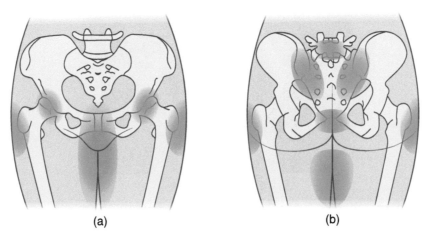

FIGURE 19.16 Possible sites of pain in pelvic girdle pain, seen anteriorly (a) and posteriorly (b). Source: https://www.thrivephysioplus.com.au/pregnancy-pelvic-girdle-pain/.

PGP's aetiology remains contested, but hormonal, mechanical and lifestyle factors are proposed. While most cases recover after birth, severe cases may persist longer term (Elden et al. 2016), especially where there is no proper treatment. It is difficult to pinpoint why some women develop PGP, but a history of previous lower back, pelvic girdle or joint pain, hypermobility syndrome and/or trauma to the pelvis may be significant. A recent review (Wuytack et al. 2020) also suggests exploring the role of age, BMI, parity and smoking for a clearer understanding.

Living with Pelvic Girdle Pain

PGP poses a challenge to physical, social, emotional and mental well-being. Some of the themes identified by the literature are represented in Figure 19.17. For many women it feels like an invisible condition, a feeling exacerbated by professional responses (Ceprnja et al. 2022). In Case 19.2, Di's request to speak to an obstetrician about the mode of delivery may reflect the fact that she needs to regain some autonomy over her care and direct conversations about mode of birth. She requires an empathic midwifery response to her requests to speak to other caregivers, a response acknowledging the effects of PGP.

Orange Flag: Psychological Considerations

Living with pain and disability, such as that caused by PGP, can exacerbate symptoms of depression and anxiety. Supporting perinatal mental health is vital, so a midwife should holistically assess a women's emotional and mental well-being alongside her physical condition. The relationship between PGP and mental well-being may be bi-directional (Algård et al. 2023); depression and anxiety frequently cause heightened pain sensitivity and may also disrupt sleep and rest.

Managing Pelvic Girdle Pain

A midwife will not be managing a woman's PGP alone. Any plan will require multidisciplinary team involvement, and discussions with/referral to specialist obstetric physiotherapy services (NICE 2021). Treatment may include manual therapy, exercise, advice on adapting activities, support belts and strategies for pain relief. In the majority of cases a vaginal birth is possible, but positions that result in excessive abduction at the hip joint such as lithotomy should be avoided. Alternative birthing positions are shown in Figure 19.18.

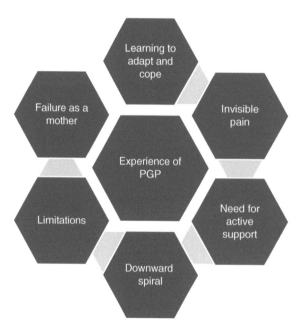

FIGURE 19.17   Themes identified from studies of women's experiences of pelvic girdle pain (PGP) in pregnancy and the puerperium.

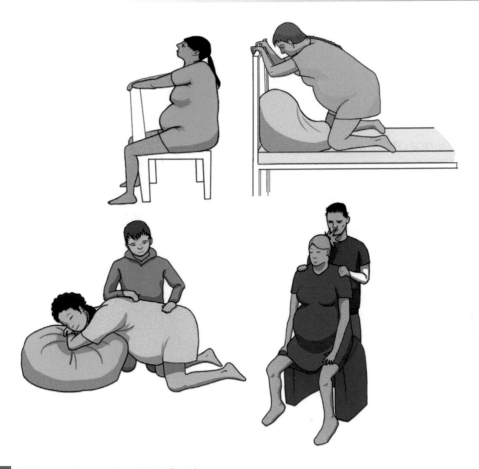

FIGURE 19.18 Birthing positions with pelvic girdle pain.

Families may worry about breastfeeding hormones prolonging PGP, but a Norwegian cohort study (2014) of 10 000+ women found no association between breastfeeding and persistent PGP. The Pelvic Partnership advises that women breastfeed in line with existing recommendations, and that PGP should not prevent them from doing so. Should she wish to breastfeed, the woman can be encouraged and supported by her midwife. It could be useful to discuss the safe use of side-lying and laid-back positions.

Red Flag

Pelvic pain can present with more serious conditions. In early pregnancy, pelvic pain may indicate an ectopic pregnancy. At any stage of pregnancy and the postnatal period, the presence of other physical symptoms such as pyrexia, unexpected bleeding, urinary frequency/urgency, bowel pain, suspected or confirmed membrane rupture or acute abdominal pain indicates a full assessment to rule out causes other than PGP.

The following conditions may present with a similar picture to PGP (Walters et al. 2018):

- **Transient osteoporosis of pregnancy**, a rare condition that typically occurs in the third trimester, affecting one hip with severe acute groin pain. It may result from pregnancy-related changes or pre-existing osteoporosis. Low BMI, first-time pregnancy, reduced calcium intake and family history of osteoporosis are risk factors. Prompt magnetic resonance imaging (MRI) and referral are needed for diagnosis and management.
- **Pubic symphysis diastasis**, a rare but serious pregnancy condition, involves the separation of the pubic symphysis due to unknown causes. Risk factors include multiple pregnancies and large babies. Diagnosis is made with a >1 cm pubic symphysis gap, detectable through clinical palpation and confirmed by imaging. Conservative measures like bed rest, pain relief and a pelvic binder are effective in most cases, while severe cases may require specialist intervention or caesarean section as the preferred mode of birth.

Carpal Tunnel Syndrome

Carpal tunnel syndrome (CTS) occurs when the median nerve is compressed as it passes through the wrist. Because the median nerve controls the muscles that move the thumb and conveys sensations in the fingers and thumb to the brain, compression causes symptoms like tingling, numbness, pain or aching. Figure 19.19 shows the median nerve, with Figure 19.20 showing the affected fingers.

The Lived Experience of Carpal Tunnel Syndrome

The prevalence of CTS in the general population is estimated to be approximately 4% (Luca Padua et al. 2016; http://carpal-tunnel.net). Pregnancy-related CTS (PRCTS) has a reported prevalence between 1% and 62%, with Meems et al. (2017) speculating that this variance is explained by women not mentioning symptoms early and healthcare professionals not asking about them. PRCTS often becomes more severe in the third trimester, but it can occur at any point and may persist into the postnatal period (Meems et al. 2017).

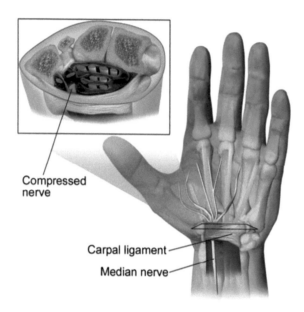

Compressed nerve

Carpal ligament

Median nerve

FIGURE 19.19   Carpal tunnel syndrome and median nerve location.

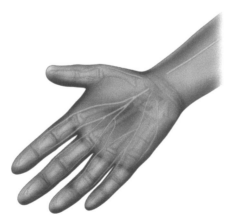

FIGURE 19.20   Area of hand served by median nerve (yellow) and affected by carpal tunnel syndrome.

Exact causes of PRCTS are unclear, but might link to the peripheral oedema experienced by around 80% of women in late pregnancy. This oedema may limit the space in the carpal tunnel and compress the median nerve, resulting in the clinical symptoms associated with CTS (Mabie 2005). Relaxin may also induce inflammation in the carpal tunnel, leading to swelling and compression. Some additional proposed risk factors include excessive gestational weight pain, gestational diabetes, higher age and previous computer-based occupation (Wright et al. 2014).

In many cases PRCTS involves lower levels of functional impairment than in the general population (Meems et al. 2017: Luca Padua et al. 2016) and severe cases appear rare. Prevalence of mild to moderate symptoms is high, however, and while functional impairment may not always be severe, it is certainly meaningful. A lack of severity does not preclude PRCTS from having an impact on quality of life (Kamysheva et al. 2009) and it often has a considerable effect on quality of sleep.

Examination Scenario

It is outside the scope of midwifery practice to diagnose MSK conditions, but it is important that holistic assessments of daily life and functioning form part of a woman-centred approach to care. While midwives do not routinely assess range of motion, they will assess pain and function loss, both commonly associated with MSK conditions. Visual pain scales, as in Figure 19.21, can help to assess pain.

For PGP, it may be possible to carefully pinpoint the site of pain during abdominal palpation. Practitioners need to exercise particular caution around measuring symphysis–fundal height and palpating the fetal head, as this may cause extreme discomfort. Midwives should also explore pain or disability associated with movements like getting up from a bed/couch, discouraging hip abduction and encouraging movements that keep the knees together.

Similarly for CTS, questions about hand and wrist pain, tingling and/or altered sensation could be easily incorporated into conversations about daily life, pre- and postnatally.

Any concerns can form part of informed conversations with specialist physiotherapists and a management plan agreed.

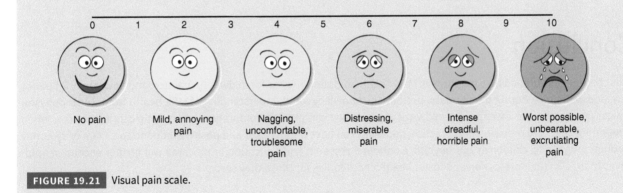

FIGURE 19.21 Visual pain scale.

Carpal Tunnel Syndrome and Breastfeeding

PRCTS may resolve after childbirth, but Luca Padua et al.'s review (2016) indicates that it can persist for 15–50% of women for up to a year. Breastfeeding can be challenging for women with CTS due to the wrist position required for an effective latch. Support should focus on finding positions with less flexion and wrist pain, like laid-back feeding or a 'rugby ball' hold, seen in Figure 19.22. Pumping milk may strain the hands and wrist, so a hands-free device can be helpful.

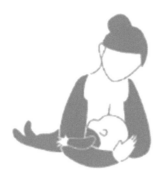
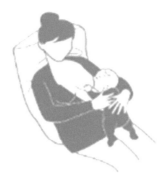

FIGURE 19.22   Alternative feeding positions with carpal tunnel syndrome.

Take-Home Points

- Midwives assess the MSK health of childbearing women, identifying any existing conditions or potential issues.
- Midwives educate and inform about MSK changes during childbearing, self-care and preventative measures.
- Where significant MSK issues develop, midwives work with other healthcare professionals for specialised assessment and individualised treatment, working in partnership with the woman and family.
- Pregnancy-related and postpartum musculoskeletal discomfort can cause distress. Midwives offer emotional support and reassurance, helping women cope with challenges.
- The midwife prepares pregnant women for labour and birth, including discussing optimal positions and movements that facilitate the birthing process and reduce strain on the musculoskeletal system.
- After birth, midwives continue to support new mothers' recovery, providing guidance to prevent long-term MSK issues.

Conclusion

This chapter has outlined how the study of MSK health holds importance for midwifery practice, and how it may influence care and well-being during the perinatal period. The knowledge and understanding of MSK health from a pathophysiological perspective are essential for midwives so that they can provide comprehensive, holistic care to women. When integrating MSK care provision into practice, midwives can have a significant and positive influence on a family's journey through pregnancy, childbirth and beyond. Continued research and education in this area will further encourage midwives to excel in their profession and foster healthier outcomes for those they serve.

References

Algård, T., Kalliokoski, P., Ahlqvist, K. et al. (2023). Role of depressive symptoms on the development of pelvic girdle pain in pregnancy: a prospective inception cohort study. *Acta Obstetricia et Gynecologica Scandinavica* 102 (10): 1281–1289.

Baird, K., Salmon, D., and White, P. (2013). A five-year follow-up study of the Bristol pregnancy domestic violence programme to promote routine enquiry. *Midwifery* 29 (8): 1003–1010.

Battaloglu, E., McDonnell, D., Chu, J. et al. (2016). Epidemiology and outcomes of pregnancy and obstetric complications in trauma in the United Kingdom. *Injury* 47 (1): 184–187.

Beynon, C.E., Gutmanis, I.A., Tutty, L.M. et al. (2012). Why physicians and nurses ask (or don't) about partner violence: a qualitative analysis. *BMC Public Health* 12: 473.

Bhandari, M., Dosanjh, S., Tornetta, P. 3rd et al. (2006). Musculoskeletal manifestations of physical abuse after intimate partner violence. *Journal of Trauma* 61 (6): 1473–1479.

Ceprnja, D., Chipchase, L., Liamputtong, P., and Gupta, A. (2022). "This is hard to cope with": the lived experience and coping strategies adopted amongst Australian women with pelvic girdle pain in pregnancy. *BMC Pregnancy Childbirth* 22 (1): 96.

Chen, S., Chen, M., Wu, X. et al. (2021). Global, regional and national burden of low back pain 1990-2019: a systematic analysis of the Global Burden of Disease study 2019. *Journal of Orthopaedic Translation* 32: 49–58.

Cieza, A., Causey, K., Kamenov, K. et al. (2021). Global estimates of the need for rehabilitation based on the Global Burden of Disease study 2019: a systematic analysis for the Global Burden of Disease study 2019. *Lancet* 396 (10267): 2006–2017.

Cooklin, A.R., Amir, L.H., Nguyen, C.D. et al. (2018). Physical health, breastfeeding problems and maternal mood in the early postpartum: a prospective cohort study. *Archives of Women's Mental Health* 21 (3): 365–374.

Corrêa, L.A., Mathieson, S., Meziat-Filho, N.A.M. et al. (2022). Which psychosocial factors are related to severe pain and functional limitation in patients with low back pain? Psychosocial factors related to severe low back pain. *Brazilian Journal of Physical Therapy* 26 (3): 100413. https://doi.org/10.1016/j.bjpt.2022.100413.

Daneau, C., Abboud, J., Marchand, A.A. et al. (2021). Mechanisms underlying lumbopelvic pain during pregnancy: a proposed model. *Frontiers in Pain Research* 2: 773988.

Downie, S., Madden, K., Bhandari, M., and Jariwala, A. (2019). Intimate partner violence in orthopaedic trauma patients: a chance to intervene? *Orthopaedic Proceedings* 101-B (Supp_7): 9.

Einhorn, T.A. and Gerstenfeld, L.C. (2015). Fracture healing: mechanisms and interventions. *Nature Reviews Rheumatology* 11 (1): 45–54.

Elden, H., Gutke, A., Kjellby-Wendt, G. et al. (2016). Predictors and consequences of long-term pregnancy-related pelvic girdle pain: a longitudinal follow-up study. *BMC Musculoskeletal Disorders* 17 (1): 276.

Florencio-Silva, R., Sasso, G.R., Sasso-Cerri, E. et al. (2015). Biology of bone tissue: structure, function, and factors that influence bone cells. *BioMed Research International* 2015: 421746.

GBD 2021 LBP Collaborators (2023). Global, regional, and national burden of low back pain, 1990-2020, its attributable risk factors, and projections to 2050: a systematic analysis of the Global Burden of Disease Study 2021. *Lancet Rheumatology* 5 (6): e316–e329.

Glazener, C.M., Abdalla, M., Stroud, P. et al. (1995). Postnatal maternal morbidity: extent, causes, prevention and treatment. *BJOG* 102: 282–287.

Hartvigsen, J., Hancock, M.J., Kongsted, A. et al. (2018). What low back pain is and why we need to pay attention. *Lancet* 391: 2356–2367.

Heesen, M. and Klimek, M. (2016). Non-obstetric anaesthesia during pregnancy. *Current Opinion in Anaesthesiology* 29 (3): 297–303.

Hoy, D., March, L., Brooks, P. et al. (2014). The global burden of low back pain: estimates from the Global Burden of Disease 2010 study. *Annals of the Rheumatic Diseases* 73: 968–974.

Kahere, M., Hlongwa, M., and Ginindza, T.G. (2022). A scoping review on the epidemiology of chronic low back pain among adults in Sub-Saharan Africa. *International Journal of Environmental Research and Public Health* 19 (5): 2964.

Kamysheva, E., Wertheim, E.H., Skouteris, H. et al. (2009). Frequency, severity, and effect on life of physical symptoms experienced during pregnancy. *Journal of Midwifery & Women's Health* 54 (1): 43–49.

Katonis, P., Kampouroglou, A., Aggelopoulos, A. et al. (2011). Pregnancy-related low back pain. *Hippokratia* 15 (3): 205.

Keynejad, R., Baker, N., Lindenberg, U. et al. (2021). Identifying and responding to domestic violence and abuse in healthcare settings. *BMJ (Clinical Research Ed.)* 373: n1047.

Komatsu, R., Ando, K., and Flood, P. (2020). Factors associated with persistent pain after childbirth: a narrative review. *British Journal of Anaesthesia* 124 (3): e117–e130.

Luca Padua, D.C., Erra, C., Pazzaglia, C. et al. (2016). Carpal tunnel syndrome: clinical features, diagnosis, and management. *Lancet Neurology* 15 (12): 1273–1284.

Mabie, W.C. (2005). Peripheral neuropathies during pregnancy. *Clinical Obstetrics and Gynecology* 48 (1): 57–66.

Meems, M., Truijens, S.E.M., Spek, V. et al. (2017). Follow-up of pregnancy-related carpal tunnel syndrome symptoms at 12 months postpartum: a prospective study. *European Journal of Obstetrics & Gynecology and Reproductive Biology* 211: 231–232.

National Institute for Health and Care Excellence (NICE) (2020). Sprains and strains. https://cks.nice.org.uk/topics/sprains-strains (accessed November 2023).

National Institute for Health and Care Excellence (NICE) (2021). Antenatal care. https://www.nice.org.uk/guidance/ng201/chapter/Recommendations#interventions-for-common-problems-during-pregnancy (accessed November 2023).

O'Doherty, L., Hegarty, K., Ramsay, J. et al. (2015). Screening women for intimate partner violence in healthcare settings. *Cochrane Database of Systematic Reviews* 2015 (7): CD007007. https://doi.org/10.1002/14651858.CD007007.pub3.

Office for Health Improvement and Disparities (2022). Guidance musculoskeletal health: applying All Our Health. https://www.gov.uk/government/publications/musculoskeletal-health-applying-all-our-health/musculoskeletal-health-applying-all-our-health (accessed December 2023).

Pierce, H., Homer, C.S., Dahlen, H.G., and King, J. (2012). Pregnancy-related lumbopelvic pain: listening to Australian women. *Nursing Research and Practice* 2012: 387428.

Schytt, E., Lindmark, G., and Waldenström, U. (2005). Physical symptoms after childbirth: prevalence and associations with self-rated health. *BJOG* 112 (2): 210–217.

Stevens, J.M., Delitto, A., Khoja, S.S. et al. (2021). Risk factors associated with transition from acute to chronic low back pain in US patients seeking primary care. *JAMA Network Open* 4 (2): e2037371.

Tarzia, L., Bohren, M.A., Cameron, J. et al. (2020). Women's experiences and expectations after disclosure of intimate partner abuse to a healthcare provider: a qualitative meta-synthesis. *BMJ Open* 10: e041339.

Taylor, J., Bradbury-Jones, C., Kroll, T., and Duncan, F. (2013). Health professionals' beliefs about domestic abuse and the issue of disclosure: a critical incident technique study. *Health & Social Care in the Community* 21 (5): 489–499.

Thomas, R., Dyer, G.S.M., Tornetta, P. III et al. (2021). Upper extremity injuries in the victims of intimate partner violence. *European Radiology* 31: 5713–5720.

Vleeming, A., Albert, H.B., Ostgaard, H.C. et al. (2008). European guidelines for the diagnosis and treatment of pelvic girdle pain. *European Spine Journal* 17 (6): 794–819.

Walters, C., West, S., and Nippita, T.A. (2018). Pelvic girdle pain in pregnancy. *Australian Journal for General Practitioners* 47: 439–443.

Williams, A., Kamper, S.J., Wiggers, J.H. et al. (2018). Musculoskeletal conditions may increase the risk of chronic disease: a systematic review and meta-analysis of cohort studies. *BMC Medicine* 16: 167.

Women's Aid (2022). What is domestic abuse? https://www.womensaid.org.uk/information-support/what-is-domestic-abuse (accessed November 2023).

World Health Organization (2022). Musculoskeletal health. https://www.who.int/news-room/fact-sheets/detail/musculoskeletal-conditions (accessed November 2023).

World Health Organization (WHO) (2021). Caring for women subjected to violence: a WHO training curriculum for health care providers. Revised ed. Geneva: WHO. https://www.who.int/health-topics/violence-against-women#tab=tab_1 (accessed November 2023).

Wright, C., Smith, B., Wright, S. et al. (2014). Who develops carpal tunnel syndrome during pregnancy: an analysis of obesity, gestational weight gain, and parity. *Obstetric Medicine* 7 (2): 90–94.

Wu, W.H., Meijer, O.G., Uegaki, K. et al. (2004). Pregnancy-related pelvic girdle pain (PPP), I: terminology, clinical presentation, and prevalence. *European Spine Journal* 13 (7): 575–589.

Wuytack, F., Begley, C., and Daly, D. (2020). Risk factors for pregnancy-related pelvic girdle pain: a scoping review. *BMC Pregnancy and Childbirth* 20 (1): 739. https://doi.org/10.1186/s12884-020-03442-5.

Zhang, M., Cooley, C., Ziadni, M.S. et al. (2023). Association between history of childbirth and chronic, functionally significant back pain in later life. *BMC Womens Health* 23 (1): 4.

Further Resources

Ceprnja, D., Chipchase, L., Liamputtong, P., and Gupta, A. (2022). 'This is hard to cope with': the lived experience and coping strategies adopted amongst Australian women with pelvic girdle pain in pregnancy. *BMC Pregnancy and Childbirth* 22: 96.

Chartered Society of Physiotherapy. www.csp.org.uk (accessed November 2023).

Heath Service Executive. Pelvic girdle pain in pregnancy. https://www2.hse.ie/conditions/pelvic-girdle-pain-pregnancy/how-it-affects-labour-and-birth/ (accessed November 2023).

Domestic Abuse Act 2021. www.gov.uk/government/publications/domestic-abuse-act-2021 (accessed November 2023).

Public Health England. Musculoskeletal health: A 5-year strategic framework for prevention across the lifecourse. https://assets.publishing.service.gov.uk/media/5d0b44eded915d0939f84803/Musculoskeletal_Health_5_year_strategy.pdf (accessed November 2023).

National Health Service. Pregnancy and Baby. http://www.nhs.uk/pregnancy-and-baby (accessed November 2023).

Glossary

Carpal tunnel syndrome	Condition caused by compression of the median nerve in the wrist, leading to tingling, numbness and pain in the hand and fingers
Coccyx	Also known as the tailbone, it is the small triangular bone at the bottom of the spine. It is relatively flexible and can shift slightly during childbirth to accommodate the passage of the baby through the birth canal
Pelvic floor muscles	A group of muscles located at the base of the pelvis, forming a hammock-like structure. They provide support to the pelvic organs and play a crucial role in childbirth and postpartum recovery. They are important for sexual function and maintaining continence. They include the levator ani muscle group (puborectalis, pubococcygeus and iliococcygeus) and the coccygeus muscle
Pelvic girdle pain (PGP)	A term used to describe pain and discomfort in the pelvic area during pregnancy, often caused by issues with the sacroiliac joint or symphysis pubis. Sometimes used interchangeably with the term symphysis pubis dysfunction (SPD)
Pubic symphysis	The joint located at the front of the pelvis that connects the two pubic bones. It can become more flexible during pregnancy to allow for easier passage of the baby during childbirth

CHAPTER 20

Fluid and Electrolyte Balance and Associated Disorders

Kate Nash

Department of Nursing and Midwifery, Faculty of Health and Wellbeing, University of Winchester, Winchester, UK

AIM

This chapter describes the importance of fluid and electrolyte balance during the perinatal period and explains key disorders associated with fluid and electrolyte balance during pregnancy and the childbearing period.

LEARNING OUTCOMES

On completion of this chapter the reader will be able to:

- Describe how fluid and electrolyte distribution within the body contribute to homeostasis
- Identify the characteristics of fluid and electrolyte balance and imbalance and their relevance for pregnancy and childbirth
- Discuss some of the pathological considerations associated with fluid and electrolyte imbalance
- Explain the associated midwifery actions relevant to maintaining fluid balance to ensure optimal care provision during the childbirth continuum

Test Your Prior Knowledge

1. List the clinical scenarios that require a fluid balance chart.
2. Provide six examples of fluid input and output that midwives would need to document on a fluid balance chart.
3. What blood tests should be taken during postpartum haemorrhage?
4. What are hot debriefs and why are they important?

Fluid balance is essential for maintaining physiological well-being. Reduced fluid intake or loss can lead to serious morbidity and mortality, whereas increased fluid input may also contribute to significant morbidity and mortality. The midwife has a crucial role in measuring fluid input and output, recognising and understanding the potential implications of significant fluid

Fundamentals of Maternal Pathophysiology, First Edition. Edited by Claire Leader and Ian Peate.

depletion or overload. This chapter will explore fluid and electrolyte distribution and function within the body, before considering key pathological conditions relating to this and the associated midwifery care and responsibilities.

Fluid and Electrolyte Distribution

Fluid and electrolytes are exchanged across cell membranes to maintain homeostasis, where the body seeks to maintain a balanced equilibrium within its internal environment (Johnson et al. 2008). The cardiovascular system is integral for the distribution of gases, nutrients and metabolites throughout the body and movement between arterioles and venous systems is regulated by endothelial capillaries (Moini 2016). Approximately 60% of an individual's total body weight is composed of water, with slightly less (approximately 52%) held within females due to increased adipose tissue and slightly more (approximately 63%) within males due to increased muscle content (Shier et al. 2016).

Body fluids contain solutes consisting of electrolytes and non-electrolytes in water that occupy different compartments within the body, separated by membranes. Extracellular compartments include all fluid held outside of cells including plasma within blood vessels and interstitial fluids found within tissue spaces outside of the vasculature of the body. Intracellular compartments include all water and electrolytes that are held within cells. Extracellular fluids comprise approximately one-third (37%) of total body water volume, with intracellular fluids consisting of approximately 63% of total body water volume (Shier et al. 2016). See Figure 20.1 regarding fluid components.

The balancing of fluid volume between the different areas within the body is a fundamental physiological requirement and the cell membrane acts as a selective barrier to determine what moves into and out of the cell (Vanputte et al. 2013). Movement across these membranes is regulated to stabilise the composition and distribution of fluids within the body. The direction of fluid exchange between intra- and extracellular compartments is mainly determined by a mixture of the relative hydrostatic and osmotic pressures of these compartments and the permeability of the capillary wall (Mathur et al. 2020).

Within the circulatory system thin capillary walls permit the movement of fluids and solutes throughout the body and hydrostatic pressure is determined by the pressure exerted by the contraction of the heart and resistance of the vessels and capillaries. When hydrostatic pressures within the capillaries are greater than the pressures within the

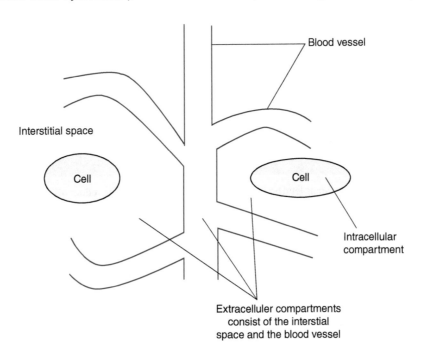

FIGURE 20.1 Fluid components.

surrounding interstitial spaces, fluid is pushed through the capillary wall into the surrounding interstitial space (Scott 2010). Plasma proteins contribute to the total osmotic pressure of the solution, referred to as colloid osmotic pressure or oncotic pressure. Because plasma proteins cannot easily cross the capillary walls, their concentration is higher within blood plasma than within the interstitial fluid. Plasma osmotic pressure and the presence of albumin act to pull water back into the intravascular circulation (Wylie and Bryce 2016).

The kidneys play a vital role in fluid and electrolyte balance and are integral to maintaining fluid balance within the body through the production and regulation of urine (Boyle and Bothamley 2018). Several hormones affect fluid balance, and prominent among these is antidiuretic hormone (ADH) produced in the hypothalamus and stored in the posterior pituitary gland. ADH acts on the kidney to regulate water retention and the production and osmolarity of urine. Disruption of the kidney and renal system are explored further in Chapter 14.

Electrolytes

Electrolytes are molecules that release ions in water and contribute to shifts in fluids between intracellular and extracellular compartments (Rankin 2017; Moini 2016). Sodium, potassium, calcium and magnesium are key electrolytes vital for optimal cellular function and impairment to neuromuscular, renal and cardiac systems can occur as a result of electrolyte imbalance. Signs of electrolyte imbalance may include lethargy, hypotension, muscle weakness, paraesthesia, blurred vision and slurred speech and gastrointestinal disturbances (Boyle and Bothamley 2018; Ahmed 2021).

Total body water content increases during pregnancy as the volume of intravascular fluid substantially rises to meet the demands of the fetal placental circulation (Rankin 2017). Serum ionic calcium and serum phosphate levels remain unchanged during pregnancy, although there is a decrease in serum total calcium due to a decrease in serum albumin because of the volume expansion of pregnancy (Ahmed 2021).

Sodium has a key role in maintaining the acid–base balance of the body along with chloride and bicarbonate ions, and is the primary electrolyte of extracellular fluid found in blood plasma and interstitial fluid. Regulation of sodium is mainly by the renin–angiotensin–aldosterone system and ADH. To maintain sodium and fluid balance, renal tubular reabsorption increases by as much as 50% during pregnancy as progesterone levels stimulate the angiotensin–renin system in the kidneys to increase aldosterone production (Rankin 2017; Wylie and Bryce 2016). Aldosterone facilitates sodium reabsorption and has an important role in maintaining blood pressure and fluid balance. Potassium levels generally remain unchanged during pregnancy despite increased urine production (Scott 2010).

Magnesium is an essential constituent of many enzyme systems and is required for more than 300 enzymatic reactions in the body (Ahmed 2021; NICE 2022). It plays a vital role in neurochemical transmission and the regulation of vasomotor tone in blood vessels (Ahmed 2021). Low magnesium levels (hypomagnesaemia) are associated with type 2 diabetes and hypertension, and cause a decrease in blood flow to the brain and cerebral vasospasm (Babys et al. 2021).

Medicines Management

Magnesium sulfate can protect the developing fetal brain and so has significant potential to reduce disability. Intravenous (IV) magnesium sulfate is offered to women in established preterm labour or who are having a planned preterm birth within 24 hours for neuroprotection of the baby (NICE 2015a). It is also recommended within a critical care setting for women with severe hypertension or severe pre-eclampsia to prevent seizures (NICE 2022).

Serum magnesium levels remain unchanged or marginally reduced in pregnancy due to haemodilution (Ahmed 2021). Pre-eclampsia and preterm birth are associated with hypomagnesaemia in pregnancy, but there is conflicting evidence about the role of oral magnesium supplementation in the prevention of preterm birth and currently routine magnesium supplementation is not recommended (Makrides et al. 2014; de Araújo et al. 2020). IV magnesium sulfate infusion is used in the management of preterm birth and severe pre-eclampsia in critical care settings (NICE 2015a, 2019).

Maintaining Fluid Balance

Normal body function depends on the body's ability to respond to changing conditions to maintain water, electrolyte levels and acid–base balance in the internal environment within the normal range. Optimal fluid balance will maintain a stable blood volume consistent with usual parameters with sufficient pressure to distribute oxygen and nutrients to the cells (Boyle and Bothamley 2018). Disruptions in fluid distribution can affect blood volume and cellular function and can ultimately be life threatening. To maintain optimal fluid balance throughout the body, fluid gained throughout the day should equal the amount that is lost.

Fluid loss can be referred to as insensible and sensible losses. Insensible fluid loss is fluid loss that cannot be measured or easily visualised and includes fluid loss through skin evaporation or exhaled through the lungs. These losses are constant, although they can be affected by factors such as body surface area and environmental humidity, which may cause increased fluid loss via sweating. Tachypnoea causes more water to be lost via the lungs and pyrexia can increase insensible losses of fluid from both the skin and lungs (Scott 2010). It is important that midwives take into consideration insensible fluid loss in their overall assessment when providing holistic care.

Sensible fluid loss refers to fluid loss that can be measured and includes loss of fluid through urination, wounds, defecation and vomit. On average an adult loses approximately 100 ml of fluid per day through defecation, although this could exceed 5000 ml/day in cases of severe diarrhoea (Scott 2010).

The usual homeostatic mechanisms of fluid balance are changed during pregnancy as blood volume increases considerably, reaching approximately 45–50% more than non-pregnant values by term (Osol et al. 2019; Sutton and Mann 2021). Despite the significant increase in cardiac output and total blood volume apparent in healthy pregnancies, systemic vascular resistance decreases during pregnancy through vasodilation and intravascular colloid osmotic pressure falls gradually during the first and second trimesters before rising after 34 weeks' gestation (Wu et al. 1983).

Conditions such as hyperemesis gravidarum, postpartum haemorrhage (PPH) and pre-eclampsia can cause considerable disturbance to fluid balance regulation. Hyperemesis gravidarum is discussed in Chapter 17 and PPH and pre-eclampsia will be considered in relation to fluid balance later in this chapter.

Measurement of Fluid Balance

383

Accurate measurement of fluid input and output is an integral part of midwifery care and assessment. Midwives are required to manage fluid and infusion pumps, monitor urine output and fluid input and maintain records of fluid balance. Indicating factors that should prompt midwives to commence a fluid balance chart are outlined in Table 20.1.

TABLE 20.1   Clinical scenarios requiring a fluid balance chart.

Vomiting and diarrhoea
Hyperemesis gravidarum
Conditions such as diabetes, renal disease and cardiac conditions
At commencement of and throughout intravenous fluids administration
At commencement of and throughout insertion of indwelling urinary catheter
Monitoring of drainage post-surgery
Post-surgery
Pre-eclampsia
Haemorrhage
Critical conditions, for example sepsis

Fluid Balance Charts

Fluid balance charts should be employed to document fluid input and output over a 24-hour period and are used to inform clinical decision-making. Figure 20.2 shows a fluid balance chart.

Red Flag

An incomplete or inaccurately completed fluid balance chart can provide misleading information, leading to incorrect diagnosis and treatment planning options.

It is important that the commencement of the fluid balance chart is clearly documented so that an accurate 24-hour balance can be achieved. Women and midwives should be educated about how to document their oral intake, for example by measuring the quantities of fluid within a glass or cup, and women should be advised to measure their urine with a jug and keep a record of their oral input and output. The importance of correct record keeping is a fundamental part of the midwife's role (NMC 2015, 2019) and incorrect recordings can result in incorrect management, leading to dehydration, fluid overload or electrolyte imbalance. Within critical care situations a fluid balance chart may be incorporated as part of the observation chart. Table 20.2 outlines the fluids that need to be documented on a fluid balance chart.

Ward:				Date:			
Surname:				Hospital Number:			
Forename:							
Date of Birth:							
	Fluid intake			**Fluid output**			
Time	**Oral**	**Intravenous**	**Other (specify)**	**Urine**	**Vomit**	**Other (specify)**	
01.00							
02.00							
03.00							
04.00							
05.00							
06.00							
07.00							
08.00							
09.00							
10.00							
11.00							
12.00							
13.00							
14.00							
15.00							
16.00							
17.00							
18.00							
19.00							
20.00							
21.00							
22.00							
23.00							
24.00							
Total							

FIGURE 20.2   Fluid balance chart.

TABLE 20.2	Examples of fluid input and output that midwives would need to document on a fluid balance chart.	
Fluid input	**Fluid output**	
Oral fluids	Urine	
Intravenous fluids	Vomiting	
Nasogastric fluids	Diarrhoea	
	Exudate from wounds (drains and dressing)	
	Blood loss	

Disturbances in Fluid Balance

Dehydration occurs when the body is using more fluid than has been taken in or when there has been excessive fluid loss. Depletion of intravascular fluid volume can occur due to prolonged vomiting, diarrhoea and excessive perspiration, or by movement of the intravascular volume of fluids to the interstitial space.

Examination Scenario

Clinical signs of dehydration may include light-headedness, thirst, dry mucus membranes, poor skin turgor, prolonged capillary re-fill of more than two minutes, headaches, raised pulse and lowered blood pressure (Boyle and Bothamley 2018). It is important that the midwife undertakes a full clinical assessment that includes careful history taking of fluid input and output, and the presence of other symptoms alongside any complicating factors. Consideration of the woman's medical, mental health and social history is important to exclude other contributory causes.

Laboratory testing is used to support or exclude diagnoses. Laboratory markers of dehydration include signs of haemoconcentration such as raised haematocrit and haemoglobin in full blood count and increased urine specific gravity (1.030) detected on urinalysis, which measures the concentration of urine. Biochemistry tests to assess renal function can be undertaken to assess sodium level, which is usually raised in dehydration. Referral to the obstetric team is necessary and oral or IV fluid and electrolyte replacement may be prescribed depending on examination and laboratory findings.

Fluid Balance and Pre-eclampsia

Fluid balance is an important consideration of the management of severe pre-eclampsia. Pre-eclampsia is a multisystem disorder that typically affects 2–5% of pregnant women (Poon et al. 2019). In 2018–2020 eight women died from hypertensive disorders of pregnancy, all either during pregnancy or up to six weeks after the end of pregnancy. The mortality rate in the United Kingdom remains low (0.38/100 000), but is four times higher than in the 2012–2014 triennium when the rate was at its lowest (Knight et al. 2022).

Early-onset pre-eclampsia arises due to abnormal placentation and maladaptation of the spiral arteries at placentation. This causes the arteries to retain their muscular layer, limiting their ability to accommodate the increased blood supply, leading to placental ischaemia and endothelial damage (Burton et al. 2019).

Generalised vasospasm reduces tissue perfusion that affects all body organs (Wylie and Bryce 2016). Endothelial damage occurs and is associated with an increase in both peripheral vascular resistance and vascular permeability, resulting in a state of relative intravascular hypovolaemia. Consequently, raised blood pressure and increased endothelial cell permeability cause depleted proteins and fluids to shift from the intravascular plasma compartment into the surrounding interstitial tissues. The management and pathophysiology of pre-eclampsia are covered in Chapter 12; this chapter will focus on fluid balance in pre-eclampsia.

Clinical Investigation

Haematological changes observed with pre-eclampsia are elevated haematocrit and haemoglobin due to haemoconcentration as plasma volume shifts from the intravascular compartment into the peripheral tissues. This may be exacerbated by diminished production of plasma proteins in the damaged liver.

Urea and electrolytes (Us and Es) are biochemical markers used to assess renal function. Increased serum creatinine and uric acid are reflective of impaired renal function. Midwives should ensure that an accurate fluid balance is maintained, and where a urinary catheter is in situ urine output is measured hourly in cases of severe pre-eclampsia to guide decision making about fluid management. Liver function tests are required to evaluate the severity of liver impairment and raised serum aspartate aminotransferase (AST) is reflective of hepatocyte damage caused by reduced hepatic blood supply (Wylie and Bryce 2016). Assessing urine protein: creatinine ratio also helps quantify loss of protein via the kidneys and assists with further evaluation of kidney function.

Fluid Therapy and Pre-eclampsia

The aim of fluid therapy is to achieve a balance between ensuring adequate renal perfusion and prevention of fluid over-load and pulmonary oedema. Pulmonary oedema is defined as the abnormal accumulation of fluid in the interstitial and alveolar spaces of the lung, leading to impaired gaseous exchange of oxygen and carbon dioxide (Farrer and Sullivan 2015). Several predisposing factors have been identified in women who develop pulmonary oedema during pregnancy, which include pre-eclampsia, iatrogenic fluid overload and cardiac disease (da Silva et al. 2021).

Examination Scenario

Symptoms of pulmonary overload often present as respiratory crackles, wheezing, lowered oxygen saturation measurements and pink frothy sputum (Boyle and Bothamley 2018). The midwife should be alert to these as part of their clinical examination, which should include careful monitoring of fluid balance, oxygen saturations, respiration rate, depth and rhythm, pulse, blood pressure and temperature.

Case Study 20.1

Martha is a 38-year-old primiparous woman being cared for on the labour ward at 34 weeks' gestation for severe pre-eclampsia, a blood pressure of 180/110 mm/Hg and significant (3+++) proteinuria. Martha received a loading dose of magnesium sulfate followed by a maintenance infusion as per local Trust guideline. During this time Martha was receiving one-to-one care from Anne, her midwife, and was under the care of the consultant obstetrician with input from the consultant anaesthetist and the senior midwife coordinator. Martha was reviewed by the multiprofessional team at each ward round or more frequently depending on the clinical findings to ensure clear communication with Martha and all team members.

Magnesium Toxicity

Because of the potential for magnesium toxicity, it is important that Anne checks Martha's respiratory rate and deep tendon reflexes every hour. If toxicity is suspected because of a respiration rate below 12/min, absent reflexes or altered conscious level, Anne should stop the infusion and immediately alert the senior obstetrician and anaesthetist (NICE 2015a). Serum magnesium levels may be requested by the obstetric team. It is important that there is a supply of calcium gluconate, the antidote for magnesium sulfate, available on the labour ward should it be required.

Red Flag

Women receiving IV magnesium sulfate infusion should be monitored for magnesium toxicity (NICE 2022). Magnesium is excreted by the kidneys and hypermagnesaemia can occur in renal failure, causing muscle weakness and arrhythmias. Calcium gluconate injection 10 mg is used for the management of magnesium toxicity (NICE 2022).

TABLE 20.3 **Key considerations for management of pre-eclampsia.**

- Record blood pressure (BP) and pulse every 15 minutes and use BP recordings to inform treatment
- Record temperature every four hours to ensure no signs of sepsis and within normal limits
- Conduct continuous pulse oximetry
- Indwelling urinary catheter and urometer in situ and urine output monitored hourly and recorded on the fluid balance chart. Usual practice is to maintain a minimum urine output of 100 ml/4 hours. A catheter stream urine (CSU) may be collected and tested for proteinuria or sent for laboratory testing
- Crystalloid infusion at 80 ml/h recorded on fluid balance chart minus the volume of infused drugs
- Maintenance infusion of magnesium via a syringe pump. Check the infusion regularly to ensure it is working properly. Check respiratory rate hourly
- Check patellar reflexes: the brisker the reflexes, the higher the risk of seizure
- IV antihypertensive labetalol via a syringe pump
- Completion of relevant documentation, including high dependency record, modified early obstetric warning score (MEOWS), drug chart and fluid balance chart
- Provide support with attending to hygiene needs and moving with a drip stand
- Check cannula sites and undertake a visual infusion phlebitis (VIP) score at regular intervals to monitor for infusion phlebitis
- Provide emotional support
- Monitor the fetal heart via electronic fetal monitoring
- Escalate and take prompt action through communicating with the multiprofessional team should the woman's condition deteriorate

---

Table 20.3 provides an overview of key aspects of care that should be provided by a midwife for a woman with pre-eclampsia. Guidance for women with severe pre-eclampsia recommends IV access and an IV fluid restriction of 80 ml/h provided there no other ongoing fluid losses such as haemorrhage (NICE 2019). Studies have suggested that restricting IV fluids is associated with reduced rates of pulmonary oedema without an increase in acute renal failure (Thornton et al. 2007; Mol et al. 2016).

It is important that fluid management should be tailored to the individual woman and informed by clinical assessment (Pretorius et al. 2018). Multidisciplinary working and clear communication are vital, along with midwife vigilance and clear documentation and communication using recognised communication tools such as Situation, Background, Assessment, Recommendation (SBAR). The usual practice of preloading IV fluids prior to epidural insertion to counteract hypotension in responsive to sympathetic nerve blockage is not recommended for women with severe pre-eclampsia (NICE 2019) because of the possible risk of fluid overload and pulmonary oedema.

Laboratory testing of platelet levels because of the potential for HELLP (haemolysis, elevated liver enzymes and low platelets) syndrome and deranged clotting prior to epidural insertion is also important and is discussed in Chapter 14.

Medicines Management: Antihypertensives – Hydralazine

Midwives must be aware of potential side effects and contra-indications associated with antihypertensives used to control blood pressure. Hydralazine, a vasodilator, can cause significant hypotension. National guidance suggests administering crystalloid fluid before or at same time as the first dose of hydralazine and the decision should be made by the senior obstetrician with input from the multiprofessional team (NICE 2019).

Pre-eclampsia and Co-existing Morbidities

The most recent confidential enquiry shone a light on the complexities of care provision of women with multiple co-morbidities. Women with pre-eclampsia and gestational diabetes share similar risk factors and coexistence of diabetes and pre-eclampsia adds complexity to women's management, particularly in relation to fluid balance, as management of the two conditions may be conflicting (Knight et al. 2022).

Women who develop gestational diabetes are at a higher risk of facing pre-eclampsia and studies have shown a correlation between diabetes and pre-eclampsia. Common risk factors between the two conditions include increased maternal age, nulliparity, multiple-gestation pregnancies and an increased pre-pregnancy body mass index (Schneider et al. 2012; Lee et al. 2017).

Pre-eclampsia management in women with diabetes during labour necessitates many IV infusions and it is vital that local policy and procedure are adhered to, with clear documentation on the fluid balance chart and patient records. Infusions may include variable-rate insulin infusion (VRII), substrate fluid, oxytocin, antihypertensives and magnesium sulfate (NICE 2015b, 2019). Midwives need to be aware of local Trust protocols and policies for fluid administration and the use of volumetric pumps to ensure safe delivery of the solutions.

Pre-eclampsia and Diabetic Ketoacidosis

Despite recent advances in the evaluation and medical treatment of diabetes in pregnancy, diabetic ketoacidosis (DKA) was highlighted in the most recent confidential inquiry (Knight et al. 2022). Untreated hyperglycaemia leads to marked glycosuria, initiating a significant osmotic diuresis. As a result, dehydration, electrolyte depletion and, if left untreated, cardiac failure and death may follow.

Learning Event

The increased fluid regimen necessitated as part of the management of DKA can also contribute to possible fluid overload, particularly in women with pre-eclampsia. The Joint British Diabetes Societies for Inpatient Care (JBDS-IP 2022) recommends early input from the critical care team and consideration of an arterial line to allow for central venous pressure monitoring for signs of fluid overload and to guide fluid management.

Fluid Balance During Labour

There is no justification for the restriction of fluids and food in labour for women at low risk of complications (Singata et al. 2013; NICE 2023), although practice among maternity units varies and oral intake has historically been restricted in many birth settings. This is mainly in response to work undertaken in the 1940s that showed increased morbidity and mortality associated with chemical pneumonitis (Mendelson 1946). Anaesthetic practices have improved considerably since then and national guidance does not discourage oral fluids during labour (NICE 2017).

Intravenous Fluids During Labour

The administration of IV fluids for hydration or the administration of drugs such as oxytocin for augmentation or induction of labour is a common aspect of midwifery intrapartum care. Midwives are expected to demonstrate proficiency in the management of IV fluids, including transfusion of blood, at registration (NMC 2019). However, IV fluid administration is one of the most poorly managed aspects of intrapartum care (Bruce et al. 2022).

Within the labour ward, crystalloids are commonly administered by midwives. These are electrolyte solutions in which the ion concentration can be altered so that they are isotonic or hypotonic with blood plasma. Isotonic fluids have equal osmotic pressure inside and outside of a cell and so there is the same ratio of solutes in the intra- and extracellular compartments. Sodium chloride 0.9% (normal saline) is comparable to the concentration of sodium in the blood and is known as an isotonic solution, which is commonly used within maternity and for first-line resuscitation of pregnant women (Royal College of Obstetricians and Gynaecologists [RCOG] 2016). Because there is equal osmotic pressure inside and outside the cell, it does not cause shifts between intra- and extra-fluid compartments.

Medicines Management: Midwives' Exemptions

Midwives and student midwives under direct supervision of a registered midwife are permitted to administer Hartmann's solution and 0.9% sodium chloride IV as part of the Midwives' Exemptions (NMC 2017). This should only be during their professional practice. In situations where women have additional complex needs, the fluid management regimen should always be led by a senior member of the obstetric or anaesthetic team.

Currently there is insufficient evidence to inform the routine use of IV fluids during labour for maternal hydration and variation in clinical practice has been reported (Dawood et al. 2013; Lindstrom et al. 2018; Bruce et al. 2022). Despite it being a widely adopted practice, there is no consensus on the type or volume of IV fluids required or whether they are necessary (Garmi et al. 2017). National guidance emphasises how many current IV fluid practices during the intrapartum period are historical and as such are not grounded in evidence-based practice (NICE 2017). It is important that midwives have a clear rationale for the administration of IV fluids during labour and understand the risks associated with IV fluid administration. Possible complications include infection of the cannulation site, fluid overload and electrolyte disturbance.

Case Study 20.2

Lois is a newly qualified midwife and is caring for Esha on the labour ward. Esha has an epidural in progress for pain relief and is receiving IV Hartmann's solution.

>   What care should Lois provide, particularly for fluid balance?
>   Care considerations can be summarised as follows:

- Ensure a fluid balance chart is commenced and maintained. Attention to bladder care is important, as the increased sympathetic and motor blockade associated with the epidural may impede bladder sensation and mobilisation.
- Provide Esha with the opportunity to empty her bladder two- to four-hourly and offer the insertion of a urinary catheter if this is not achieved.
- Observe the catheter for free drainage of clear urine and record this on the fluid balance chart. Should no urine be observed, Lois should check the bladder tubing for kinking that may prevent drainage.
- IV hydration is recommended with epidural analgesia because of the hypotensive effect due to vasodilation associated with sympathetic blockade. This should be recorded on the fluid balance chart.
- Any concerns should be escalated immediately to the midwife in charge, anaesthetist and senior obstetrician.

Insertion of a urinary catheter with epidural analgesia may be recommended to prevent complications associated with bladder distension. Urinary retention is a known side effect of epidural analgesia (Anim-Somuah et al. 2018). However, the evidence around urinary catheter insertion is inconclusive, and no difference has been found between intermittent and continuous catheterisation in the incidence of postpartum urinary tract infection, urinary retention and haemorrhage (Li et al. 2019). Midwives should encourage women to pass urine spontaneously in the first instance and advise urinary catheter insertion to ensure an empty bladder if this is not accomplished.

Hyponatraemia

Excessive oral and IV fluid intake is associated with hyponatraemia, low serum sodium levels. Approximately one in four women who take in more than 2.5 l of fluid (orally and IV) during labour will become hyponatraemic (Moen et al. 2009). It is important that midwives document and review the fluid input and output of women they provide care for in the intrapartum period. Women should not be encouraged to drink excessively during labour and routine IV hydration is not recommended.

Hypovolaemia

Absolute hypovolaemia can be defined as a reduction in total circulating blood volume that may be related to blood loss (haemorrhage) or plasma loss (gastrointestinal, renal, cutaneous, extravasation into interstitial tissues). It occurs from direct loss of whole blood or body fluid. Relative hypovolaemia occurs from fluid shifts within the body. In the case of relative hypovolaemia, fluid or blood has moved out of the intravascular space and begun pooling elsewhere. Relative hypovolaemia can occur in patients with conditions such as ascites or peritonitis.

Postpartum Haemorrhage

PPH can cause acute hypovolaemia, leading to hypovolaemic shock. Hypovolaemic shock presents with a deterioration in vital signs in a non-pregnant individual, but these signs can be masked in pregnancy, which can hinder early recognition and delay treatment. The pathophysiology of PPH is discussed in Chapter 10 and fluid balance management in relation to haemorrhage and hypovolaemia will be the focus of this section.

PPH refers to an estimated blood loss of 500 ml or more from the genital tract after the birth of the baby (World Health Organization [WHO] 2020) or any amount that adversely affects the mother. Primary PPH occurs 24 hours after birth, whereas secondary PPH occurs after 24 hours and before the end of the puerperium.

RCOG (2016) further defines PPH as minor pertaining to blood loss from 500 to 1000 ml and the absence of maternal compromise, and major referring to blood loss over 1000 ml or the presence of maternal compromise. This is further defined as moderate (1000–2000 ml) and severe (2000 ml or more) (RCOG 2016). Midwives must be aware of their local guidelines for the management and documentation of PPH.

Learning Event

Factors such as haemoglobin levels, previous history, cause of bleeding, body weight and maternal response are integral to the assessment process and a lower level of blood loss may be clinically significant for women weighing less than 60 kg (RCOG 2016).

Fluid Replacement

Fluid replacement is a critical component of the response to PPH and the rapid administration of warmed fluids is vital for resuscitation (RCOG 2016). Ensuring fluids are warmed helps prevent against hypothermia, which could cause further deterioration in the mother's condition.

The fundamental objectives during the management of PPH are to restore blood volume and oxygen-carrying capacity, arrest bleeding and stabilise the mother (RCOG 2016). Accurate measurement of blood loss is a fundamental component of the treatment of fluid loss and restoration of blood volume. The recording of an accurate and contemporaneous fluid balance chart will guide management and further treatment with IV fluids (Lilley et al. 2015). The visual estimation of blood loss is not sufficient and can lead to an inaccurate recording of fluid balance, as midwives considerably underestimate the amount of blood loss at birth (Hancock et al. 2019). It is important that blood loss is measured to avoid overestimation of blood loss and the prevention of fluid overload and unnecessary transfusion.

Expert Midwife

Accurate measurement of blood loss is vital and leads to timely recognition, escalation, management and resuscitation, which in turn result in a reduction of complications of major PPH. Midwives and other health professionals are known to underestimate blood loss in up to 60% of cases with visual estimation and therefore accurate weighing of blood loss is recommended. It is vital to speak out and ensure that blood loss is measured frequently during the management of PPH and cumulative blood loss is accurately documented on the fluid balance chart or proforma and communicated to the multidisciplinary team. Women's weight should also be considered, as smaller women have a lower circulatory blood volume therefore their ability to tolerate blood loss can be reduced.

Jemma Walker, Midwife, Lecturer and PROMPT trainer

Continuous physiological monitoring is essential and there should be continual re-evaluation and re-assessment of the mother's overall condition, considering blood loss, fluid balance, vital signs and overall demeanour.

The midwife has a key role to play in assessing blood loss and urine output, running through intravenous fluids, administration of uterotonics and undertaking appropriate actions such as the rubbing up of a contraction and expelling of blood clots to assist with the correction of uterine atony, the commonest cause of PPH.

Consent for venepuncture is important as fluid management will be guided by serum haematology, biochemistry and clotting factors. The following venous bloods should be taken:

- Full blood count
- Cross-match
- Clotting including fibrinogen
- Urea and electrolytes to assess kidney and electrolyte function
- Liver function tests

An indwelling urinary catheter should be inserted with consent and hourly urine measurements taken and recorded to further assess renal function and fluid balance. Bladder emptying is important in the first-line management of PPH. A full bladder can impede myometrial contraction, and often the bladder is not completely emptied during labour.

A combination of clear fluids, red blood cells and blood products is given to replace blood loss. Traditional recommendations are up to 3.5 l of clear fluids, which should include 2 l of warmed crystalloids followed by 1.5 l of warmed colloids if blood products are still not available (RCOG 2016). The WHO recommends the use of crystalloids over colloids and studies have shown that resuscitation with colloids is not associated with an improvement in survival (Perel et al. 2013).

Midwives on the labour ward work as part of a multidisciplinary team under the leadership of the consultant obstetrician and labour ward coordinator, with close input from the anaesthetic, haematology and blood transfusion team to

Orange Flag

Communication with women and their partners is important following an emergency to provide reassurance, offer opportunities for questions and facilitate planning for future pregnancies.

Further research is needed to understand the psychological and emotional impacts of PPH and to understand whether better information and follow-up can improve outcomes.

In addition, providing the opportunity for communication with team members following an emergency is an important part of checking staff well-being and ensuring time for reflection and learning.

Source: Adapted from Dunning et al. (2016).

guide fluid management. Clear leadership is vital in emergency situations with closed-loop communication to check understanding, completion of actions and accuracy of communication (Siassakos et al. 2011).

Expert Midwife

Hot debriefs are interactive structured team dialogues that take place either immediately or very shortly after a major clinical incident. Their aim is to assist the whole team to learn from the experience, reflect on what went well, identify team strengths or difficulties, and consider ways to improve future performance. Further support can then be provided by the Professional Midwifery Advocate team if required.

Liz Macleod, Head of Midwifery and Professional Midwifery Advocate

Red Flag

Hypothermia from tissue hypoperfusion and inadequately warmed fluids is a serious complication of haemorrhage and can affect transfusion coagulopathy, impair oxygen delivery, and decrease heart rate and cardiac output. Shivering can also lead to lactic acidosis.

Senior critical care and anaesthetic input is important to manage fluid balance and ensure the woman remains haemodynamically stable. There is a risk of fluid overload and haemodilutional coagulopathy with the transfusion of large volumes of crystalloids, colloids or red blood cells (RCOG 2016). Haematology and blood transfusion expertise is required for the transfusion of fresh frozen plasma, platelets and cryoprecipitate. The insertion of a central venous pressure line can enable accurate measurement of central venous pressure to guide fluid management and early involvement of the critical care team is essential (RCOG 2016). It is recommended that women who are actively bleeding have regular assessment of their fibrinogen levels to check for underlying clotting disorders that may contribute to continued bleeding and to manage the management and replacement of blood and clotting factors (Klein et al. 2016). Point-of-care testing is recommended alongside a locally agreed treatment algorithm within maternity (RCOG 2016).

Take-Home Points

- The midwife has a crucial role in measuring fluid input and output, and recognising and understanding the potential implications of significant fluid depletion or overload. Incorrect recordings can result in incorrect management, leading to dehydration, fluid overload or electrolyte imbalance.
- Fluid management should be tailored to the individual woman and informed by clinical assessment. Midwives need to be aware of local Trust protocols and policies for fluid administration and the use of volumetric pumps to ensure safe delivery of the solutions.
- Multidisciplinary working and clear communication are essential, along with midwife vigilance, accurate documentation and communication using recognised communication tools.
- Accurate measurement of blood loss is vital and leads to timely recognition, escalation, management and resuscitation, which in turn result in a reduction of complications of major PPH.
- Midwives and other health professionals are known to underestimate blood loss in up to 60% of cases with visual estimation and therefore accurate weighing of blood loss is important.

Conclusion

This chapter has described fluid and electrolyte distribution and function within the body and considered some of the key pathological conditions relating to fluid and electrolyte imbalance during the perinatal period and the associated midwifery care and responsibilities.

References

Ahmed, A. (2021). Fetomaternal acid–base balance and electrolytes during pregnancy. *Indian Journal of Critical Care Medicine* 25 (Suppl. 3): S193–S199. https://doi.org/10.5005/jp-journals-10071-24030.

Anim-Somuah, M., Smyth, R.M.D., Cyna, A.M., and Cuthbert, A. (2018). Epidural versus non-epidural or no analgesia for pain management in labour. *Cochrane Database of Systematic Reviews* (5): CD000331. https://doi.org/10.1002/14651858.CD000331.pub4.

de Araújo, C.A.L., Ray, J.G., Figueiroa, J.N., and Alves, J.G. (2020). BRAzil magnesium (BRAMAG) trial: a double-masked randomized clinical trial of oral magnesium supplementation in pregnancy. *BMC Pregnancy and Childbirth* 20 (1): 234. https://doi.org/10.1186/s12884-020-02935-7.

Babys, D., Idris, I., and Prihantono (2021). Differences in serum magnesium levels, folic acid, and infant outcomes in severe preeclampsia: a literature review. *Medicina Clínica Práctica* 4 (Supplement 1): 100221. https://doi.org/10.1016/j.mcpsp.2021.100221.

Boyle, M. and Bothamley, J. (2018). *Critical Care Assessments by Midwives*. London: Routledge.

Bruce, B., Hartz, D., Tracy, S. et al. (2022). The administration of intravenous fluids to nulliparous women in labour: a retrospective clinical chart review and fluid balance documentation audit. *Collegian* 29 (3): 364–369. https://doi.org/10.1016/j.colegn.2021.10.002.

Burton, G.J., Redman, C.W., Roberts, J.M., and Moffett, A. (2019). Pre-eclampsia: pathophysiology and clinical implications. *BMJ* 366: l2381. https://doi.org/10.1136/bmj.l2381.

Dawood, F., Dowswell, T., and Quenby, S. (2013). Intravenous fluids for reducing the duration of labour in low risk nulliparous women. *Cochrane Database of Systematic Reviews* (6): CD007715. https://doi.org/10.1002/14651858.CD007715.pub2.

Dunning, T., Harris, J.M., and Sandall, J. (2016). Women and their birth partners' experiences following a primary postpartum haemorrhage: a qualitative study. *BMC Pregnancy and Childbirth* 16: 80. https://doi.org/10.1186/s12884-016-0870-7.

Farrer, J. and Sullivan, J.T. (2015). Pulmonary edema in pregnancy. In: *Maternal Medicine* (ed. L.D. Pacheco, G.R. Saade, and G.V. Hankins). New York: McGraw Hill, ch. 8. https://obgyn.mhmedical.com/content.aspx?bookid=1580&sectionid=96349517.

Garmi, G., Zuarez-Easton, S., Zafran, N. et al. (2017). The effect of type and volume of fluid hydration on labor duration of nulliparous women: a randomized controlled trial. *Archives of Gynecology and Obstetrics* 295: 1407–1412. https://doi.org/10.1007/s00404-017-4381-1.

Hancock, A., Weeks, A.D., and Tina, L.D. (2019). Assessing blood loss in clinical practice. *Best Practice & Research. Clinical Obstetrics & Gynaecology* 61: 28–40. https://doi.org/10.1016/j.bpobgyn.2019.04.004.

Johnson, J., Lyons, E., and Vaughans, B. (2008). *Fluids and Electrolytes Demystified*. New York: McGraw Hill Medical.

Joint British Diabetes Societies for Inpatient Care (JBDS-IP) (2022). *Managing Diabetes and Hyperglycaemia During Labour and Birth (JBDS 12)*. London: JBDS-IP.

Klein, A.A., Arnold, P., Bingham, R.M. et al. (2016). AAGBI guidelines: the use of blood components and their alternatives 2016. *Anaesthesia* 71: 829–842. https://doi.org/10.1111/anae.13489.

Knight, M., Bunch, K., Patel, R. et al. (ed.) (2022) on behalf of MBRRACE-UK). *Saving Lives, Improving Mothers' Care Core Report – Lessons Learned to Inform Maternity Care from the UK and Ireland Confidential Enquiries into Maternal Deaths and Morbidity 2018–20*. Oxford: National Perinatal Epidemiology Unit, University of Oxford.

Lee, J., Ouh, Y.-t., Ahn, K.H. et al. (2017). Preeclampsia: a risk factor for gestational diabetes mellitus in subsequent pregnancy. *PLoS One* 12 (5): e0178150. https://doi.org/10.1371/journal.pone.0178150.

Li, M., Xing, X., Yao, L. et al. (2019). The effect of bladder catheterization on the incidence of urinary tract infection in laboring women with epidural analgesia: a meta-analysis of randomized controlled trials. *International Urogynecology Journal* 30: 1419–1427. https://doi.org/10.1007/s00192-019-03904-1.

Lilley, G., Burkett-St-Laurent, D., Precious, E. et al. (2015). Measurement of blood loss during postpartum haemorrhage. *International Journal of Obstetric Anesthesia* 24: 8–14.

Lindstrom, H., Kearney, L., Massey, D. et al. (2018). How midwives manage rapid pre-loading of fluid in women prior to low dose epidurals: a retrospective chart review. *Journal of Advanced Nursing* 74: 2588–2595. https://doi.org/10.1111/jan.13783.

Makrides, M., Crosby, D.D., Bain, E., and Crowther, C.A. (2014). Magnesium supplementation in pregnancy. *Cochrane Database of Systematic Reviews* 4: CD000937. https://doi.org/10.1002/14651858.CD000937.pub2.

Mathur, A., Johnston, G., and Clark, L. (2020). Improving intravenous fluid prescribing. *Journal of the Royal College of Physicians of Edinburgh* 50 (2): 181–187. https://doi.org/10.4997/JRCPE.2020.224.

Mendelson, C.L. (1946). The aspiration of stomach contents into the lungs during obstetric anaesthesia. *American Journal of Obstetrics and Gynecology* 52: 191–205.

Moen, V., Brudin, L., Rundgren, M., and Irestedt, L. (2009). Hyponatremia complicating labour – rare or unrecognised? A prospective observational study. *BJOG* 116 (4): 552–561. https://doi.org/10.1111/j.1471-0528.2008.02063.x.

Moini, J. (2016). *Anatomy and Physiology for Health Professionals*, 2e. Burlington, MA: Jones and Bartlett Learning.

Mol, B.W.J., Roberts, C.T., Thangaratinam, S. et al. (2016). Pre-eclampsia. *Lancet* 387 (10022): 999–1011. https://doi.org/10.1016/S0140-6736(15)00070-7.

National Institute for Health and Care Excellence (NICE) (2015a). Preterm labour and birth. NICE guideline NG25. https://www.nice.org.uk/guidance/ng25/chapter/Recommendations (accessed November 2023).

National Institute for Health and Care Excellence (NICE) (2015b). Diabetes in pregnancy: management from preconception to the postnatal period. NICE guideline NG3. https://www.nice.org.uk/guidance/ng3/chapter/Recommendations#intrapartum-care (accessed November 2023).

National Institute for Health and Care Excellence (NICE) (2017). Intravenous fluid therapy in adults in hospital. NICE guideline CG174. https://www.nice.org.uk/CG174 (accessed November 2023).

National Institute for Health and Care Excellence (NICE) (2019). Hypertension in pregnancy: diagnosis and management. NICE guideline NG133. https://www.nice.org.uk/guidance/ng133 (accessed November 2023).

National Institute for Health and Care Excellence (NICE) (2022). BNF treatment summaries: Magnesium imbalance. https://bnf.nice.org.uk/treatment-summaries/magnesium-imbalance (accessed November 2023).

National Institute for Health and Care Excellence (NICE) (2023). Intrapartum care. NICE guideline NG235. https://www.nice.org.uk/guidance/ng235 (accessed November 2023).

Nursing and Midwifery Council (NMC) (2015). The Code: professional standards of practice and behaviour for nurses, midwives and nursing associates. https://www.nmc.org.uk/globalassets/sitedocuments/nmc-publications/nmc-code.pdf (accessed November 2023).

Nursing and Midwifery Council (NMC) (2017). Practising as a midwife in the UK. https://www.nmc.org.uk/globalassets/sitedocuments/nmc-publications/practising-as-a-midwife-in-the-uk.pdf (accessed November 2023).

Nursing and Midwifery Council (NMC) (2019). Standards of proficiency for midwives. https://www.nmc.org.uk/globalassets/sitedocuments/standards/standards-of-proficiency-for-midwives.pdf (accessed November 2023).

Osol, G., Ko, N.L., and Mandalà, M. (2019). Plasticity of the maternal vasculature during pregnancy. *Annual Review of Physiology* 81: 89–111. https://doi.org/10.1146/annurev-physiol-020518-114435.

Perel, P., Roberts, I., and Ker, K. (2013). Colloids versus crystalloids for fluid resuscitation in critically ill patients. *Cochrane Database of Systematic Reviews* (2): CD000567. https://doi.org/10.1002/14651858.CD000567.pub6.

Poon, L.C., Shennan, A., Hyett, J.A. et al. (2019). The International Federation of Gynecology and Obstetrics (FIGO) initiative on pre-eclampsia: a pragmatic guide for first-trimester screening and prevention. *International Journal of Gynecology & Obstetrics* 145: 1–33. https://doi.org/10.1002/ijgo.12802.

Pretorius, T., van Rensburg, G., Dyer, R.A. et al. (2018). The influence of fluid management on outcomes in preeclampsia: a systematic review and meta-analysis. *International Journal of Obstetric Anesthesia* 34: 85–95.

Rankin, J. (2017). *Physiology in Childbearing with Anatomy and Related Biosciences*, 4e. Edinburgh: Elsevier.

Royal College of Obstetricians and Gynaecologists (RCOG) (2016). Prevention and management of postpartum haemorrhage. Green-top guideline no. 52. https://obgyn.onlinelibrary.wiley.com/doi/epdf/10.1111/1471-0528.14178 (accessed November 2023).

Schneider, S., Freerksen, N., Rohrig, S. et al. (2012). Gestational diabetes and preeclampsia—similar risk factor profiles? *Early Human Development* 88 (3): 179–184.

Scott, W.N. (2010). *Fluids and Electrolytes Made Incredibly Easy!* Philadelphia: Lippincott Williams & Wilkins.

Shier, D., Butler, J., and Lewis, R. (2016). *Holes Human Anatomy and Physiology*, 14e. New York: McGraw-Hill Education.

Siassakos, D., Bristowe, K., and Draycott, T. (2011). Clinical efficiency in a simulated emergency and relationship to team behaviours: a multisite cross-sectional study. *BJOG* 118: 596–607.

da Silva, W.A., Pinheiro, A.M., Lima, P.H., and Malbouisson, L.M.S. (2021). Renal and cardiovascular repercussions in preeclampsia and their impact on fluid management: a literature review. *Brazilian Journal of Anesthesiology* 71 (4): 421–428. https://doi.org/10.1016/j.bjane.2021.02.052.

Singata, M., Tranmer, J., and Gyte, M.L. (2013). Restricting oral fluid and food intake during labour. *Cochrane Database of Systematic Reviews* (8): CD003930. https://doi.org/10.1002/14651858.CD003930.pub3.

Sutton, C. and Mann, D. (2021). Physiology of pregnancy. In: *Anesthesia for Maternal-Fetal Surgery: Concepts and Clinical Practice* (ed. O. Olutoye), 1–16. Cambridge: Cambridge University Press https://doi.org/10.1017/9781108297899.002.

Thornton, C., Hennessy, A., von Dadelszen, P. et al. (2007). An international benchmarking collaboration: measuring outcomes for the hypertensive disorders of pregnancy. *Journal of Obstetrics and Gynaecology Canada* 29 (10): 794–800.

Vanputte, C., Regan, J., and Russo, A. (2013). *Seeley's Essential Anatomy and Physiology*, 8e. New York: McGraw-Hill.

World Health Organization (WHO) (2020). WHO recommendation on routes of oxytocin administration for the prevention of postpartum haemorrhage after vaginal birth. Geneva: World Health Organization. https://www.who.int/publications/i/item/9789240013926 (accessed November 2023).

Wu, P.Y., Udani, V., Chan, L. et al. (1983). Colloid osmotic pressure: variations in normal pregnancy. *Journal of Perinatal Medicine* 11 (4): 193–199. https://doi.org/10.1515/jpme.1983.11.4.193.

Wylie, B. and Bryce, H. (2016). *The Midwives' Guide to Key Medical Conditions*, 2e. Edinburgh: Elsevier.

Further Resources

SBAR communication tool: situation, background, assessment, recommendation. www.england.nhs.uk/wp-content/uploads/2021/03/qsir-sbar-communication-tool.pdf (accessed November 2023).

Visual Infusion Phlebitis score. www.vipscore.net (accessed November 2023).

Glossary

Term	Definition
Albumin	The main protein in human blood, important for regulating the osmotic pressure of blood
Aldosterone	A hormone released by adrenal glands, involved with blood pressure regulation through managing serum sodium and potassium levels
Angiotensin–renin system	A hormone system within the body that is essential for the regulation of blood pressure and fluid balance
Antidiuretic hormone (ADH)	Also known as vasopressin, a small peptide hormone that regulates the body's retention of water
Antidote	A medicine taken or given to counteract a particular poison or drug toxicity
Colloid osmotic pressure	Osmotic pressure exerted by plasma proteins, responsible for moving fluid into the blood and preventing excess fluid loss between blood capillaries and the interstitial fluid, therefore helping to maintain blood volume and blood pressure
Diabetic ketoacidosis (DKA)	A life-threatening complication of diabetes that results from increased levels of ketones in the blood
Electrolytes	Minerals that carry an electric charge, vital for many essential bodily processes
Homeostasis	An organism's process of maintaining a stable internal environment
Hydrostatic pressure	The force of the fluid volume against a membrane
Hypothalamus	A region of the forebrain that organises the autonomic nervous system and pituitary gland activity. It has an essential role in controlling body temperature, thirst, hunger and other homeostatic systems, and is involved in sleep and emotional activity
Interstitial spaces	The fluid-filled areas that surround the cells of a given tissue; also known as tissue space
Pituitary gland	A major gland of the endocrine system that secretes hormones that control the actions of other endocrine organs and various tissues around the body
Tachypnoea	Rapid breathing

CHAPTER 21

Mental Health and Well-being

Maria Noonan

Department of Nursing and Midwifery, University of Limerick, Ireland

AIM

This chapter aims to explore perinatal mental health and well-being, as well as risk factors for and consequences of mental health conditions for the woman, baby, partner and family.

LEARNING OUTCOMES

On completion of this chapter the reader will be able to:

- Explain the definition of perinatal mental health and describe the usual psychological transitions occurring during pregnancy and postnatally
- Discuss the psychosocial factors that may affect the woman's perinatal mental health
- Describe the impact that an experience of a perinatal mental health condition may have for everyone involved
- Outline the spectrum of perinatal mental health conditions

Test Your Prior Knowledge

1. Define perinatal mental health.
2. List five protective factors that may decrease a woman's risk of developing a mental health condition during pregnancy.
3. Discuss five strategies a woman may implement to optimise her perinatal mental well-being.
4. Describe the impact of poor perinatal mental health for the woman and family unit.

Perinatal mental health refers to the mental health of women during pregnancy and up to one year after birth. Transitioning to parenthood involves major changes in the psychological, social and biological domains, which vary widely across time and from woman to woman (Felder et al. 2014) and can be particularly complex and challenging for women susceptible to severe mental illness (Jones et al. 2014). One in five women may experience a range of perinatal mental health conditions that affect her mood, thinking and behaviour. Mental health conditions, most commonly mood and anxiety disorders, may occur for the first time during the perinatal period or be a continuation or relapse of a pre-existing illness.

Usual Perinatal Emotional/Psychological Transitions

It is important that midwives are aware of the usual psychological transitions to avoid pathologising these emotions, which may result in over-referral to resource-dependent services. In addition, midwives have a role in supporting women to navigate typical psychological transitions and to recognise when their symptoms are not normal. Psychological transitions are influenced by changes in hormones, adjustments to this major life event and available supports.

In the first trimester of pregnancy, a woman may experience mixed feelings ranging from happiness and excitement to ambivalence or transient feelings of anxiety and fear about the pregnancy. They may worry about their new role of becoming a mother/parent, changes in relationships, work, finances and problems with the pregnancy or baby. These emotional transitions are accompanied by physical symptoms including fatigue, difficulty sleeping and changes in libido.

The second trimester brings an improvement in physical symptoms for many women, who begin to experience increased energy levels accompanied by feelings of relief and increased attachment to the fetus. The last trimester is characterised by feelings of anticipation and worry about their baby's health and the birth of the baby.

During the postnatal period the woman recovers from childbirth and adjusts to parenthood, renegotiating roles at work and friendship and intimate partner relationships (Felder et al. 2014). Women may experience mood changes in the first three to five days after the birth, known as 'postnatal blues' or 'the baby blues'. Research suggests that 50–80% of women experience this normal transitory adjustment state (Raynor and Oates 2014), which may last up to two weeks. During this time the woman may experience a range of emotions such as sadness, tearfulness, despair, irritability, isolation, vulnerability, loneliness, euphoria and laughter, commonly referred to a 'rollercoaster of emotions' (Felder et al. 2014). The exact cause is not known, however hormonal changes (e.g. alteration in oestrogen, progesterone and prolactin) and lack of sleep have been implicated in the cause of baby blues. This is self-limiting and resolves spontaneously with support from healthcare professionals, partner, family and friends.

Maintaining Mental Health and Well-being

Through the provision of supportive and holistic care, midwives have a role in optimising perinatal mental health and supporting women to adjust to the psychological changes of pregnancy and parenthood. Midwives can incorporate perinatal mental well-being conversations with the woman at booking and at each perinatal encounter and involve her significant other(s). It may be appropriate to sensitively explore the woman's feelings about the pregnancy, previous birth experiences and current sources of stress for her and her family (Glover 2020).

The midwife can work with parents to identify potential suggestions that optimise mental health and well-being, including the importance of eating a well-balanced diet (Li et al. 2017; Sparling et al. 2017). The woman is encouraged to engage in regular physical activity, which releases feel-good endorphins and distracts the woman from a cycle of negative thoughts that may lead to depression and anxiety. Other suggestions include the importance of adequate sleep, talking to and seeking out help from partner, family, friends or other pregnant couples (American College of Obstetricians and Gynecologists [ACOG] 2022) and practising meditation and mindfulness (Yan et al. 2022) The development of a well-being plan is endorsed by the National Institute for Health and Care Excellence (NICE 2014) and helps parents to start thinking about how they may feel emotionally and what support they might need in the perinatal period.

Health Promotion

A well-being plan template can be downloaded from the charity Tommy's website, http://www.tommys.org/pregnancy-information/health-professionals/free-pregnancy-resources/wellbeing-plan.

Teaching women techniques like breathing exercises and hypnobirthing may support relaxation. Other strategies include attuning to fetal movements, music and the use of complementary therapies. The midwife can encourage expectant parents to build a support network to connect with other parents to prevent feelings of isolation.

However, the unique physiological, psychological and social changes that occur can reveal a biological vulnerability to a changed mental state (Anderson 2022) and approximately 20% of women will experience a perinatal mental health condition. The causes and risk factors associated with poor perinatal mental health will be explored next.

Causes of Perinatal Mental Health Conditions

The causes of poor perinatal mental health are diverse, multifactorial and specific to the perinatal mental health condition (Ayers et al. 2016). An integrated model of risk and protective factors may best explain the complex interplay of psychological, biological and psychosocial processes that increase the woman's risk of experiencing a perinatal mental health condition (Felder et al. 2014).

Learning Event

Take some time to think about and list the psychosocial risk factors that may increase the woman's or partner's chances of experiencing poor perinatal mental health.

Risk Factors

A knowledge of risk factors for perinatal mental health conditions may raise awareness of individuals requiring additional perinatal mental health support. The presence of some risk factors will require referral to the specialist perinatal mental health services (SPMHS); for example, women with a history of bipolar disorder, schizophrenia, psychosis or severe depression are at increased risk of severe postpartum episodes. Of women with pre-existing bipolar disorder, 20% experience a severe postnatal episode (i.e. psychosis, mania and/or hospitalisation) and relapse rates are significantly higher among those who are not on antenatal pharmacological treatment (Wesseloo et al. 2016). In addition, women with a family history of a first-degree relative with bipolar disorder or puerperal psychosis have an increased risk of developing a postpartum psychosis episode.

It is estimated that approximately 10–20% of pregnant women with a history of depression may experience a relapse of their depression (Stevens et al. 2019). Furthermore, an experience of antenatal depression increases women's risk of postnatal depression (Felder et al. 2014). Women with personality disorder, obsessive-compulsive disorder (OCD), post-traumatic stress disorder (PTSD) and birth trauma will also be offered referral to the SPMHS.

The primary risk factor for perinatal mental health conditions is a history of experiencing a mental health condition. However, women with other psychosocial risk factors may require additional support for their perinatal mental health needs, including referral to the SPMHS.

Orange Flag

Women are at increased risk of perinatal anxiety and depression (Howard et al. 2014) if they have:

- A history of adverse childhood experiences.
- Perceived poor quality of their relationship with their mother in childhood.
- Recent stressful events, such as a death in the family or a relationship ending.
- Current interpersonal stress, including high life stress.
- Poor partner relationships, including intimate partner violence (IPV) (Yang et al. 2022).
- Lack of family and social support that leads to isolation and loneliness.

Language and cultural barriers may exacerbate social isolation experienced by women of migrant background (Fellmeth et al. 2017; COPE 2017).

Perinatal substance use may lead to poor perinatal mental health or be taken to reduce negative affective states, including anxiety and depression. Substance use is known to increase the risk of perinatal suicide (Knight et al. 2021).

Personality styles such as neuroticism (a general tendency towards negative emotions), vulnerable personality styles and trait anxiety have been found to be associated with postpartum depression (PPD) (Puyané et al. 2022). Furthermore, perinatal depression and anxiety are significantly associated with perfectionism (Evans et al. 2022).

Persons who identify as lesbian, gay, bisexual, transgender, queer, questioning or intersex (LGBTQI*) are more likely to experience mental health conditions (Steele et al. 2008). Psychosis and suicidal thoughts are more common in ethnic minorities communities (Knight et al. 2021).

Age has been identified as a potential risk factor in some studies. Adolescents (Siegel and Brandon 2014) and young women (15–25 years) (Estrin et al. 2019) are more likely to be single, experience an unplanned pregnancy, IPV, isolation and insecure employment, and are at increased risk of poor mental health. Perinatal suicide is 11/100 000 among teenagers (Knight et al. 2021).

Obstetric complications such as gestational diabetes (Arafa and Dong 2019), preterm birth (de Paula Eduardo et al. 2019) and pre-eclampsia (Caropreso et al. 2019) increase the risk of PPD. Pre-eclampsia and diabetes are associated with obstetric complications that have been linked to a higher risk of PPD. Furthermore, pre-eclampsia may lead to the woman experiencing psychological symptoms such as increased worry, grief, acute stress and symptoms of trauma, which may increase vulnerability to PPD and anxiety (Caropreso et al. 2019). An experience of perinatal bereavement through miscarriage, stillbirth, neonatal death or the child being taken into care increases vulnerability to mental illness. Women who have experienced an infertility journey are at increased risk of perinatal anxiety and depression.

Orange Flag

Other risk factors include lower educational attainment, unplanned/unwanted pregnancy, termination of pregnancy, low self-esteem, migrant status (including refugees, asylum seekers), women from ethnic minority groups, women detainees, women with poor sleep patterns that may influence emotional regulation and those who experience poor socioeconomic circumstances.

Source: Adapted from Yang et al. (2022).

Maternal depression, marital and parental distress, gender role stress, IPV, and mismatched expectations of pregnancy and childbirth are risk factors that may affect a partners' perinatal mental health (Chhabra et al. 2020).

Evidence suggests that factors such as the quality of fetal and infant attachment, maternal care giving, sensitive mothering, quality parenting, partner support and emotional, social, practical and financial support can moderate the effects of perinatal stress (Howard and Khalifeh 2020).

Risk factors for poor perinatal mental health are not static and a woman's mental health state may change. The perinatal period is associated with significant life changes that may lead to anxiety and chronic stressors, such as changes in the dynamics of partner and family relationships and financial changes (Raynor and Oates 2014). Women with multiple vulnerabilities require additional support. However, women with no apparent risk factors or triggers can still develop perinatal mental health conditions. Therefore, it is important essential that midwives enquire about the woman and her partner's mental health and well-being throughout the perinatal period. Furthermore, it is important that information is provided to women and their significant other that the presence of psychosocial risk factors may increase the woman's likelihood of experiencing a perinatal mental health condition (Centre of Perinatal Excellence [COPE] 2017) so that they can identify preventative support (protective factors) and seek early additional support and interventions when required (COPE 2017).

Symptoms of Perinatal Mental Health Conditions

Symptoms will depend on the specific perinatal mental health condition and a symptom or behaviour is not an automatic sign of mental or psychological distress, as women may experience these symptoms naturally in a variety of situations (Anderson 2022). Diagnosis is made based on significant impairment in personal, family, social, educational and occupational behaviour and in function (Anderson 2022). Symptoms do not differ significantly from the symptoms of mental health conditions that occur at any other time in the woman's life, but the content of the symptoms may be focused on the pregnancy or the newborn, such as anxiety or negative thoughts about the pregnancy or the baby (Anderson 2022). Women may be unaware of the significance of the symptoms they are experiencing, and it is important to consult with and listen to partners, family or close friends who may notice and report significant change in the woman's baseline behaviour because of a change in mental state or report that the woman is acting out of character. Symptoms are explored under each perinatal mental health condition.

Red Flag

The following symptoms require immediate referral to the SPMHS:

- Recent significant changes in mental state or emergence of new symptoms.
- Women presenting with uncharacteristic symptoms and marked changes to normal functioning, including confusion, general perplexity or unusual or overvalued ideas (ideas that seem out of context or extreme).
- New thoughts or acts of violent self-harm (suicidal ideas, intent or actions).
- Violence and aggression set in the context of psychosis.
- Specific items such as command hallucinations, delusional misidentification and grandiose delusions.
- Increased substance use.
- New and persistent expressions of incompetence as a mother or estrangement from the infant.

Source: Adapted from Gloucestershire Health & Care NHS Foundation Trust (n.d.); Anderson (2022); Knight et al. (2021).

Consequences of Poor Perinatal Mental Health

Perinatal mental health conditions are associated with a myriad of adverse effects on maternal and immediate family outcomes. Adverse outcomes depend on timing and severity of symptoms and on the specific type of mental health condition (Stein et al. 2014). In addition, given the high level of co-morbidity between perinatal depression and anxiety, researchers have been challenged to separate the differential effects of one versus the other on children (Anderson 2022). Biologically mediated effects of antenatal mental health conditions (through in utero effects) are specific to mothers, whereas genetic and postnatal effects may occur if either parent is affected by a mental health condition (Glover 2015).

The levels of psychological distress associated with perinatal mental health conditions may influence the development of depression, anxiety, conduct disorders and emotional dysregulation in offspring, which may persist through adolescence into early adulthood (Madigan et al. 2018). Mechanisms whereby perinatal mental health conditions adversely affect fetal, infant and child health outcomes are complex, not completely understood and likely include direct disease effects such as alterations to the intrauterine environment (elevated cortisol, decreased dopamine and serotonin), behavioural factors and co-morbidities (Glover 2015; Glover et al. 2018).

An association between new and recurrent antenatal depression and anxiety and adverse birth outcomes such as an increased risk for preterm birth (PTB) and for low birth weight (LBW) has been identified (Grote et al. 2010). Several explanations for this finding have been postulated, including elevated maternal cortisol levels that are linked to restricted fetal growth, LBW and PTB, and decreased attendance for perinatal care and practising of recommended health behaviours during pregnancy (Grote et al. 2010).

Women with poor perinatal mental health are at a higher risk of perinatal and infant mortality including stillbirth, although the mechanisms are unclear (Adane et al. 2021). Behavioural factors and unhealthy lifestyles are correlated with perinatal mental health conditions for some women and include poor help-seeking behaviour, late and less frequent attendance for antenatal care and increased exposure to environmental factors associated with adversity, including smoking, alcohol, substance use, poverty and poor nutrition, which are all common risk factors for perinatal morbidity and mortality (Adane et al. 2021). Prenatal mental health conditions may continue postnatally and compromise the quality of parenting, which may contribute to an increased infant mortality risk.

There is some evidence that physical symptoms of life-threatening complications are attributed to mental health conditions in women (Howard and Khalifeh 2020). Suicide remains a leading cause of maternal death (2.64/100 000 births) (Knight et al. 2021) and is particularly related to perinatal depression. It is most likely to occur in the second half of the first postpartum year when women are not receiving treatment or in contact with perinatal services (Howard and Khalifeh 2020). Women from lower socioeconomic groups and those who experience IPV, use substances and are known to social services are at higher risk of suicide (Knight et al. 2021). Infanticide is a rare outcome of severe perinatal mental health conditions.

The link between perinatal mental health conditions and adverse maternal and child outcomes are correlational, do not prove cause-and-effect relationships and acknowledge that other explanatory confounding factors may exist in these relationships, such as placental functioning, environmental toxins, socioeconomic status and effects of programming (Howard and Khalifeh 2020). Collectively, a knowledge of the consequences of experiencing a perinatal mental health condition for parents underscores the need for comprehensive perinatal awareness campaigns, screening to identify women and partners who require additional support, and appropriate referral to SPMHS to ensure early access to evidence-based treatment interventions for women and their partners who experience poor mental health (Felder et al. 2014).

Learning Event

Read Sanah Ahsan's article in the *Guardian*, 'I'm a psychologist – and I believe we've been told devastating lies about mental health' and think about the link between perinatal mental health and social conditions.
https://www.theguardian.com/commentisfree/2022/sep/06/psychologist-devastating-lies-mental-health-problems-politics

Diagnosing a Mental Health Condition

A midwife who identifies parents with risk factors or current symptoms of perinatal mental ill health will refer the woman ideally to a psychiatrist specialising in perinatal mental health, who will make a diagnosis based on a variety of information sources including structured clinical interviews, screening tools, psychological assessments, laboratory tests and

TABLE 21.1   Two systems for diagnosing mental health conditions.

Diagnostic and Statistical Manual of Mental Disorders, fifth edition (DSM-5)	International Classification of Diseases, 11th Revision (ICD-11)
A reference handbook published by the American Psychiatric Association (APA) to guide mental health clinicians to diagnose, classify and identify mental health conditions	A global categorisation of physical and mental illnesses published by the World Health Organization (WHO)
Focused on North America and primarily used in the United States	Used internationally

physical exams. This information will be utilised to make a diagnosis based on diagnostic criteria and those from the *Statistical Manual of Mental Disorders*, fifth edition (DSM-5) or the *International Classification of Diseases*, 11th Revision (ICD-11). Before treatment, medical causes of symptoms (e.g. hypothyroidism may cause depression symptoms) must be excluded. See Table 21.1 for information on diagnostic systems used to categorise specific perinatal mental health conditions.

Perinatal Mental Health Conditions

Some common mental health conditions that women may experience in the perinatal period are now explored.

Perinatal Depression

Perinatal depression is a mood disorder and Gavin et al. (2005) estimated point prevalence rates for depression to be 11% in the first trimester, 9% in the remaining trimesters and 19% in the first three months postpartum. The prevalence of paternal perinatal depression is approximately 10% (Paulson and Bazemore 2010) and 3.18% of couples may concurrently experience perinatal depression (Smythe et al. 2022).

Learning Event

Check out this video: https://youtu.be/IyHDoEL59ho.
After you've watched it, list the signs of perinatal depression.

Screening

International guidelines recommend screening for perinatal depression (O'Connor et al. 2016; NICE 2014; WHO 2015). Table 21.2 highlights recommendations for screening for perinatal depression.

Learning Event

Investigate the EPDS: https://perinatology.com/calculators/Edinburgh%20Depression%20Scale.htm.

Treatment of Perinatal Depression

Treatment needs to be tailored to women with different types and severity of perinatal depression (Putnam et al. 2017).

TABLE 21.2 Recommendations for screening for perinatal depression.

Questions to ask at the booking visit and during the early postnatal period	If a woman responds positively to either of the depression identification questions, is at risk of developing a mental health problem or there is clinical concern
During the past month, have you often been bothered by feeling down, depressed or hopeless?	Use the appropriately translated version of the Edinburgh Postnatal Depression Scale (EPDS) or the Patient Health Questionnaire (PHQ-9) with culturally relevant cut-off scores as part of a full assessment
During the past month, have you often been bothered by having little interest or pleasure in doing things?	*or* Refer the woman to her GP or, if a severe mental health problem is suspected, to a mental health professional for a diagnostic mental health assessment

Source: Adapted from NICE (2014).

Pharmacological and Non-pharmacological Treatment

Treatment options for perinatal depression include pharmacological – selective serotonin reuptake inhibitors (SSRIs), tricyclic anti-depressants (TCAs); psychological – cognitive behavioural therapy (CBT), interpersonal therapy (IPT); mindfulness-based interventions (MBI), facilitated self-help, parenting interventions and behavioural interventions (nutrition, exercise).

Source: Adapted from NICE (2014); Adina et al. (2022).

Perinatal Anxiety

It is usual for women to have concerns about various aspects of pregnancy and a certain level of stress and anxiety is thought to be protective, as women are more likely to engage in health-promoting behaviours. However, when anxiety interrupts thoughts and interferes with everyday life, including the person's ability to function, relationships or employment, it is classified as an anxiety disorder (Anderson 2022). Reviews report prevalence rates of 15–20% for antenatal anxiety and 10% for postnatal anxiety (Dennis et al. 2017). In addition, women may experience co-morbid anxiety and depression (Ayers et al. 2015). Diagnostic categories for anxiety include generalised anxiety disorder, panic disorder, specific phobia (e.g. needles), pregnancy-specific anxiety (e.g. fear of childbirth), social anxiety disorder, substance/medication-induced anxiety disorder and obsessive compulsive disorder (Ayers et al. 2014).

Learning Event

Listen to Professor Agnes Higgins discuss perinatal anxiety: https://youtu.be/8MYGCuSTYco.
After you've watched the video, list the signs of perinatal anxiety.

Screening
NICE (2014) guidelines recommend inquiring about anxiety using the two-item Generalized Anxiety Disorder scale (GAD-2) at a woman's booking visit and during the early postnatal period (see Table 21.3). Ayers et al. (2014) recommend repeating screening to avoid over-pathologising transient distress.

Treatment of Perinatal Anxiety
Management of perinatal anxiety is tailored to the individual woman's needs and may involve a combination of psychosocial interventions (non-directive counselling, psychoeducation, support groups), psychological therapy (e.g. CBT) (Li et al. 2022) and pharmacological treatment (SSRIs, TCAs).

TABLE 21.3   Recommendations for screening for perinatal anxiety: the Generalized Anxiety Disorder scale (GAD-2).

Questions to ask	Question to ask if a woman scores less than 3 on the GAD-2 scale, but you are still concerned she may have an anxiety disorder
Over the last two weeks, how often have you been bothered by feeling nervous, anxious or on edge? Over the last two weeks, how often have you been bothered by not being able to stop or control worrying?	Do you find yourself avoiding places or activities and does this cause you problems?
Scoring	**Action to take**
An answer of 'not at all' scores 0; 'several days' scores 1; 'more than half the days' scores 2; 'nearly every day' scores 3	If the woman responds positively, consider using the GAD-7 scale for further assessment or referring the woman to her GP or, if a severe mental health problem is suspected, to a mental health professional

Source: Adapted from NICE (2014).

Medicines Management: SSRIs for Perinatal Depression and Anxiety

Low serotonin system activity has been linked to the development of depression and anxiety. Therefore, SSRIs, which regulate serotonin levels in the brain and help elevate mood, are identified as a pharmacological treatment intervention for perinatal mood and anxiety disorders (NICE 2014). SSRIs are associated with a risk of persistent pulmonary hypertension in the newborn and transient self-limiting neonatal withdrawal (NICE 2014). Data from observational studies suggest that the use of SSRIs during the month before birth may result in a small increased risk of postpartum haemorrhage due to the serotonergic effect impairing platelet aggregation (Jiang et al. 2016).

Perinatal Post-Traumatic Stress Disorder

Yildiz et al. (2017) found a 3.35% prevalence rate of post-traumatic stress disorder (PTSD) in pregnancy in community samples and 18.95% in high-risk samples. PTSD in pregnancy may develop in response to a traumatic pregnancy experience (e.g. diagnosis of fetal anomaly, pregnancy complication) or other traumatic events such as accidents, interpersonal violence or a history of adverse childhood experiences (Yildiz et al. 2017). Women may also experience birth-related PTSD (Case Study 21.1).

Case Study 21.1

Thirty-year-old Salem gave birth to her first baby by an emergency caesarean section undertaken for shoulder dystocia. At her six-week GP postnatal check-up, Salem discloses that she is experiencing intrusive symptoms associated with her birth, including re-experiencing the traumatic birth through nightmares, intrusive thoughts and flashbacks; persistent avoidance of reminders of the event (e.g. visits to hospital); numbing of general responsiveness; as well as increased arousal such as hypervigilance, irritability, difficulty concentrating and negative alterations in cognitions and mood.

Salem's GP referred her to the SPMHS, where the psychiatrist conducted a clinical interview that is recognised as the gold standard for identifying PTSD. Salem was also requested to complete the City Birth Trauma Scale (City BiTS), a self-report questionnaire specifically assessing PTSD following childbirth symptoms in postpartum women according to the DSM-5 (Ayers et al. 2018).

Salem was diagnosed with birth-related PTSD, which is defined as 'A woman's experience of interactions and/or events directly related to childbirth that caused overwhelming distressing emotions and reactions; leading to short and/or long-term negative impacts on a woman's health and wellbeing' (Leinweber et al. 2022, p. 1). Approximately 3–5% of women meet the diagnostic criteria for birth-related PTSD and 12.3% of mothers experience birth-related post-traumatic stress symptoms (Heyne et al. 2022). The DSM-5 outlines the specific requirements that must be met for a diagnosis of birth-related PTSD (Heyne et al. 2022).

Salem was referred to the perinatal psychologist for focused CBT and eye movement desensitisation and reprocessing (EMDR) therapy (NICE 2014).

Postpartum Psychosis

Postpartum psychosis (PP; also known as puerperal psychosis or postnatal psychosis) is a rare acute mood disorder that affects one to two of every 1000 women after birth and occurs when a person loses touch with reality and may start to see, hear and/or believe things that are not true (VanderKruik et al. 2017). It is a psychiatric emergency and in rare cases the illness can result in suicide and, infrequently, infanticide (Jones et al. 2014)

Symptoms usually start suddenly within the first 14 days after birth – sometimes within hours, or between days 1 and 3 of giving birth (Heron et al. 2008), and more rarely several weeks after childbirth. The most severe symptoms tend to last 2–12 weeks and recovery can take between 6 and 12 months or more (Jones et al. 2014) (see Table 21.4). Differential diagnosis for other cerebral or systemic conditions (sepsis, eclampsia, delirium, thyroid disorders) causing psychosis is important, as misattribution of symptoms to psychiatric disorders has led to several deaths in new mothers (Jones et al. 2014).

Treatment of Postpartum Psychosis

PP can be an overwhelming and frightening experience for the woman, her partner and the family. The midwife should stay with the woman and make an urgent referral to the SPMHS (Oates 2014). The woman will usually require admission ideally to a mother and baby unit (MBU), where she will receive pharmacological and psychological (CBT) treatment interventions (Tinkelman et al. 2017).

Pre-conceptual Care

For some women the episode of psychosis is an isolated, one-off occurrence. However, there is a 50% risk of a reoccurrence, and some women may be diagnosed with bipolar disorder (Oates 2014). Pre-conceptual care will include conversations around the risk of recurrence of PP. Women pregnant with a history of PP will be referred to the SPMHS during pregnancy and an integrated care plan developed through a coordinated team approach. A pre-birth planning meeting is scheduled for around 32 weeks of pregnancy with the multidisciplinary team involved in the woman's perinatal care and with the woman and her family or carer.

TABLE 21.4 **Symptoms of postpartum psychosis.**

Intense shifts in moods that can quickly go from depression to elation
Intense confusion and disorientation
Intrusive thoughts about the baby's safety
Hallucinations

Conditions Associated with Perinatal Mental Health

The following is a list of perinatal mental health conditions. Take some time and write notes about each of the conditions. Think about interventions that may be used to treat them. Remember to include aspects of care. If you are making notes about people you have offered care and support to, you must ensure that you have adhered to the rules of confidentiality.

The condition	Your notes
Perinatal depression	
Perinatal anxiety	
Psychosis	
Post-traumatic stress disorder	
Others	

Take-Home Points

- Midwives require knowledge of the usual perinatal psychological adjustments that women may experience.
- Midwives can support awareness of perinatal mental health and provide information to women on strategies they can use to promote optimal perinatal mental well-being.
- It is important that midwives know the risks and protective factors for poor perinatal mental health, which supports recognition of women requiring additional support.
- Midwives need to be aware of the potential impact poor perinatal mental has for the woman and her immediate family.
- Knowing the spectrum of mental health conditions that women may experience supports the midwife to identify risk factors and symptoms of specific conditions.

Conclusion

During the perinatal period, which spans pregnancy through to the first year after the birth of the baby, some women will experience poor mental health that may have consequences for them and their immediate family. Midwives have an important role in promoting emotional and mental well-being, identifying risk factors and current symptoms that may indicate that the woman requires additional support with her mental health and linking women to early support and evidence-based interventions.

References

Adane, A.A., Bailey, H.D., Morgan, V.A. et al. (2021). The impact of maternal prenatal mental health disorders on stillbirth and infant mortality: a systematic review and meta-analysis. *Archives of Women's Mental Health* 24 (4): 543–555.

Adina, J., Morawska, A., Mitchell, A.E., and McBryde, M. (2022). Effect of parenting interventions on perinatal depression and implications for infant developmental outcomes: a systematic review and meta-analysis. *Clinical Child and Family Psychology Review* 25 (2): 316–338. https://doi-org.proxy.lib.ul.ie/10.1007/s10567-021-00371-3.

American College of Obstetricians and Gynecologists (ACOG) (2022). Anxiety and pregnancy. https://www.acog.org/womens-health/faqs/anxiety-and-pregnancy (accessed November 2023).

Anderson, M. (2022). *Midwifery Essentials: Perinatal Mental Health*, vol. 9. London: Elsevier Health Sciences.

Arafa, A. and Dong, J.-Y. (2019). Gestational diabetes and risk of postpartum depressive symptoms: a meta-analysis of cohort studies. *Journal of Affective Disorders* 253: 312–316. https://doi.org/10.1016/j.jad.2019.05.001.

Ayers, S., Baum, A., McManus, C. et al. (2014). *Cambridge Handbook of Psychology, Health and Medicine*, 2e. Cambridge: Cambridge University Press.

Ayers, S., Bond, R., Bertullies, S., and Wijma, K. (2016). The aetiology of posttraumatic stress following childbirth: a meta-analysis and theoretical framework. *Psychological Medicine* 46 (6): 1121–1134. https://doi.org/10.1017/S0033291715002706.

Ayers, S., Wright, D.B., and Thornton, A. (2018). Development of a measure of postpartum PTSD: the city birth trauma scale. *Frontiers in Psychiatry* 9: 409.

Caropreso, L., de Azevedo Cardoso, T., Eltayebani, M., and Frey, B.N. (2019). Preeclampsia as a risk factor for postpartum depression and psychosis: a systematic review and meta-analysis. *Archives of Women's Mental Health* 23 (4): 493–505. https://doi.org/10.1007/s00737-019-01010-1.

Centre of Perinatal Excellence (COPE) (2017). Effective mental health care in the perinatal period: Australian COPE clinical practice guideline. https://cope.org.au/wp-content/uploads/2017/10/Final-COPE-Perinatal-Mental-Health-Guideline.pdf (accessed November 2023).

Chhabra, J., McDermott, B., and Li, W. (2020). Risk factors for paternal perinatal depression and anxiety: a systematic review and meta-analysis. *Psychology of Men & Masculinity* 21 (4): 593–611. https://doi.org/10.1037/men0000259.

Dennis, C.L., Falah-Hassani, K., and Shiri, R. (2017). Prevalence of antenatal and postnatal anxiety: systematic review and meta-analysis. *British Journal of Psychiatry* 210: 315–323. https://doi.org/10.1192/bjp.bp.116.187179.

Estrin, G.L., Ryan, E.G., Trevillion, K. et al. (2019). Young pregnant women and risk for mental disorders: findings from an early pregnancy cohort. *British Journal of Psychiatry Open* 5: e21.

Evans, C., Kreppner, J., and Lawrence, P.J. (2022). The association between maternal perinatal mental health and perfectionism: a systematic review and meta-analysis. *British Journal of Clinical Psychology* 61 (4): 1052–1074. https://doi-org.proxy.lib.ul.ie/10.1111/bjc.12378.

Felder, J.N., Abigail, M., Lindemann, A.M., and Dimidjian, S. (2014). Perinatal depression. In: *The Oxford Handbook of Depression and Comorbidity* (ed. C.S. Richards and M.W. O'Hara), 476–492. New York: Oxford University Press.

Fellmeth, G., Fazel, M., and Plugge, E. (2017). Migration and perinatal mental health in women from low- and middle-income countries: a systematic review and meta-analysis. *BJOG: An International Journal of Obstetrics and Gynaecology* 124 (5): 742–752. https://doi.org/10.1111/1471-0528.14184.

Gavin, N.I., Gaynes, B.N., Lohr, K.N. et al. (2005). Perinatal depression: a systematic review of prevalence and incidence. *Obstetrics and Gynecology* 106 (5 Pt 1): 1071–1083. https://doi.org/10.1097/01.AOG.0000183597.31630.db.

Gloucestershire Health & Care NHS Foundation Trust (n.d.). Perinatal red flags and risk indicators. https://ghc.nhs.uk/wp-content/uploads/Perinatal-red-flags-and-risk-indicators.pdf (accessed November 2023).

Glover, V. (2015). Prenatal stress and its effects on the fetus and the child: possible underlying biological mechanisms. *Advances in Neurobiology* 10: 269–83.

Glover, V. (2020). Prenatal mental health and the effects of stress on the foetus and the child. Should psychiatrists look beyond mental disorders? *World Psychiatry* 19 (3): 331–332. https://doi.org/10.1002/wps.20777.

Glover, V., O'Donnell, K.J., O'Connor, T.G., and Fisher, J. (2018). Prenatal maternal stress, fetal programming, and mechanisms underlying later psychopathology—A global perspective. *Development and psychopathology* 30 (3): 843–854. https://doi.org/10.1017/S095457941800038X.

Grote, N.K., Bridge, J.A., Gavin, A.R. et al. (2010). A meta-analysis of depression during pregnancy and the risk of preterm birth, low birth weight, and intrauterine growth restriction. *Archives of General Psychiatry* 67 (10): 1012–1024. https://doi.org/10.1001/archgenpsychiatry.2010.111.

Heron, J., McGuinness, M., Blackmore, E.R. et al. (2008). Early postpartum symptoms in puerperal psychosis. *BJOG* 115: 348–353.

Heyne, C.-S., Kazmierczak, M., Souday, R. et al. (2022). Prevalence and risk factors of birth-related posttraumatic stress among parents: a comparative systematic review and meta-analysis. *Clinical Psychology Review* 94: 102157–102157. https://doi.org/10.1016/j.cpr.2022.102157.

Howard, L.M. and Khalifeh, H. (2020). Perinatal mental health: a review of progress and challenges. *World Psychiatry* 19: 313–327.

Howard, L.M., Molyneaux, E., Dennis, C.L. et al. (2014). Non-psychotic mental disorders in the perinatal period. *Lancet* 384 (9956): 1775–1788.

Jiang, H., Xu, L., Li, Y. et al. (2016). Antidepressant use during pregnancy and risk of postpartum hemorrhage: A systematic review and meta-analysis. *Journal of Psychiatric Research* 83: 160–167. https://doi.org/10.1016/j.jpsychires.2016.09.001.

Jones, I., Chandra, P.S., Dazzan, P., and Howard, L.M. (2014). Bipolar disorder, affective psychosis, and schizophrenia in pregnancy and the post-partum period. *Lancet* 384 (9956): 1789–1799. https://doi.org/10.1016/S0140-6736(14)61278-2.

Knight, M., Bunch, K., Tuffnell, D. et al. (eds) (2021). Saving lives, improving mothers' care: lessons learned to inform maternity care from the UK and Ireland confidential enquiries into maternal deaths and morbidity 2017–19. MBRRACE-UK. https://www.npeu.ox.ac.uk/assets/downloads/mbrrace-uk/reports/maternal-report-2021/MBRRACE-UK_Maternal_Report_2021_-_FINAL_-_WEB_VERSION.pdf (accessed November 2023).

Leinweber, J., Fontein-Kuipers, Y., Thomson, G. et al. (2022). Developing a woman-centred, inclusive definition of traumatic childbirth experiences–a discussion paper. *Birth* 49 (4): 687–696. https://doi.org/10.1111/birt.12634.

Li, Y., Lv, M.-R., Wei, Y.-J. et al. (2017). Dietary patterns and depression risk: a meta-analysis. *Psychiatry Research* 253: 373–382. https://doi.org/10.1016/j.psychres.2017.04.020.

Li, X., Laplante, D.P., Paquin, V. et al. (2022). Effectiveness of cognitive behavioral therapy for perinatal maternal depression, anxiety and stress: a systematic review and meta-analysis of randomized controlled trials. *Clinical Psychology Review* 92: 102129. https://doi-org.proxy.lib.ul.ie/10.1016/j.cpr.2022.102129.

Madigan, S., Oatley, H., Racine, N. et al. (2018). A meta-analysis of maternal prenatal depression and anxiety on child socioemotional development. *Journal of the American Academy of Child and Adolescent Psychiatry* 57 (9): 645–657.e8. https://doi.org/10.1016/j.jaac.2018.06.012.

National Institute for Health and Care Excellence (NICE) (2014). Antenatal and postnatal mental health: clinical management and service guidance. Clinical guideline CG192. https://www.nice.org.uk/guidance/CG192 (accessed November 2023).

Oates, M.R. (2014). Perinatal psychiatric conditions. In: *Myles Textbook for Midwives*, 16e (ed. J. Marshall and M. Raynor), 531–553. Edinburgh: Churchill Livingstone.

O'Connor, E., Rossom, R.C., Henninger, M. et al. (2016). Primary care screening for and treatment of depression in pregnant and postpartum women: evidence report and systematic review for the US Preventive Services Task Force. *JAMA* 315: 388–406.

de Paula Eduardo, J.A.F., de Rezende, M.G., Menezes, P.R., and Del-Ben, C.M. (2019). Preterm birth as a risk factor for postpartum depression: a systematic review and meta-analysis. *Journal of Affective Disorders* 259: 392–403. https://doi.org/10.1016/j.jad.2019.08.069.

Paulson, J.F. and Bazemore, S.D. (2010). Prenatal and postpartum depression in fathers and its association with maternal depression: a meta-analysis. *JAMA* 303 (19): 1961–1969.

Putnam, K.T., Wilcox, M., Robertson-Blackmore, E. et al. (2017). Clinical phenotypes of perinatal depression and time of symptom onset: analysis of data from an international consortium. *Lancet Psychiatry* 4 (6): 477–485. https://doi.org/10.1016/S2215-0366(17)30136-0.

Puyané, M., Subirà, S., Torres, A. et al. (2022). Personality traits as a risk factor for postpartum depression: a systematic review and meta-analysis. *Journal of Affective Disorders* 298 (Part A): 577–589. https://doi-org.proxy.lib.ul.ie/10.1016/j.jad.2021.11.010.

Raynor, M.D. and Oates, M.R. (2014). Perinatal mental health. In: *Myles Textbook for Midwives*, 16e (ed. J. Marshall and M. Raynor), 531–553. Edinburgh: Churchill Livingstone.

Regier, D.A., Kuhl, E.A., and Kupfer, D.J. (2013). The DSM-5: classification and criteria changes. *World Psychiatry* 12 (2): 92–98. https://doi.org/10.1002/wps.20050.

Siegel, R.S. and Brandon, A.R. (2014). Adolescents, pregnancy, and mental health. *Journal of Pediatric & Adolescent Gynecology* 27 (3): 138–150. https://doi.org/10.1016/j.jpag.2013.09.008.

Smythe, K.L., Petersen, I., and Schartau, P. (2022). Prevalence of perinatal depression and anxiety in both parents: a systematic review and meta-analysis. *JAMA Network Open* 5 (6): e2218969. https://doi-org.proxy.lib.ul.ie/10.1001/jamanetworkopen.2022.18969.

Sparling, T.M., Henschke, N., Nesbitt, R.C., and Gabrysch, S. (2017). The role of diet and nutritional supplementation in perinatal depression: a systematic review. *Maternal & Child Nutrition* 13 (1): https://doi.org/10.1111/mcn.12235.

Steele, L.S., Ross, L.E., Epstein, R. et al. (2008). Correlates of mental health service use among lesbian, gay, and bisexual mothers and prospective mothers. *Women & Health* 47 (3): 95–112. https://doi.org/10.1080/03630240802134225.

Stein, A., Pearson, R.M., Goodman, S.H. et al. (2014). Effects of perinatal mental disorders on the fetus and child. *Lancet* 384 (9956): 1800–1819. https://doi.org/10.1016/S0140-6736(14)61277-0.

Stevens, A.W.M.M., Goossens, P.J.J., Knoppert-van der Klein, E.A.M. et al. (2019). Risk of recurrence of mood disorders during pregnancy and the impact of medication: a systematic review. *Journal of Affective Disorders* 249: 96–103. https://doi.org/10.1016/j.jad.2019.02.018.

Tinkelman, A., Hill, E.A., and Deligiannidis, K.M. (2017). Management of new onset psychosis in the postpartum period. *Journal of Clinical Psychiatry* 78 (9): 1423–1424. https://doi.org/10.4088/JCP.17ac11880.

VanderKruik, R., Barreix, M., and Chou, D. (2017). The global prevalence of postpartum psychosis: a systematic review. *BMC Psychiatry* 17 (1): 272. https://doi.org/10.1186/s12888-017-1427-7.

Wesseloo, R., Kamperman, A.M., Munk-Olsen, T. et al. (2016). Risk of postpartum relapse in bipolar disorder and postpartum psychosis: a systematic review and meta-analysis. *American Journal of Psychiatry* 173 (2): 117–127. https://doi.org/10.1176/appi.ajp.2015.15010124.

World Health Organization (WHO) (2015). *WHO Recommendations on Health Promotion Interventions for Maternal and Newborn Health*. Geneva: WHO https://www.who.int/publications/i/item/9789241508742.

Yan, H., Wu, Y., and Li, H. (2022). Effect of mindfulness-based interventions on mental health of perinatal women with or without current mental health issues: a systematic review and meta-analysis of randomized controlled trials. *Journal of Affective Disorders* 305: 102–114. https://doi-org.proxy.lib.ul.ie/10.1016/j.jad.2022.03.002.

Yang, K., Wu, J., and Chen, X. (2022). Risk factors of perinatal depression in women: a systematic review and meta-analysis. *BMC Psychiatry* 22: 63. https://doi-org.proxy.lib.ul.ie/10.1186/s12888-021-03684-3.

Yildiz, P.D., Ayers, S., and Phillips, L. (2017). The prevalence of posttraumatic stress disorder in pregnancy and after birth: a systematic review and meta-analysis. *Journal of Affective Disorders* 208: 634–645. https://doi.org/10.1016/j.jad.2016.10.009.

Further Resources

National Institute for Health and Care Excellence (2020). Antenatal and Postnatal Mental Health: Clinical Management and Service Guidance. https://www.nice.org.uk/guidance/cg192 (accessed January 2024).

Royal College of Midwives (ND) Specialist Mental Health Midwives. https://www.rcm.org.uk/media/2370/specialist-mental-health-midwives-what-they-do-and-why-they-matter.pdf (rcm.org.uk) (accessed January 2024).

Glossary

Term	Definition
Antenatal anxiety	Anxiety experienced during pregnancy, which might be related to concerns about the pregnancy, birth or impending motherhood
Antenatal depression	Depression that occurs during pregnancy, affecting the expectant mother's mental health
Cognition	Refers to a range of mental processes relating to the acquisition, storage, manipulation and retrieval of information
Command hallucinations	Auditory hallucinations that instruct a person to act in specific ways; these commands can range in seriousness from innocuous to life-threatening
Delusional misidentification	A group of complex, monothematic delusional phenomena in which subjects hold a belief that the identity of a familiar person, object, location or self has been altered or replaced
Grandiose delusions	Unfounded or inaccurate beliefs that one has special powers, wealth, mission or identity
Infant attachment	The emotional connection and attachment that a mother develops with her baby during pregnancy and after birth
Maternal mental health	The emotional, psychological and mental well-being of pregnant women and new mothers during pregnancy and the postpartum period
Networks	Support networks, the social connections and resources that provide emotional, practical and psychological support to new parents and others, helping to alleviate stress and enhance mental well-being
Perinatal post-traumatic stress disorder	A type of anxiety disorder, also known as birth trauma
Postnatal anxiety	Intense feelings of worry, fear and anxiety that occur in the postpartum period, often involving excessive concerns about the baby's well-being
Postnatal depression	A mood disorder characterised by persistent feelings of sadness, hopelessness and a lack of interest or pleasure in activities after childbirth
Postnatal psychosis	A rare but severe mental health condition that involves hallucinations, delusions and disorganised thoughts, typically occurring within the first weeks after childbirth
Self-harm	Occurs when a person hurts themselves as a way of dealing with very difficult feelings, painful memories or overwhelming situations and experiences

Index

Fundamentals of Maternal Pathophysiology, First Edition. Edited by Claire Leader and Ian Peate.
© 2024 John Wiley & Sons Ltd. Published 2024 by John Wiley & Sons Ltd.
Companion website: www.wiley.com/go/leader/maternalpatho